PLUMER'S PRINCIPLES & PRACTICE OF

INTRAVENOUS THERAPY

EIGHTH EDITION

Sharon M. Weinstein, MS, RN, CRNI, FAAN

President, Global Education Development Institute, Lake Forest, Illinois

Assistant Clinical Professor, The University of Illinois College of Nursing
Department of Administrative and Public Health Nursing and
Institute for Healthcare Innovation
Chicago, Illinois

Infusion Therapy Consultant
Former Faculty, Department of Surgery
Rosalind Franklin University of Medicine and Health Sciences
North Chicago, Illinois

Director Member, Infusion Nurses Certification Corporation Board of Directors

Past President, Infusion Nurses Society, Inc.

Leader, Intravenous Therapy Delegations to People's Republic of China,
Austria, Germany, Commonwealth of Independent States, and Egypt

Lippincott Williams & Wilkins
a Wolters Kluwer business
Philadelphia · Baltimore · New York · London
Buenos Aires · Hong Kong · Sydney · Tokyo

Senior Acquisitions Editor: Margaret Zuccarini
Editorial Assistant: Katherine Rothwell
Director of Nursing Production: Helen Ewan
Production Project Manager: Cynthia Rudy
Senior Managing Editor/Production: Erika Kors

Art Director: Doug Smock
Manufacturing Coordinator: Karin Duffield
Production Services/Compositor: TechBooks
Printer: R. R. Donnelley–Crawfordsville

8th Edition

Library of Congress Cataloging-in-Publication Data
Weinstein, Sharon.
    Plumer's principles & practice of intravenous therapy / Sharon M.
Weinstein. — 8th ed.
        p. ; cm.
    Includes bibliographical references and index.
    ISBN 13: 978-0-7817-5944-1
    ISBN 10: 0-7817-5944-7
    1. Intravenous therapy.   I. Plumer, Ada Lawrence.   II. Title.
III. Title: Plumer's principles and practice of intravenous therapy.
IV. Title: Principles & practice of intravenous therapy.   V. Title:
Principles and practice of intravenous therapy.
    [DNLM: 1. Infusions, Intravenous—methods.   2. Infusions,
Intravenous—nursing.   3. Evidence-Based Medicine.   4. Fluid Therapy
—methods.   5. Nurse's Role.   6. Parenteral Nutrition—methods.
WB 354 W424p 2007]
RM170.P57 2007
615'.6—dc22   2006000877

Care has been taken to confirm the accuracy of the information presented and to describe generally accepted practices. However, the author, editors, and publisher are not responsible for errors or omissions or for any consequences from application of the information in this book and make no warranty, express or implied, with respect to the content of the publication.

The author, editors, and publisher have exerted every effort to ensure that drug selection and dosage set forth in this text are in accordance with the current recommendations and practice at the time of publication. However, in view of ongoing research, changes in government regulations, and the constant flow of information relating to drug therapy and drug reactions, the reader is urged to check the package insert for each drug for any change in indications and dosage and for added warnings and precautions. This is particularly important when the recommended agent is a new or infrequently employed used drug.

Some drugs and medical devices presented in this publication have Food and Drug Administration (FDA) clearance for limited use in restricted research settings. It is the responsibility of the health care provider to ascertain the FDA status of each drug or device planned for use in his or her clinical practice.

LWW.com

CONTRIBUTORS

Anne Marie Frey, BSN, RN, CRNI
IV Nurse Clinician
Children's Hospital of Philadelphia
Philadelphia, Pennsylvania
Chapter 21

Mary Hagle, PhD, RN, AOCN
Director/Nursing Practice Specialist
Center for Nursing Research and Practice
Aurora Health Care
Milwaukee, Wisconsin
Chapters 14, 16, 17, 19

Barbara St. Marie, RN, CNP
Pain Specialist
University of Minnesota/Fairview Health
   System
Minneapolis, Minnesota
Chapter 20

Marianne Valentine, BSN, RN, CRNI
Assistant Director of Clinical Services
Option Care of Cumberland
Cumberland, Maryland
Chapter 23

The following individuals assisted Mary Hagle in preparing her chapter updates:

Chapter 14

Beth P. Johnson, MS, RN
Clinical Nurse Specialist
St. Michael Hospital
Covenant Healthcare
Milwaukee, Wisconsin

Nora Ladewig, MSN, RN, CNRN, CCNS
Clinical Nurse Specialist
Aurora St. Luke's Medical Center
Aurora Health Care
Milwaukee, Wisconsin

Dianne Montenero, MSN, RN
Clinical Nurse Specialist–Oncology
Covenant Healthcare
Milwaukee, Wisconsin

Terri Pawlak, RN, CRRN
Staff Nurse–Rehabilitation
Chairperson, Metro Nursing Practice Council
Aurora Sinai Medical Center
Aurora Health Care
Milwaukee, Wisconsin

Chapter 16

Deborah Gentile, MSN, RN
Nursing Education Specialist
Aurora Health Care
Milwaukee, Wisconsin

Stephanie Kassulke, RN, ADN, CPAN
Staff Nurse–Surgical Services
Aurora Sinai Medical Center
Aurora Health Care
Milwaukee, Wisconsin

Kristine Laack, RD, CD, CNSD
Clinical Dietitian; Nutritional Support–
    Critical Care
West Allis Memorial Hospital
Aurora Health Care
West Allis, Wisconsin

Bruce Yale, RPh, CNSP
Pharmacy Supervisor; Nutritional
    Support–Critical Care
Aurora St. Luke's South Shore
Aurora Health Care
Milwaukee, Wisconsin

Chapter 17

Sara Grant, MSN, RN, CEN
Nurse Case Manager
Care Management–Metro
Aurora Health Care
Milwaukee, Wisconsin

Lee Jeske, MSN, RN
Clinical Nurse Specialist
Aurora St. Luke's Medical Center
Aurora Health Care
Milwaukee, Wisconsin

Connie Teichert, BSN, RN
Staff Nurse–Ambulatory Surgery
Aurora Sinai Medical Center
Aurora Health Care
Milwaukee, Wisconsin

Chapter 19

Carrie Bilicki, BSN, RN, OCN
Vince Lombardi Cancer Center
Aurora St. Luke's Medical Center
Aurora Health Care
Milwaukee, Wisconsin

Kerry Twite, MSN, RN, AOCN
Clinical Nurse Specialist–Oncology
Aurora St. Luke's Medical Center
Aurora Health Care
Milwaukee, Wisconsin

Sol A. Yoder, PharmD, RPH, BCOP
Oncology Pharmacy Clinical Coordinator
Aurora St. Luke's Medical Center
Aurora Health Care
Milwaukee, Wisconsin

REVIEWERS

Brenda Dugger, RN, MS, CRNI, CAN
Vice President of Nursing, Chief
  Nursing Officer
St. Mary's Health Care System
Athens, Georgia

Judy Hankins, RN, CRNI, BSN
IV Admixture Coordinator
Moses H. Cone Memorial Hospital
Greensboro, North Carolina

Elizabeth A. Krzywda, ANP, MSN
Adult Nurse Practitioner
Medical College of Wisconsin
Milwaukee, Wisconsin

Roxanne Perucca, MS, CRNI
Nurse Manager
University of Kansas Hospital
Kansas City, Kansas

Anne Swanson, MSN, RNC
Clinical Education Manager
Medex, Inc.
Carlsbad, California

ACKNOWLEDGMENTS

Plumer's Principles & Practice of Intravenous Therapy, Eighth Edition, is the result of the collaborative efforts of its original authors, Ada Lawrence Plumer and Faye Cosentino; and the contributions of veteran authors Anne Marie Frey and Barbara St. Marie, and myself. This edition welcomes the contributions of new authors Mary Hagle and a team of collaborators from Aurora Health Care, as well as home infusion specialist Marianne Valentine. I am so grateful to them for their valuable contributions to this text, and for the contributions that they have individually and collectively made to our professional practice. I would also like to thank the manufacturers of infusion products and equipment for their information and assistance, as well as the authors and publishers who permitted use of their copyrighted materials in producing this text.

A special thank you to Margaret Zuccarini, Senior Acquisitions Editor at Lippincott Williams & Wilkins, Katherine Rothwell, and Doug Smock for their encouragement, support, and technical assistance in developing a superior manuscript—one that readily supports the Plumer name.

Thanks are extended to William Eudailey, PharmD, and to the late David Blaess, RPh, who served as my mentors, and who taught me to apply the principles gleaned from Plumer's book to my daily practice. Men of vision, they gave me the opportunity to explore the world of infusion therapy.

There are so many professionals in the infusion specialty whose names are synonymous with quality; these individuals are seasoned professionals as well as novices. You will continue to generate passion for infusion therapy in those with whom you work for years to come. You may have been taught by one of your mentors or colleagues; you, in turn, have the responsibility to teach others. We must develop future generations of leaders in the infusion specialty practice; we must think globally with a vision for the future. Thus, all proceeds from the eighth edition of Plumer will go to the Global Education Development Institute, an organization whose mission is to foster the professional and personal growth of nurse leaders in developing countries.

And so, to the countless numbers of infusion specialty nurses throughout the world who promote quality outcomes each and every day of their lives, regardless of the clinical setting in which care is delivered, this book is for you.

Finally, thanks to my husband Steve, and to my family, for delighting in and acknowledging my continuing passion for infusion therapy.

SMW

SPECIAL ACKNOWLEDGMENT

As Plumer's reaches nearly 40 years as the *premier* source of information in infusion therapy, it is appropriate to recognize the woman who first penned this text. The name Ada Plumer is synonymous with infusion therapy. A leader, pacesetter, and cofounder of the professional society, Plumer set the tone for our professional practice, served as a mentor to many nurses, and encouraged excellence in the delivery of intravenous nursing care.

From my first entry into this rapidly changing field to today, I have used Plumer's book as a reference, a guide, and a bible for professional practice. Plumer's retains its position today as the only complete source of information available to the practicing clinician, student, and educator. The success of the current edition is attributed to Plumer . . . the growth of our practice is likewise a result of her initial efforts. Many thanks from all of us in whom you have instilled a passion for excellence in intravenous nursing practice.

PREFACE

For nearly 40 years, *Plumer's Principles & Practice of Intravenous Therapy* has retained its position as the most reliable, complete source of information addressing intravenous therapy for practicing clinicians, educators, and students. Completely updated and revised to meet the changing needs of our professional practice, this eighth edition, like its predecessors, provides the most current base of knowledge available to those who share the responsibility of ensuring high-quality infusion care to patients in diverse clinical settings.

The practice of infusion therapy is a multifaceted one. Infusion therapy is at the core of patient care. Our practice continually changes as a result of changing patient care delivery systems, the impact of managed care, re-engineering of the health care system, and the impact of integrated health care delivery systems. These changes have had a dramatic impact on our professional practice as we move on the continuum from care delivered in the acute care environment to care delivered in alternative sites. One thing remains unchanged, however, and that is the continuous need for an unprecedented high level of expertise for delivering infusion therapy.

Plumer's Principles & Practice of Intravenous Therapy, Eighth Edition, has been updated and reorganized to produce a resource that clearly exceeds these needs. The addition of even more boxes, tables, legal issues, step-by-step directions, nursing alerts, tables, and references to the World Wide Web and evidence-based practice create an easy-to-use format and easy-to-access references. The CD-ROM contains an updated IV drug list and 11 appendices, two of them new. A more integrated approach to content results in a streamlined five-section organization. Unit 1 reviews the history of infusion therapy, risk reduction and performance improvement, legal safeguards, nursing role and responsibilities, and application of the Infusion Nurses Society Standards of Practice. New content addresses shared governance models, knowledge-sharing, mentoring, applications for Magnet Recognition, and the future of infusion nursing.

Unit 2 has undergone extensive change. Now addressing assessment and monitoring, this section has been expanded to encompass fluid and electrolyte balance, principles of parenteral fluid administration, relevant anatomy and physiology, laboratory data, ongoing monitoring, and local and systemic complications. A new section on sentinel events and reflex sympathetic dystrophy (RSD) discusses the challenging clinical outcomes that we now face.

Unit 3 has been renamed Clinical Decision Making. In this section, we present current information about infusion equipment and safety; methods for assessing product and equipment needs; short peripheral lines; central vascular access; and alternate access, which encompasses intra-arterial, Ommaya reservoir, and intraosseous approaches. New contributing authors have created a user-friendly section that meets your continuous learning needs.

Patient-specific therapies are addressed in the revamped Unit 4. A plethora of talented contributing authors has created the most current and complete source of information available today. Mary Hagle and a team of clinical nurse specialists, dieticians, and pharmacists from Aurora Health System have revised the chapter on parenteral nutrition. Mary also led the team that completely updated the section on transfusion therapy, including Factor II and Factor V Leiden disorders, consistent with the dramatic changes in practice and the revised standards. Mary's expertise as an Oncology Nurse Specialist and a contributor to the ONS Core Curriculum prepared her to co-author the chapter on antineoplastics. Once again, Barbara St. Marie, a renowned expert in pain management, has updated the chapter on pain, emphasizing practical aspects of care, IV conscious sedation, and continuous local anesthesia. The chapter on pharmacology applied to infusion therapy has been updated with an emphasis on therapeutic monitoring and drug level ranges.

Unit 5 addresses special applications. Ann Marie Frey has updated the information on pediatric infusion therapy. New author Marianne Valentine edited the section on alternate clinical settings and cost factors, bringing the voice of experience to home care, long-term, and subacute environments. Infusion therapy in the older adult patient remains a focus. And finally, a new chapter on global applications for infusion nurses rounds out an expanded, updated, and state-of-the-art eighth edition.

Revised to meet the needs of the clinician responsible for delivering high-quality infusion care, regardless of the clinical setting in which care is provided, *Plumer's Principles & Practice of Intravenous Therapy*, Eighth Edition, retains its place as the most essential tool available in intravenous practice today. May you enjoy it and gain value from it.

Sharon M. Weinstein, MS, RN, CRNI, FAAN

CONTENTS

LIST OF TABLES

UNIT 1

Overview of Infusion Therapy

CHAPTER 1

History of Infusion Therapy

KEY TERMS

Hypotonicity

Parenteral

Pyrogens

Quill and Bladder

Standards of Practice

Early History and Methodology

Almost 400 years have passed since the discovery of blood circulation. William Harvey's 1628 research stimulated increased experimentation, and he found that the heart is both a muscle and a pump.

Renaissance Period

In 1656, Sir Christopher Wren, the famed architect of St. Paul's Cathedral in London, injected opium intravenously into dogs. Wren, known as the father of modern intravenous (IV) therapy, used a **quill and bladder.** In 1662, Johann Majors made the first successful injection of unpurified compounds into human beings, although death resulted from infection at the injection site.

In 1665, an animal near death from loss of blood was saved by the infusion of blood from another animal. In 1667, a 15-year-old Parisian boy was the first human to receive a transfusion successfully; lamb's blood was administered directly into the boy's circulation by Jean Baptiste Denis, physician to Louis XIV (Cosnett, 1989). The enthusiasm aroused by this success led to promiscuous transfusions of blood from animals to humans with fatal results, and in 1687, by an edict of church and parliament, animal-to-human transfusions were prohibited in Europe. Nearly 150 years passed before serious attempts were again made to inject blood into people.

The 19th Century

James Blundell, an English obstetrician, revived the idea of blood transfusion. In 1834, saving the lives of many women threatened by hemorrhage during child-birth, he proved that animal blood was unfit to inject into humans and that only human blood was safe. Nevertheless, complications persisted, with infections developing in donors and recipients. With the discovery of the principles of anti-sepsis by Pasteur and Lister, another obstacle was overcome, although reactions and deaths continued.

The first recorded attempt to prevent coagulation during transfusion was in 1821 by Jean Louis Prévost, a French physician who, with Jean B. A. Dumas, used defibri-nated blood in animal transfusions (Cosnett, 1989).

In the middle to late 19th century, increased knowledge of bacteriology, phar-macology, and pathology led to new approaches. Ignaz Semmelweis, a Viennese obstetrician, was the first to correlate the effect of hand washing on prevention of infection. Semmelweis is credited with a 90% reduction of maternal deaths between 1846 and 1848. Meanwhile, chemist Louis Pasteur was proving that bacteria were liv-ing microorganisms, although his ideas were challenged by many researchers and practitioners.

In 1889, William Halsted of the Johns Hopkins Hospital, in cooperation with Goodyear Rubber Company, introduced the use of surgical gloves in the operating theater. Ten years later, the use of rubber gloves was widely accepted as a means of protecting patients and physicians (Sutcliff, 1992).

French physiologist Claude Bernard is credited with experimental injection of sugar solutions into dogs. The precursor to modern nutritional support, Bernard's experiments were followed by the subcutaneous injection of fat, milk, and camphor by Menzel and Perco in Vienna. Work in nutritional support remained at a standstill for many years.

20th-Century Advances

In the 20th century, IV therapy advanced rapidly. Blood transfusions and **parenteral** fluids, which bypass the intestines, were administered, and parenteral nutrition became possible as well. Moreover, nurses became skilled both in administering and monitoring infusions.

TRANSFUSION THERAPY

In 1900, Karl Landsteiner proved that not all human blood is alike when he identified four main classifications. In 1914, sodium citrate was found to prevent blood from clotting (Cosnett, 1989), and since then, rapid advances have been made (Table 1-1).

TABLE 1–1   20th- and 21st-Century Progress in Infusion Therapy

Year	Significant Advancement
1900	Karl Landsteiner discovered three of four main blood groups.
1914	Sodium citrate was first used to preserve blood.
	Hydrolyzed protein and fats were administered to animals.
1925	Dextrose was used as an infusate.
1935	Marriot and Kekwick introduced slow-drip method of transfusion.
1937	Rose identified amino acids essential for growth.
1940	Disposable plastic administration sets were developed.
1945	Flexible intravenous (IV) cutdown catheter was introduced.
1950	Rochester needle was introduced.
1960	Peripherally inserted catheter lines were introduced in intensive care areas.
1963–65	First success with hyperalimentation at the University of Pennsylvania.
1970	Centers for Disease Control (CDC) guidelines for IV therapy were published.
	First edition of *Plumer's Principles and Practice of Intravenous Therapy* was published.
1972	Access of implanted ports was introduced.
1973	The National Intravenous Therapy Association (NITA) was founded.
	Broviac tunneled catheter was introduced.
1976	Fat emulsions were used for nutritional support.
1980	NITA Standards of Practice was published.
	NITA National Office opened.
	IV Nurse Day was recognized by U.S. House of Representatives.
1981	CDC Guidelines were revised and published.
1982	Implantable ports were used for long-term access.
	First IV teaching program in People's Republic of China.
1983	Home blood transfusion initiated.
	Osteoport was developed.
1984	First edition of *Core Curriculum for Intravenous Nursing* was published.
1985	Intravenous Nurses Certification Corporation offered its first credentialing examination (CRNI).
1986	Use of patient-controlled analgesia increased.
1987	NITA changed its name to the Intravenous Nurses Society (INS).
1990	Safe Medical Device Act and Food and Drug Administration Device Reporting regulations published.
	INS Revised Standards of Practice published.
1992	U.S. Food and Drug Administration issued alert concerning needlestick injuries.
1995	Occupational Safety and Health guidelines for handling cytotoxic drugs published.
1996	LPNI examination offered to LPN/LVNs by INS.
	CDC Guidelines revised and published.
1998	INS celebrated its 25th Anniversary (Houston, TX).
1999	*Journal of Intravenous Nursing* offered CE/recertification units.
2000	*Core Curriculum for Intravenous Nursing*, 2nd edition, published.
	Revised Standards of Practice published.
	INS Policies and Procedures Manual published.
	CRNI Exam Preparation Guide & Practice Questions published.
	First public member added to the INS board of directors.
2003	*Core Curriculum for Infusion Nursing*, 3rd edition, published.
	Infusion Nurses Society celebrates its 30th year.
2004	*Infusion Nurses Society Standards for Adult Patients* published.
2005	Revised Infusion Nurses Standards of Practice published.
2006	*Plumer's Principles and Practice of Intravenous Therapy*, 8th edition, published.

In 1911, Dr. Ottenberg of New York demonstrated the use of donor blood; his theory that safe transfusion was possible from a donor whose serum agglutinated the recipient's red blood cells was readily accepted. Dr. Ottenberg further suggested that it was unsafe to use a donor whose red blood cells were acted on by the recipient's serum. These research findings evolved into the universal donor concept still valid today.

Hugh Leslie Marriot and Alan Kekwick, English physicians, introduced the continuous slow-drip method of blood transfusion; their findings were published in 1935 (Cosnett, 1989).

The Rh factor was discovered in 1940, and the American Association of Blood Banks was formed in 1947. The invention of the first cell separator in 1951 introduced component therapy (for more information, see Chap. 19).

PARENTERAL FLUIDS

Administration of parenteral fluids by the IV route has been widely used only since the late 1950s. The difficulty in accepting this procedure resulted from the lack of safe fluids. The fluids then in use contained substances called **pyrogens,** proteins that are foreign to the body and not destroyed by sterilization. These caused chills and fever when injected into the circulation. The 1923 discovery and elimination of pyrogens led to safer and more frequent IV administration of parenteral fluids. In 1925, the most frequently used parenteral fluid was normal saline (0.9% sodium chloride). Because of its **hypotonicity,** water could not be administered IV and had to be made isotonic. A certain percentage of sodium chloride added to water achieved this effect (Cosnett, 1989). After 1925, dextrose was used extensively to make isotonic fluids and provide a source of calories.

INFUSION NURSING

Massachusetts General Hospital is credited with many firsts in medical history. The first nurse to hold the title "IV nurse" is known to have practiced at this Boston hospital. That nurse, Ada Plumer was a founder of the National Intravenous Therapy Association, now known as the Infusion Nurses Society; she was also the original author of this text. Early on, IV nurses were responsible for phlebotomy, transfusion therapy, venipuncture, and maintaining equipment. Emphasis was placed on the technical responsibility of maintaining the infusion and keeping the needle and tubing apparatus patent. The sole requisite for being an IV nurse was the ability to perform a venipuncture skillfully.

At the time, IV therapy was limited to use in surgery and treating dehydration. Infusates were administered through rubber administration sets and 16- to 18-gauge steel needles strategically placed in the antecubital fossa and secured with an arm board.

As knowledge of electrolyte and fluid therapy grew, more parenteral fluids became available, and additional knowledge was then needed to monitor the fluid and electrolyte status of the patient. The nurse assigned to the patient in need of IV therapy was expected to have a working knowledge of fluid and electrolyte balance and to assess the "whole" patient in terms of fluid needs. Normal saline was no longer the only electrolyte fluid. Today, more than 200 commercially prepared IV fluids are available to meet patients' needs.

PARENTERAL NUTRITION

W. C. Rose identified amino acids in 1937, leading to the development of protein hydrolysates for human infusion. A whole new approach to IV therapy and a respite to the starving patient evolved between 1963 and 1965, when members of the Harrison Department of Surgical Research at the University of Pennsylvania showed that sufficient nutrients could be given to juvenile beagles to support normal growth and development (Cosnett, 1989). This led to what is known today as *total parenteral nutrition* (TPN).

In the mid-1960s, as a result of animal TPN research, Stanley Dudrick developed the first formula for parenteral nutrition, a method by which sufficient nutrients are administered into the central vein to support life and maintain growth and development. Home TPN was introduced in 1983. Research into the use of antioxidants, the role of amino acids, and indications for medium-, short-, and long-chain triglycerides in TPN continues today (Grant, 1992).

EARLY INTRAVENOUS DEVICES AND EQUIPMENT

Cutdown procedures were performed frequently until 1950, with the introduction of the Rochester needle, a resinous catheter on the outside of a steel introducer needle. On successful insertion, the catheter was slipped off the needle into the vein and the needle was removed. Desert Pharmaceutical Co. introduced the Intracath in 1958, minimizing the need for surgical cutdown. McGaw Laboratories introduced the first small vein set with foldable wings in 1957; this product is known today as a winged infusion needle.

Since the 1980s, tunneled catheters have enhanced central venous access. Totally implanted access devices are now used routinely (for more information, see Chap. 14).

The first IV fluid containers were made of glass. Plastic bags were introduced in the 1970s. Because they do not require air venting, these containers reduced the risks of air embolism and airborne contamination. Today, plastic is the primary container for IV fluids, whereas glass containers are used when the fluid stability in plastic is a concern.

In the mid-1940s, disposable plastic IV administration sets became available and eventually replaced the reusable rubber tubings. Manufacturers have continued to keep pace with demands for technologically advanced products that ensure patient safety and reliability in the delivery of infusion therapy.

Progress in Clinical Practice

In the 1970s, tremendous scientific, technologic, and medical advances occurred, and IV therapy gained recognition as a highly specialized field. Nurses performed many of the functions formerly reserved for the medical staff—intra-arterial therapy, neonatal therapy, and antineoplastic therapy. Professional societies were established to provide a forum for the exchange of ideas, knowledge, and experiences, with the ultimate goal of raising standards and increasing the level of patient care.

On October 1, 1980, the United States House of Representatives recognized the profession and declared an official day of honor for IV nurses: "Resolved, that IV Nurse Day be nationally celebrated in honor of the National Intravenous Therapy Association, Inc., on January 25 of each year." The proclamation was presented by the Honorable Edward J. Mackey from the Fifth Congressional District of the Commonwealth of Massachusetts (Gardner, 1982).

The Infusion Nurses Society, Inc.

The Infusion Nurses Society, Inc. has continued to grow worldwide. Educational offerings have expanded to include advanced studies in an effort to meet the needs of the advanced practitioner.

Credentialing

The Infusion Nurses Certification Corporation has credentialed thousands of nurses across the country. Professional IV nurses are encouraged to prepare for the credentialing process through DVD and CD presentations, a revised core curriculum, educational programs, the society's professional journal, clinical textbooks, and published **Standards of Practice.**

Because delivery of IV therapy permeates all clinical settings, the role of the IV nurse is now well established as integral to multidisciplinary, high-quality care in all practice settings (Baranowski, 1995). The growth of this specialty practice has expanded the roles of IV nurses nationally and internationally. IV nurses are constantly striving to find new and more efficient ways to perform their services in an integrated health care environment.

Infusion Nursing in the 21st Century

Nurses continue to lead the labor sector throughout the United States, and advanced-practice nursing has grown dramatically (Kalisch & Kalisch, 1995). In one study (Coffman and Spetz, 1999), the authors demonstrated the need for 43,000 additional registered nurses by the year 2010 to keep pace with the local population growth. Data on national trends in nursing school enrollment indicate that nurse educators are in general quicker than educators in other fields to adjust enrollment in response to market signals (Salsberg, Wing, & Brewer, 1998). With new graduates producing a relatively new workforce in many institutions, there will be an increasing need for IV resource experts.

The challenge for nurses is to effect health policy through use of their knowledge and skills. Wakefield (1999) stated that the value assigned to nursing will be based on a standard that measures how the profession effects access and achieves the highest-quality care at the lowest cost.

References and Selected Readings

Asterisks indicate references cited in text.

*Baranowski, L. (1995). Presidential address: Take ownership. *Journal of Intravenous Nursing, 18*(4), 163.

*Coffman, J., & Spetz, J. (1999). Maintaining an adequate supply of RNs in California. *Image: Journal of Nursing Scholarship, 31*, 389–391.

*Cosnett, J.E . (1989). Before our time: The origins of intravenous fluid therapy. *Lancet, 4*, 768–771.

*Gardner, C. (1982). United States House of Representatives honors the National Intravenous Therapy Association, Inc. *Journal of the National Intravenous Therapy Association, 5*(1), 14.

*Grant, J.P. (1992). *Handbook of total parenteral nutrition* (3rd ed., pp. 21–29). Philadelphia: W.B. Saunders.

Griffith, J.M., Thomas, N., & Griffith, L. (1991). MDs bill for these routine nursing tasks. *American Journal of Nursing, 90*(10), 65–73.

*Kalisch, P.A., & Kalisch, B.J. (1995). *The advance of American nursing* (3rd ed.). Philadelphia: J.B. Lippincott.

*Salsberg, E., Wing, P., & Brewer, C. (1998). Projecting the future supply and demand for registered nurses. In: E. O'Neil & J. Coffman (Eds.), *Strategies for the future of nursing*. San Francisco: Jossey-Bass.

*Sutcliff, J. (1992). *A history of medicine*. New York: Barnes & Noble.

*Wakefield, M. (1999). Nursing's future in health care policy. In: E. Sullivan (Ed.), *Creating nursing's future* (pp. 41–49). St. Louis, MO: Mosby.

Review Questions

Note: Questions below may have more than one right answer.

1. The clinical use of amino acids led to the development of which of the following?

   A. Antioxidants

   B. Home total parenteral nutrition

   C. Protein hydrolysates

   D. Triple-mix fluid

2. The initial role of the IV specialist included which of the following?

   A. Phlebotomy

   B. Crossmatching of blood

   C. Maintaining equipment

   D. Maintaining IV lines

3. Three of the four main blood groups were discovered by:

   A. Karl Landsteiner

   B. Florence Seibert

   C. William Halsted

   D. W. C. Rose

4. The first national certification examination for nurses was offered in:

   A. 1983

   B. 1985

   C. 1988

   D. 1991

5. Primary fluids in use in the mid-1950s included:

   A. Lactated Ringer's injection

   B. 5% Dextrose in water

   C. 0.9% Sodium chloride (normal saline)

   D. 0.45% Sodium chloride (half-normal saline)

CHAPTER 2

Minimizing Risk and Improving Performance

KEY TERMS

Assault

Battery

Benchmarking

Civil Law

Criminal Law

Malpractice

Performance Improvement

Plan of Corrective Action

Regulating Agencies

Tort

Unusual Occurrence Report

Professional Nursing and Legal Safeguards

The law and its interpretation lead to doubts and questions regarding the legal rights and obligations of nurses to administer infusion (IV) therapy. Legal standards are an integral component of a **performance improvement** (PI) program. As IV therapy becomes more complex and specialized, and as infusion experts gain national acceptance, nurses are becoming more involved in procedures formerly performed solely by physicians. Because violation of the Medical Practice Act is a criminal offense, infusion nurses need to be well versed on the subject and the law, not only to protect themselves but also to ensure safe, high-quality care for their patients.

To clarify the roles of nurses and physicians in various aspects of health care, joint policy statements have been issued by the medical societies and nursing associations on a number of procedures, including infusion therapy. See Box 2–1 for strategies for reducing risks related to IV therapy.

BOX 2–1   Strategies for Reducing Risks Related to IV Therapy

- Keep abreast of laws and regulations governing practice.
- Stay up to date on defined standards of practice and their clinical application.
- File incident reports and record sentinel events (unforeseen outcomes resulting in a negative response to treatment) as appropriate.
- Ensure that informed consent is obtained and on file as needed.
- Participate in product evaluation processes and ensure safe use by providing internal product education.
- Maintain continued competency in your professional practice; ensure that you meet credentialing criteria.
- Monitor patients' responses and unforeseen reactions to treatment; document these events appropriately and in a timely manner.
- Ensure that safety standards are maintained; be aware of Occupational Safety and Health Administration (OSHA) regulations; practice risk management.
- Participate in the quality improvement process in your institution.

Regulating Agencies

Regulating agencies issue mandates that directly or indirectly impact the role of the health care professional, in this case, the infusion nurse. These agencies include the Food and Drug Administration (FDA), the Occupational Safety and Health Administration (OSHA), the Joint Commission on Accreditation of Healthcare Organizations (JCAHO), state regulatory boards, and professional organizations.

Federal Statutes

Federal statutes are laws enacted by Congress and published in the *Federal Register*. Such laws relevant to IV nursing include those addressing occupational health and safety, infection control, environmental hazards, medical device safety, control of drug abuse, federally funded insurance programs, and patient self-determination acts (Table 2–1).

Applying Law to Practice

In hospitals and states in which no written opinion relevant to IV therapy exists, nurses are legally required to perform any nursing or medical procedure they are directed to carry out by a duly licensed physician unless they have reason to believe harm will result to the patient from doing so. To meet their legal responsibilities to patients, nurses must be qualified by knowledge and experience to execute the procedure; otherwise, they may properly refuse to perform it.

In cases in which the nurse finds no medical reason to question a physician's order, the nurse's failure to carry out such an order subjects him or her to liability for any consequent harm to the patient. It has been established by law that in a question of

TABLE 2–1   Sources of Standards of Care Related to IV Therapy

Source	Agency	Examples of Standard
Federal statutes	Occupational Safety and Health Administration (OSHA)	• Hazard Communication Standard Practice Guidelines for Handling Cytotoxic Drugs • Occupational Safe Exposure to Bloodborne Pathogens
	United States Food and Drug Administration (FDA)	Safe Medical Device Act of 1990
	Drug Enforcement Agency (DEA)	Controlled Substances Act
State statutes	Department of Health	Licensure of health care facilities
	Board of Nursing	Nurse Practice Act
	Board of Regents	
Private/professional bodies	Joint Commission for the Accreditation of Hospitals and Healthcare Organizations (JCAHO)	• Accreditation manual for hospitals and health care organizations • Accreditation manual for home health care
	American Nurses Association	Standards of Nursing Practice
	Infusion Nurses Society (INS)	Infusion Nursing Standards of Practice
	American Association of Blood Banks (AABB)	Technical manual
	ECRI	Health devices standard nomenclature
Institutional bodies	Infusion Therapy or Nursing Department	Job descriptions; nursing policies and procedures

negligence, individuals are not protected because they have "carried out the physician's orders." Rather, they are held liable in relation to their knowledge, skill, and judgment.

Currently, several states recommend that schools of professional nursing include an IV therapy course in the curriculum. The course should provide the student nurse with clinical instruction and experience in IV therapy. Infusion nursing specialists have been instrumental in developing the content for such programs.

ROLES OF CONTRACTED PERSONNEL

Among the dramatic changes in today's health care environment are the decreasing numbers of private duty nurses and contracted (agency) personnel. However, cyclic staff shortages continue to create a market niche for these patient care providers. Thus, nurses working in institutions that use private duty and contracted nurses as well as nurses whose employers are contracted agencies must be aware of their own accountability for their actions and practice in addition to their accountability to their employers, patients, and colleagues.

PRIVATE DUTY NURSE

A private duty nurse, who works under the direction, supervision, and control of a hospital and private physician, is subject to the rules and regulations of the hospital concerning all matters relating to nursing care. The institution's joint policy statement may note that the private duty nurse who has complied with the criteria applicable to the administration of IV therapy may give an IV infusion.

AGENCY NURSE

Nationwide, temporary staffing agencies provide valuable assistance during shortages of licensed professional personnel. When given responsibility for the administration of intravascular therapies, agency personnel must be oriented to the health care facility's policies and procedures and the functions performed by specialized department personnel. When the facility must use agency staff, every effort should be made to ensure patient safety, public protection, and viability of the IV therapy program.

Guarding Against Malpractice

The IV nurse's risk of involvement in **malpractice** suits is increasing with the increasing complexity of therapy and delegation of responsibility for infusion therapy in some institutions to less qualified paraprofessionals. In many cases, the professional nurse is legally responsible for the work performed by non-licensed assistive personnel. Therefore, many of the functions performed by the nurse have important legal consequences. An understanding of the legal principles and guidelines involved is necessary if daily professional actions are not to result in unwanted malpractice suits. Terminology related to potential litigation is presented in Box 2–2.

If the hospital or involved professional person (or both) is to be charged with malpractice resulting from injury to a patient, the patient's representative should be able to demonstrate that

1. A standard of care or duty can be established.
2. The standard of care or duty was not met.
3. The patient was harmed or injured because the standard was not met.
4. It was possible to foresee that injury or harm would result from not meeting the standards (depending on state law).

BOX 2–2   Legal Terms

- **Criminal law**—Actions judged under criminal law include violation of the Nurse Practice Act, which is prosecuted by a government authority and punishable by fine or imprisonment, or both. An example of a criminal act is unlawful administration of IV therapy.
- **Civil law**—Actions judged under civil law relate to conduct affecting the legal rights of the private person. According to civil law, the guilty party is responsible for damages (*compensation*).
- **Tort**—A private wrongful act (of omission or commission) for which relief may be obtained by injunction or damages. Examples of a **tort** include assault, battery, negligence, slander, libel, false imprisonment, and invasion of privacy. **Assault** includes anticipation of harm; **battery** is the actual infliction of harm.
- **Malpractice**—Negligent conduct of professionals characterized by not acting in a prudent manner and resulting in damage to another person or property.

Personal Liability and Protective Measures

The rule of personal liability states that "every person is liable for his [or her] own tortious conduct" (his own wrongdoing). No physician can protect a nurse from an act of negligence by bypassing this rule with verbal reassurances. The nurse cannot avoid legal liability even though another person may be sued and held liable. For example, the physician who orders placement of a peripherally inserted central catheter (PICC) cannot assume responsibility for the nurse who is negligent in implementing the action. If harm occurs as a result of the action, the nurse is held liable for this wrongdoing.

The rule of personal liability is relevant to medication errors as well. Medication errors are a common cause of malpractice claims against nurses. Negligence results from the administration of a drug to the wrong patient, at the wrong time, in an incorrect dosage, or in an improperly prescribed manner. If the physician writes an incomplete or partially illegible order and the nurse fails to clarify it before administration and harm results, the nurse is liable for negligence. The same applies to the administration of IV fluids. Nurses have a legal and professional responsibility to know the purpose and effect of the IV fluids and medications they administer. They must ensure that patients receive the prescribed volume of fluid at the prescribed rate of flow.

The rule of personal liability applies to directors of nursing and to nurses under their supervision. Although directors/nurse managers usually are not held liable for the negligence of nurses under their supervision (because every person is liable for his or her own wrongdoing), a director is expected to know if the nurse is competent to perform assigned duties without supervision.

On the other hand, directors who are negligent in the assignment of an inexperienced nurse or a nurse who requires supervision may be held liable for the acts of the nurse. Floating nurses to units to provide direct patient care when they are not experienced at the assigned level is a good example. Some institutions float nurses only to like intensive care units.

Observe Carefully

Nursing today requires a strong knowledge base and good observation skills. The act of observation is the legal and professional responsibility of the nurse. Frequent observation is imperative for the early detection and prevention of complications. Undetected complications that are allowed to increase in severity because of failure to observe the patient constitute an act of negligence on the part of the nurse (see Chap. 10).

Establish Therapeutic Relationships

Nurse–patient relationships play a significant role in influencing patients to initiate legal liability against nurses. Nurses performing IV therapy must be particularly aware of and attentive to the emotional needs of their patients, particularly when patients experience pain and apprehension during such procedures as catheter insertion. Clearly, specialists must foster appropriate interpersonal relationships. Nurses who are impersonal, aloof, and so busy with the technical process of starting an IV infusion that they have no time for establishing kindly relationships are the suit-prone nurses whose personalities may initiate resentment and later malpractice suits.

Patients most likely to sue are those who are resentful, frequently hostile, uncooperative, and dissatisfied with the nursing care. By demonstrating respect, care, and concern for all patients, as well as rendering skilled, efficient nursing care, nurses may avoid malpractice claims.

REVIEW AND CLARIFY CURRENT POLICIES AND PROCEDURES

Policies and procedures should be detailed, and all nurses practicing infusion therapy should be required to know them and review them periodically. Policies and procedures should follow national guidelines established by the Centers for Disease Control and Prevention (CDC) and Standards of Practice established by the Infusion Nurses Society (INS). These guidelines provide a model for IV nurses and foster optimal care for the patient receiving IV therapy.

KEEP CREDENTIALS UP TO DATE

Credentialing of IV nurses nationwide began with the first certification examination in 1985. The credentialing process consists of three components: licensure, accreditation, and certification.

Licensure represents the entry into practice level afforded to all professional nurses who successfully complete the registered nurse examination.

Accreditation establishes that a program or service meets established guidelines. Accreditation is offered to facilities, agencies, and other health care providers by such groups as JCAHO, which is an accrediting body that evaluates (rates) the programs of hospitals and home care agencies.

Certification is the highest level attainable by the professional IV nurse. It is the process by which society attests to the professional and clinical competence of the person who successfully completes the process.

PRESERVE CONFIDENTIALITY

Health Insurance Portability and Accountability Act (HIPAA) regulations have impacted confidentiality in all clinical settings. Confidentiality of patient information consists of three related components: privacy, confidentiality, and security (Conner, 1999). With current advances in communication, such as electronic mail (e-mail) and other communication systems, including fax machines, cellular or cordless telephones, answering machines, and voice mail, nurses need to be aware and vigilant in preventing the misdirection, printing, interception, rerouting, or reading of information by unintended recipients.

Technology alone cannot ensure the legal and ethical use of e-mail and other communications in the health care environment. The e-mail message, for example, accurately documents communication and, as such, is part of the medical record and a legal document.

Expert security sources recommend the use of multilevel, individual passwords for all e-mail users, as opposed to generic group sign-ons and systems that require a single pass code (Dorodny, 1998). Monitored audit trails and increased accountability of caregivers to their patients should be established (Connor, 1999). Health information has become a commodity over the Internet, and every precaution should be taken to maintain the confidentiality of electronic additions to the clinical record.

PERFORMANCE EVALUATIONS

A standard must be carefully defined for the health care institution or the nurse to evaluate adequate performance. Tools useful in guiding this process include the following:

- Standards of Practice (INS, 1998, 2000, 2005)
- State Board of Nursing regulations for registered nurses and licensed practical/vocational nurses
- American Nurses Association Standards of Nursing Practice
- Policies and procedures of the employing health care institution or agency

Professional Nursing and Performance Improvement

The complexity of infusion therapy practice today mandates a higher level of expertise and training than ever before. An illustration of this point involves the issues associated with placement of a long-term catheter, such as the PICC.

Qualified Personnel

The placement of a PICC requires special training and demonstrated competency on the part of the professional registered nurse. Each state sets its own practice guidelines, and not all states consider the placement of PICC catheters to be within the scope of professional nursing practice. The INS assembled a task force to standardize the usage, terminology, and adjunctive guidelines for the insertion of PICCs. A teaching program has also been developed (see Chaps. 12 through 14). Still, the institution or facility should contact the respective state Board of Nursing to determine policy. Each health care facility must establish criteria that qualify nurses to insert a PICC. The criteria should be within the institution's own legal guidelines. Such a program should address

- Indications
- Care and maintenance
- Advantages
- Legal issues
- Placement technique
- Product education
- Complications

Minimal standards for successful completion of an educational program include

- Satisfactory performance during initial probationary/review period
- Successful completion of in-house IV certification course
- Clinical competency evidenced by actual practice
- Successful completion of in-house requirements for PICC insertion

Risk Reduction

Given the continued growth of infusion therapy practice and the shift to alternative care settings, the potential for associated risks is higher than ever before. The institution is responsible for the quality of care delivered by its agents.

REPORT PRODUCT PROBLEMS

Because risk may be increased as a result of inappropriate use of medical devices, the U.S. Food and Drug Administration evaluates approximately 2,000 medical devices monthly. The evaluation assesses

- Good manufacturing controls
- Application for a device existing before 1976 (in current use)
- Implantable or hazardous devices

Nurses and other health care providers are encouraged to report problems with equipment and other medical devices (see Chap. 12) directly to Medical Device and Laboratory Product Problem Reporting Program (PRP), United States Pharmacopeia, 12601 Twinbrook Parkway, Rockville, MD 20853; (800) 638-6725.

FILE UNUSUAL OCCURRENCE REPORTS

A report is required for any accident or error resulting in actual or potential injury or harm. The report should contain only factual statements regarding the incident. Each report must be immediately followed by a full investigation into all possible causes, and corrective action must be taken immediately to prevent its recurrence.

Unusual occurrence reports should be routinely filed when there is a deviation from the standards. These reports are used as an internal reporting mechanism for a facility's quality assurance program. Components of the report may be found in Box 2–3. This type of report may also be used to help identify problem patterns and institute corrective actions. Surveillance programs documented by such reports can be effective in preventing unsafe or insecure environments that can result in injuries to the patient.

Safety

Leape (Buerhaus, 1999), a health policy analyst, suggests in a study in the *Harvard Medical Practice Journal* that nearly 4% of people who are hospitalized have an adverse event. The study further states that at least two thirds of the events are preventable,

---

BOX 2–3   Components of an Unusual Occurrence Report

- Admitting diagnosis
- Date of occurrence
- Patient's room number/location
- Patient's age
- Location of occurrence
- Type of occurrence (medication error, policy and procedure)
- Factual description
- Patient's prior clinical condition
- Results/interventions

---

meaning that approximately 1 million preventable injuries and 120,000 preventable deaths from injury occur annually. Based on the findings, Leape asserts that the cost of adverse events to health care facilities in 1998 was approximately $100 billion. Much of the increase in adverse events is attributed to a more complex health care system and to the acuity of the patient population at the turn of the century.

The National Patient Safety Foundation, established in 1997 by the American Medical Association, brought together representatives from nursing, pharmacy, medicine, and patient advocacy groups to examine ways to improve safety in health care across the health care continuum. On a hospital-wide level, organizations have continued to emphasize quality improvement processes.

Performance Improvement Process

The JCAHO previously mandated an ongoing program for monitoring quality-based outcomes. The trend continues to be toward process improvement, which involves pursuing opportunities to improve the quality of care and to ensure positive patient outcomes. Typically, quality assurance has focused on

- Identification of deficiencies or problem areas
- Analysis and interpretation
- Plans for corrective action
- Evaluation of the outcome of corrective action
- Resolution

This assessment process has typically been useful in improving the quality of care to patients receiving IV therapies (see Chap. 10).

IDENTIFY DEFICIENCIES OR PROBLEM AREAS

Data may be collected by interview, observation, or visual inspection. Problems and deficiencies may be readily identified through incident reports, patient complaints, employee complaints, questionnaires, patient satisfaction surveys, and suggestions from patients, visitors, or other staff. Determine the cause of the deficiency by comparing actual care with established standards. In assessing the need for further investigation, the facility should determine the character of the problem or deficiency, which in most cases involves noncompliance with standards of care. Examples of questions to ask include the following:

- Does the deficiency/problem relate to the quality of patient care?
- Does the deficiency/problem occur frequently enough to require correction?
- Can the deficiency/problem be solved?
- Do the potential benefits to patient care warrant the cost of investigation and resolution?

Methods and instruments used for evaluation may include criterion-based studies, interviews with patients and staff members, surveys, and observations. Experimental research designs can be an excellent method for assessing and collecting meaningful data about the problem, although such designs can be complex and costly. First, however, study methodology and criteria must be established before data can be collected, analyzed, and interpreted. The Standards of Practice of the INS and guidelines of the CDC, American Association of Blood Banks (AABB), and JCAHO may all be beneficial in developing criteria for IV practice standards by which to assess problems and measure performance (INS, 1998, 2000, 2005; AABB, 1999; CDC, 1998; JCAHO, 1999).

ANALYZE AND INTERPRET

In collecting, analyzing, and interpreting data related to meeting the standards of practice and care, *compliance* refers to those situations in which the criteria are met. *Noncompliance* refers to the situations in which the criteria are not met. Both compliance and noncompliance are usually expressed in percentages. The expected compliance rate should be reasonable and achievable.

In most studies, findings are compiled statistically. These statistics provide a meaningful and concise description of the deficiency or problem. The data can then be used to calculate the average result, the difference between individual results and the average, and the relationship between the average result on one part of the study and the average result on another part.

PLAN CORRECTIVE ACTION

Once the findings are compiled, analyzed, and interpreted, a **plan of corrective action** can be developed. Two major forms of deficiencies require corrective action: knowledge and performance (Alexander and Corrigan, 2004). Components of the plan may address

- Changes that the environment can best accommodate
- Potential barriers or constraints
- Areas of potential support
- Needed resources

The best method of corrective action depends on the particular problem and individual situation. Methods may include revision of policies or procedures, change of equipment such as inclusion of tamper-proof nonpermeable sharps containers in patients' rooms, at shoulder height, and emptied regularly and as needed (Alexander and Corrigan, 2004), creation of a new information system, continuous monitoring, and on-site education.

RE-EVALUATE

After corrective action has been implemented, a re-evaluation is necessary to determine whether the applied corrective action resolves the problem. Frequently, re-evaluation is performed by repeating the first evaluation and comparing preaction data with postaction data.

RESOLUTION

The final step in the process is resolution, which involves developing a plan to ensure the maintenance of the quality of care achieved with the corrective action. Periodic or continuous screening may be required.

Continuous Quality Improvement

The influence of Deming and others, who introduced the concept of total quality improvement—also called continuous quality improvement (CQI)—has had a great impact on quality in health care organizations. CQI provides a mechanism for examining the process, rather than the individual involved, and encourages participation across interdepartmental lines to improve the process itself. Quality improvement teams in an organization are appointed and study areas are identified. Process improvement is the direct result of the CQI program (see Box 2–4 for more information).

Measurement of Outcomes and Improvement

Interest in patient outcomes and their improvement continues to escalate. One reason for this is mounting evidence of wide and perplexing variations in outcomes of care, use of resources, and costs of care.

Outcome Improvement

Patient outcomes may include physiologic values (vital signs, chemical results), physical values (ability to self-administer IV therapy), mental or psychologic terms (cognitive skill, affective interactions), social terms (ability to assume responsibility for self-care), and other health-related quality-of-life parameters (pain level, energy, sleep).

PROCESS IMPROVEMENT

The quality assurance technique operates on the assumption that the professional or institution is the sole cause of adverse outcomes and ignores the reality that sources

---

BOX 2–4   Deming's 14-Point System for Managing Quality

- Create consistency of purpose for continuous product improvement.
- Adopt the new philosophy across the organization.
- Cease dependence on inspection; improve the *process*.
- Avoid awarding business on price alone.
- Constantly seek to improve.
- Provide opportunities for training and staff development.
- Institute leadership; recognize the difference between management and leadership.
- Eliminate fear; fear inhibits innovation.
- Eliminate barriers among staff.
- Eliminate slogans; involve workers in the identification of new methods.
- Eliminate numerical quotas.
- Empower workers.
- Institute a broad-based education program to engage support.
- Be proactive in achieving transformation.

Adapted from Walton, M. (1991). *Deming management at work.* New York: Putnam.

---

of adverse outcomes are complex and include variations in policies, procedures, equipment, and techniques, as well as people (patients, professionals, support staff) and their interactions. In many cases, process improvement may be measured by developing a flowchart (*flowcharting*) to identify patterns related to the basic process, the detailed process, errors and corrective measures, and redesigns (Batalden, Nelson, & Roberts, 1994).

The flowchart begins with the basic process at admission to the institution; the flowchart continues the detailed process by highlighting areas of possible duplication, complexity, and sources of error (Batalden et al., 1994). Using the flowchart as a basic tool, many institutions have developed ways to manage the improvement process by incorporating the model known as the plan-do-check-act (PDCA) improvement trial. Those who use this model proceed through the following sequence: state aim, identify measures of improvement, plan and do a pilot test, check and study results, act to improve, and reflect on learning (Batalden et al.):

- Aim—What are we trying to accomplish?
- Measure—How will we know that a change is an improvement?
- Possible changes—What changes can we make that we predict will lead to improvement?
- Plan—How shall we plan the pilot? Who does what? When? And with what tools and training? What baseline data need to be collected?
- Do—What are we learning as we do the pilot?
- Check—As we check and study what happened, what have we learned?
- Act—As we act to hold the gains or to abandon the pilot, what needs to be done? (Batalden et al.)

A multidisciplinary quality council may be appointed within an organization to determine the best institution-wide approach to managing quality. A technique such as process management—consisting of merging comparative data analyses, operational and clinical analyses, **benchmarking** (comparing an institution with the best institutions nationwide), quality methods, and simulation methods—results in improvements in quality.

Some responsible and progressive hospitals and health networks have committed themselves to seeking significant improvements yearly. One goal, for example, is specific improvement in medication management by a certain year or other time frame. To achieve the overall outcome, the collaborative group may design an ideal plan for improved medication management. Some examples of the goals of the plan may be reducing medication errors within the respective facilities by 50% over a 3-year period; deploying an advanced adverse drug event detection technique in 100% of the collaborating systems; and introducing one breakthrough technology per year.

References and Selected Readings

Asterisks indicate references cited in text.

*Alexander, M., & Corrigan, A.M. (2004) Core curriculum for infusion nursing (pp. 428–230). Philadelphia: Lippincott Williams and Wilkins.

Alspach, G. (1998). Nurse-to-nurse recognition. *Critical Care Nurse, 18*(3), 6–9.

*American Association of Blood Banks. (1999). *Technical manual* (13th ed.). Bethesda, MD: Author.

*Batalden, P.B., Nelson, E.C., & Roberts, J.S. (1994). Linking outcomes measurement to continual improvement: The serial "V": Way of thinking about improving clinical care. *Journal on Quality Improvement, 20*(4), 168–169.

*Buerhaus, P.I. (1999). Lucian Leape on the causes and prevention of errors and adverse events in health care. *Image: Journal of Nursing Scholarship, 31*(3), 281–286.

*Centers for Disease Control and Prevention. (1998). Guidelines for prevention of intravascular infection. *Federal Register, 60*(187), 49978–50006.

*Conner, V.W. (1999). Patient confidentiality in the electronic age. *Journal of Infusion Nursing, 22,* 199–201.

*Dorodny, V. (1998). The highwire act of medical records security. *Advice for Health Information Executives, 2,* 24–32.

Institute of Medicine of the National Academies. (1999). Report on preventing medical errors: To err is human: Building a safer health system. [On-line]. Available at http://www.ashp.org/public/news/breaking/IOM.num.

*Infusion Nurses Society. (1998). Revised infusion nursing standards of practice. *Journal of Infusion Nursing, 21*(Suppl. 1), 517, 525.

*Infusion Nurses Society. (2000). Revised standards of practice. *Journal of Infusion Nursing, 23*(Suppl. 1).

*Infusion Nurses Society. (2005). Revised Standards of practice. *Journal of Infusion Nursing, 28*(Suppl. 1).

*Joint Commission on Accreditation of Hospitals and Healthcare Organizations. (1999). *Accreditation manual for hospitals.* Chicago: Author.

Premier, Inc. (1999, December 21). Internal communications: Executive express (p. 1). San Diego, CA.

Spielberg, A.R. (1998). Sociohistorical, legal and ethical implications of e-mail for the patient-physician relationship. *Journal of the American Medical Association, 280*(15), 1353–1357.

Weinstein, S. (1996). Legal implications/risk management. *Journal of Infusion Nursing, 19*(3 Suppl), S16–S18.

Review Questions

Note: Questions below may have more than one right answer.

1. The statement, "every person is liable for his own tortious conduct" is known as the rule of:
   A. Negligent action
   B. Personal liability
   C. Tortious conduct
   D. Wrongdoing act

2. A nurse inserts an IV cannula against the wishes of a coherent adult patient. In this situation, the nurse could be charged with:
   A. Assault
   B. Battery
   C. Assault and battery
   D. Malpractice

3. Which of the following is not a component of the credentialing process?
   A. Accreditation
   B. Certification
   C. Diploma
   D. Licensure

4. Confidentiality of patient information involves all of the following except:
   A. Audits
   B. Communication
   C. Privacy
   D. Security

5. Process improvement begins with which of the following patterns?
   A. Developing a basic flowchart
   B. Identifying/reworking errors
   C. Redesigning flow chart
   D. Updating policies and procedures

6. Researchers who have affected the quality improvement process include:
   A. Conner
   B. Evanson
   C. Deming
   D. Dorodny

7. Benchmarking is the process of comparing:
   A. Institution to like institutions
   B. Institution to the best institutions
   C. Practitioner to practitioner
   D. Practitioner to the best practitioner

8. Quality improvement programs examine:
   A. Individuals
   B. Processes
   C. A only
   D. A and B

9. The Food and Drug Administration inspects devices on which of the following levels?
   A. Good manufacturing controls
   B. Application for a device existing before 1976 (still in common use)
   C. Implantable or hazardous device
   D. Nurse-inserted devices

10. Electronic patient records may include which of the following?
    A. E-mail
    B. Fax documents
    C. Computerized records
    D. Voice mail

CHAPTER 3

Nursing Role and Responsibilities

KEY TERMS

Anesthesia   Mentor
Blood Bank   Pharmacist
Infusion Nurse Specialist   Resource Personnel
Infusion Nursing Team   Shared Governance
Knowledge-sharer   Staff Nurse
Magnet Recognition

Collaborative Role of the Nurse

Administration of safe, high-quality infusion therapy today depends on a collaborative practice environment in which many members of the health care team play a key role. The nurse, in particular, plays a primary role in collaborating with other health care providers to maintain an infusion and to protect the patient from the hazards and complications associated with routine infusion (IV) therapy. Policies regarding the responsibilities of a **staff nurse** in relation to therapy vary significantly among health care institutions and are often influenced by the presence or absence of a full-service infusion team.

An essential component of the collaborative practice setting is the flexibility of the infusion nurse in adapting to changing institutional environments. Expanded roles might include mentor, knowledge-sharer, Magnet Team member, and researcher. The global role of the infusion nurse is addressed in this chapter.

Role of Infusion Nursing Teams

Research findings show that an **infusion nursing team** enhances the level of care that an organization provides. To ensure that the team approach provides safe IV care, the role of the team and the delineation of responsibilities must be part of the orientation program and ongoing education for all nurses. Specialized teams of infusion nurses provide clinical expertise and cost-effective care. In the ideal setting, registered nurses with clinical and theoretic expertise should be responsible for administering infusion therapy. This improves the quality of patient care because specialized nurses, freed from other responsibilities, can focus their attention on developing a high standard of performance. Such nurses, aware of the inherent risks of therapy, are vigilant and meticulous in performing and maintaining IV therapy. Their advanced skills promote trauma-free venipunctures, conserve veins for future use, and reduce routine complications. The knowledge, skills, and abilities of these specialized nurses ensure patient safety. Infusion nursing teams succeed in those institutions in which their value is recognized and appreciated.

Resource Nurse

In lieu of a full-service infusion team, the health care facility may use the services of one or more IV nurse specialists as **resource personnel**. In such situations, the infusion specialist may serve as educator, clinician, or team leader to a number of integrated health care organizations or home care agencies. The role for the infusion nurse specialist is continually evolving. Changes in clinical practice and in the practice setting direct this process (Lozins Miller, 1998).

Mentor

The infusion nurse specialist has a unique responsibility and opportunity to **mentor** others. This responsibility transcends the nursing department as well as members of the infusion nursing team. Considerations for potential mentors may be found in Box 3–1.

Educator and Knowledge-Sharer

One of the challenges of knowledge management is that of convincing people to share their knowledge. Why should people give up their hard-won knowledge when it is one of their key sources of personal advantage? In some organizations, sharing is natural. In others, the old dictum, knowledge is power, reigns. In this chapter, we explore some of the barriers and offer some pointers in overcoming them. The infusion nurse is a knowledge expert with a broad spectrum of knowledge to be shared with others.

The role of the **knowledge-sharer** involves cultural change, cooperation, and commitment (David J. Skyrme www.skyrme.com/updates/u64_f1.htm; accessed October 5, 2005). According to Skyrme, culture change is never easy and takes time.

BOX 3–1   Mentoring

Here for your consideration are some potential benefits of your becoming a mentor. Maybe one or two of them will influence you to venture forth.

1. **Mentees need your expertise.**
   You have a wealth of life experience no matter what your age. You know how to listen, plan a project, make things happen, study and evaluate situations, talk to individuals and groups, influence others to take steps, bargain, write documents, parent, handle aging parents, express your feelings, and telecommute, among a multitude of other skills. Many individuals could benefit from grasping at least one thing you know.

2. **Mentees need your particular slant on your expertise.**
   Mentees need more than just the general expertise you possess; they need your particular version of it. How do you do it differently from others? What are the unwritten rules you've learned on how to do it better, faster, more enjoyably, or with more sensitivity? No one but you knows this, and it will end with you if you don't pass it on.

3. **Mentoring is less time intensive and mentor managed than it used to be.**
   Remember when mentoring was a lengthy, very involved one-way process? Mentors did all the choosing, pushed mentees to reach goals the mentors had in mind, and kept mentees under their wings sometimes for years and decades. The good news is that mentoring has changed drastically in the past 10 years.
   Mentees now manage the relationships, or at least take a major share of responsibility for setting goals, making sure meetings happen, monitoring their progress, and asking for and providing feedback. A little mentoring goes a long way. Even 1 to 2 hours per month of focused contact time with a mentee over 6 to 12 months can make a large positive difference in the mentee's life, career, and self-confidence.

4. **Mentoring is a way to leave a legacy.**
   Are you a parent or guardian? If so, you have a natural way to leave a legacy to the world through your children. You can also leave an important legacy through the work you do, what you create, improve, and influence that makes the world and the people in it better for having you in it. Mentoring at least one person well is another powerful legacy you can leave. A part of you, your experience, and your character will be a part of that person's journey, which in turn is likely to be a part of someone else's. Mentors really can change the world one person at a time.

5. **You will learn from your mentees.**
   We hear a lot of buzz these days about reverse mentoring. This means that the person normally thought of as the mentor is the receiver of guidance and learning from the person normally thought of as the mentee. An example of reverse mentoring is in the corporate world where older mentors are learning computer tips and tricks from their younger counterparts. No matter what your mentees know and can do, you'll learn something from them about their worlds and experiences.

6. **It is satisfying to see someone shine.**
   As a psychologist who has worked with a variety of clients on issues ranging from shness and relationship problems to achieving career excellence and healing from past sexual abuse, I know there is nothing quite as exhilarating as seeing a person get beyond a difficulty and become better than she or he ever thought possible. It's truly a high! This doesn't *always* happen when we reach out and try to help another, or at least it doesn't always happen in our presence. But we can help them start the process and pass them on in time to another mentor who takes them further. If we are fortunate, we will see at least one person flourish. That, quite frankly, is the best payoff of mentoring.

But, cultures can be changed once the term *culture* is clearly defined. Culture is defined in many ways, such as "commonly held beliefs, attitudes, and values," "the collective programming of the mind that distinguishes one group from another" and in many other ways that also embrace rituals, artifacts, and other trappings of the work environment. Cooperation is an essential component of knowledge-sharing; we are both competitive and cooperative. In today's complex world, we need help from others with whom we compete in order to achieve our goals.

And commitment is based on culture and cooperation. Organizations need to create a commitment to culture, to change, to challenge, to compete, and to cooperate. If, as is often the case, time pressure leads to poor knowledge sharing, then there must be a commitment to allow time for it to happen. Commitment to knowledge sharing must be demonstrated throughout the organization. It is inherent in the behaviors of infusion nurse specialists who consistently share knowledge with others even if it is not formally part of their job (Skyrme, www.skyrme.com/updates/u64_f1.htm).

Magnet Team Member

The **Magnet Recognition** Program was developed by the American Nurses Credentialing Center (ANCC) to recognize health care organizations that provide the very best in nursing care and uphold the tradition within nursing of professional nursing practice. The program provides a vehicle for disseminating successful practices and strategies among nursing systems.

The Magnet Recognition Program is based on quality indicators and standards of nursing practice as defined in the American Nurses Association's *Scope and Standards for Nurse Administrators* (2003). The Magnet designation process includes the appraisal of both qualitative and quantitative factors in nursing. (See Box 3–2 for the findings of independent research on magnet-designated facilities.)

Recognizing quality patient care and nursing excellence, the Magnet Recognition Program provides consumers with the benchmark for measuring the quality of care

---

BOX 3–2   Independently Sponsored Research Concerning Magnet-Designated Facilities

- Consistently outperform non-Magnet organizations
- Deliver better patient outcomes
- Experience increased time spent at the bedside of patients
- Have shorter patient stays
- Have lower patient mortality rates
- Have lower incidence of needlestick injuries
- Enjoy increased nurse retention and recruitment rates

that they can expect to receive. As a natural outcome of this, the program elevates the reputation and standards of the nursing profession. One such standard recognizes the number of credentialed nurses in a health care organization. The Infusion Nurses Credentialing Corporation (INCC) credentials infusion nurse specialists whose accomplishments are included in the evidence developed to support this standard. (See Chap. 2; also see Appendix B, on the CD-ROM in the front of this book.)

Shared Governance

A modern nursing shortage is revitalizing **shared governance**. This innovative organizational model gives staff nurses control over their practice and can extend their influence into administrative areas previously controlled only by managers (Hess, 2004). Shared governance in nursing is more than a new organizational chart or committee configuration; structures can be deceiving. The key factors are those who make up the membership. The meaning of success in terms of shared governance and patient care should be the control of practice leading to better patient outcomes. Shared governance is a frequent model within Magnet facilities, and research related to Magnet-designated hospitals indicates a clear correlation between status and outcome. In nursing, shared governance models have always focused on nurses controlling their professional practice. Shared governance is an ongoing journey moving from past orientations where the few rule to an orientation where many learn to make consensual decisions. Such institutions are in a constant state of growth, renewal, and revival. The infusion nurse specialist is an important part of that process.

Role as a Leader

Traditionally, the responsibility for IV therapy is allocated to the director of the **blood bank,** the **pharmacist,** or the **anesthesia** department. Infusion nurses fulfill several important functions. Not only do they administer blood and blood components, but they are in close alliance with the pharmacy. IV nurses administer infusions of which 50% to 80% contain additives. Moreover, they execute many of the functions performed by the anesthesiologist.

In some health care settings, IV departments may also function as self-contained cost centers within an institution's infrastructure. The infusion team has become an integral part of the nursing department, engaging in increased interaction and collaboration with nursing colleagues, especially as they seek Magnet Recognition (see Chap. 5).

IV Department Considerations

In organizing a department, the first consideration should be to establish a philosophy and the objectives necessary to support such a philosophy (Box 3–3). Next, the functions to be performed must be delineated (Box 3–4).

BOX 3–3 Example of Mission and Objectives of an IV Department

Mission

To administer safe and successful infusion therapy in the best interests of the patient, the hospital, and the nursing profession

Objectives

The objectives of an IV department are as follows:

1. To develop skills and impart knowledge that will provide a high level of safety in the practice of infusion nursing
2. To encourage further education and knowledge in the field of IV therapy
3. To assist in keeping the nursing staff educated in the maintenance of IV therapy and other nursing needs relevant to IV therapy
4. To collaborate with other personnel in the development and implementation of continuing education in infusion therapy
5. To develop nursing judgment and critical thinking in infusion therapy
6. To keep abreast of the latest scientific and medical advances and their implications in the practice of IV therapy
7. To attain and maintain certification

Departmental Policies and Procedures

Policies and procedures play a vital role in the functioning of the department, serving as a guide to its operations, providing the nurse with adequate instruction, and ensuring the patient a high level of nursing care. They may also provide legal protection in determining whether a person involved in negligent conduct has had adequate instruction in performing the procedure.

Policies and procedures should comply with state and federal laws, and national guidelines should be followed. The Joint Commission on Accreditation of Hospitals and Healthcare Organizations (JCAHO) publishes manuals for hospital, home care, ambulatory, and long-term care accreditation. The American Association of Blood Banks (AABB) provides a technical manual with standards for care and administration of blood and component therapy. The Centers for Disease Control and Prevention (CDC) and the Infusion Nurses Society (INS) provide guidelines as well as Standards of Practice (CDC, 1998; INS, 1998, 2000, 2005; see Chapters 2 and 4 for more information).

Policies describing the responsibilities of the IV nurse vary significantly among facilities and should be outlined to prevent confusion or misunderstanding. Examples of such policies are found in Box 3–5.

Delineation of IV Nurse Qualifications

Because infusion therapy involves specialized judgment and skills, the infusion nurse must be qualified to meet the job requirements and scope of practice (CDC, 1998; INS,

BOX 3–4   Functions of an IV Department

Infusion Administration

Parenteral fluids
Blood and blood components
Total parenteral nutrition
Antineoplastic therapy
Intra-arterial therapy
Pain management

IV Access and Monitoring

Peripheral lines
Pediatrics
Administration set and dressing changes
Therapeutic phlebotomy
Venous sampling
Peripherally inserted central catheters
Ommaya reservoirs
Other alternative access devices

Patient/Family Education

Self-care
Home therapy

Preparation

Drugs in solution

Collaborative Practice

Safety committee
Quality improvement
Code team
Product evaluation
Development of policies and procedures
Magnet preparation

1998, 2000, 2005). The success of the department depends on the selection of its personnel. Ideally, a credentialed **infusion nurse specialist** meets this goal.

These nurses must be not only meticulous in their actions, but also conscientious and dedicated to the specialty practice. There is no margin for error. Collaboration and teamwork are essential to the success of the department.

Mental and emotional stability are equally important to the nurse's success as an IV specialist. Manual dexterity, necessary in administering an IV, is greatly affected by the mental and emotional attitude of the nurse. Moreover, the performance of few

---

BOX 3–5   Examples of Policies Describing Infusion Nurse's Responsibilities

Administration of Parenteral Fluids

- Infusion nurses will, on written order, initiate all IVs, with the exception of those not approved for administration by the nurse.
- No more than two attempts at venipuncture will be allowed.
- Venipunctures should be avoided in the lower extremities except when the patient's condition may necessitate this use and this location has specifically been ordered by the physician.

Preparation and Administration of IV Drugs

- Nurses will, on written order, prepare and administer only those solutions, medications, and combinations of drugs approved in writing by the pharmacy and the therapeutics committee.
- Nurses must check the patient's clinical record and question the patient regarding sensitivity to drugs that may cause anaphylaxis. They must observe the patient after initial administration of such drugs.

Nursing Care Plan

- A nursing care plan should be established within 24 hours of date/time of admission.

Peripheral Catheter Selection

- The catheter selected should be of the smallest gauge and shortest length to accommodate the prescribed therapy.
- Only radiopaque catheters may be used.

---

other procedures is so easily affected by stress as a difficult venipuncture. Outstanding verbal and written communication skills are other assets necessary to the success of the nurse and the department.

Nursing Process Model

A study in the *Journal of Infusion Nursing* (Pierce and Baker, 2004) referred to the design and application of a nursing process model that illustrates infusion procedures performed in an outpatient setting. The effort aspect of the model may be applied to other clinical settings and involves parameters for before, during, and after service. During the therapy administration phase, reconstitution of a drug or solution may occur in a hospital-based admixture service, and greet-and-escort responsibilities refer to the outpatient setting. The study further details time and motion studies associated with infusion therapy and cost-justification. (See Chapter 23.)

Requests for Service

A system for receiving calls must be developed, with special emphasis on emergency calls. The size of the hospital, number of patients, size and location of the department, and the functions to be performed must be considered when deciding which system would be most appropriate. Voice mail may be used for routine scheduling and non-emergencies. Pagers are effective, as are facsimile (fax) transmissions to ensure accuracy and save time.

Preparation of Equipment

To maximize safety and minimize response time, the facility may choose to set up an equipment cart (Box 3–6) or designated supply cabinet on each patient care unit. Such equipment should comply with safety standards and infection control guidelines (see Chapters 9 and 11).

Before using the equipment, the professional infusion nurse ascertains the accuracy of the physician's order and then assembles the needed supplies from the cart if it is maintained on each nursing unit, or from supply storage areas located elsewhere. Regardless of the method of obtaining equipment for venipuncture, the IV nurse has a crucial role in determining the accuracy of the order, assembling the appropriate equipment consistent with the therapy that has been ordered, and using the equipment in a safe manner.

During their hospital stay, patients with IVs in progress may visit ancillary hospital departments, including medical imaging, nuclear medicine, and surgery. To ensure the success and viability of an IV department or team, other departments in the institution must be oriented to the team's functions. If orders are written early in the day, it will be easier to meet all requests and ensure timely delivery of therapy to each patient under the team's care (Lozins Miller, 1998; INS, 1998, 2000, 2005).

Educational Approach

Today's methods of health care delivery demand excellence in the administration of complex infusion skills and the application of critical thinking (Hammer and Souers,

---

BOX 3–6   Components of the Infusion Cart

The cart contains all necessary, single-use equipment for parenteral administration, including the following:

- Infusate
- Skin prep
- Venous access devices
- Syringes
- IV securement devices
- Administration sets
- IV start kits
- IV filters
- Transparent dressings
- Tape and gloves

2004). An adequate teaching program and criteria for evaluating the infusion nurse specialist must be established. The program curriculum and performance criteria depend on the role of the IV nurse as dictated by hospital policies. The nurse's competency must be evaluated and maintained, particularly when the infusion nurse receives on-the-job training.

The length of time involved in teaching depends on the individual and may range from 6 to 8 weeks. Box 3–7 provides a suggested outline for teaching IV, drug, and transfusion therapy. The outline is consistent with that defined in the Core Curriculum for Infusion Nursing (Alexander and Corrigan, 2004; Corrigan, Pelletier, & Alexander, 2000). The nursing faculty should incorporate active learning principles while teaching clinical skills. Clinical simulation allows students to learn and practice critical thinking skills in a controlled setting while ensuring patient safety.

Impact of Cost Containment on Teams

In today's health care environment, it is becoming increasingly difficult for established infusion teams to justify their existence and for new teams to gain approval. The health care setting has changed dramatically; fiscal constraints are often overwhelming, forcing institutions to scrutinize methods of IV delivery for efficiency and cost effectiveness (see Chapter 23).

As a result, hospitals have downsized, restructured the workplace, and developed new patient care delivery models. Such models have had a significant impact on IV teams because ancillary services are not regarded as appropriate to the new, centralized, unit-based approach to patient care. In all practice settings, IV teams must be innovative and adaptable while maximizing capabilities and analyzing complementary practice roles and multidisciplinary care. The teams must work with their professional society to lead the way toward designing new directions for intravenous nursing practice.

The CDC document "Guidelines for Prevention of Intravascular Device-Related Infections: An Overview" and part 2, "Recommendations for Prevention of Intravascular Device-Related Infections," published in *Infection Control and Hospital Epidemiology* and the *American Journal of Infection Control,* suggested that eliminating infusion teams downgrades patient care by raising the risk of infection (CDC/Federal Register, 1998). Lozins Miller (1998) studied the use of IV clinicians to maintain high-quality venous access care in a health care system involved in downsizing its ranks. Reassigning the role of the infusion team member to an IV nurse clinician added new skill sets and an expanded role (Table 3–1).

The Future of Infusion Nursing

This chapter addressed many expanding roles of the infusion nurse specialist; enhanced role models create a solid future for infusion practice. Teambuilding, partnering, outreach, collaboration—all terms of this millennium—suggest a continuing trend in health care. As the health care environments in which infusion care

BOX 3–7   Suggested Teaching Outline for IV Team Nurses

I. Legal implications of IV therapy
 A. State and institutional policy: review of state rulings and joint policies related to infusion therapy
 B. Health institution or agency policy
  1. Responsibilities of nurse in administering infusion therapy
  2. List of fluids and drugs delineated for administration by the nurse
 C. National guidelines and published standards
  1. Centers for Disease Control and Prevention
  2. Infusion Nurses Society
 D. Legal requirements
  1. Qualification by education and experience
  2. Adherence to institutional policy
  3. Knowledge base and skills sets
  4. Order by licensed physician for specific patient
  5. Skilled judgment
 E. Review of policy and procedure books
  1. Policy statements do not provide immunity if the nurse is negligent.
  2. The nurse is legally responsible for own actions.

II. Equipment
 A. Review all types of equipment, their characteristics, and usage.
 B. Review procedures for the proper handling of equipment, changing of administration sets, and safe use of products.
 C. Adhere to established infection control procedures and safety guidelines.

III. Anatomy and physiology applied to IV therapy

IV. Safety
 A. Choice of catheter (steel needle, catheter)
 B. Hazards and complications (observing the patient, reporting reactions, and taking measures to prevent complications are the nurse's legal and professional responsibilities)
  1. Systemic complications, including infection (septicemia, fungemia)
  2. Local complications, including phlebitis (mechanical, chemical, and septic)
  3. Preventive measures:
   a. Do not use veins located over an area of joint flexion.
   b. Anchor catheters well to prevent motion and reduce the risk of introducing micro-organisms into puncture wound.
   c. Adequately dilute medications.
   d. Use a catheter relatively smaller than the vein.
   e. Use aseptic and antiseptic technique.
   f. Remove catheter within 48 hours or consistent with institutional policy.
   g. Remove catheter for:
    (1) Erythema
    (2) Induration
    (3) Tenderness by palpation of venous cord
    (4) Nonfunctioning needle
    (5) Infiltration (recognize extravasation): Check questionable extremity against normal extremity, then apply a tourniquet tightly enough to restrict venous flow proximal to the injection site. If continues regardless of this venous obstruction, extravasation is evident.

BOX 3–7   Suggested Teaching Outline for IV Team Nurses   *(Continued)*

   C. Intra-arterial therapy
     1. Arterial puncture
     2. Constant arterial pressure monitoring
     3. Arterial blood gases
     4. Swan-Ganz catheter
       a. Basic knowledge
       b. Insertion
       c. Complications

V. Rationale of fluid and electrolyte therapy
   A. Fundamentals of fluid and electrolyte metabolism
     1. Body fluid compartments
     2. Electrolyte composition
     3. Acid–base balance
   B. Principles of fluid therapy
     1. Deficit
     2. Maintenance
     3. Replacement
   C. Infusion fluids: classification and effect

VI. Drug therapy
   A. Hazards
     1. Incompatibilities
     2. Vascular trauma
     3. Speed shock
     4. Bacterial and fungal contamination
     5. Particulate contamination
     6. Medication errors
   B. Knowledge of the drug
     1. Dose and effect
     2. Recommended rate of infusion
     3. Reactions
     4. Contraindications
   C. Factors controlling stability and compatibility of admixtures
   D. Preparation of admixture
     1. Procedure for transcribing orders on medication label
     2. Frequency with which medication order should be renewed
     3. Reconstitution of drug using aseptic and antiseptic technique
     4. Procedure for adding drug to fluid container
     5. Stability of the admixture
     6. Labeling
   E. Administration of drugs
     1. Verify identity of patient and admixture.
     2. Check for sensitivities of patient to any drug that may cause anaphylaxis.
     3. Observe patient for untoward reactions when administering an initial dose of an antibiotic.

(Continued)

BOX 3–7   Suggested Teaching Outline for IV Team Nurses   *(Continued)*

   4. Patients known to be sensitive to a drug require the presence of a physician.
   5. Inspect admixture each time before administration.
   6. Record drug, dosage, and amount of fluid on fluid intake chart and medication sheet.
VII. **Transfusion therapy**
   A. Principles of immunohematology
   B. Blood and blood components

is delivered continue to expand, encompassing tertiary care, home care, outpatient clinics, and work sites, the need to align with strategic partners escalates. The complex process of providing infusion care requires collaboration among a diverse group of professionals with a diverse group of skills, including, but not limited to, the following: infusion nurses, infection control, oncology, pharmacy, education, quality improvement, and medicine, as well as the patients and families they serve (Weinstein, 2004).

Partnering and collaboration are the hallmark of many successful models implemented by practice and academic healthcare settings worldwide. Strategic partnering, within and beyond institutions, provides opportunities for personal and professional growth, outreach, and collaboration. Within the global nursing community, cross-national partnerships represent a vehicle for extending knowledge sharing, using on-site visits, teleconferencing and videoconferencing, electronic mail, and other resources. The World Wide Web has opened doors to distance learning programs that were once only a dream. The future of infusion nursing is evolving each and every day in settings around the country and across the globe (see Chapter 24).

TABLE 3–1   Reassessing the Role of the Infusion Team

Reassessment Objective	Time Frame	Accountability
Reduce IV team full-time equivalents (FTEs)	60 days	Task force
Develop and implement training plan for staff nurse generalists	30 days	IV team leader, nurse educator, IV resource clinician
Transfer 3.0 FTEs to staff nurse positions	30 days	Chair, co-chair, nurse recruiter
Develop clinical practice guidelines for infusion therapy based on Infusion Nurses Society Standards of Practice	60 days	Task force
Establish advanced practice skills with 2.0 FTEs determined by caseload	60 days	IV team leader, nurse educator, medical director
Maintain level of quality	Ongoing	Task force

Adapted from Lozins Miller, P.K. (1998). Downsizing. *Journal of Infusion Nursing, 21*(2), 107.

References and Selected Readings

Asterisks indicate references cited in text.

*Alexander, M., & Corrigan, A.M. (Eds.). (2004). *Infusion Nurses Society core curriculum for infusion nursing* (3rd ed.). Philadelphia: Lippincott Williams & Wilkins.

*Baranowski, L. (1995). Presidential address: Take ownership. *Journal of Infusion Nursing, 18*(4), 163.

*Centers for Disease Control and Prevention. (1998). Guidelines for prevention of intravascular infection. *Federal Register, 60*(187), 49978–50006.

*Corrigan, A.M., Pelletier, G., & Alexander, M. (Eds.). (2000). *Infusion Nurses Society core curriculum for infusion nursing* (2nd ed.). Philadelphia: Lippincott Williams & Wilkins.

*Hess, R. (January 31, 2004). From Bedside to Boardroom – Nursing Shared Governance. Online *Journal of Issues in Nursing, 9*(1), Manuscript 1. Available at www.nursingworld.org/ojin/topic23/tpc23_1.htm; accessed October 5, 2005.

*Infusion Nurses Society. (2003). Revised infusion nursing standards of practice. *Journal of Infusion Nursing, 21*(Suppl. 1), S8–11.

*Infusion Nurses Society. (2005). Revised infusion nursing standards of practice. *Journal of Infusion Nursing. 28,* (Suppl. 1).

*Lozins Miller, P.K. (1998). Downsizing. *Journal of Infusion Nursing, 21*(2), 105–112.

National Electronic Library for Health. *The Knowledge Worker*. National Health Service. Available at: http://www.nelh.nhs.uk; accessed October 5, 2005.

Skyrme, D. www.skyrme.com/updates; accessed October 2, 2005.

*Weinstein, S.M. (2004) Strategic partnerships: Bridging the collaboration gap. *Journal of Infusion Nursing, 27*(5), 297–301.

Review Questions

Note: Questions below may have more than one right answer.

1. Infusion specialists may provide clinical support in which of the following settings?

   A. Home care

   B. Acute care

   C. Infusion centers

   D. All of the above

2. Research about Magnet facilities demonstrates which of the following?

   A. Shorter patient stays

   B. Lower mortality rates

   C. Lower incidence of needlestick injuries

   D. All of the above

3. Policies and procedures should comply with which of the following?

   A. State and federal laws

   B. Hospital handbook

   C. County rules and regulations

   D. Local law

4. The first step in developing an infusion department is to:

   A. Establish philosophy

   B. Define objectives

   C. Order supplies

   D. Create requisitions

5. A catheter selected for peripheral therapy should be:

   A. Largest gauge and longest length

   B. Smallest gauge and shortest length

   C. Largest gauge and shortest length

   D. Smallest gauge and longest length

6. All of the following statements are true about mentoring *except*:

   A. Mentoring is not time-intensive

   B. Mentees need your expertise

   C. You learn from mentees

   D. You leave a legacy

7. The infusion nurse specialist may have an essential role in which of the following?

A. Shared governance models

B. Magnet recognition

C. Mentoring programs

D. All of the above

8. The infusion nurse specialist must have which of the following attributes?

A. Mental and emotional stability

B. Manual dexterity

C. Verbal and written communication skills

D. All of the above

9. A nursing care plan should be established within how many hours of admission?

A. 6

B. 12

C. 18

D. 24

10. The infusion specialist may serve as:

A. Resource nurse/clinician

B. Educator

C. A and B

D. A only

CHAPTER 4

Application of Infusion Nurses Society Standards of Practice

KEY TERMS

Competencies
Educational Requirements
Practice Criteria

Scope of Practice
Standards of Practice

The Standards

The Infusion Nurses Society (INS) has established the **scope of practice, competencies,** and **educational requirements** for the administration of infusion therapy and has set forth **Standards of Practice.** In 1998, the INS revised the Standards and published the revision as a supplement to the *Journal of Infusion Nursing* (INS, 1998, 2000).

Because infusion (IV) practice changes continually, practice standards are updated to reflect those changes. The latest edition of the Standards, for example, eliminates the procedural aspects of IV practice; however, a Policy and Procedures Manual, also developed by INS, can be used as a companion to the Standards to complete the information base (INS, 2000).

Policies, Procedures, and Infusion Therapy

Each nurse in an organization must be cognizant of the policies and procedures relevant to infusion therapy and familiar with the nurse's responsibilities to provide a safe level of care for the patient. All nurses responsible for administering IV therapy should be familiar with established Standards of Practice.

The INS Standards of Practice establishes the educational, experiential, and technical criteria required to perform successfully at various levels in the specialty practice of infusion therapy. The Standards systematically direct practice and provide guidelines for assessing competency.

Competencies in Practice

The Standards allow for those inside and outside the profession to judge the competency of nurses practicing infusion therapy. The recently drafted edition of the Standards provides a framework for nurses to evaluate patient outcomes. Tools used for evaluation include nursing plans of care, assessment and monitoring processes, appropriate IV site selection and assessment, and various criteria for safe and effective clinical management of infusion therapy. Key standards and the **practice criteria** related to them are summarized in the following sections. (*Standards are printed in italics;* practice criteria are not in italics.) How well the nurse integrates the Standards and practice criteria is one way to evaluate competence in specialty IV nursing practice.

Care Planning and Practice Criteria

Care plans shall be established upon completion of the initial nursing assessment of the patient.

The methodology for content and construction of care plans should be defined in organizational policy and procedure and should reflect collaboration with the physician, pharmacist, dietitian, and appropriate others. The plan should set forth measurable goals and time frames as a means to evaluate the patient's progress and the effectiveness of nursing care (INS, 2000).

Assessment and Practice Criteria

Patient assessment by the registered nurse shall be an ongoing process to determine the appropriateness of infusion therapy and to ensure desired patient outcomes.

The use of infusion therapy assessment and monitoring tools should be established in policy and procedure. Initial assessment of the patient for whom IV therapy has been ordered includes the patient's primary medical diagnosis, nursing diagnosis, medical and surgical histories, allergies, vascular access history, patient preferences regarding vascular access device types and site locations, and long-range plans for infusion therapy when appropriate. It is essential that information obtained during the assessment and monitoring process be communicated to other health care professionals responsible for patient care (INS, 2000).

Clinical Management: Standards Applied

SITE SELECTION AND PRACTICE CRITERIA

Site selection for vascular access includes assessment of the patient's condition, age, and diagnosis; vascular condition, size, and location; and type and duration of therapy. The vascular

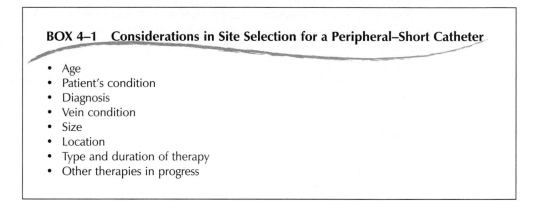

BOX 4–1 Considerations in Site Selection for a Peripheral–Short Catheter

- Age
- Patient's condition
- Diagnosis
- Vein condition
- Size
- Location
- Type and duration of therapy
- Other therapies in progress

---

site should accommodate the gauge and length of the cannula required by the prescribed therapy.

Specific practice criteria address peripheral sites, midline sites, peripherally inserted central catheters (PICCs), and central and arterial lines. Procedures have been developed for peripheral-short, peripheral-midline, arterial, peripherally inserted central, and central catheterizations. The method and choice should be clearly delineated in organizational policy. The application of this standard is essential in producing positive patient outcomes. Considerations in the catheterization of a peripheral vein are featured in Boxes 4–1 and 4–2 (INS, 2005).

CATHETER SELECTION AND PRACTICE CRITERIA

The catheter (or cannula) shall be the smallest gauge and shortest length to accommodate the prescribed therapy.

BOX 4–2 Considerations in Site Selection for Peripherally Inserted Central Catheters (PICC)

- Patient's condition
- Age
- Diagnosis
- Vein condition
- Size
- Location
- Type and duration of therapy
- Anatomic measurements to ensure full advancement of the catheter and catheter tip placement in a central vein

---

Note: Site selection of central catheters, other than for peripherally inserted central catheters, is a medical *responsibility.*

The tip of central vascular access catheters shall reside in the superior vena cava. Femorally placed central vascular access catheters shall have the distal tip residing in the inferior vena cava. Midline catheters shall have the distal tip residing in or at the junction of the axillary vein. All catheters shall be radiopaque.

Defined practice criteria identify the properties of a peripheral, midline, PICC, central, and arterial line (INS, 2005).

HAIR REMOVAL AND PRACTICE CRITERIA

Excess hair shall be removed by clipping with scissors or clippers.

Using a razor may potentially cause microabrasions of the skin that increase the risk of infection. Depilatories should not be used because of the potential for allergic reaction or irritation (INS, 2000).

INSERTION SITE PREPARATION AND PRACTICE CRITERIA

Prior to placement, the intended insertion site shall be cleaned with antimicrobial solution(s) using aseptic technique.

Maximum barrier precautions, including sterile gown and gloves, mask, surgical scrub, and large sterile drapes and towels, should be used for midline, PICC, arterial, and central line insertions. Talc-free sterile gloves should be used as well. Antimicrobial solutions include

- 2% tincture of iodine
- 70% isopropyl alcohol
- 10% povidone–iodine
- chlorhexidine (INS, 2005)

CATHETER PLACEMENT AND PRACTICE CRITERIA

Placement of catheters shall reflect the state Nurse Practice Act. Catheters should be placed for definitive therapeutic and/or diagnostic purposes. Cannulas should be used one time only. The placement of central catheters other than PICCs shall be considered a medical act. (The Standard also addresses the appropriate location of the PICC tip.)

Practice criteria address the need for a comprehensive understanding of human anatomy and physiology, vein assessment techniques, and insertion techniques specific to the device being used. The criteria further stress the need to consider manufacturer's recommendations for product use, including any modifications to be made to the catheter tip (INS, 2005).

ADD-ON DEVICES, JUNCTION SECUREMENT, AND PRACTICE CRITERIA

The revised Standard emphasizes the need for aseptic technique and standard precautions in the use of all add-on devices.

A method of securing the catheter should be used at the juncture points of administration sets and add-on devices. All add-on devices should have a Luer-lock device. The criteria define add-on devices as stopcocks, extension sets, manifold sets, extension loops, solid catheter caps, infection/access ports, needle/needleless systems, and filters (INS, 2005).

DRESSINGS AND PRACTICE CRITERIA

A sterile dressing, gauze, or transparent semipermeable membrane (TSM) should be applied and maintained on all vascular access devices.

The use of dressings and frequency of dressing changes should be established in organizational policy and procedure (INS, 2005).

BIOHAZARDOUS WASTE HANDLING

Improper disposal and use of needles/stylets (sharps) increase potential risk to the practitioner, patient, and community (Pugliese & Salahuddin, 1999).

Needles and stylets should be disposed of in nonpermeable tamperproof containers. Needles and stylets (sharps) should not be broken, bent, or recapped with two hands. Safety products that are consistent with Occupational Safety and Health Administration (OSHA) guidelines should be utilized (see Chap. 11; OSHA, 1999).

The practice criteria clearly suggest that all needles or other sharp devices have a safety device engineered to protect the nurse or other professional health care provider from injury. This is consistent with the recommendations for product selection found in Chapter 11, and in Appendix K on the CD-ROM in the front of this book.

INFUSION ADMINISTRATION SET CHANGE AND PRACTICE CRITERIA

The Standards address primary and secondary continuous lines and the need to change the sets every 72 hours and immediately on suspected contamination or when the integrity of the product has been compromised.

> **SAFE PRACTICE ALERT** An organization may consider extending the maximum 72-hour interval for routine primary administration set change for peripheral catheters if a consistent monthly phlebitis rate of 5% or less is achieved for a minimum of 3 consecutive months.

Again, the criteria suggest defining rules for set changes in organizational policy and procedure, and identifying the need to maintain an ongoing phlebitis rate of less than 5% with administration set changes after 72 hours or reducing the time factor to 48 hours in the presence of redness, infiltration, or any ongoing phlebitis >5%.

RESEARCH ISSUES: What Is the Phlebitis Rate?

A potential area of research is a study of the phlebitis rate in your organization and the impact that application of Standards of Practice has on patient outcomes.

TABLE 4–1   Infiltration Scale

Grade	Criteria (Indicators)
0	No symptoms
1	Skin blanched Edema <1 inch Affected area cool to touch
2	Skin blanched Edema 1–6 inches Affected area cool to touch Patient may or may not have pain
3	Skin blanched, translucent Gross edema >6 Affected area cool to touch Patient may have mild to moderate pain Possible numbness
4	Skin blanched, translucent Skin tight, leaking Gross edema >6 Deep-pitting tissue edema Circulatory impairment Patient may have moderate to severe pain

To calculate the infiltration grade of any amount of blood product, irritant, or vesicant, use the following formula:

$$\frac{\text{Number of infiltration indicators}}{\text{Total number of IV peripheral lines} \times 100 + \% \text{ peripheral infiltration}}$$

INFILTRATION AND PRACTICE CRITERIA

Infiltration is the inadvertent administration of a nonvesicant solution or medication into surrounding tissue (Tables 4–1 and 4–2).

The practice criteria clearly articulate the need to discontinue the infusion with an observed infiltration incident and to maintain statistical records including frequency, severity, and type of infusate for all such occurrences.

TABLE 4–2   Recognizing and Managing Infiltration or Inflammation

	Infiltration	Inflammation
Characteristics	Damage to tissue (limits access to vessel in the future)	Presence of erythema, induration, tenderness
Intervention	Delay treatment	Obtain sterile equipment and select opposite extremity for replacement site.
Verification	Confirm by tourniquet, not backflow of blood[*]	Send a sample of catheter and infusate to the laboratory for culture. Record lot numbers of catheter and infusate.

* An infusion has infiltrated if swelling occurs about the catheter site or a tourniquet applied above the catheter does not stop the flow of fluid. In small veins, the catheter may approach the side of the vein, occluding the lumen and obstructing blood flow; the solution flows undiluted so that no backflow of blood is obtained. The catheter may have punctured the vein, causing an infiltration, and at the same time be within the lumen of the vein, or the bevel may be only partially within the lumen of the vein, causing a swelling and still producing a backflow of blood on test.

CHANGE OF FLUID CONTAINERS

Air embolism and blood embolism are significant hazards of infusion therapy and may be associated with delay in changing solution containers. Subsequent solutions should be added before the level of fluid falls in the drip chamber. Failure to do this results in some of the serious problems that follow.

Plugged Catheter

Infusion fluids flow into the vein by means of gravity. Once the fluid level has dropped in the tubing to approximately the level of the patient's chest, blood is forced back into the catheter, occluding its lumen.

An occluded catheter should be removed, not irrigated. Fibrinous material injected into the vein can propagate a thrombus, possibly resulting in an infarction. Irrigation may embolize small, infected catheter thrombi, which could result in septicemia. Aspiration efforts aimed at dislodging the fibrin may cause the vein to collapse around the catheter point, traumatizing the vessel wall.

Trapped Air

If the bottle (in an air-venting system) is changed after the level of fluid drops in the tubing and before the catheter plugs, air becomes trapped in the tubing. The pressure of the fresh fluid then forces the trapped air into the patient, and fatal air embolism can result. Using plastic fluid bags, containers that contain no air, and administration

---

KEY INTERVENTIONS: Managing a Stopped Infusion

Avoid potential complications of infusion therapy by knowing what to do when the infusion stops:

1. Check for infiltration.
2. Check the fluid level in the bottle.
3. Check for kinking of the tubing.
4. Open the clamp.
5. Check air vent.
6. Check the catheter for patency by kinking the tubing a few inches from the catheter while pinching and releasing the tubing between the catheter and the kinked tubing. Resistance, if encountered, should be treated with caution because a clot may have plugged the catheter. If the patient complains of pain, a sclerosed vein may be causing the cessation of flow. In either case, the catheter must be removed.
7. Consider whether the catheter is in line with the vein or up against the wall of the vein. A slight adjustment, by moving the catheter, may remedy the problem.
8. Consider the possibility of a venous spasm, which may result from cold IV fluid (e.g., blood). Heat placed directly on the vein relieves the spasm and increases the flow of the infusion.
9. If the infusion is blood, check the filter; heavy sediment may be slowing the flow. Replace the filter if necessary.
10. Increase the height of the bottle to increase gravity.
11. If flow does not resume after following the preceding procedures, restart the infusion.

sets that have no junctions through which air can leak has reduced the risk of introducing air into the patient's veins.

Air can be introduced at the beginning of an infusion, however, if the administration set is not completely cleared of air, or when containers are changed. Infusions administered through a central venous catheter carry an even greater risk of air embolism than do those administered through a peripheral vein. Air embolism can occur during tubing changes involving the central venous catheter.

It has been suggested, through animal experimentation, that a normal adult can tolerate air embolism of as much as 200 mL, but for people in poor health, smaller amounts may be fatal; <10 mL might be fatal in a gravely ill person (INS, 1998, 2005; see Chap. 11).

Nonfunctioning (leaking or plugged) sets should be removed. In functioning sets, the old fluid should be replaced with fresh fluid before the flow ceases and the bottle empties. The following procedure should be used:

1. Vent a fresh bottle if venting is required.
2. Kink the tubing to prevent air from being introduced into the flowing fluid.
3. Change the fluid container, hanging the infusion bottle before unkinking the tubing.
4. Readjust flow rate if necessary.

FILTERS AND PRACTICE CRITERIA

Filters prevent the passage of undesirable substances into the vascular system.

Particulate matter filters should be used when preparing infusion medications for administration, and blood filters should be used to filter blood or its components (see Chap. 17).

Air-eliminating filters, such as a 0.2-μm filter, protect the patient from air embolism, bacteria, and particulate matter. The INS advocates using 0.2-μm air-eliminating filters for routine administration of IV fluids as follows:

1. The filter should be placed at the terminal end of the administration set, that is, as close to the catheter as possible.
2. The filter should be changed at the time of administration set change.
3. Lipid emulsions, blood, and blood products should not be administered through the filter.
4. Follow the manufacturer's recommendations regarding administration, particularly when infusing certain drugs whose dosage may be affected by the filter.
5. The pounds per square inch (psi) of the filter must be compatible with the electronic infusion device in use (INS, 2005).

MONITORING AND PRACTICE CRITERIA

Ongoing monitoring provides information regarding a patient's response to the prescribed therapies.

Patients receiving IV therapies should be monitored at frequent, established intervals based on practice setting, prescribed therapy, condition, and age. Monitoring should

- Follow established policies and procedures
- Minimize risk of potential complications of routine IV therapy
- Include documentation of the catheter site, flow rate, clinical data, and patient response (INS, 1998, 2005; Perucca, 1995)

DOCUMENTATION AND PRACTICE CRITERIA

Documentation of care provides a mechanism to record and retrieve information.
Documentation of IV therapy should include the following:

- Catheter
- Site
- Patient's response to treatment
- Type of treatment
- Date and time
- Name of the professional providing care

Documentation should provide sufficient information to identify procedures, prescribed treatments, complications, and nursing interventions (INS, 2005).

DISCONTINUATION OF THERAPY, CATHETER REMOVAL, AND PRACTICE CRITERIA

The patient's need for and/or response to therapy determine discontinuation of therapy.
To discontinue an infusion, the following procedure should be used:

1. Stop flow by clamping off tubing.
2. Remove all tape from catheter. Do not use scissors, which could accidentally cut the tubing.
3. With a dry, sterile sponge held over the injection site, remove the catheter. The catheter must be removed nearly flush with the skin. This prevents the point from damaging the posterior wall of the vein, thus encouraging the process of thrombosis.
4. Visually ascertain that the length of the catheter removed corresponds with the length inserted, and note this information in the record.
5. Apply pressure instantly and firmly. Do not rub. A hematoma may result from catheters carelessly removed, thereby rendering veins useless for future catheterization.

Small adhesive bandages, such as Band-Aids, should not be used unless specifically ordered. An adhesive strip does not stop bleeding, nor does it take the place of pressure. When used, it should be applied only after pressure has been applied and the bleeding stopped (INS, 2005).

References and Selected Readings

*Infusion Nurses Society. (1998). Revised infusion nursing standards of practice. *Journal of Infusion Nursing, 21*(Suppl. 1).

*Infusion Nurses Society. (2005). Draft revised infusion nursing standards of practice. *Journal of Infusion Nursing.*

Mazzola, J.R., Schott-Baer, D., & Addy, L. (1999). Clinical factors associated with the development of phlebitis after insertion of a peripherally inserted central catheter. *Journal of Infusion Nursing, 22*, 36.

Miller, J.M., Goetz, A.M., Squier, C., et al. (1996). Reduction in nosocomial infusion device-related bacteremias after institution of an infusion therapy team. *Journal of Infusion Nursing, 19*, 103–106.

*Occupational Safety and Health Administration. (1999, November). *Revised compliance directive.* Washington, DC: Author.

*Perucca, R. (1995). Changing and discontinuing infusion therapy. In: J. Terry, L. Baranowski, R.A. Lonsway, & C. Hedrick (Eds.). *Infusion therapy: Clinical principles and Journal infusion nursery practice* (pp. 400–405). Philadelphia: W.B. Saunders.

*Pugliese, G., & Salahuddin, M. (1999). *Sharps injury prevention program: A step-by-step guide.* Chicago: American Hospital Association.

Reed, T., & Phillips, S. (1996). Management of central venous catheter occlusion and repairs. *Journal of Infusion Nursing, 19*, 289–292.

Smith, R.L., & Sheperd, M. (1995). Central venous catheter infection rates in an acute care hospital. *Journal of Infusion Nursing, 18*, 255.

Zaragoza, M., Salles, M., Gomez, J., Bayas, J. M., & Trilla, A. (1999). Handwashing with soap or alcoholic solution? *American Journal of Infection Control, 27*(3), 258–261.

Review Questions

Asterisks indicate references cited in text.

Note: Questions below may have more than one right answer.

1. The INS Standards document was most recently revised in:
   A. 1995
   B. 1996
   C. 1998
   D. 2005

2. Which of the following statements is true of standards?
   A. They provide a framework for evaluation of outcomes.
   B. They must be implemented institution wide.
   C. They are applicable throughout a facility.
   D. They should regularly be compared with existing policies.

3. Which of the following is *not* true about care plans?
   A. They are an integral component of the nursing process.
   B. They reflect nursing diagnosis.
   C. They should be established before assessment.
   D. They include time frames for goal achievement.

4. Antimicrobial solutions suitable for skin preparation include which of the following?
   A. Tincture of iodine 1% to 2%
   B. Iodophors
   C. 70% Isopropyl alcohol
   D. Chlorhexidine

5. The 0.2-μm filter protects the patient from which of the following?
   A. Air
   B. Bacteria
   C. Particulate matter
   D. All of the above

6. Junction securement devices include:
   A. Luer-lock devices
   B. Tape
   C. Clasps
   D. Needleless systems

7. Which of the following is *not* a sign of infusion phlebitis?
   A. Swelling
   B. Redness
   C. Tenderness
   D. Raised wheal

8. An organization may consider extending the interval for routine primary administration set changes beyond 72 hours for peripheral catheters in the presence of a consistent monthly phlebitis rate of:
   A. Less than 1%
   B. 3% or less
   C. 5% or less
   D. Less than 7.5%

9. Hematoma is the result of:
   A. Careless removal of catheters
   B. Lack of patient compliance
   C. A only
   D. A and B

UNIT 2

Assessment and Monitoring

CHAPTER 5

Anatomy and Physiology Applied to Infusion Therapy

KEY TERMS

Aberrant Artery
Arterial Spasm
Arteriovenous Anastomosis
Integument
Radiopaque

Superficial Fascia
Tunica
Valves
Vascular System
Vasovagal Reaction

Vascular Anatomy and Therapeutic Goals

Because infusion therapy involves the administration of fluids, blood, and drugs directly into the **vascular system**—that is, into arteries, bone marrow, and veins—the nurse and others responsible for administering therapy need to understand the anatomy and physiology of vascular structures and related systems.

Although the *veins*, because of their abundance and location, provide the most readily accessible route for infusion therapies, the arteries and bone marrow are also used. *Arteries* provide the route for introducing **radiopaque** material for diagnostic purposes, such as in arteriograms to detect cerebral disorders, blood pressure monitoring, determinations of arterial blood gas levels, and administration of chemotherapy. The dangers of **arterial spasm** and subsequent gangrene present problems that make this route of therapy hazardous for therapeutic use. The *bone marrow*, because of its venous plexus, is used for infusion therapy by the intraosseous route.

The primary goal of infusion (IV) therapy is to provide a positive outcome for the patient. Painless and effective therapy is desirable, promoting the patient's comfort, well-being, and often complete recovery from disease or trauma. An integral part of this goal is the recognition and prevention of complications. To achieve the goal and minimize the risk of complications, the IV nurse needs a solid knowledge of vascular anatomy and physiology.

Integration of Knowledge With Practice

By studying the superficial veins, for example, the nurse learns to discriminate the best veins to use for IV therapy. Factors to be considered in selecting a vein include size, location, and resilience. In addition, understanding the reaction of veins to the nervous stimulation of the vasoconstrictors and vasodilators enables the clinician to increase the size and visibility of a vein before attempting venipuncture and to relieve venous spasm and thus assist in infusion maintenance.

By studying the superficial veins of the lower extremities, the nurse becomes alert to the dangers resulting from their use. Avoiding venipunctures in veins susceptible to varicosities and sluggish circulation decreases the likelihood of complications, such as phlebitis and thrombosis, and reduces the secondary risk of pulmonary embolism.

Common Venous Complications

Phlebitis and thrombosis are by far the most common complications resulting from parenteral therapy (see Chap. 9). Although seemingly mild, phlebitis and thrombosis may have serious consequences. First, they cause moderate to severe discomfort, often taking many days or weeks to subside. Second, they limit the veins available for future therapy. Injury to the endothelial lining of the vein contributes to these local complications.

Crucial to recognizing and preventing complications is a solid knowledge of the characteristics that differentiate veins from arteries and the positions of each. Understanding this helps the nurse avoid the complications of an inadvertent arterial puncture. The knowledge also helps to reduce the risk of necrosis and gangrene and to recognize the existence of an **arteriovenous anastomosis,** a congenital or traumatic abnormality in which blood flows directly from the artery into the vein.

Failure to recognize an arteriovenous anastomosis results in repeated and unsuccessful venipunctures performed in an attempt to initiate the infusion. Repeated punctures compound the trauma to the inner lining of the vein and increase the risk of the local complications already described, any one of which limits the number of available veins, interrupts the course of therapy, and causes unnecessary pain or, possibly, dire consequences for the patient.

Systems and Organs Involved in Infusion Therapy

Among the organs and systems closely associated with infusion therapy are the integumentary, neurologic, cardiovascular, and respiratory systems, as well as individual circulatory organs and structures.

Integumentary System and Connective Tissue

The **integument,** or skin, is the first organ affected in IV access. It protects the body from the environment and is a natural barrier to external forces. The skin is made up of two layers, the epidermis and the dermis.

EPIDERMIS AND DERMIS

The epidermis is the uppermost layer, which forms a protective covering for the dermis. Its thickness varies in different parts of the body. It is thickest on the palms of the hands and the soles of the feet and thinnest on the inner surface of the limbs. Its thickness also varies with age. In an elderly patient, for example, the skin on the dorsum of the hand may be so thin that it does not adequately support the vein for venipuncture when parenteral infusions are required.

The dermis, or underlayer, is highly sensitive and vascular. It contains many capillaries and thousands of nerve fibers (Fig. 5–1).

SUPERFICIAL FASCIA

The **superficial fascia,** or subcutaneous areolar connective tissue, lies below the two layers of skin and is, itself, another covering. The superficial veins are located in this fascia, which varies in thickness. When a catheter is inserted into this fascia, there is free movement of the skin above. Great care and meticulous aseptic technique must be observed because an infection in this loose tissue spreads easily. Such an infection is called *cellulitis* (Williams, Warwick, Dyson, & Bannister, 1995).

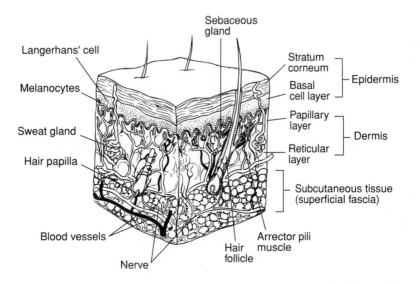

FIGURE 5–1. Layers of the skin. The epidermis protects the highly vascular dermis that lies above the superficial fascia (subcutaneous tissue).

Neurologic System

The human nervous system responds to changes in the environment through sensory organs. The nervous system is responsible for the following:

- Sensory function, transmitting information from tactile, visual, and auditory receptors
- Motor functions, controlling skeletal and smooth muscle
- Autonomic function, controlling glands and smooth muscle

Nerve fibers under the skin include those that react to temperature, touch, pressure, and pain. The number of nerve fibers varies in different areas of the body. Some areas of the skin are highly sensitive; other areas are only mildly sensitive. The insertion of a needle in one area may cause a great deal of pain, yet another area may be virtually insensitive to pain. The inner aspect of the wrist is a highly sensitive area. Venipunctures are performed here only when other veins have been exhausted.

The anatomic divisions of the nervous system are the central nervous system (brain and spinal cord) and peripheral nervous system (12 cranial and 31 spinal nerves). The vagus nerve, which innervates the heart, is of prime importance. Stimulation of the vagus nerve produces a depressant effect on cardiac muscle, resulting in clinical signs such as bradycardia and hypotension. This condition is known as a **vasovagal reaction** or vasovagal syncope.

Cardiovascular System

The heart is encased in the pericardium, which has two layers. The outer, fibrous layer is composed of strong collagen fibers and covers the aorta, superior vena cava, right and left pulmonary arteries, and the four pulmonary veins. The inner, serous layer is further divided into the parietal and visceral layers. A thin film of fluid between these two layers enables the heart to move.

The superior vena cava returns blood from the upper part of the body and has no valve. The inferior vena cava returns blood from the lower part of the body and has a semilunar valve near the opening into the atrium. The atrium, in its role as reservoir, has sufficient capacity to move blood through the tricuspid valve into the right ventricle.

Cardiac output is regulated by changes in the volume of blood flowing into the heart and control of the heart by the autonomic nervous system.

Respiratory System

Parenteral fluid administration affects the trachea, bronchi, and lungs. Blood flows into the lungs from the pulmonary arteries, which carry deoxygenated blood. These arteries follow the path of the bronchi. Undissolved particles in infusates may enter the microcirculation of the lungs, which may lead to emboli (see Chap. 11).

Circulatory System

The blood volume and distribution, for which the circulatory system is responsible, result from complex interactions between cardiac output, excretion of fluids and electrolytes by the kidneys, and hormonal and nervous system factors. Total blood volume may be enhanced by pregnancy, large varicose veins, polycythemia, and inability of the heart to pump enough blood to perfuse the kidneys (see Chap. 17).

The circulatory system is divided into two main systems, the pulmonary and the systemic, each with its own set of vessels. The pulmonary system directs the blood flow from the right ventricle of the heart to the lungs, where it is oxygenated and returned to the left atrium.

The systemic circulatory system, the larger of the two, is the one that concerns the IV nurse. It consists of the aorta, arteries, arterioles, capillaries, venules, and veins through which the blood must flow.

The blood leaves the left ventricle, flows to all parts of the body, and returns to the right atrium of the heart through the vena cava. Systemic veins are categorized as superficial and deep.

SUPERFICIAL VEINS

The superficial or cutaneous veins are used in venipuncture. Located just beneath the skin in the superficial fascia, these veins and the deep veins sometimes unite, especially in the lower extremities. For example, the small saphenous vein, a superficial vein, drains the dorsum of the foot and the posterior section of the leg; it ascends the back of the leg and empties directly into the deep popliteal vein.

Superficial Veins of the Lower Extremities

Before the small saphenous vein terminates in the deep popliteal, it sends out a branch that, after joining the great saphenous vein, also terminates in a deep vein, the femoral vein. Because of these deep connections, great concern arises when it becomes necessary to use the veins in the lower extremities. Thrombosis may occur, which could easily extend to the deep veins and cause pulmonary embolism. Understanding this, the nurse should refrain from using these veins.

Varicosities in the lower extremities, although readily available to venipuncture, are not a satisfactory route for parenteral administration. The relatively stagnant blood in such veins is likely to clot, resulting in a superficial phlebitis. Medication injected below a varicosity may result in another potential danger: a collection of the infused drug as a result of stagnated blood flow. This pocket of infused medication may delay the effect of the drug when immediate action is desired. Another concern is the danger of untoward reactions to the drug, which may occur when this accumulation finally reaches the general circulation.

Superficial Veins of the Upper Extremities

The superficial veins of the upper extremities are shown in Figures 5–2 and 5–3. They consist of the digital, metacarpal, cephalic, basilic, and median veins (Table 5–1).

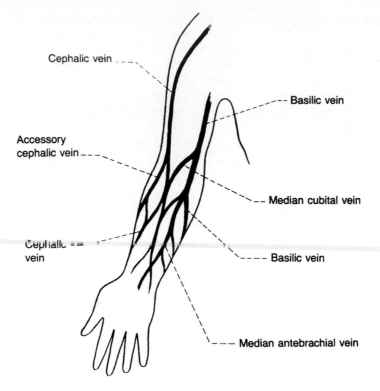

FIGURE 5–2. Superficial veins of the forearm.

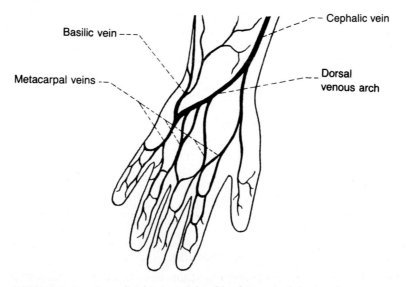

FIGURE 5–3. Superficial veins of the dorsal aspect of the hand.

TABLE 5–1   Determining the Appropriate Peripheral Venipuncture Site

Vein	Location	Advantages	Disadvantages
Digital	Along lateral–distal portion of fingers	Ideal for short-term use	Fingers may require splinting and immobilization. Catheterization may create patient discomfort.
Metacarpal	On dorsum of hand; formed by the union of digital veins between the knuckles	Easily accessible; lies flat on the back of the hand	Wrist movement is decreased unless a short catheter is used. Insertion is painful because of increased nerve endings. Site may become phlebitic.
Accessory cephalic	Along radial bone	Large vein ideal for venipuncture; readily accepts large-bore needle; easily stabilized	May be difficult to align catheter hub flush with the patient's skin. Catheter may impair patient mobility if placed over a point of flexion.
Cephalic	Along radial side of forearm–upper arm	Excellent large vein; readily accessible; does not impair mobility	Proximity to elbow may compromise joint movement; site must be stabilized properly before venipuncture.
Medial antebrachial	Arises from palm and runs along ulnar side of forearm	Easily accommodates winged infusion needle access	Proximity to nerve endings; inherent danger of infiltration
Basilic	Along ulnar side of forearm–upper arm	Accommodates large-gauge needle; appropriate for large-gauge devices	May be difficult to position patient comfortably during insertion; penetration of dermal layer of skin and proximity of site to nerve endings may cause pain.
Antecubital	In the antecubital fossa: median cephalic (radial side); median basilic (ulnar side); median cubital (in front of elbow joint)	Large veins facilitate blood sampling; good for emergency use	Median cephalic crosses in front of brachial artery; scarred vessels owing to frequent blood draws; difficult to stabilize properly

DEEP VEINS

Deep veins are usually enclosed in the same sheath with the arteries. Occasionally an arteriovenous anastomosis may occur congenitally or as the result of past penetrating injury of the vein and adjacent artery. When such trauma occurs, the blood flows directly from the artery into the vein. As a result, the veins draining an arteriovenous fistula are overburdened with high-pressure arterial blood. These veins appear large and tortuous. In these unusual circumstances, the nurse's quick recognition of an arteriovenous fistula may prevent pain, complications, and loss of time resulting from repeated unsuccessful attempts to start the infusion.

DIFFERENCES BETWEEN ARTERIES AND VEINS

Possibly the most dramatic difference between arteries and veins is that arteries pulsate and veins do not. Less apparent differences involve location and structure. Although arteries and veins are similar in structure—both comprise three layers of tissue—a close examination of these layers reveals their differentiating characteristics.

Tunica Intima: The Inner Layer

The first vascular layer is known as the **tunica** intima. It consists of an inner elastic endothelial lining, which also forms the valves in veins. Although these valves are absent in arteries, the endothelial lining is identical in the arteries and the veins, consisting of a smooth layer of flat cells.

This smooth surface allows the cells and platelets to flow through the blood vessels without interruption under normal conditions. Care must be taken to avoid roughening this surface when performing a venipuncture or removing a needle from a vein. Any trauma that roughens the endothelial lining encourages thrombin formation, a result of cells and platelets adhering or aggregating to the vessel wall.

Many veins contain **valves,** which are semilunar folds of the endothelium. Found in the larger veins of the extremities, these valves function to keep the blood flowing toward the heart. Where muscular pressure would cause a backup of the blood supply, these valves play an important role. They are located at points of branching and often cause a noticeable bulge in the veins. Applying a tourniquet to the extremity impedes the venous flow. When suction is applied, as occurs in the process of drawing blood, the valves compress and close the lumen of the vein, preventing the backward flow of blood. Thus, these valves interfere with the process of withdrawing blood. Recognizing the presence of a valve, the nurse may resolve the difficulty by slightly readjusting the needle.

These valves are absent in many of the small veins. However, if a thrombus obstructs an ascending vein, a small vein may be used instead. The catheter may be inserted below the thrombosis, directed toward the distal end of the extremity; this results in a rerouting of the fluid and avoidance of the thrombosed portion.

Tunica Media: The Middle Layer

The second layer consists of muscular and elastic tissue. The nerve fibers, both vasoconstrictors and vasodilators, are located in this middle layer. These fibers, which constantly receive impulses from the vasoconstrictor center in the medulla, keep the vessels in a state of tonus. They also stimulate both arteries and veins to contract or relax.

The middle layer is not as strong and stiff in the veins as it is in the arteries. Therefore, the veins tend to collapse or distend as the pressure within falls or rises. Arteries do not collapse.

Stimulation by a change in temperature or by mechanical or chemical irritation may produce spasms in the vein or artery. For example, interrupting a continuous infusion to administer a pint of cold blood may produce vasoconstriction; this results in spasm, impedes the flow of blood, and causes pain. Application of heat to the vein promotes vasodilation, which relieves the spasm, improves the flow of blood, and relieves the pain. The same results are obtained by heat when an irritating drug has caused vasoconstriction. In this situation, heat relieves the spasm, increases the blood flow, and protects the vessel wall from inflammation caused by the medication. With heat dilating the vein and increasing the flow of blood, the drug becomes more diluted and less irritating. The use of heat to achieve vasodilation is also helpful when the nurse must use a small or poorly filled vein.

Spasms produced by a chemical irritation in an artery may have dire consequences. A single artery supplies circulation to a particular area. If this artery is damaged, the related area experiences impaired circulation, with the possible development of necrosis and gangrene. If a chemical agent is introduced into the artery, the result may be a spasm—a contraction that could shut off the blood supply completely. This problem is not as serious when veins are used because many veins supply a particular area; if one is injured, others maintain the circulation.

Tunica Adventitia: The Outer Layer

The third layer, which consists of areolar connective tissue, surrounds and supports the vessel. In arteries, this layer is thicker than in veins because it is subjected to greater pressure from the force of blood.

Arteries require more protection than veins and are placed where injury is less likely to occur. Whereas veins are superficially located, most arteries lie deep in the tissues and are protected by muscle. Occasionally an artery is located superficially in an unusual place; this artery is then called an **aberrant artery**. An aberrant artery must not be mistaken for a vein. If a chemical that causes spasm is introduced into an aberrant artery, permanent damage may result.

References and Selected Readings

Asterisks indicate references cited in text.

Terry, J. (2001). *Infusion therapy: Clinical principles and practice.* 2nd ed. Philadelphia: W.B. Saunders.

*Williams, P.L., Warwick, R., Dyson, M., & Bannister, L.H. (1995). *Gray's anatomy*, 39th ed. London: Churchill Livingstone.

Review Questions

Note: Questions below may have more than one right answer.

1. Blood volume and distribution result from which of the following interactions?

   A. Interaction between cardiac output and excretion of excessive amounts of fluids and electrolytes

   B. Excretion of excess fluids and electrolytes by the kidneys, and hormonal and nervous system

   C. A only

   D. A and B

2. Total fluid volume may be enhanced by:

   A. Pregnancy

   B. Large varicose veins

   C. Polycythemia

   D. Inability of the heart to pump enough blood to perfuse the kidneys

3. Which of the following statements is *not* true about valves?

   A. They may be found in many veins.

   B. They are semilunar folds of the endothelium.

   C. They are found in smaller veins of the extremities.

   D. They keep the blood flowing toward the heart.

4. Stimulation of which nerve produces a depressant effect on cardiac muscle?

   A. Vagus

   B. Brachial

   C. Ulnar

   D. Radial

5. All of the following statements are true about the epidermis *except*:

   A. It is the uppermost layer.

   B. It forms a protective covering.

   C. Its thickness varies.

   D. It is thinnest on the palms of the hands.

6. Which of the following veins is appropriate for peripheral access (short-term)?

   A. Digital

   B. Brachial

   C. Ulnar

   D. Femoral

7. Which vein is located on the surface of the hand?

   A. Ulnar

   B. Radial

   C. Metacarpal

   D. Brachial

8. Which of the following statements is true of an aberrant artery?

   A. It requires more protection than a vein.

   B. It lies deep in tissue.

   C. It is protected by muscle.

   D. It is located superficially in an unusual place.

9. A working knowledge of the anatomy and physiology of which systems enables the IV clinician to practice?

   A. Peripheral vasculature

   B. Neurologic and cardiopulmonary systems

   C. A only

   D. A and B

10. Which of the following contributes to arterial spasm?

   A. Chemical irritation

   B. Impaired circulation

   C. Intra-arterial injection

   D. Necrosis

CHAPTER 6

Laboratory Tests and Values

KEY TERMS

Factor V Leiden
Glycolysis
Hematoma
Hemoconcentration
Herbal Remedies
International Normalized
Ratio (INR)

Peak Level
Postprandial
Reference Range
Trough Level
Venous Blood Samples

Reference Range

Although some laboratory tests offer a simple yes or no answer, ie, whether the culture was positive or negative, other results depend on their context. Results are reported in ranges, and those ranges are established by testing a large number of healthy people and observing what appears to be normal for them. The term *reference range* is preferred over *normal range* because the reference population can be clearly defined. What is normal for one group may not appear normal for another, ie, the changes that occur during pregnancy alter the body's chemistry and thus test results (Lab Tests Online).

Peak and Trough Testing

The value of drug level testing is enhanced when those levels are obtained at the most appropriate times. The actual time the specimen was obtained must be known to interpret the level, whether the specimen was drawn at the optimal sampling time or not. The actual time of draw should be entered on the requisition by the person obtaining the specimen. This will ensure that the draw time is entered into the patient's clinical record along with the serum concentration. The lab request should also indicate whether the draw is a peak or trough. For greatest utility, the best time to draw a **trough level** is just before the next dose. For convenience, trough levels may be obtained from 0 to 30 minutes before the dose, provided the actual time of draw is indicated on the requisition. Except where otherwise indicated, **peak levels** should be drawn 30 minutes after an IV dose and 1 to 2 hours after an oral dose. (See chapter on Pharmacology.)

Collection of Venous Blood

Safety

Safety is the first priority in obtaining, handling, and processing of blood samples (Chapter 11). In the past, infusion departmental responsibilities included the collection of **venous blood samples**. Although collection of venous blood now is usually delegated to a team of laboratory phlebotomists or technologists, in many instances the IV nurse will be involved in the following situations:

- When the patient is in an intensive care unit
- When veins have become exhausted
- When the patient is to receive an IV infusion
- When the specimen is to be obtained from a central venous catheter that is to be removed, from a multilumen central venous catheter, or from an implanted vascular access device

Role of Infusion Nurse

Advantages are gained when the IV department is involved in collecting venous blood. First, the nurse, understanding the importance of preserving veins for infusion therapy, is cautious when choosing veins and in applying blood-drawing techniques. Second, the IV nurse is skilled at using a single venipuncture to permit both the withdrawal of blood and the initiation of an infusion, thereby preserving veins, reducing discomfort, and avoiding undue patient distress. Third, patient–blood identification is of paramount importance in preventing the error of infusing incompatible blood. Because the IV department assumes responsibility for patient–blood identification before transfusion and is aware of existing hazards, its personnel are well qualified and trained in the collection of samples for typing and crossmatching.

Significance of Blood Collection for Testing

The nurse in any clinical setting is often charged to collect blood in a specified amount and in a specified type of tube. This chapter is intended primarily to provide the nurse with information concerning the most commonly performed laboratory tests—their purpose and normal values—and the collection and proper handling of blood samples. Laboratory procedures are not explained.

Practice Standards in Testing

The nurse is responsible for maintaining the practice standard in diagnostic testing (Table 6–1). The collection of blood samples for certain tests must meet special requirements. Some tests call for whole blood, whereas others require components such as plasma, serum, or cells. The requirements must be met correctly to prevent erroneous or misleading laboratory analysis. Practice standards cover a wide range of test procedures, techniques, and circumstances, such as those that follow.

TABLE 6–1   Standards for Diagnostic Testing*

Source and Standard	Applications to Testing
American Nurses Association (ANA) Council on Cultural Diversity and Nursing Practice prescribes culturally competent care.	The nurse serves as an advocate for the patient, communicates and collaborates with health care team from a cultural perspective. The nurse tailors instructions and care to patient's cultural needs.
Individual agency has a policy statement for specimen collection and procedure statement for monitoring patient after an invasive diagnostic procedure; policy for unusual witnessed consent situations.	The nurse observes universal precautions when handling any body fluid specimens. Labeled biohazard bags are used for transport of specimens. The nurse monitors and records vital signs for specific times before, during, and after completion of certain procedures. The nurse documents any deviations from basic consent policies and employs measures to obtain appropriate consents for the procedure.
U.S. Department of Transportation requires alcohol testing in emergency rooms in special situations.	The properly trained emergency room nurse performs blood and breath alcohol testing in unresponsive people and accident victims.
Occupational Safety and Health Administration (OSHA) standards apply to preventing transmission of hepatitis B and C and human immunodeficiency virus, safe work practices, vaccinations, and minimizing exposure to hazardous and toxic materials.	Nurses are exposed to bloodborne pathogens in the course of their work and are trained to observe universal precautions. Tasks and procedures in which occupational exposure may occur include the following: phlebotomy, injections, immunizations; handling contaminated materials, wastes, body fluids, and sharps; performing laboratory tests on body fluids; invasive procedures; vaginal exams and procedures; starting IVs; spinal taps; wound care; surgical procedures; cleaning.

*Nurses are accountable for safeguarding their patients within reasonable and prudent professional limits of practice.
(From Fischbach, F. [2002]. Nurse's quick reference to common laboratory and diagnostic tests [3rd ed.]. Philadelphia: Lippincott Williams & Wilkins.)

COLLECTING BLOOD AND BLOOD COMPONENTS

Serum consists of plasma minus fibrinogen and is obtained by drawing blood in a dry tube and allowing the blood to coagulate. Serum is required for most of the laboratory tests in common use.

Plasma consists of the stable components of blood minus the cells and is obtained by using an anticoagulant to prevent the blood from clotting. Several anticoagulants are available in color-coded tubes. Choice of the anticoagulant depends on the test to be performed. Most of the anticoagulants, including sodium or potassium oxalate, citrate, and ethylenediamine tetra-acetic acid (EDTA), prevent coagulation by binding the serum calcium. Other anticoagulants, such as heparin, are valuable in specific tests but are not commonly used. Heparin prevents coagulation for only limited periods.

Whole blood is required for many tests, including blood counts and bleeding time. Potassium oxalate is commonly used to preserve whole blood.

> **⚠ SAFE PRACTICE ALERT** *Hemoconcentration* through venous stasis should be avoided to avoid inaccurate results in some tests. Hemoconcentration, which occurs when a tourniquet is applied, increases proportionally with the length of time the tourniquet is in use. Once the venipuncture has been made, the tourniquet should be removed. This is a simple but important precaution, ignored by many.

Carbon dioxide and pH are examples of tests in which results are affected by hemoconcentration. If the tourniquet is required to withdraw the blood, it should be noted on the requisition that the blood was drawn with stasis.

Hemolysis causes serious errors in many tests in which lysis of the red blood cells (RBCs) permits the substance being measured to escape into the serum. When erythrocytes, which are rich in potassium, rupture, the serum potassium level rises, giving a false measurement. See Box 6–1 for a summary of special precautions for avoiding hemolysis.

BOX 6–1   Avoiding Hemolysis When Drawing a Blood Sample

1. Use dry syringes and dry tubes.
2. Avoid excess pressure on the plunger of the syringe. Such pressure collapses the vein and may cause air bubbles to be sucked from around the hub of the needle into the blood.
3. Do not shake clotted blood specimens unnecessarily.
4. Avoid using force when transferring blood to a container or tube. Force of the blood against the tube results in rupture of the cells. In transferring blood to a vacuum tube, use no needle larger than 20 gauge.

EFFECT OF INFUSION FLUIDS ON BLOOD SAMPLE

Infusion fluids may contribute to misleading laboratory interpretations. Blood samples should never be drawn proximal to an infusion but preferably from the contralateral extremity. If the fluid contains a substance that may affect the analysis, an indication of its presence should be made on the requisition—for example, "potassium determination during infusion of electrolyte solution."

SPECIAL HANDLING

Some samples require special handling when a delay is unavoidable. Some determinations, such as the pH, must be done within 10 minutes after the blood is drawn. When a delay is inevitable, the sample is placed in ice, which partially inhibits **glycolysis**—the production of lactic acid by the glycolytic enzymes of the blood cells—resulting in a rapid lowering of pH on standing.

Samples for blood gas analyses also require special handling and must be analyzed as soon as blood is collected. When the carbon dioxide content of serum is to be determined, the blood must completely fill the tube or carbon dioxide will escape. Several procedures are currently in use; in each, the escape of carbon dioxide must be prevented.

FASTING

Because absorption of food may alter blood composition, test results often depend on the patient fasting. Blood glucose and serum lipid levels are increased by ingestion of food. Serum inorganic phosphorus values are depressed after meals.

TIMELY EXAMINATION

Immediate dispatch of blood samples to the laboratory is vital to accuracy of findings in some blood tests. Promptness in examining blood samples is necessary in the analysis of labile constituents of blood. In certain tests (eg, those involving potassium), the substance being measured diffuses out of the cells into the serum being examined. The result is a false measurement. To prevent this rise in serum concentration, the cells must be separated from the serum promptly.

INFECTED SAMPLES

Special caution must be observed in the care of all blood samples because blood from all patients is considered infective. Blood samples should not be allowed to spill on the outside of the containers. Contaminated material should be placed in bags and treated according to institutional policies for disposal of infectious material. Catheters should not be recapped or broken but disposed of intact in catheter-proof containers. All personnel handling blood should wear gloves.

EMERGENCY TESTS

Blood for tests ordered on an emergency basis must be sent directly to the laboratory. Red cellophane tape or other special markings, according to the facility's preference, may be used to indicate a state of emergency. Tests most likely to be designated as emergency tests include amylase, blood urea nitrogen (BUN), carbon dioxide, potassium, prothrombin, sodium, glucose, and blood typing.

Effective Equipment: Vacuum System

Infusion nurses are often involved in venous sampling from peripheral or long-term vascular access devices. The vacuum system, which has increased the efficiency of the blood sampling process, consists of a plastic holder into which screws a sterile, disposable, double-ended needle. A rubber-stoppered vacuum tube slips into the barrel. The barrel has a measured line denoting the distance the tube is inserted into the barrel; at this point, the needle becomes embedded in the stopper. The stopper is not punctured until the needle has been introduced into the vein. Advancing technology has made this process relatively bloodless and consistent with Occupational Safety and Health Administration and Centers for Disease Control and Prevention safety standards.

After entry into the vein, the rubber-stoppered tube is pushed the remaining distance into the barrel. As the needle is pushed into the vacuum tube, a rubber sheath covering the shaft is forced back, allowing the blood to flow. The tourniquet is released and several blood specimens may be obtained by simply removing the tube containing the sample and replacing it with another tube. As the tube is removed, the rubber sheath slips back over the needle, preventing blood from dripping into the holder.

If the vein is not located, removing the tube before the needle is withdrawn preserves the vacuum in the tube.

It sometimes is necessary to draw blood from small veins. If suction from the vacuum tube collapses the vein, drawing the blood becomes difficult. By pressing a finger against the vein beyond the point of the needle or by placing the bevel of the needle lightly against the wall of the vein, suction is reduced and the vein is allowed to fill. In the latter process, the nurse should exercise particular caution to prevent injury to the endothelial lining of the vein. The pressure is intermittently applied and released, filling and emptying the vein. A small-gauge winged infusion needle with vacuum adapter may also be used; the smaller needle reduces the amount of suction and may prevent collapse of the vein. A syringe is often used to draw blood from small veins because the amount of suction can be more easily controlled.

Skillful Technique

PERIPHERAL VENIPUNCTURES

When skillfully executed, a venipuncture causes the patient little discomfort. The numerous blood determinations necessary for diagnosis and treatment make good technique imperative. The one-step entry technique should be avoided because too often it results in through-and-through punctures, contributing to hematoma formation. The needle should be inserted under the skin and then, after relocation of the vein, into the vessel.

The veins most commonly used are those in the antecubital fossa. The median antecubital vein, although not always visible, is usually large and palpable. Because it is well supported by subcutaneous tissue and least likely to roll, it is often the best choice for venipuncture. Second choice is the cephalic vein. The basilic vein, although often the most prominent, is likely to be the least desirable. This vein rolls easily, making the venipuncture difficult, and a hematoma may readily occur if the patient is allowed to flex the arm, which squeezes the blood from the engorged vein into the tissues.

Sufficient time should be spent in locating the vein before attempting venipuncture. Whenever the veins are difficult to see or palpate, the patient should lie down. If the patient is seated, the arm should be well supported on a pillow.

CENTRAL ACCESS DEVICES: BLOOD WITHDRAWAL

Occasionally, venous samples must be drawn from a central line, especially because these catheters are commonly placed in patients with limited venous access. A dual-lumen catheter may facilitate this process. When multiple-lumen catheters are used for central venous blood sampling, the proximal lumen is the preferred site from which to draw the specimen. Aseptic technique is vital in preventing the introduction of bacteria into the catheter. A sterile IV catheter cap (Luer locking) reduces the risk of bacterial invasion. A recommended method is highlighted in Procedure 6–1. Manufacturers have kept pace with our demands for technologically advanced products that enhance the sampling process, maintain the integrity of the sample, and ensure safety for both patient and caregiver.

Complications Resulting From Venipuncture

Complications related to venipuncture include hematomas, clotting, bloodborne diseases, syncope, and other problems.

HEMATOMAS

Hematomas are the most common complication of routine venipuncture for withdrawing blood, and they contribute more to the limitation of available veins than any other complication. They may result from through-and-through puncture to the vein or from incomplete insertion of the needle into the lumen of the vein, which allows the blood to leak into the tissues through the bevel of the needle. In the latter case, advancing the needle into the vein corrects the situation. At the first sign of uncontrolled bleeding, the tourniquet should be released and the needle withdrawn.

Hematomas also result from the application of the tourniquet after an unsuccessful attempt to draw blood. The tourniquet should never be applied to the extremity immediately after a venipuncture.

Hematomas most frequently result from insufficient time spent in applying pressure and from the bad habit of flexing the arm to stop the bleeding. Once the venipuncture is completed, the patient should be instructed to elevate the arm; elevation causes a negative pressure in the vein, collapsing it and facilitating clotting. With patients who have cardiac disease, elevation of the arm should be avoided.

PROCEDURE 6.1
Steps for Obtaining Blood Samples From a Central Venous Catheter

Equipment
To collect a blood sample from a central venous catheter when the patient is not receiving medications, obtain the following:

    Gloves

    Alcohol wipes or other appropriate cleansing agent

    Sterile 2" × 2" gauze sponge

    Collection tubes

    Vacutainer equipment or syringes as needed

    Labels

Action	*Rationale*
Wash hands, put on gloves, and clamp the infusion line.	Ensures aseptic technique
Aseptically cleanse infusion port or injection cap.	Ensures closed system
Withdraw 4 mL blood and discard.	First sample contains flush solution, which may alter test results.
Withdraw required quantity of blood; then raise the patient's arm to shoulder level.	Reduces axillary pressure on catheter
Open clamp. Follow manufacturer's recommendations for preparing and using diluent. Then flush the line with the designated amount.	Maintains patency
Adjust flow at prescribed rate.	Ensures compliance with therapeutic regimen
Wash hands and dispose *properly* of all sharps and *any contaminated equipment.*	*Promotes safety and infection control*

Constant pressure is maintained until the bleeding stops. The pressure is applied with a dry, sterile sponge because a wet sponge encourages bleeding. Adhesive strips do not take the place of pressure and, if ordered, are not applied until bleeding stops. Ecchymoses on the arm indicate poor or haphazard technique.

BLOODBORNE DISEASE

Special caution must be exercised in caring for needles used to draw blood from patients suspected of harboring micro-organisms. Contaminated needles should be placed immediately in a separate container for disposal, and standard precautions should be followed. A vacuum tube with stopper provides adequate protection against accidental puncture from the contaminated needle until proper disposal can be made. Any needle puncture should be reported at once. See Chapter 11 for more information about equipment.

OTHER COMPLICATIONS

Other complications of venipuncture include syncope, continued bleeding, and thrombosis of the vein. Syncope is rarely encountered when the clinician is confident and skillful and when patient teaching has preceded the venipuncture process. Continued bleeding is a complication that may affect the patient receiving anticoagulants, the patient with a blood dyscrasia, or the oncology patient undergoing chemotherapy. To prevent bleeding and to preserve the vein, pressure to the site may be required for an extended period. The nurse should remain with the patient until the bleeding stops.

Thrombosis in routine venipuncture occurs from injury to the endothelial lining of the vein during the venipuncture. Antecubital veins may be used indefinitely if the clinician uses good technique.

Common Laboratory Tests

Laboratory tests are performed for several reasons:

- To indicate relatively common disorders
- To make a diagnosis
- To follow the course of a disease
- To regulate therapy

Standard laboratory values are listed in Table 6–2; examples of conversions of those values to Système International (SI) units are given in Table 6–3.

Blood Cultures

Blood cultures are performed to identify the causative micro-organism when a bacteremia is suspected. Isolation of the organism facilitates appropriate treatment. Blood cultures are performed during febrile illnesses or when the patient is having chills with spiking fever. Intermittent bacteremia accompanies such infections as pyelonephritis, brucellosis, cholangitis, osteomyelitis, and others. In such cases, repeated blood cultures are usually ordered when the fever spikes.

In other infections, such as subacute bacterial endocarditis, the bacteremia is more constant during the 4 to 5 febrile days. Usually four or five cultures are

(text continues on p. 76)

TABLE 6–2 Selected Laboratory Values

Parameter	Normal values
Blood chemistry/electrolytes	
Blood urea nitrogen (BUN)	10–20 mg/dL
Serum creatinine	0.7–1.5 mg/dL
Creatinine clearance	Male: 110–150 mL/min Female: 105–132 mL/min
BUN:creatinine ratio	10:1
Hematocrit	Male: 44%–52% Female: 39%–47%
Hemoglobin	Male: 13.5–18.0 g/dL Female: 12.0–16.0 g/dL
Red blood cells	Male: 4600–6000/mm³ Female: 4200–5400/mm³
Mean corpuscular volume	80–95 mm³
Mean corpuscular hemoglobin	26–34 pg
Mean corpuscular hemoglobin concentration	32%–36%
Complete blood count	
Total leukocytes	4500–11,000/mm³
Myelocytes	0
Band neutrophils	150–400/mm³ (3%–5%)
Segmented neutrophils	3000–5800/mm³ (54%–62%)
Lymphocytes	1500–3000/mm³ (25%–33%)
Monocytes	300–500/mm³ (3%–7%)
Eosinophils	50–250/mm³ (1%–3%)
Basophils	15–50/mm³ (0%–0.75%)
Platelets	150,000–300,000/mm³
Reticulocytes	0.5%–1.5%
Red cell volume	Male: 20–36 mL/kg Female: 19–31 mL/kg

Parameter	Normal values
Blood chemistry/electrolytes	
Magnesium	1.3–2.1 mEq/L or 1.8–3.0 mg/dL
Chloride	97–110 mEq/L
Carbon dioxide	24–30 mmol/L
Phosphate	Adults: 2.5–4.5 mg/dL (1.8–2.6 mEq/L) Children: 4.0–7.0 mg/dL (2.3–4.1 mEq/L)
Zinc	77–137 µg/dL (by atomic absorption)
Lithium	0.8 mEq/L (therapeutic level 8–12 h after administration)
Serum proteins	
Total	6.0–8.00 g/dL
Albumin	3.5–5.5 g/dL
Globulin	1.5–3.0 g/dL
Lactate (arterial blood)	4.5–14.4 mg/dL
Serum ketones	Often >50 mg/dL in diabetic ketoacidosis. Usually <20 mg/dL in salicylate intoxication
Serum salicylates	Therapeutic range: 20–25 mg/dL Toxic range: >30 mg/dL
Anion gap	12–15 mEq/L
Aspartate aminotransferase (AST)	5–40 U/L
Alanine aminotransferase (ALT)	10–60 U/L
Alkaline phosphatase (ALP)	Varies with testing method

Plasma volume	Male: 25–43 mL/kg Female: 28–45 mL/kg
Clotting time	8–18 min
Prothrombin time	11–15 s
Iron	60–90 µg/dL
Total iron-binding capacity (TIBC)	250–420 µg/dL
Serum transferrin	>200 mg/dL (measured directly)
Partial thromboplastin time	Standard: 68–82 s Activated: 32–46 s
Fibrinogen	160–415 mg/dL
Serum osmolality	280–295 mOsm/kg
Serum amylase	25–125 U/L
Serum glucose	70–110 mg/dL
Serum electrolytes	
Sodium	135–145 mEq/L
Potassium	3.5–5.0 mEq/L
Calcium	Total: 8.9–10.3 mg/dL or 4.6–5.1 mEq/L Ionized: 4.6–5.1 mg/dL
Serum bilirubin	
Total	0.3–1.1 mg/dL
Direct	0.1–0.4 mg/dL
Indirect	0.2–0.7 mg/dL (total minus direct)
Lactate dehydrogenase (LDH)	100–190 mµ/mL
Urine chemistry/electrolytes*	
Sodium	80–180 mEq/24 h (varies with Na^+ intake)
Potassium	40–80 mEq/24 h (varies with dietary intake)
Chloride	100–250 mEq/24 h
Calcium	100–150 mg/24 h (if on average diet; varies with dietary intake)
Osmolality	Typical urine is 500–800 mOsm/L (extreme range is 50–1400 mOsm/L); usually about $1\frac{1}{2}$–3 times greater than serum osmolality
Specific gravity (SG)	1.002–1.030 (most random samples have an SG of 1.012–1.025)
pH	4.5–8.0
Arterial blood gases	
pH	7.35–7.45
PaO_2	80–100 mm Hg
$PaCO_2$	38–42 mm Hg
Bicarbonate	22–26 mEq/L
Base excess	−2 to +2

*Measurement of electrolytes may be of limited value because of recent administration of diuretics or lack of knowledge of dietary intake.

TABLE 6–3   Examples of Conversions to Système International (SI) Units

Component	System	Present Reference Intervals	Present Unit	Conversion Factor	SI Reference Intervals	SI Unit
Alanine aminotransferase (ALT)	Serum	5–40	U/L	1.0	5–40	U/L
Albumin	Serum	3.9–5.0	mg/dL	10	39–50	g/L
Alkaline phosphatase	Serum	35–110	U/L	1.00	35–110	U/L
Aspartate aminotransferase (AST)	Serum	5–40	U/L	1.00	5–40	U/L
Bilirubin	Serum					
Direct		0–0.2	mg/dL	17.10	0–4	μmol/L
Total		0.1–1.2	mg/dL	17.10	2–20	μmol/L
Calcium	Serum	8.6–10.3	mg/dL	0.2495	2.15–2.57	mmol/L
Carbon dioxide, total	Serum	22–30	mEq/L	1.00	22–30	mmol/L
Chloride	Serum	98–108	mEq/L	1.00	98–108	mmol/L
Cholesterol	Serum					
Age <29 y		<200	mg/dL	0.02586	<5.15	mmol/L
30–39 y		<225	mg/dL	0.02586	<5.80	mmol/L
40–49 y		<245	mg/dL	0.02586	<6.35	mmol/L
>50 y		<265	mg/dL	0.02586	<6.85	mmol/L
Complete blood count	Blood					
Hematocrit						
Men		42–52	%	0.01	0.42–0.52	1
Women		37–47	%	0.01	0.37–0.47	1
Hemoglobin						
Men		14.0–18.0	g/dL	10.0	140–180	g/L
Women		12–16	g/dL	10.0	120–160	g/L
Red cell count						
Men		$4.6–6.2 \times 10^8$	/mm^3	10^6	$4.6–6.2 \times 10^{12}$/L	
Women		$4.2–5.4 \times 10^8$	/mm^3	10^6	$4.2–5.4 \times 10^{12}$/L	
White cell count		$4.5–11.0 \times 10^3$	/mm^3	10^6	$4.5–11.0 \times 10^9$/L	
Platelet count		$150–300 \times 10^3$	/mm^3	10^6	$150–300 \times 10^9$/L	
Cortisol	Serum					
8 AM		5–25	μg/dL	27.59	140–690	nmol/L
8 PM		3–13	μg/dL	27.59	80–360	nmol/L
Cortisol	Urine	20–90	μg/24 h	2.759	55–250	nmol/24 h
Creatine kinase (CK)	Serum					
High CK group (Black men)		50–520	U/L	1.00	50–520	U/L
Intermediate CK group (non-Black men, Black women)		35–345	U/L	1.00	35–345	U/L
Low CK group (non-Black women)		25–145	U/L	1.00	25–145	U/L

TABLE 6–3   Examples of Conversions to Système International (SI) Units   (*Continued*)

Component	System	Present Reference Intervals	Present Unit	Conversion Factor	SI Reference Intervals	SI Unit
Creatinine kinase isoenzyme, MB fraction	Serum	>5	%	0.01	>0.05	1
Creatinine	Serum	0.4–1.3	mg/dL	88.40	35–115	μmol/L
Men		0.7–1.3	mg/dL	88.40	60–115	μmol/L
Women		0.4–1.1	mg/dL	88.40	35–100	μmol/L
Digoxin, therapeutic	Serum	0.5–2.0	ng/mL	1.281	0.6–2.6	nmol/L
Erythrocyte indices	Blood					
Mean corpuscular volume (MCV)		80–100	μm^3	1.00	80–100	fL
Mean corpuscular hemoglobin concentration (MCHC)		27–31	pg	1.00	27–31	pg
Mean corpuscular hemoglobin concentration (MCHC)		32–36	%	0.01	0.32–0.36	1
Ferritin	Serum					
Men		12–300	ng/mL	1.00	29–438	μg/L
Women		12–150	ng/mL	1.00	9–219	μg/L
Folate	Serum	2.5–20.0	ng/mL	2.266	6–46	nmol/L
Follicle-stimulating hormone (FSH)	Serum					
Children		≤ 12	mIU/mL	1.00	≤ 12	IU/L
Men		2.0–10.0	mIU/mL	1.00	2.0–10.0	IU/L
Women, follicular		3.2–9.0	mIU/mL	1.00	3.2–9.0	IU/L
Women, midcycle		3.2–9.0	mIU/mL	1.00	3.2–9.0	IU/L
Women, luteal		2.0–6.2	mIU/mL	1.00	2.0–6.2	IU/L
Gases, arterial	Blood					
P_{O_2}		80–95	mm Hg	0.1333	10.7–12.7	kPa
P_{CO_2}		37–43	mm Hg	0.1333	4.9–5.7	kPa
Glucose	Serum	62–110	mg/dL	0.05551	3.4–6.1	mmol/L
Iron	Serum	50–160	μg/dL	0.1791	9–29	μmol/L
Iron-binding capacity (IBC)	Serum					
Total IBC		230–410	μg/dL	0.1791	41–73	μmol/L
Saturation		15–55	%	0.01	0.15–0.55	1
Lactic dehydrogenase	Serum	120–300	U/L	1.00	120–300	U/L
Luteinizing hormone	Serum					
Men		4.9–15.0	mIU/mL	1.00	4.9–15.0	IU/L
Women, follicular		5.0–25	mIU/mL	1.00	5.0–25	IU/L
Women, midcycle		43–145	mIU/mL	1.00	43–145	IU/L
Women, luteal		3.1–31	mIU/mL	1.00	3.1–31	IU/L

(*Continued*)

TABLE 6–3   Examples of Conversions to Système International (SI) Units   *(Continued)*

Component	System	Present Reference Intervals	Present Unit	Conversion Factor	SI Reference Intervals	SI Unit
Magnesium	Serum	1.2–1.9	mEq/L	0.4114	0.50–0.78	mmol/L
Osmolality	Serum	278–300	mOsm/kg	1.00	278–300	mmol/kg
Osmolality	Urine	None defined	mOsm/kg	1.00	None defined	mmd/kg
Phenobarbital, therapeutic	Serum	15–40	μg/mL	4.306	65–175	μmol/L
Phenytoin, therapeutic	Serum	10–20	μg/mL	3.964	40–80	μmol/L
Phosphate (phosphorus, inorganic)	Serum	2.3–4.1	mg/dL	0.3229	0.75–1.35	mmol/L
Potassium	Serum	3.7–5.1	mEq/L, g/mL	1.00	3.7–5.1	mmol/l
Protein, total	Serum	6.5–8.3	g/dL	10.0	65–83	g/L
Sodium	Serum	134–142	mEq/L	1.00	134–142	mmol/L
Theophylline, therapeutic	Serum	5–20	μg/mL	5.550	28–110	μmol/L
Thyroid-stimulating hormone (TSH)	Serum	0–5	μIU/mL	1.00	0–5	mIU/L
Thyroxine	Serum	4.5–13.2	μg/dL	12.87	58–170	nmol/L
T_3 uptake ratio	Serum	0.88–1.19	—	1.00	0.88–1.19	—
Tri-iodothyronine (T_3)	Serum	70–235	ng/mL	0.01536	1.1–3.6	nmol/L
Triglycerides	Serum	50–200	mg/dL	0.01129	0.55–2.25	mmol/L
Urate (uric acid)	Serum					
Men		2.9–8.5	mg/dL	59.48	170–510	μmol/L
Women		2.2–6.5	mg/dL	59.48	130–390	μmol/L
Urea nitrogen	Serum	6–25	mg/dL	0.3570	2.1–8.9	mmol/L
Vitamin B_{12}	Serum	250–1000	pg/mL	0.7378	180–740	pmol/L

(From Fischbach, F.T. [2000]. *A manual of laboratory and diagnostic tests* [6th ed., pp. 1138–1141]. Philadelphia: Lippincott Williams & Wilkins.)

obtained over a span of 1 to 2 days, and antimicrobial therapy is initiated once it is established that most cultures harbor the offending micro-organism. If antimicrobial therapy is administered before the blood culture or before the patient's admittance to the hospital, the bacteremia may be suppressed, rendering isolation difficult.

Penicillinase may be ordered to be added to the blood culture medium to neutralize the existing penicillinemia and recover the organism. Antimicrobial therapy usually must be withheld to await report of culture to make a precise diagnosis. The penicillinase is added to the culture medium before or immediately after the blood sample is drawn.

Some bacteriology laboratories routinely culture blood under both aerobic and anaerobic conditions. If this is not done routinely and the clinician suspects bacteremia with strict anaerobes, the laboratory should be notified because a special culture broth is necessary.

Extreme care should be taken in ensuring a sterile field for venipuncture; the skin is a fertile field for bacterial growth. Colonization of organisms at the insertion site is associated with a high incidence of catheter-related infections. *Staphylococcus epidermidis,* diphtheroids, and yeast (common skin or environment contaminants) usually indicate contamination, whereas *Staphylococcus aureus* presents a greater problem, indicating either a contaminant or another serious pathogen.

Electrolyte Measurements

Electrolyte imbalances are serious complications in the critically ill patient and must be recognized and corrected at once. Electrolyte determinations frequently are ordered on an emergency basis. Accurate measurement is essential and to a large degree depends on the proper collection and handling of blood specimens.

POTASSIUM LEVEL

Potassium is an electrolyte essential to body function. Approximately 98% of all body potassium is found in the cells; only small amounts are contained in the serum.

The kidneys normally do not conserve potassium. When large quantities of body fluid are lost without potassium replacement, a severe deficiency occurs. Chronic kidney disease and the use of diuretics may cause a potassium deficit. Adrenal steroids play a major role in controlling the concentration of potassium: hyperadrenalism causes increased potassium loss, with deficiency resulting; steroid therapy promotes potassium excretion.

An elevated potassium level results from potassium retention in renal failure or adrenal cortical deficiency. Hypoventilation and cellular damage also result in an elevated potassium level.

Because intracellular ions are not accessible for measurement, determination must be made on the serum. Because the concentration of potassium in the cells is roughly 15 times greater than that in the serum, the blood for potassium determination must be carefully drawn to prevent hemolysis.

Blood Collection

Blood (2 mL) is drawn in a dry tube and allowed to clot or, preferably, placed under oil, which minimizes friction and hemolysis of the RBCs. The blood should be sent to the laboratory immediately because potassium diffuses out of the cells and gives a falsely high reading.

Test Result

Normal serum range is 3.5 to 5.0 mEq/L (Fischbach, 2002).

SODIUM LEVEL

The main role of sodium is the control of the distribution of water throughout the body and the maintenance of a normal fluid balance.

The excretion of sodium is regulated mainly by the adrenocortical hormone aldosterone. Water excretion is regulated by antidiuretic hormone, and as long as these two systems are in harmony, the sodium and water remain in isosmotic proportion. Any change in the normal sodium concentration indicates that the loss or gain of water and sodium is in other than isosmotic proportion. Increased sodium levels may be caused by excessive infusions of sodium, insufficient water intake, or excess loss of fluid without a sodium loss, as in tracheobronchitis. Decreased sodium levels may be caused by excessive sweating accompanied by intake of large amounts of water by mouth, adrenal insufficiency, excessive infusions of nonelectrolyte fluids, or gastrointestinal suction accompanied with water by mouth.

Blood Collection

Blood (3 mL) is drawn carefully to prevent hemolysis and placed in a dry tube or a tube with oil.

Test Result

Normal serum range is 135 to 145 mEq/L.

CHLORIDE LEVEL

Chlorides are usually measured along with other blood electrolytes. The measurement of chlorides is helpful in diagnosing disorders of acid–base balance and water balance of the body. Chloride reciprocally increases or decreases in concentration whenever changes in concentration of other anions occur. In metabolic acidosis, a reciprocal rise in chloride concentration occurs when the bicarbonate concentration drops.

Elevation in the blood chloride level occurs in such conditions as Cushing's syndrome, hyperventilation, and some kidney disorders. A decrease in blood chloride levels may occur in diabetic acidosis and heat exhaustion and after vomiting and diarrhea.

Blood Collection

Venous blood (5 mL) is withdrawn and placed in a dry tube to clot.

Test Result

Normal serum range is 97 to 110 mEq/L.

CALCIUM LEVEL

Calcium, an essential electrolyte of the body, is required for blood clotting, muscular contraction, and nerve transmission. Only ionized calcium is useful, but because it cannot be satisfactorily measured, the total amount of body calcium is determined; 50% of the total is believed to be ionized (Metheny, 2000). In acidosis, there is a higher level of ionized calcium; in alkalosis, a lower level.

Hypocalcemia (decrease in blood calcium) occurs whenever impairment of the gastrointestinal tract, such as with sprue or celiac disease, prevents absorption. Deficiency, which also occurs in hypoparathyroidism and in some kidney diseases, is characterized by muscular twitching and tetanic convulsions.

Hypercalcemia (excess of calcium in the blood) occurs in hyperparathyroidism and in respiratory disturbances in which the carbon dioxide blood content is increased, such as in respiratory acidosis.

Blood Collection

Venous blood (5 mL) is placed in a dry tube and allowed to clot. Analysis is performed on the serum.

Test Result

Normal serum range in adults is 8.9 to 10.3 mg/100 mL. The range is slightly higher in children.

PHOSPHORUS LEVEL

Phosphorus metabolism is related to calcium metabolism, and the serum level varies inversely with calcium.

Phosphorus concentrations may be increased in conditions such as hypoparathyroidism, kidney disease, or excessive intake of vitamin D. Decreased concentrations may occur in hyperparathyroidism, rickets, and some kidney diseases.

Blood Collection

Because RBCs are rich in phosphorus, hemolysis must be avoided. Analysis is performed on the serum; 4 mL blood is placed in a dry tube to clot.

Test Result

Normal serum range is 2.5 to 4.5 mg/100 mL (Metheny, 2000). In infants in the first year, the upper limit of the range rises to 6.0 mg/100 mL.

Venous Blood Measurements of Acid–Base Balance

The body's major buffer system is the bicarbonate (HCO_3)-carbonic acid (H_2CO_3) buffer system. Normally, there are 20 parts of bicarbonate to one part of carbonic acid. When deviations occur in the normal ratio, the pH changes. The change is accompanied by a change in bicarbonate concentration.

CARBON DIOXIDE CONTENT

Carbon dioxide content is the measurement of the free carbon dioxide and bicarbonate content of the serum, which provides a general measure of acidity or alkalinity. An increase in carbon dioxide content usually indicates alkalosis; a decrease indicates acidosis. This test, along with clinical findings, is helpful in determining the severity and nature of the disorder. Measurement of pH is necessary for accuracy—a change in carbon dioxide does not always signify a change in pH because pH depends on the buffer ratio and not the carbon dioxide content. When the carbon dioxide and pH are known, the buffer ratio can be determined.

An elevated carbon dioxide content is present in metabolic alkalosis, hypoventilation, loss of acid secretions (such as occurs in persistent vomiting or drainage of the stomach), and excessive administration of corticotropin or cortisone. A low carbon dioxide content usually occurs in loss of alkaline secretions such as in severe diarrhea, certain kidney diseases, diabetic acidosis, and hyperventilation.

Blood Collection

Several procedures are now used to collect blood: collection in a heparinized syringe with immediate placement on ice, collection in a heparinized vacuum tube, or collection in a dry tube without an anticoagulant. The procedure used depends on the laboratory. The containers must always be filled with blood to prevent carbon dioxide from escaping.

 SAFE PRACTICE ALERT   In all methods, it is important that the patient avoid clenching his or her fist; excess muscular activity of the arm can increase the carbon dioxide level in the blood.

Test Result

Normal serum range is 22 to 31 mEq/L.

BLOOD PH

The pH, a measure of acidity, indicates the serum concentration of hydrogen ions. The pH becomes lower in acid conditions, such as hypoventilation, diarrhea, and diabetic acidosis. The pH rises in alkaline conditions, such as hyperventilation and excessive vomiting.

Blood Collection

The blood is collected without stasis in a heparinized 2-mL syringe; the syringe is then capped. The blood may be drawn with a small-vein needle, the needle discarded, and the tubing tied off. The specimen is left in the syringe and packed in ice. Loss of carbon dioxide from contact with the air is thus avoided and excess production of lactic acid by enzymic reaction reduced. Blood (5 mL) may also be collected in a green-stoppered vacuum tube containing heparin.

Test Result

Normal blood pH ranges between 7.35 and 7.45.

Enzyme Analyses

AMYLASE

Amylase determination is helpful in the diagnosis of acute pancreatitis or the acute recurrence of chronic pancreatitis. Amylase is secreted by the pancreas; a rise in the serum level occurs when outflow of pancreatic juice is restricted. This test is usually performed on patients with acute abdominal pain or on surgical patients in whom injury may have occurred to the pancreas. Amylase levels usually remain elevated for only a short time (3 to 6 days).

Blood Collection
Venous blood (6 mL) is allowed to clot in a dry tube.

Test Result
Normal serum range is 4 to 25 U/mL. The range may depend on the normal values established by clinical laboratories because the method may be modified.

LIPASE

Lipase determination is used for detecting damage to the pancreas and is valuable when too much time has elapsed for the amylase level to remain elevated. When secretions of the pancreas are blocked, the serum lipase level rises.

Blood Collection
The test is performed on serum from 6 mL of clotted blood.

Test Result
Normal serum level is 2 U/mL or less.

ACID PHOSPHATASE

Acid phosphatase levels are useful in determining metastasizing tumors of the prostate. The prostate gland and prostatic carcinoma are rich in phosphatase, but do not normally release the enzyme into the serum. Once the carcinoma has spread, it starts to release acid phosphatase, increasing the serum concentration. In addition to carcinoma of the prostate, other conditions that produce increased serum acid phosphatase levels are Paget's disease, hyperparathyroidism, metastatic mammary carcinoma, renal insufficiency, multiple myeloma, some liver disease, arterial embolism, myocardial infarction, and sickle cell crisis.

Blood Collection
Blood (5 mL) is allowed to clot in a dry tube. Hemolysis should be avoided. Analysis should be immediate, or the serum should be frozen.

Test Result
Normal serum range is 0 to 3, 1 ng/mL

ALKALINE PHOSPHATASE

Alkaline phosphatase is a useful test in diagnosing bone diseases and obstructive jaundice. In bone diseases, the small amount of alkaline phosphatase usually present in the serum rises in proportion to the number of new bone cells. When excretion of alkaline phosphatase is impaired, as in some disorders of the liver and biliary tract, the serum level rises and may give some evidence of the degree of blockage in the biliary tract.

Blood Collection

Blood (5 mL) is drawn and the test is performed on the serum. Sodium sulfobromophthalein dye should be avoided.

Test Result

Normal serum range is 13 to 39 U/mL.

ASPARTATE AMINOTRANSFERASE

The transaminases are enzymes found in large quantities in the heart, liver, muscle, kidney, and pancreas cells. Any disease that damages these cells results in an elevated serum transaminase level. Clinical signs and other tests are used in diagnosis.

The aspartate aminotransferase (AST; formerly known as serum glutamic-oxaloacetic transaminase) level is used to distinguish between myocardial infarction and acute coronary insufficiency without infarction. It is also useful as a liver function test to follow the progression of liver damage or ascertain when the liver has recovered.

Blood Collection

The test is performed on serum from 5 mL clotted blood.

Test Result

Normal serum range is 10 to 40 U/mL. In myocardial infarction, the level is increased 4 to 10 times, whereas in liver involvement a high of 10 to 100 times normal may occur. The serum level remains elevated for approximately 5 days.

ALANINE AMINOTRANSFERASE

The alanine aminotransferase (formerly known as serum glutamic-pyruvic transaminase) level is more specific for hepatic malfunction than the AST value.

Blood Collection

The test is performed on 5 mL of serum.

Test Result

Normal serum range is 10 to 60 U/L.

SERUM LACTATE DEHYDROGENASE

The transaminase lactate dehydrogenase is present in all tissues and in large quantities in the kidney, heart, and skeletal muscles. Elevated serum levels usually parallel AST levels. Elevation occurs in myocardial infarction and may continue through the sixth day. Elevations have been found in lymphoma, disseminated carcinoma, and some cases of leukemia.

Blood Collection

Blood (3 mL) is collected and allowed to coagulate. Care must be taken to avoid hemolysis because only a slight degree may give an incorrect reading.

Test Result

Normal serum range is 60 to 120 U/mL.

LIVER FUNCTION TESTS

Liver function tests measure albumin, globulin, total protein levels, and the albumin/globulin ratio. These tests may be useful in diagnosing kidney and liver disease or in judging the effectiveness of treatment. The chief role of serum albumin is to maintain osmotic pressure of the blood; globulin assists. The globulin molecule, because it is larger than the albumin, is less efficient in maintaining osmotic pressure and does not leak out of the blood. With the loss of albumin through the capillary wall, the body compensates by producing more globulin. The osmotic pressure is reduced, which may result in edema. Certain conditions, such as chronic nephritis, lipoid nephrosis, liver disease, and malnutrition, result in a lowered albumin concentration.

Blood Collection

The test is performed on serum from 6 mL of clotted blood.

Test Result

Normal serum ranges:

- Total protein: 6.0 to 8.0 g/100 mL
- Albumin: 3.2 to 5.6 g/100 mL
- Globulin: 1.3 to 3.5 g/100 mL

BILIRUBIN (DIRECT AND INDIRECT)

The bilirubin test, which is becoming less common, differentiates between impairment of the liver by obstruction and hemolysis. Bilirubin arises from the hemoglobin liberated from broken-down RBCs. It is the chief pigment of the bile, excreted by the liver. Impairment by obstruction of the excretory function of the liver leads to an excess of free (non–protein-bound) circulatory bilirubin. Measurement of free bilirubin (direct) usually indicates obstruction.

When increased RBC destruction (hemolysis) occurs, the increased bilirubin is believed to be bound to protein (indirect).

A total bilirubin determination detects increased concentration of bilirubin before jaundice appears.

Blood Collection

The test is performed on serum from 5 mL of clotted blood.

Test Result

Normal serum range is 0.1 to 1.0 mg/100 mL.

CHOLESTEROL

Cholesterol, a normal constituent of the blood, is present in all body cells. In various disease states, the cholesterol concentration in the serum may rise or fall. Cholesterol is transported in the blood by the low-density lipoproteins (LDLs; 60% to 75%) and high-density lipoproteins (HDLs; 15% to 35%). A high level of HDL indicates a healthy metabolic system in a patient free of liver disease. Very-low-density lipoproteins (VLDLs) are major carriers of triglyceride. Degradation of VLDL is a major source of LDLs.

Cholesterol measurements may be part of a total lipid profile or an absolute test value. A lipid profile includes total cholesterol count.

Blood Collection

The test is performed on serum from 5 mL of clotted blood.

Test Result

Normal serum range is 120 to 260 mg/100 mL.

PROTHROMBIN TIME AND INTERNATIONAL NORMALIZED RATIO (INR)

The prothrombin time (PT) is a screening test used to assess the activity of factors in the extrinsic pathway of the coagulation system and to monitor oral anticoagulant therapy. The extrinsic pathway includes factors VII, X, V, II (prothrombin), and I (fibrinogen). Long considered one of the most important screening tests in coagulation studies, PT indirectly measures the ability of the blood to clot. During the clotting process, prothrombin is converted to thrombin. It is thought that when the prothrombin level falls below normal, the tendency for the blood to clot in the blood vessel decreases. The prothrombin time is an important guide to drug therapy and is commonly used when anticoagulants are prescribed. The prothrombin content is reduced in liver diseases.

The lack of uniformity for the reporting of PT results along with variations in thromboplastin (PT reagent) sensitivities, instrumentation, and methodologies have led to interlaboratory variations in patient's PT results.

The World Health Organization (WHO) developed a protocol to standardize PT results internationally. All PT reagents and methodologies are compared with the WHO reference thromboplastin and laboratory method. The International Sensitivity Index (ISI) is a number derived from the comparison of the PT reagent with the

WHO reference PT reagent. The ISI is used by the laboratory to calculate the **international normalized ratio (INR).** The INR is the PT ratio that would have been obtained using the WHO reference PT reagent. As a result, a patient on oral anticoagulant therapy could be accurately monitored anywhere in the world providing the INR is calculated and reported. (See Box 6–2.)

BOX 6–2   Use of the CoaguChek Plus System to Assess INR

The CoaguChek Plus System is a photometric system for measuring prothrombin times on whole blood. The system is activated by inserting a reagent cartridge, encoded for calibration and test identity. The reagent cartridge contains a sample application area, a reaction chamber containing the PT reagent, and a molded capillary pathway. After applying whole blood to the sample site, capillary action draws the sample through the cartridge. A coherent laser light is focused through the reaction chamber so that the blood flowing through the cartridge causes an interference pattern. The interference pattern is measured by a photo detector and converted to an electrical signal. The instrument measures the optical patterns from the time of application of blood to the cessation of flow. The biochemical reactions of the assay create an alteration in the optical interference pattern detected, resulting in a change in the photo detectors electronic signal. This change in electronic signal is converted to a quantitative result shown on the liquid crystal display.

Specimen Requirements

1. Whole blood collected using the finger stick method or whole blood collected in a syringe
2. Test sample immediately after collection.

Interferences

1. Do not test anti-coagulated samples or serum.
2. Do not test clotted samples. If the sample clots before testing, collect another sample.

Linearity

1. If PT result is ,<8 seconds or >.32 seconds, collect a citrate tube and send to the Core Laboratory for testing.

Reference Range

INR = 0.98–1.08	INR range for normal patient
INR = 2.00–3.00	INR range for anticoagulant therapy
INR = 2.50–3.50	INR range for high-intensity anticoagulant therapy for patients with mechanical valves

---

Adapted from www.ohsu.edu/pathology/POC/procedures/inrwholeblood.html.
Accessed December 31, 2004.

Blood Collection

Venous blood (4 mL) is collected, added to the coagulant, and quickly mixed. It is important to avoid clot formation and hemolysis. The blood should be examined as soon as possible.

Test Result

The normal value is between 11 and 18 seconds, depending on the type of thromboplastin used.

FACTOR V LEIDEN DEFICIENCY

Factor V Leiden is the most common hereditary blood coagulation disorder in the United States. It is present in 5% of the White population and 1.2% of the Black population. Factor V Leiden increases the risk of venous thrombosis 3- to 8-fold for heterozygous (one bad gene inherited) and substantially more, 30- to 140-fold, for homozygous (two bad genes inherited) individuals. (See Table 6–4 and Chapter 17.)

The prothrombin 20210 mutation is the second most common inherited clotting abnormality. It is more common than protein S and C deficiency and antithrombin deficiency combined; 2% of the general population is heterozygous. It is only a mild risk factor for clots, but together with other risk factors (such as oral contraceptives, surgery, trauma, high blood pressure, obesity, smoking, etc) or combined with other clotting disorders (like Factor V Leiden), the risk of clotting increases dramatically (www.fvleiden.org/).

TABLE 6–4   Recommended Laboratory Evaluation for Patients Suspected of Having an Underlying Hypercoagulable State

Screening Tests	Confirmatory Tests
• Activated protein C resistance	• Factor V Leiden PCR
• Prothrombin G20210A mutation testing by PCR	• Antigenic assays for antithrombin, protein C, and/or protein S
• Antithrombin, protein C, and protein S activity (functional) levels	• Confirmatory tests for lupus anticoagulants*
• Factor VIII activity level	
• Screening tests for lupus anticoagulants (sensitive aPTT, aPTT mixing studies, dilute Russell viper venom time)	
• Anticardiolipin antibody testing by ELISA	
• Fasting total plasma homocysteine level	

*Include at least one of the following: platelet neutralization procedure, hexagonal phase phospholipids, Textarin/Ecarin test, platelet vesicles, DVV confirm.
PCR, polymerase chain reaction; aPTT, activated partial thromboplastin time; ELISA, enzyme-linked immunosorbent assay.
(From The Cleveland Clinic Foundation. Available at www.clevelandclinicmeded.com/diseasemanagement/hematology/hyperco/hypercotables.htm Accessed October 11, 2005.)

Factor V Leiden can be associated with the following complications:

- Venous thrombosis in veins, such as:
    - Deep vein thrombosis (DVT), veins in arms and legs
    - Superficial thrombophlebitis
    - Sinus vein thrombosis, veins around the brain
    - Mesenteric vein thrombosis, intestinal veins
    - Budd-Chiari syndrome, liver veins
- Pulmonary embolism (PE), blood clots in the lungs
- Arterial clots (stroke, heart attack) in selected patients (some smokers)
- Possibly with stillbirth or recurrent unexplained miscarriage
- Pre-eclampsia and/or eclampsia (toxemia while pregnant)

Kidney Function Tests

CREATININE

The creatinine test measures kidney function. Creatinine, the result of the breakdown of muscle creatine phosphate, is produced daily in a constant amount in each person. A disorder of kidney function prevents excretion, and an elevated creatinine value gives a reliable indication of impaired kidney function. A normal serum creatinine value does not indicate unimpaired renal function, however. Baseline creatinine should be determined.

Blood Collection

The test is performed on serum from 6 mL of clotted blood.

Test Result

Normal serum range is 0.6 to 1.3 mg/100 mL.

BLOOD UREA NITROGEN

The BUN is a measure of kidney function. Urea, the end product of protein metabolism, is excreted by the kidneys. Impairment in kidney function results in an elevated concentration of urea nitrogen in the blood. Rapid protein metabolism may also increase the BUN above normal limits. The nonprotein nitrogen is a similar test for measuring kidney function.

Blood Collection

The test is performed on blood or serum. Blood (5 mL) is added to an oxalate tube and shaken, or placed in a dry tube to clot.

Test Result

Normal range is 10 to 20 mg/100 mL.

BLOOD GLUCOSE TESTS

The tests for blood glucose detect a disorder of glucose metabolism, which may result from any one of several factors, including inability of pancreatic islet cells to produce insulin, inability of the intestines to absorb glucose, and inability of the liver to accumulate and break down glycogen.

An elevated blood glucose level may indicate diabetes, chronic liver disease, or overactivity of the endocrine glands. A decrease in blood glucose concentration may result from an overdose of insulin, tumors of the pancreas, or insufficiency of various endocrine glands.

A fasting blood glucose test requires that the patient fast for 8 hours.

Blood Collection

Venous blood (3 to 5 mL) is collected in an oxalate tube and shaken to prevent microscopic clots.

Test Result

Normal serum range is 70 to 100 mg/100 mL (true blood glucose method). The normal value depends on the method of determination. Values >120 mg/100 mL on several occasions may indicate diabetes mellitus.

POSTPRANDIAL BLOOD GLUCOSE DETERMINATIONS

The **postprandial** blood glucose test, which is performed approximately 2 hours after the patient has eaten, is helpful in diagnosing diabetes mellitus. If the blood glucose value is above the upper limits of normal for fasting, a glucose tolerance test is performed.

The glucose tolerance test is indicated for the following conditions:

- When the patient has glycosuria
- When the fasting or 2-hour blood glucose concentration is only slightly elevated
- When Cushing's syndrome or acromegaly is a suspected diagnosis
- When the cause of hypoglycemia needs to be determined

Blood Collection

First, a sample of blood is drawn from the fasting patient. The patient then drinks 100 g of glucose in lemon-flavored water (some laboratories use 1.75 g glucose/kg of ideal body weight). Blood and urine samples are then collected at 30, 60, 90, 120, and 180 minutes after ingestion of glucose.

Test Result

Normal (true blood glucose) values are:

- Fasting blood glucose <100 mg/100 mL
- Peak <160 mg/100 mL in 30 or 60 minutes

The values depend on the standards used.

Blood Group Identification

Blood typing, which is one of the most common tests performed on blood, is required for all donors and for all patients who may need blood. The ABO system denotes four main blood groups: O, A, B, and AB. The designations refer to the particular antigen present on the RBCs: group A contains RBCs with the A antigen, B with B antigen, AB with A and B antigens, and O erythrocytes contain neither A nor B antigens.

When erythrocytes containing antigens are placed with serum containing corresponding antibodies under favorable conditions, agglutination (clumping) occurs. Therefore, an antigen is known as an agglutinogen and an antibody as an agglutinin.

A person's serum contains antibodies that react with corresponding antigens not usually found on the person's own cells. For instance, serum of group O contains antibodies A and B, which react with the corresponding antigens A and B found on the RBCs of group AB.

Although agglutination occurs in antigen–antibody reactions in the laboratory, hemolysis occurs in vivo; antibody attacks RBCs, causing rupture with liberation of hemoglobin. Hemolysis results from infusion of incompatible blood and may lead to fatal consequences.

Rh Factor and Blood Collection

The antigens belonging to the Rh system are D, C, E, c, and e. They are found in conjunction with the ABO group. The strongest of these factors is the Rho(D) factor, found in approximately 85% of the White population. Therefore, the Rho(D) factor is often the only factor identified in Rh typing. When the Rho(D) factor is not present, further typing may be done to identify the less common Rh factors.

Venous blood is collected and allowed to clot. Usually one tube (10 mL) sets up 4 to 5 U blood. Positive patient identification must be made before the blood is drawn; the name and number on the identification bracelet must correspond with that on the requisition and label. The label is placed on the blood tube at the patient's bedside.

Blood Typing

Various methods are used in typing blood, but all involve the same general principle. The patient's cells are mixed in standard saline serum samples of anti-A and of anti-B. The type of serum, A or B, that agglutinates the patient's cells indicates the blood group. As a double check, the patient's serum is mixed with saline suspensions of A and of B erythrocytes. The ABO group is determined on the basis of agglutination or absence of agglutination of A and of B cells (see Chapter 17).

Coombs' Test

Not all antibodies cause agglutination in saline; some merely coat the RBCs by combining with the antigen, which is not a visible reaction. Coombs' test is performed to detect antibodies that cannot cause agglutination in saline; these are known as incomplete antibodies. Anti–human globulin serum is used. This serum is obtained by the immunization of various animals, usually rabbits, against human gamma globulin by the injection of human serum, plasma, or isolated globulin. This antiserum, when added to sensitized RBCs (erythrocytes coated with incomplete antibody), causes visible agglutination.

Direct Method

Coombs' test is performed in two ways. The direct Coombs' test is performed when the patient's RBCs have become coated in vivo. This test is a valuable procedure in diagnosing the following:

- Erythroblastosis fetalis. The erythrocytes of the infant are tested for sensitization.
- Acquired hemolytic anemia. The patient may have produced an antibody that coats his or her own cells.
- Investigating reactions. The patient may have received incompatible blood that sensitizes the RBCs.

Indirect Method

The indirect Coombs' test detects incomplete antibodies in the serum of patients sensitized to blood antigens. It tests the patient's serum, in contrast to the patient's RBCs in the direct Coombs' test. When pooled, normal erythrocytes containing the most important antigens are exposed in a test tube to the patient's serum and to Coombs' serum; the RBCs agglutinate, indicating the presence of incomplete antibody. This test is valuable in the following:

- Detecting incompatibilities not found by other methods
- Detecting weak or variant antigens
- Typing with certain antiserums, such as anti-Duffy or anti-Kidd, which require Coombs' serum to produce agglutination
- Detecting anti-agglutinins produced by exposure during pregnancy

Herbal Preparations and Effect on Drug Levels

Herbal remedies have reached their highest usage since the FDA's decision to categorize them as food supplements in 1990. Estimates of annual herbal medicine sales have skyrocketed to between $2 and $3 billion. In 1997, a survey suggested that nearly 60 million Americans use herbal medicines. Estimates suggest that one fourth of this population or 15 million people use vitamins or herbal medicines together with prescription medications. As a result, many patients are at risk for having an herb–drug interaction. Furthermore, estimates suggest that 47% to 72% of patients fail to report herbal medicine use to health care professionals. This may result in increased harm to patients, especially if they are using herbal and prescription medicines that have latent interactions. These interactions can go unnoticed until a patient is hurt or a serious life-threatening event occurs.

Currently, there is very little information published on herb–drug interactions. This challenges health care professionals to discern appropriate action during patient visits or counseling sessions. Health care professionals must continue to educate themselves and patients about herb–drug interactions to provide the best possible patient care and guard patients from choosing inappropriate and unsafe herbal medicines in relation to their current medical conditions and prescription medications. The purpose of this section is to enhance health care professional knowledge about

TABLE 6–5   Clinically Important Interactions of St. John's Wort (SJW; *Hypericum perforatum*). Patients taking drugs listed in the table should not start taking SJW preparations.

Drug	Effect of Interaction on Drug	Suggested Management of Patients Already Taking SJW Preparations
HIV protease inhibitors (indinavir, nelfinavir, ritonavir, saquinavir)	Reduced blood levels with possible loss of HIV suppression	Measure HIV RNA viral load and stop SJW.
HIV non-nucleoside reverse transcriptase inhibitors (efavirenz, nevirapine, delavirdine)	Reduced blood levels with possible loss of HIV suppression	Measure HIV RNA viral load and stop SJW.
Cyclosporin, tacrolimus	Reduced blood levels with risk of transplant rejection	Check cyclosporin or tacrolimus blood levels and stop SJW. Levels may increase on stopping SJW. The dose may need adjusting.
Warfarin	Reduced anticoagulant effect and need for increased warfarin dose	Check INR and stop SJW. Monitor INR closely as this may rise on stopping SJW. The dose of warfarin may need adjusting.
Digoxin	Reduced blood levels and loss of control of heart rhythm or heart failure	Check digoxin levels and stop SJW. Digoxin levels may increase on stopping SJW. The dose of digoxin may need adjusting.
Theophylline	Reduced blood levels and loss of bronchodilator effect	Check theophylline levels and stop SJW. Theophylline levels may increase on stopping SJW The dose of theophylline may need adjusting.
Anticonvulsants (carbamazepine, phenobarbitone, phenytoin)	Reduced blood levels with risk of seizures	Check anticonvulsant levels and stop SJW. Anticonvulsant levels may increase on stopping SJW. The dose of anticonvulsant may need adjusting.

Note: The action of many other drugs depends on their rate of metabolism, and thus other drugs may also interact with St. John's wort preparations.

known and potential herb–drug interactions by providing a review of documented and potential herb–drug interactions, as well as discussing counseling and monitoring issues concerning the use of herbal and prescription medications. (See Table 6–5.)

 SAFE PRACTICE ALERT Herbal medicines may affect clinical laboratory testing. Abnormal laboratory results owing to the use of herbal medicine may be classified in three categories:
1. Abnormal test results owing to direct interference of a component of the herbal medicine with the assay
2. Unexpected concentration of a therapeutic drug owing to drug–herb interactions
3. Abnormal test results owing to toxic effects of the herbal product.

Herbal medicines are used widely in the United States, and according to a recent survey, most people who use herbal medicines do not inform their physicians about their use. Herbal medicines can cause abnormal test results and confusion in proper diagnosis. Herbal medicines can alter test results by direct interference with certain immunoassays. Drug–herb interactions can result in unexpected concentrations of therapeutic drugs. For example, low concentrations of several drugs (eg, cyclosporine, theophylline, digoxin) can be observed in patients who initiated self-medication with St John's wort. Herbal medicines can alter physiology, and these changes can be reflected in abnormal test results. For example, kava-kava can cause drug-induced hepatitis, leading to unexpected high concentrations of liver enzymes. Use of toxic herbal products such as ma huang (an ephedra-containing herbal product), Chan Su, and comfrey may cause death. Other toxic effects of herbal medicines include cardiovascular toxic effects, hematologic toxic effects, neurotoxic effects, nephrotoxic effects, carcinogenic effects, and allergic reactions (www.medceu.com/tests/herbal.htm).

References and Selected Readings

Asterisks indicate references cited in text.

*www.medceu.com/tests/herbal.htm. Accessed October 11, 2005.
*www.fvleiden.org. Accessed October 11, 2005.
*The Cleveland Clinic Foundation (2004) *Hypercoagulable states.* www.clevelandclinicmeded.com/diseasemanagement/hematology/hyperco/hypercotables.htm
*Fischbach, F. (2002). Nurse's quick reference to common laboratory and diagnostic tests (3rd ed.). Philadelphia: Lippincott Williams & Wilkins.
*Fischbach, F.T. (2000). *A manual of laboratory and diagnostic tests* (6th ed.). Philadelphia: Lippincott Williams & Wilkins.
*Williamson, E.M. Drug interactions between herbal and prescription medicines (2005). Accessed October 1, 2005 online at www.ncbi.nih/gov/entrez/query.fcgi?cmd
*Lab Tests Online (2004) Reference ranges and what they mean. www.labtestsonline.org/understanding/features/ref ranges-2.html. Accessed October 11, 2005.

Lambrecht, J., Hamilton, W., Rabinovich, A. A review of herb-drug interactions: Documented and theoretical. www.uspharmacist.com/oldformat.asp?url=newlook/files/comp/aug00alt.htm. Accessed October 11, 2005.
*Metheny, N.M. (2000). *Fluid and electrolyte balance* (3rd ed.). Philadelphia: Lippincott-Raven Publishers.
National Institute for Occupational Safety and Health. (1997). *NIOSH alert: Preventing allergic reactions to natural rubber latex in the workplace* (NIOSH Publication 97–135). Washington, DC: Author.
*Williamson, E.M. Drug interactions between herbal and prescription medicines (2005). Accessed October 1, 2005 online at www.ncbi.nih/gov/entrez/query.fcgi?cmd
*Yale Clinical Medicine. http://info.med.yale.edu/labmed/clinical/labman/D011.html. Accessed January 1, 2005.

Review Questions

Note: Questions below may have more than one right answer.

1. A glucose tolerance test is indicated in which of the following clinical situations?
   A. When the patient shows glycosuria
   B. When fasting or 2-hour blood glucose concentration is only slightly elevated
   C. When Cushing's syndrome or acromegaly is a suspected diagnosis
   D. To establish the cause of hypoglycemia

2. Venous sampling through the central vein may be required in which of the following situations?
   A. When it is difficult to obtain an adequate vein
   B. When the practitioner wants to minimize patient stress
   C. When frequent sampling is required
   D. When the patient requests it

3. Which of the following statements is true of creatinine?

   A. Elevated creatinine level is a reliable indication of impaired kidney function.

   B. Normal serum creatinine level does not indicate normal renal function.

   C. Normal serum creatinine level indicates normal renal function.

   D. Decreased creatinine level is a reliable indication of impaired kidney function.

4. Measurement of chlorides is effective in diagnosing which of the following types of disorders?

   A. Acid–base

   B. Water balance

   C. Anion concentration

   D. Hypoventilation

5. Which of the following is true of blood glucose and serum lipid levels?

   A. They are increased by ingestion of food.

   B. They are depressed after meals.

   C. A only

   D. B only

6. To prevent an elevated serum potassium concentration, which of the following is true?

   A. Samples must be processed in a timely manner.

   B. False measurements must be avoided.

   C. Potassium should be allowed to diffuse from the cells.

   D. Cells must be separated.

7. Complications of venipuncture (for venous sampling) include which of the following?

   A. Syncope

   B. Continued bleeding

   C. Thrombosis

   D. All of the above

8. Coombs' test is valuable in which of the following clinical situations?

   A. Detecting incompatibilities not found by other methods

   B. Detecting weak or variant antigens

   C. Detecting anti-agglutinins produced by exposure during pregnancy

   D. All of the above

9. All of the following statements about prothrombin are true *except*:

   A. Prothrombin indirectly measures the ability of the blood to clot.

   B. Prothrombin is converted to thrombin during the coagulation cascade.

   C. A low level of prothrombin increases the blood's tendency to clot.

   D. Prothrombin is reduced in liver disease.

10. Urea is an end product of which metabolism?

   A. Carbohydrate

   B. Fat

   C. Protein

   D. Mineral

CHAPTER 7

Fluid and Electrolyte Balance

KEY TERMS

Dehydration
Glycosuria
Homeostatic Mechanisms
Hyperkalemia
Hypernatremia
Hyponatremia

Hypovolemia
Metabolic Acidosis
Metabolic Alkalosis
Respiratory Acidosis
Respiratory Alkalosis
Stress Response

Overview of Physiology

An imbalance of fluid or electrolyte levels is recognized as a threat to life. Never before has the nurse's responsibility for fluid and electrolyte administration and monitoring been more intense, regardless of the clinical setting in which care is provided. Patient outcomes depend in large part on specialty practice skills (see Chap. 10), which are based on a sound knowledge of physiology, in particular of fluid and electrolyte interplay.

Dehydration

Dehydration lowers the blood volume, decreasing renal blood flow, and the kidneys produce less of the ammonia needed to maintain acid–base balance. Severe dehydration may lower the blood volume enough to cause circulatory shock and oliguria.

The body loses water from the lungs, skin, gastrointestinal tract, and kidneys on a regular basis. There is a small, but significant, amount of water lost in the stool in normal conditions. The renal and stool loss of water is known traditionally as *sensible water loss*. Although the kidney can minimize the loss of fluid, it can never totally conserve water (Klotz, 1998).

The evaporative water loss that occurs through the lungs and skin is known as *insensible water loss*. Insensible water loss is independent of the body water and solute (electrolytes) and content. It does, however, depend on the patient's body surface area and environmental temperature (Adelman & Solhung, 1996).

At least 80% of all fluids administered today contain some electrolytes. Because electrolyte therapy is often a life-saving procedure, its safe and successful administration is essential. Knowledge of the fundamentals of fluid and electrolyte metabolism contributes to safe electrolyte therapy.

Abnormalities of body fluid and electrolyte metabolism present therapeutic problems. Treatment is complex when the mechanisms that normally regulate fluid volume, electrolyte composition, and osmolality are impaired. An understanding of these metabolic abnormalities enables the nurse to recognize the problems involved. Such clinical challenges arise in patients with renal insufficiency, adrenal insufficiency, adrenal hyperactivity, and other kinds of impaired organ function.

The two following examples illustrate how knowledge of fluid and electrolyte metabolism contributes to safe, successful therapy in the critically ill patient. Correction of a severe potassium deficit resulting from vomiting and diarrhea presents a problem in the dehydrated patient. Potassium replacement is imperative. However, potassium administered to patients with renal insufficiency results in potassium toxicity because the kidneys are unable to excrete electrolytes. The adverse effects of excess potassium on the heart muscle are arrhythmia and heart block. The nurse must recognize the importance of both hydrating the patient before potassium can be administered safely and watching for diminished diuresis that could necessitate a change in therapy. Once antidiuresis occurs, the potassium infusion must be interrupted and the physician notified.

Another example relates to therapeutic problems in patients with impaired liver function. When excessive loss of gastric fluid occurs, replacement fluid is necessary. Most deficits caused by gastric suction, unless severe, are treated with 0.9% sodium chloride in 5% dextrose in water or 0.33% sodium chloride in 5% dextrose in water. However, severe loss may call for gastric replacement fluids containing ammonium chloride, which can be potentially dangerous when administered to patients with impaired liver function. Ammonium chloride administered to a patient with severe liver damage may result in ammonia intoxication because of the liver's inability to convert ammonia to hydrogen ions and urea.

Fluid Content of the Body

The total body water content of a person varies with age, weight, and sex. The amount of water depends on the amount of body fat. Body fat is essentially water-free; the greater the fat content, the lower the water content.

In contrast to infants, who have a high body fluid content (approximately 70% to 80% of body weight), approximately 60% of a typical adult's weight consists of fluid

FIGURE 7–1.   Total body fluid is 60% of body weight.

(water and electrolytes; Fig. 7–1). After 40 years of age, mean values for total body fluid in percentage of body weight decrease for both men and women; a sex differentiation, however, remains. After 60 years of age, the percentage may decrease to 52% in men and 46% in women. With aging, lean body mass decreases in favor of fat (Metheny, 2000).

Fluid Compartments

The total body fluid is functionally allocated into two main compartments: the intracellular and the extracellular compartments (Fig. 7–2). The intracellular compartment consists of the fluid inside the cells and comprises approximately two thirds of the body fluid, or 40% of the body weight. The extracellular compartment consists of the fluid outside the body cells—the plasma, representing 5% of the body weight, and the interstitial fluid (fluid in tissues), representing 15% of the body weight (Metheny, 2000).

In newborn infants, the proportion is approximately three-fifths intracellular and two-fifths extracellular. This ratio changes and reaches the adult level by the time the infant is approximately 30 months of age.

There is one additional compartment, the transcellular compartment. The transcellular fluid is the product of cellular metabolism and consists of secretions such as gastrointestinal secretions and urine. An analysis of the secretions may assist the practitioner in tracing lost electrolytes and prescribing proper fluid and electrolyte replacement. Excessive fluid and electrolyte loss must be replaced to maintain fluid and electrolyte balance in the two main compartments. The amount of body water loss is easily computed by weighing the patient and noting loss of weight: 1 L body water is equivalent to 1 kg, or 2.2 lb, of body weight. Up to 5% weight loss in a child or adult may signify moderate fluid volume deficit—>5% may indicate severe fluid volume deficit. Weight changes are also valuable as indicators of body water gains—acute weight gain may indicate water excess.

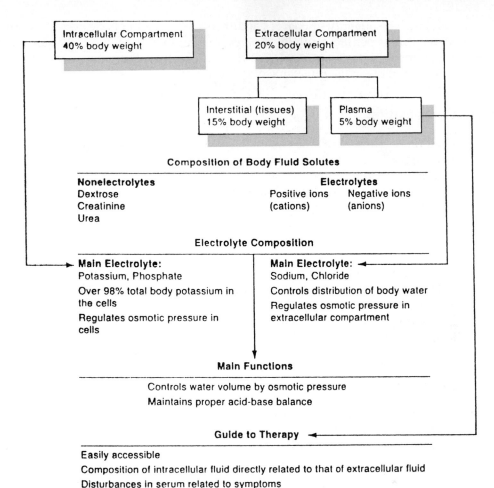

FIGURE 7–2.   Total body water composition.

Body Fluid Composition

Body fluid contains two types of solutes (dissolved substances): the electrolytes and the nonelectrolytes. Electrolytes serve two main purposes: to act in controlling body water volume by osmotic pressure and to maintain the proper acid–base balance of the body. The nonelectrolytes are molecules that do not break into particles in solution, but remain intact. They consist of dextrose, urea, and creatinine.

Electrolytes are molecules that break into electrically charged particles called *ions*. The ion carrying a positive charge is called a *cation*, and the ion with a negative charge is called an *anion*. Potassium chloride is an electrolyte that, dissolved in water, yields potassium cations and chloride anions. Chemical balance is always maintained; the total number of positive charges equals the total number of negative charges. The quantity of charges and their concentration is expressed as milliequivalents (mEq) per liter of fluid. Because the number of negative charges must equal the number of positive charges for chemical balance, the milliequivalents of cations must equal the milliequivalents of anions.

Electrolyte Composition

Each fluid compartment has its own electrolyte composition. The extracellular compartment (plasma and interstitial fluid) contains a high concentration of sodium, chloride, and bicarbonate and a low concentration of potassium. The composition of the intracellular fluid is quite different; the concentrations of potassium, magnesium, and phosphate are high, whereas the sodium and chloride concentrations are relatively low.

Electrolyte composition of the intracellular fluid is in part related to electrolyte composition of the plasma and interstitial fluids. Disturbances in the extracellular fluid are reflected in the patient's symptoms; this information, combined with an analysis of plasma, is thus a valuable guide to therapy.

Occasionally, however, the electrolyte determination of plasma may be misleading. For example, the concentration of potassium in plasma may be high while there is a body deficit. This surplus is due to the shift of potassium from intracellular to extracellular fluid in the process of large potassium losses through the kidneys. Determination of plasma sodium may also present a false picture. In the case of an edematous cardiac patient, the plasma concentration may be low despite excess body sodium because total body sodium is equal to the sum of the products of volume times concentration in the various compartments.

Characteristics of Fluids

Fluids are described in various ways. Significant characteristics of fluids include their concentration, or osmolality, as well as their acidity or alkalinity (pH).

OSMOLALITY

Osmolality is the total solute concentration and reflects the relative water and total solute concentration; it is expressed per liter of serum. Osmotic pressure is determined by the amount of solutes in solution. If the extracellular fluid contains a relatively large number of dissolved particles and the intracellular fluid contains a small amount of dissolved particles, the osmotic pressure causes water to pass from the less concentrated fluid to the more concentrated. Therefore, fluid from the intracellular compartment passes into the extracellular compartment until the concentration becomes equal.

The unit of osmotic pressure is the osmole, and values are expressed in milliosmoles (mOsm). Normal blood plasma has an osmolality of approximately 290 mOsm/kg water. The determination of serum osmolality is sometimes used to detect dehydration or overhydration. Measurement of sodium concentration also indicates the water needs of the body. At times, the osmolality reading may falsely indicate dehydration. Because the osmolality is the total solute concentration, non-electrolytes are included in the reading. An elevated blood urea level can therefore increase the osmolality without exerting osmotic pressure. A determination of blood urea nitrogen (BUN) may supply a correction to the osmolality reading in cases of increased serum urea.

Concentration as a Metric Value

Concentrations of solutes may be expressed in several ways in addition to milliequivalents per liter, such as, milligrams per deciliter (mg/dL) or millimoles per liter (mmol/L). Each of these units of measure may be used in a clinical setting. A milliequivalent of an ion is its atomic weight expressed in milligrams divided by the valence. This is the measure most often used for expressing small concentrations of electrolytes in body fluids because it emphasizes the principles that ions combine milliequivalent for milliequivalent.

Concentration as an SI Value

Milligrams per 100 mL (deciliter) expresses the weight of the solute per unit volume. In the International System of Units (Système Internationale, SI), electrolyte content in body fluids is expressed in millimoles. For practical purposes, one mole (mol) of a substance has a mass equal to its atomic weight, expressed in grams. For example, a mole of sodium has a mass of 23 g (the atomic weight of sodium is 23). A millimole is one-thousandth of a mole, or the molecular or atomic weight expressed in milligrams. Therefore, a millimole of sodium equals 23 mg. Sometimes it is necessary to convert from millimoles per liter to milliequivalents per liter (Fig. 7–3). The following formula applies:

$$mEq/L = mmol/L \times valence$$

ACID–BASE BALANCE

The acidity or alkalinity of a solution depends on the degree of hydrogen ion concentration. An increase in the hydrogen ions results in a more acid solution; a decrease results in a more alkaline solution. Acidity is expressed by the term *pH*, which refers to the amount of hydrogen ion concentration. A solution having a pH of 7 is regarded as neutral.

FIGURE 7–3.   Millimoles versus milliequivalents for univalent and divalent ions.

The extracellular fluid has a pH ranging from 7.35 to 7.45 and is slightly alkaline. When the pH of the blood is >7.45, an alkaline condition exists; when <7.35, an acid condition exists.

The biologic fluids, both extracellular and intracellular, contain a buffer system that maintains the proper acid–base balance. This buffer system consists of fluid with salts of a weak acid or weak base. A base or hydroxide neutralizes the effect of an acid. These weak acids and bases maintain pH values by soaking up surplus ions or releasing them; acids yield hydrogen ions, bases accept hydrogen ions.

The carbonic acid–sodium bicarbonate system is the most important buffer system in the extracellular compartment. The normal ratio is 1 part of carbonic acid to 20 parts of base bicarbonate, which represents 1.2 mEq carbonic acid to 24 mEq base bicarbonate.

ACID–BASE IMBALANCE

Acid–base imbalances are normally the result of an excess or a deficit in either base bicarbonate or carbonic acid. Deviations of pH from 7.35 to 7.45 are combatted by the buffer system and by the respiratory and renal regulatory mechanisms. Two types of disturbance can affect the acid–base balance: respiratory and metabolic. A diagrammatic presentation of these disturbances is presented in Figure 7–4.

Respiratory Disturbances

Respiratory disturbances affect the carbonic side of the balance by increasing or decreasing carbonic acid; when carbon dioxide unites with extracellular fluid, carbonic acid is produced.

Respiratory alkalosis results when excess carbon dioxide is exhaled during rapid or deep breathing. Carbonic acid is depleted because of the carbon dioxide loss. Respiratory alkalosis may occur as the result of emotional disturbances, such as anxiety and hysteria, and also from lack of oxygen or from fever (Metheny, 2000).

Symptoms are convulsions, tetany, and unconsciousness. Laboratory determination is a urinary pH >7 and a plasma bicarbonate concentration <24 mEq/L. The body attempts to restore the ratio to normal by depressing the bicarbonate to compensate for the deficit in the carbonic acid.

Respiratory acidosis occurs when exhalation of carbon dioxide is depressed and the excess retention of carbon dioxide increases the carbonic acid. It may occur in conditions that interfere with normal breathing, such as emphysema, asthma, and pneumonia. Symptoms are weakness, disorientation, depressed breathing, and coma. Urinary pH is below 6 and plasma bicarbonate concentration is above 24 mEq/L. The bicarbonate increase is due to the body's attempt to restore the carbonic acid–bicarbonate ratio.

Metabolic Disturbances

Metabolic disturbances affect the bicarbonate side of the balance. Kidney function controls the bicarbonate concentration by regulating the amount of cations (hydrogen, ammonium, and potassium) in exchange for sodium ions to combine with the reabsorbed bicarbonate in the distal tubular lumen. As hydrogen ions are excreted,

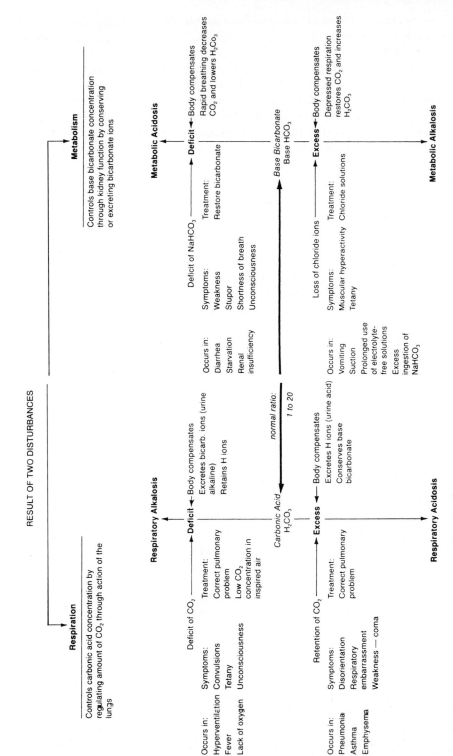

FIGURE 7–4. Acid–base imbalances resulting from respiratory or metabolic disturbances.

bicarbonate is generated, maintaining the proper acid–base balance of the blood. Ammonia excretion is increased in response to a high acidity; bicarbonate replaces the ammonia.

Metabolic alkalosis is a condition associated with excess bicarbonate; it occurs when chloride is lost. Chloride and bicarbonate are both anions, and the total number of anions must equal the total number of cations. When chloride anions are lost, the deficit must be made up by an equal number of anions to maintain electrolyte equilibrium; bicarbonate increases in compensation and alkalosis occurs.

Metabolic alkalosis is also associated with decreased levels of intracellular potassium. Potassium escapes from the cell into the extracellular fluid and is lost through the transcellular fluid. When body potassium is lost, the shift of sodium and hydrogen ions from the extracellular fluid causes alkalosis, whereas the increase of hydrogen ions in the intracellular fluid causes cellular acidosis.

Muscular hyperactivity, tetany, and depressed respiration are symptoms of metabolic alkalosis. Muscular hyperactivity and tetany are symptoms of the deficit in ionized calcium that exists in alkalosis. Laboratory determinations are urinary pH >7, plasma pH >7.45, and bicarbonate level >24 mEq/L.

Treatment consists of the administration of fluids containing chloride to replace bicarbonate ions. An excess of bicarbonate ions is accompanied by potassium deficiency, so potassium must also be replaced.

Metabolic acidosis is a condition associated with a deficit in the bicarbonate concentration. This occurs when

- Excessive amounts of ketone acids accumulate, as in uncontrolled diabetes or starvation.
- Inorganic acids, such as phosphate and sulfate, accumulate, as in renal disease.
- Excessive losses of bicarbonate occur from gastrointestinal drainage or diarrhea.

Acidosis may occur also from infusion (IV) administration of excessive amounts of sodium chloride or ammonium chloride, causing chloride ions to flood the extracellular fluid.

Stupor, shortness of breath, weakness, and unconsciousness are the symptoms of metabolic acidosis, and laboratory determinations of metabolic acidosis are a urinary pH <6, plasma pH <7.35, and plasma bicarbonate concentration <24 mEq/L.

Treatment and clinical management consist of increasing the bicarbonate level. Solutions of sodium lactate are often used, but because lactate ion must be oxidized to carbon dioxide before it can affect the acid–base balance, it is advisable to use sodium bicarbonate solutions, which are effective even when the patient is suffering from oxygen lack.

Homeostatic Mechanisms

The body uses regulating mechanisms called **homeostatic mechanisms** to maintain the constancy of body fluid volume, electrolyte composition, and osmolality. These mechanisms function through the renocardiovascular, endocrine (adrenal, pituitary, and parathyroid), and respiratory systems. The kidneys, skin, and lungs are the main regulating agents (Metheny, 2000).

KIDNEY FUNCTION

The kidney plays a major role in fluid and electrolyte balance. To function adequately, the kidney depends on its own soundness as well as on the coordination of all the regulating organs. The distal renal tubules in the kidney are important in regulating body fluid. They selectively retain or reject electrolytes and other substances to maintain normal osmolality and blood volume. Sodium is retained and potassium is excreted (Baxter Healthcare, 1999).

The kidneys also play an important part in acid–base regulation. The distal tubule has the ability to form ammonia and exchange hydrogen ions (in the form of ammonia) for bicarbonate to maintain the carbonic acid–bicarbonate ratio.

SKIN AND LUNG FUNCTION

The skin and lungs play an important role in fluid balance—the skin in loss of fluid through insensible perspiration and the lungs in loss of fluid by expiration. Normal intake of 2,500 mL from all sources delivers a loss of approximately 1,000 mL in breath and perspiration, 1,400 mL in urine, and 100 mL in feces.

FUNCTIONS OF OTHER SYSTEMS AND ORGANS

The renocardiovascular system maintains fluid balance by regulating the amount and composition of urine. Plasma must reach the kidneys in sufficient volume to permit regulation of water and electrolyte balance. Renal disease, cardiac failure, shock, postoperative stress, and alarm impair this regulating mechanism.

The adrenal glands influence the retention or excretion of sodium, potassium, and water. These glands secrete aldosterone, a hormone that increases the reabsorption of sodium from the renal tubules in exchange for potassium, thus maintaining normal sodium concentration. Any stress, such as surgery, increases the secretion of aldosterone, thus increasing the reabsorption of sodium bicarbonate. Adrenal hyperactivity also increases the secretion of aldosterone and causes excess sodium retention. Excess loss of sodium occurs with adrenal insufficiency.

The pituitary gland is another important organ in the control of fluid and electrolyte balance. The posterior lobe of the pituitary releases antidiuretic hormone (ADH), which inhibits diuresis by increasing water reabsorption in the distal tubule. Increased concentration of sodium in the extracellular fluid stimulates the pituitary to release ADH. This hormone increases the reabsorption of water to dilute the sodium to the normal level of concentration. Increased body fluid osmolality, decreased body fluid volume, stress, and shock are conditions that increase ADH secretion. Increased body fluid volume, decreased osmolality, and alcohol inhibit ADH secretion.

The parathyroid glands, pea-sized glands embedded in the corners of the thyroid gland, regulate calcium and phosphate balance by means of parathyroid hormone (PTH). When the calcium level is low, PTH secretion is stimulated. This acts on bone to increase reabsorption of bone salts, releasing large amounts of sodium into extracellular fluid (ECF). When the extracellular calcium concentration is too high, PTH secretion is depressed so that almost no bone reabsorption occurs (Metheny, 2000).

The pulmonary system regulates acid–base balance by controlling the concentration of carbonic acid through exhalation or retention of carbon dioxide.

Electrolytes of Biologic Fluids

Electrolyte content of the intracellular fluid differs from that of extracellular fluid. Because specialized techniques are required to measure electrolyte concentration in the intracellular fluid, it is customary to measure the electrolytes in the extracellular fluid, chiefly plasma. Plasma electrolyte concentrations may be used to assess and manage patients with a diversity of electrolyte imbalances. Although some tests are performed on serum, the terms *serum electrolytes* and *plasma electrolytes* are used interchangeably. Table 7–1 identifies intracellular and extracellular concentrations and serum values. Table 7–2 lists plasma electrolyte values.

POTASSIUM

Potassium is one of the most important electrolytes in the body. An excess or deficiency of potassium can cause serious impairment of body function and even result in death. Potassium is the main electrolyte in the intracellular compartment, which houses more than 98% of the body's total potassium. The healthy cell requires a high potassium concentration for cellular activity. When the cell dies, there is an exchange of potassium into the extracellular fluid with a transfer of sodium into the cell. This process also occurs to some degree when cellular metabolism is impaired, as in catabolism (breaking down) of cells from a crushing injury.

Serum concentration of potassium is 3.5 to 5.0 mEq/L. In the cell, the normal concentration is 115 to 150 mEq/L fluid. Variations from either of these levels can produce critical effects. When the potassium level is repeatedly >5 to 6 mEq/L, a potassium excess is indicated; renal impairment usually is shown by renal function studies.

High serum concentrations have an adverse effect on the heart muscle and may cause cardiac arrhythmias. Serum potassium levels that are elevated two to three times

TABLE 7–1   Intracellular and Extracellular Concentrations and Related Serum Values

	Normal Concentrations and Values		
	Intracellular	**Extracellular**	**Serum Laboratory Value**
Elements:			
Na$^+$	10 mEq/L	142 mEq/L	135–145 mEq/L
K$^+$	140 mEq/L	4 mEq/L	3.5–5.2 mEq/L
Ca^{2+}	>1 mEq/L	5 mEq/L	8.5–10.5 mg/dL
Mg^{2+}	58 mEq/L	3 mEq/L	1.5–3.5 mEq/L
Cl$^-$	4 mEq/L	103 mEq/L	100–106 mEq/L
HCO$_3^-$	10 mEq/L	28 mEq/L	24–31 mEq/L
pH	7.0	7.4	7.35–7.45
Osmolality			280–294 mOsm/kg

TABLE 7–2 Plasma Electrolytes

Electrolytes	mEq/L
Cations	
Sodium (Na^+)	142
Potassium (K^+)	5
Calcium (Ca^{2+})	5
Magnesium (Mg^{2+})	2
Total cations	154
Anions	
Chloride (Cl^-)	103
Bicarbonate (HCO_3^-)	26
Phosphate (HPO_4^{2-})	2
Sulfate (SO_4^{2-})	1
Organic acids	5
Proteinate	17
Total anions	154

(From Metheny, N.M. [2000]. *Fluid and electrolyte balance* [4th ed., p. 115]. Philadelphia: Lippincott Williams & Wilkins.)

normal may result in cardiac arrest. The electrocardiogram (ECG) may detect signs of potassium excess with peaked and elevated T waves, later disappearance of P waves, and finally, decomposition and prolongation of the QRS complex (Metheny, 2000).

Hypokalemia

Hypokalemia refers to a serum potassium level below normal, whereas **hyperkalemia** denotes a serum potassium level above normal. Hypokalemia, or a serum potassium level <4 mEq/L, may result when either of the following conditions occurs:

- Total body potassium is below normal.
- Concentration of potassium in cells is below normal.

Hypokalemia and hyperkalemia are often caused by variations in the intake or output of potassium. A decreased intake of potassium from prolonged fluid therapy (lacking potassium replacement) may result in hypokalemia. Hypokalemia also may occur during a "starvation diet" because the kidneys do not normally conserve potassium. An increased loss of potassium usually results from polyuria, vomiting, gastric suction (prolonged), diarrhea, and steroid therapy.

Potassium deficiency may be unrelated to intake and output. It can be caused by a sudden shift of potassium from extracellular to intracellular fluid, such as that occurring from anabolism (building up of cells), healing processes, or the use of insulin and glucose in the treatment of diabetic acidosis. The shifts resulting from anabolism and healing processes are not usually of severe consequence unless accompanied by intervening factors. During treatment of diabetic acidosis, for example, the potassium shift may occur suddenly with grave consequences. When cells are anabolized, potassium shifts into the cells. When glucose is used in the treatment of diabetic acidosis, the glucose in the cells is quickly metabolized into glycogen for storage, causing a sudden shift of potassium from the extracellular to the intracellular fluid. This process results in hypokalemia.

The signs and symptoms of hypokalemia are malaise, skeletal and smooth muscle atony, apathy, muscular cramps, and postural hypotension. Treatment consists of administration of potassium orally or parenterally.

Hyperkalemia

Hyperkalemia may result from renal failure with potassium retention or from excessive or rapid administration of potassium in fluid therapy. It may also occur in conditions unrelated to retention or excessive intake. A sudden shift of potassium from intracellular to extracellular fluid results when catabolism of cells occurs, as in a crushing injury; potassium shifts from cells to plasma.

The signs and symptoms of hyperkalemia are similar to those of hypokalemia. In addition to the signs already listed, the patient may experience tingling or numbness in the extremities, and the heart rate may be slow. A serum potassium level >5.5 mEq/L confirms the diagnosis.

Treatment consists of stopping the potassium intake. Dialysis may be necessary for a long-term renal problem. If the cause is a shift of potassium from cells to plasma, glucose and insulin therapy may be used.

SODIUM

Sodium is the main electrolyte in the extracellular fluid; its normal concentration is 135 to 145 mEq/L plasma. The main role of sodium is to control the distribution of water throughout the body and maintain a normal fluid balance. Alterations in sodium concentration markedly influence the fluid volume: the loss of sodium is accompanied by water loss and dehydration; the gain of sodium, by fluid retention.

The body, by regulating urine output, normally maintains a constant fluid volume and isotonicity of the plasma. Urine output is controlled by ADH, secreted by the pituitary gland. If a hypotonic concentration results from a low sodium concentration, the fluid is drawn from plasma into the cells. The body attempts to correct this process; the pituitary inhibits ADH and diuresis results, with a loss of extracellular fluid. This loss of fluid increases sodium concentration to a normal level.

If a hypertonic concentration results from increased concentration of extracellular sodium, fluid is drawn from the cells. Again the body reacts, and the pituitary is stimulated to secrete ADH. This causes a retention of fluid that dilutes sodium to normal concentrations.

Therefore, increased sodium concentration stimulates the production of ADH, with retention of water, thus diluting sodium to the normal level; a decrease in sodium concentration inhibits the production of ADH, resulting in a loss of water, which raises the concentration of sodium to the normal level.

In the kidneys, sodium is reabsorbed in exchange for potassium. Therefore, with an increase in sodium there is loss of potassium; with a loss of sodium, there is an increase in potassium.

Hyponatremia

A sodium deficit (**hyponatremia**) may be present when the plasma sodium concentration falls below 135 mEq/L. It is caused by excessive sweating combined with a large intake of water by mouth (salt is lost and fluid increased, thus reducing the sodium concentration), excessive infusion of nonelectrolyte fluids, gastrointestinal suction plus water by mouth, and adrenal insufficiency, which causes a large loss of electrolytes.

The symptoms of a sodium deficit are apprehension, abdominal cramps, diarrhea, and convulsions. Dehydration results from loss of sodium and leads to peripheral circulatory failure. When sodium and water are lost from the plasma, the body attempts to replace them by a transfer of sodium and water from the interstitial fluid. Eventually water is drawn from the cells and circulation fails; plasma volume cannot be sustained.

Hypernatremia

Sodium excess (**hypernatremia**) may be present when the plasma sodium rises >145 mEq/L. Its causes are excessive infusions of saline, diarrhea, insufficient water intake, diabetes mellitus, and tracheobronchitis (excess loss of water from lungs because of rapid breathing). The symptoms of sodium excess are dry, sticky mucous membranes, oliguria, excitement, and convulsions.

CALCIUM

Calcium is an electrolyte constituent of the plasma present in a concentration of approximately 4.6 to 5.1 mg/dL ionized calcium. The total calcium range is 8.5 to 10.5 mg/dL. Calcium serves several purposes. It plays an important role in formation and function of bones and teeth. As ionized calcium, it is involved in normal clotting of the blood and regulation of neuromuscular irritability.

The parathyroid glands control calcium metabolism. By acting on the kidneys and bones, PTH regulates the concentration of ionized calcium in the extracellular fluid. Impairment of this regulatory mechanism alters the calcium concentration. Hyperparathyroidism typically elevates the serum calcium level and decreases the serum phosphate level.

Hypocalcemia

Calcium deficit may occur in patients who have diarrhea or problems in gastrointestinal absorption, extensive infections of the subcutaneous tissue, or burns. This deficiency can result in muscle tremors and cramps, excessive irritability, and even convulsions.

Calcium ionization is influenced by pH; it is decreased in alkalosis and increased in acidosis. With no loss of calcium, a patient in alkalosis may have symptoms of calcium deficit (e.g., muscle cramps, tetany, and convulsions). This is due to the decreased ionization of calcium caused by the elevated pH.

A patient in acidosis may have a calcium deficit with no symptoms because the acid pH has caused an increased ionization of available calcium. Symptoms of calcium deficit may appear if acidosis is converted to alkalosis.

Hypercalcemia

It is estimated that 98% of patients with hypercalcemia, or calcium excess, have cancer or hyperparathyroidism, or they use thiazide diuretics. Characteristics of hypercalcemia include muscular weakness, tiredness, lethargy, constipation, anorexia, polyuria, polydipsia, shortened QT interval on the ECG, and a serum calcium concentration >10.5 mg/dL.

OTHER ELECTROLYTES

The primary role of magnesium is in enzyme activity, where it contributes to the metabolism of both carbohydrates and proteins. Its serum concentration is 1.3 to 2.1 mEq/L. A magnesium deficit is a common imbalance in critically ill patients. Deficits may also occur in less acutely ill patients, such as those experiencing withdrawal from alcohol and those receiving parenteral or enteral nutrition after a period of starvation. Neuromuscular irritability, disorientation, and mood changes are indicative of hypomagnesemia. Hypermagnesemia is uncommon, but it may be seen in patients with advanced renal failure. Magnesium is excreted by the kidneys; therefore, diminished renal function results in abnormal renal magnesium retention.

Chloride, the chief anion of the extracellular fluid, has a plasma concentration of 97 to 110 mEq/L. A deficiency of chloride leads to a deficiency of potassium, and vice versa. There is also a loss of chloride with a loss of sodium, but because this loss can be compensated for by an increase in bicarbonate, the proportion differs.

Phosphate is the chief anion of the intracellular fluid. Its normal level in plasma is 1.7 to 2.3 mEq/L.

Objectives of Fluid and Electrolyte Therapy

Parenteral therapy has three main objectives: to maintain daily body fluid requirements, to restore previous body fluid losses, and to replace present body fluid losses.

Maintenance

Maintenance therapy is aimed at providing all the nutrient needs of the patient: water, electrolytes, dextrose, vitamins, and protein. Of these needs, water is the most important. The body may survive for a prolonged period without vitamins, dextrose, and protein, but without water, dehydration and death occur.

WATER

The body needs water to replace the insensible loss that occurs with evaporation from the skin and from expired air. An average adult loses from 500 to 1,000 mL water per 24 hours through insensible loss. The skin loss varies with the temperature and humidity. Water balance is closely correlated to energy expenditure (Klotz, 1998).

Water is essential for kidney function. The amount needed depends on the amount of waste products to be excreted as well as the concentrating ability of the kidneys. Protein and salt increase the need for water.

A person's fluid requirements are based on age, height, weight, and amount of body fat. Because fat is water free, a large amount of body fat contains a relatively low amount of water; as body fat increases, water decreases in inverse proportion to body weight. The normal fluid and electrolyte requirements based on body surface area are more constant than when expressed in terms of body weight. Many of the essential physiologic processes such as heat loss, blood volume, organ size, and respiration have a direct relationship to the body surface area.

Fluid and electrolyte requirements are also proportionate to surface area, regardless of the patient's age. These requirements are based on square meters of body surface area and are calculated for a 24-hour period. Nomograms are available for determining surface area (see Chap. 11). Table 7–3 highlights maintenance requirements based on body weight (assuming that renal function, gastrointestinal status, and temperature are normal).

Balanced electrolyte fluids are available for maintenance. The average requirements of fluid and electrolytes are estimated for a healthy person and applied to a patient. The balanced fluids contain electrolytes in proportion to the daily needs of the patient, but not in excess of the body's tolerance, as long as adequate kidney function exists. When a patient's water needs are provided by these maintenance fluids, the daily needs of sodium and potassium are also met. For maintenance, 1,500 mL/m^2 body surface area is administered over a 24-hour period.

GLUCOSE

Because it is converted into glycogen by the liver, thereby improving hepatic function, glucose has an important role in maintenance. By supplying necessary calories for energy, it spares body protein and minimizes the development of ketosis caused by the oxidation of fat stores for essential energy in the absence of added glucose.

The basic daily caloric requirement of a 70-kg adult at rest is approximately 1,600 calories. However, the administration of 100 g glucose a day is helpful in minimizing the ketosis of starvation; 100 g is contained in 2 L of 5% dextrose in water or 1 L 10% dextrose in water (Terry et al., 1995).

TABLE 7–3 Fluid and Electrolyte Maintenance Requirements*

Weight Range	Required Volume
Premature infant (<3 kg)	60 mL/kg
Younger patient	
0–10 kg	100 mL/kg/d
10–20 kg	1,000 mL + 50 mL/kg/d
21 kg to average adult weight	1,500 mL + 20 mL/kg/d
Adult (nonpregnant)	30–35 mL/kg/d

*Based on body weight.

PROTEIN

Protein is another nutrient important to maintenance therapy. Although a patient may be adequately maintained on glucose, water, vitamins, and electrolytes for a limited time, protein may be required to replace normal protein losses over an extended period. Protein is necessary for cellular repair, wound healing, and synthesis of vitamins and some enzymes. The usual daily protein requirement for a healthy adult is 1 g/kg body weight. Protein is available as amino acid. Taken orally, protein is broken down into amino acids before being absorbed into the blood.

VITAMINS

Vitamins, although not nutrients in the true sense of the word, are necessary for the utilization of other nutrients. Vitamin C and the various B complex vitamins are the most frequently used in parenteral therapy. Because these vitamins are water soluble, they are not retained by the body but lost through urinary excretion. Because of this loss, larger amounts are required parenterally to ensure adequate maintenance than may be required when administered orally. The B complex vitamins play an important role in the metabolism of carbohydrates and in maintaining gastrointestinal function. Vitamin C promotes wound healing and is frequently used for surgical patients. Vitamins A and D are fat-soluble vitamins, better retained by the body and not usually required by the patient on maintenance therapy.

Restoration of Previous Losses

Restoration of previous losses is essential when past maintenance has not been met—that is, when output exceeds intake. Severe dehydration may occur from failure to replace these losses. Therapy consists of replacing losses from previous deficits in addition to providing fluid and electrolytes for daily maintenance. Kidney status must be considered before electrolyte replacement and maintenance can be initiated; urinary suppression may result from decreased fluid volume or renal impairment. A hydrating fluid such as 5% dextrose in 0.2% (34.2 mEq) sodium chloride solution is administered. Urinary flow is restored if the retention is functional. The patient must be rehydrated rapidly to establish adequate urine output. Only after kidney function proves adequate can large electrolyte losses be replaced.

Replacement of Present Losses

Replacement of present losses of fluid and electrolytes is also an objective of therapy. Accurate measurement of all intake and output is a significant means of calculating fluid loss. Fluid loss may be estimated by determining loss of body weight; 1 L body water equals 1 kg, or 2.2 lb, body weight. An osmolality determination may indicate the water needs of the body. If necessary, a corrective BUN determination may be performed with the osmolality evaluation.

The type of replacement depends on the type of fluid being lost. A choice of appropriate replacement fluids is available. For example, excessive loss of gastric fluid may be replaced by fluids resembling the fluid lost, such as gastric replace-

TABLE 7–4   Differentiating Acidosis from Alkalosis

Cause	Physiology	Symptoms	Intervention
Alkalosis			
Loss of NaCl/KCl gastric fluid	Concentration of bicarbonate gastric ions; anions must equal cations.	Slow shallow respiration, pallor	Administer appropriate replacement fluids.
	Ammonia is converted into urea and hydrogen ion. If liver fails to convert ammonia to urea, ammonia retention and toxicity result.	Sweating, tetany, coma	
Acidosis			
Excess fluid is alkaline	Intestinal secretions contain excessive bicarbonate ions; with loss, chloride ion	Shortness of breath; rapid breathing	Administer base salts; ie, sodium lactate or sodium.

ment fluids. Excessive loss of intestinal fluid must be replaced by an intestinal replacement fluid. Examples of conditions that may result from current losses are alkalosis and acidosis (Table 7–4).

Fluid and Electrolyte Disturbances in Specific Patients

Understanding how the endocrine system responds to stress helps the nurse better understand the imbalances and problems associated with stress. It also contributes to safe and successful parenteral therapy. The nurse anticipates what to expect, knows the possible dangers of imbalances, and recognizes early symptoms.

The Surgical Patient

The neuroendocrine response stimulated by many anesthetic agents is further heightened by surgical stress. Apprehension, pain, and duration and severity of trauma give rise to surgical stress and contribute to an increased endocrine response during the first 2 to 5 days after surgery.

The **stress response** is normal and is nature's way of protecting the body from hypotension resulting from trauma and shock. Correction is often unnecessary and may, in fact, be harmful.

The two major endocrine homeostatic controls affected by stress are pituitary gland and adrenal gland function (Fig. 7–5). The posterior pituitary controls quantitative secretions of ADH. The anterior pituitary controls secretions of corticotropin, which stimulates the adrenal gland to increase mineralocorticoid secretions (aldosterone) and glucocorticoid secretions (hydrocortisone). The adrenal medulla secretes vasopressors (epinephrine and norepinephrine) to help maintain the blood pressure.

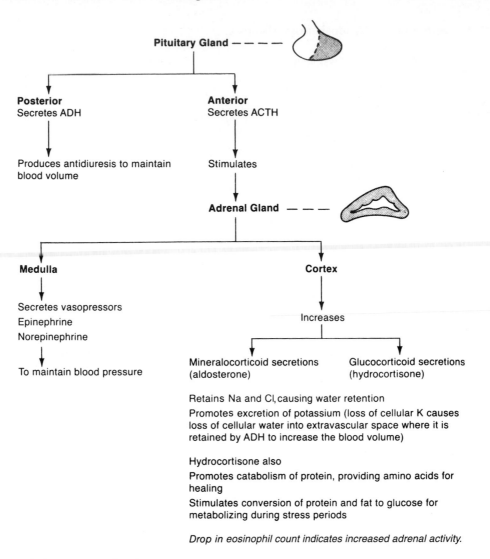

FIGURE 7–5.   Endrocrine response to stress.

A direct physiologic effect occurs when stress increases the secretions of these various hormones. When the posterior pituitary increases ADH secretions, antidiuresis is effected, thus helping maintain blood volume. When the anterior pituitary increases corticotropin secretions, the adrenal gland is stimulated to increase aldosterone.

FLUID REPLACEMENT MECHANISMS

Adrenal hormones help maintain blood volume by causing the retention of sodium ions and chloride anions, thereby causing water retention and promoting the excretion of potassium (loss of cellular potassium ions causes loss of cellular water into extracellular space, where it is retained by ADH to maintain blood volume).

Hydrocortisone also promotes the catabolism of protein to provide necessary amino acids for healing and stimulates the conversion of protein and fat to glucose for metabolism during the stress period. This metabolic activity may elevate the blood glucose level, a finding that may mistakenly suggest diabetes mellitus. A drop in the eosinophil count and an elevated level of serum 17-hydroxycorticosteroid hormones indicate increased adrenal activity.

FLUID NEEDS

Accurate records of intake and output are important for assessing fluid requirements and preventing serious fluid imbalances during the early postoperative period. The daily requirement of 1,500 to 2,000 mL varies with the patient's needs. Caution must be taken not to overhydrate the patient—the intake should be adequate but should not exceed the fluid losses.

The adrenocortical secretions, increased by trauma and stress of surgery, cause some water and sodium retention. This retention may be severe enough to present a false picture of oliguria. Excessive quantities of nonelectrolyte fluids (such as 5% dextrose in water) administered at a time when antidiuresis is occurring may cause hyponatremia, a serious electrolyte imbalance.

In hyponatremia, the serum sodium concentration is lower than normal. Water-yielding fluids, infused in excess of the body's tolerance, expand the extracellular compartment, lowering the electrolyte concentration. By osmosis, water invades the cells, with a resulting excess accumulation of intracellular fluid. Usually there is no edema because edema is the result of an excess accumulation of fluid in the extracellular compartment.

Symptoms of water excess include confusion, hallucinations, delirium, weight gain, hyperventilation, muscular weakness, twitching, and convulsions. If these occur during the early postoperative stages, the nurse should suspect water excess. This is of particular concern in young and elderly patients. Serious consequences, even death, can result.

Restricting the fluid intake may correct mild water excess, but for more severe cases, the administration of high concentrations of sodium chloride may be indicated. The electrolyte concentration of the plasma, increased by the concentrated saline, causes an increase in the osmotic pressure, drawing fluid from the cells for excretion by the kidneys.

Parenteral therapy during the stress period often consists of administering conservative amounts of 5% dextrose in water. Because some sodium retention results from the endocrine response to stress, care must be taken to avoid administering excessive quantities of saline at a time when there is an interference in the elimination of salt. During this early period, the physician frequently gives 5% dextrose in quarter- or half-strength saline to avoid sodium excess.

In hypernatremia, the serum sodium concentration is higher than normal. This excess may expand extracellular fluid volume or cause edema and possible disruption of cellular function (in potassium-depleted patients, the sodium may replace the intracellular potassium).

Symptoms of sodium excess include flushed skin, elevated temperature, dry and sticky mucous membranes, thirst, and a decreased or absent urine output. Treatment consists of reducing the salt and water intake and promoting diuresis to eliminate the excess salt and water from the plasma.

NUTRIENT NEEDS

Among the various nutrients needed by postsurgical patients are carbohydrates, proteins, fats, potassium, and vitamins.

Carbohydrates

Carbohydrates provide an indispensable source of calories for the postoperative patient unable to receive food orally. When carbohydrate supplies are inadequate, the body uses its own fat to supply calories; the by-products are ketone bodies. These acid bodies neutralize bicarbonate and produce metabolic acidosis. The only by-products excreted in the metabolism of carbohydrates are water and carbon dioxide.

By providing calories for essential energy, carbohydrates also reduce catabolism of protein. During the stress response, the renal excretion of nitrogen (from the catabolism of protein) exceeds the intake. By reducing the protein breakdown, glucose helps prevent a negative nitrogen balance.

Carbohydrates do not provide adequate calories for the patient receiving prolonged therapy. Approximately 1 L of 5% dextrose in water provides 170 calories. Many liters, a volume too great for most patients to tolerate, would be required to provide a patient with 1,600 calories. Greater concentrations of glucose, 20% and 50%, may be administered to provide calories for patients unable to tolerate large volumes of fluid (e.g., patients with renal insufficiency). The concentrated fluids must be administered slowly for glucose utilization to occur. Rapid administration results in diuresis; the concentrated glucose acts as a diuretic, drawing interstitial fluid into the plasma for excretion by the kidneys.

Alcohol

Alcohol fluids may be administered to the postoperative patient for nutritional and physiologic benefits. Nutritionally, the alcohol supplements calories provided by the glucose, with 1 g ethyl alcohol yielding 6 to 8 calories. Because alcohol is quickly and completely metabolized, it provides calories for essential energy, sparing fat and protein. Metabolized in preference to glucose, alcohol allows the infused glucose to be stored as glycogen.

Physiologically, alcohol produces a sedative effect, reducing pain; 200 to 300 mL of a 5% solution per hour produces sedation without intoxication in the average adult. Alcohol also inhibits the secretion of ADH, promoting water excretion.

Fluids containing alcohol, particularly hypertonic fluids, can cause phlebitis. These fluids, if allowed to infiltrate, may cause tissue necrosis. The IV catheter should be carefully inserted within the lumen of the vessel and inspected frequently to detect any infiltration.

Protein

Patients who receive parenteral fluid therapy for a prolonged time require protein for cellular repair, wound healing, and growth. Stress states accompanying surgical procedures and trauma frequently result in protein deficiency.

During the stress period, increased secretions of glucocorticoids from the adrenal cortex cause protein breakdown and the conversion of protein and fat to glucose for energy. More urinary nitrogen is lost than normal. When nitrogen loss exceeds intake, the patient is said to be in a negative balance. This response to stress is normal. However, protein losses must be counteracted; preservation of body cell mass is essential. A depleted body cell mass can be restored only by hyperalimentation. Approximately 1 g/kg body weight is required by a healthy adult to replace normal protein loss.

Because of their high ammonia level, extreme caution is required if proteins are administered to patients with hepatic insufficiency or emaciation. Organ-specific formulas have been developed for the patient with renal or hepatic disease.

 SAFE PRACTICE ALERT Supplemental medications added to the fluid may result in incompatibilities. Always check with the pharmacist before adding any medication to fluids.

Fluids, once opened, must be used immediately. Storing a partially used container of fluid in the refrigerator for future use provides a culture medium for the growth of bacteria. No fluids that are cloudy or contain precipitate should be used.

Lipid Emulsions

Lipid emulsions offer calories and essential fatty acids for metabolic processes. They are rich in calories, yielding 9 kcal/g, compared with 4 kcal/g from carbohydrates.

Potassium

Once the stress period passes, adrenal activity decreases and diuresis begins. At this time, usually after the second to the fifth postoperative day, potassium is given daily to prevent a deficit. Potassium is not conserved by the body but is lost in the urine. Electrolyte maintenance fluids may be used or potassium may be added to parenteral fluids. When potassium is added to parenteral fluids, the container, bag, or bottle should be thoroughly shaken to mix and dilute the potassium. Potassium should never be added to a hanging container while the infusion is running. Such an action could result in a bolus injection of the drug. Rapid injection, which increases the drug concentration in the plasma, can result in trauma to the vessel wall and even in cardiac arrest. Potassium should never be given by IV push or bolus administration.

The status of the kidneys must be considered. If kidney function is inadequate, the patient must be rehydrated. During this infusion, the nurse must watch for diminished diuresis and notify the physician if antidiuresis occurs.

SAFE PRACTICE ALERT Potassium chloride must be used with considerable caution and is considered potentially dangerous if administered when renal function is impaired. A buildup of potassium, caused by the kidney's inability to excrete salts, can prove hazardous; arrhythmia and heart block can result from the effect of excess potassium on the heart muscle.

An amount of 40 mEq/L usually is sufficient to replace normal potassium loss. It is usually infused over an 8-hour period. Premixed potassium replacement fluids are available in a variety of strengths.

In extreme cases of hypokalemia, when the serum potassium concentration is <2.0 mEq/L, the nurse may need to infuse potassium at a much faster rate—but not faster than 40 mEq/hour. When the serum potassium concentration reaches 2.5 mEq/L and ECG manifestations of hypokalemia diminish, the rate should be decreased to no more than 10 mEq/hour, using a fluid that contains no more than 30 mEq/L.

Continuous ECG monitoring is required when high doses of potassium are infused. The fluid containing potassium should be conspicuously labeled and must never be used when positive pressure is indicated—rapid infusion may result in cardiac arrest.

Potassium is irritating to the vein and may cause a great deal of discomfort, especially if infused into a vein where a previous venipuncture has been performed. Slowing the rate may decrease the pain.

Vitamins

The B complex vitamins and vitamin C are usually added to parenteral fluids if, after 2 or 3 days, the patient cannot take fluids orally. Vitamin C is important in promoting healing in the surgical patient, and B complex vitamins aid carbohydrate metabolism.

NURSING DIAGNOSES

Nursing diagnoses for the postsurgical patient should address relevant fluid and electrolyte disturbances. Table 7–5 lists selected nursing diagnoses.

The Burn Patient

The patient with burns presents special clinical challenges (Table 7–6). The rule of nines (Table 7–7) is commonly used to estimate burned area. The body's surface area is divided into sections equal to 9% or multiples of 9% of total body area. The portion of the areas sustaining second- or third-degree burns is identified, and the percentages are totaled to represent the full percentage of body surface area burned. This method may be inaccurate in children, and other charts are available for accurately determining percentage of body surface area burned.

FORMULAS FOR FLUID REPLACEMENT

Fluid requirements for the first 24 hours after burn injury range from 2 to 4 mL/kg body weight depending on percentage of body surface area burned. Several factors must be considered, including age of the patient, size and depth of the burn, type of fluid, and complication factors such as inhalation injury, electrical burns, or multiple trauma. Numerous formulas have been developed for this purpose, but an ideal rate of infusion is one that maintains perfusion, as reflected by a urinary output of 0.5 mL/kg body weight per hour in the adult patient.

TABLE 7–5   Selected Nursing Diagnoses for Postoperative Patient After Abdominal Surgery

Nursing Diagnosis	Etiologic Factors	Defining Characteristics
Fluid volume deficit related to actual fluid loss and third-space fluid shift during surgical procedure	Vomiting after reaction to anesthesia GI suction Third-space fluid shift at surgical site	Postural tachycardia Postural hypotension initially; later, low blood pressure in all positions Decreased skin turgor Decreased capillary refill time Oliguria (<30 mL/h in adult) Weight change depends on cause (decreased if actual fluid loss, as in GI suction; usually increased if fluid loss is due to third-space shift, provided parenteral fluids are given in an attempt to correct hypovolemia)
Altered tissue perfusion (renal) related to hypotension during surgical procedure	Hypotensive effects of anesthesia Hypovolemia due to direct or indirect loss of fluid Hypovolemia due to inadequate parenteral fluid replacement	Oliguria or polyuria in presence of elevated serum creatinine
Alteration in sodium balance (hyponatremia) related to excessive ADH activity	Major surgery with its premedication, anesthesia, decreased blood volume, and postoperative pain results in increased ADH release (causing water retention with sodium dilution)	Serum sodium <135 mEq/L May be asymptomatic if Na >120 mEq/L Lethargy, confusion, nausea, vomiting, anorexia, abdominal cramps, muscular twitching
Alteration in acid–base balance (metabolic alkalosis) related to vomiting or gastric suction	Vomiting after reaction to anesthesia Gastric suction, particularly if patient is allowed to ingest ice chips freely	Tingling of fingers, toes, and circumoral region, due to decreased calcium ionization pH >7.45, bicarbonate above normal, chloride below normal
Altered nutrition (less than body requirements) related to negative nitrogen balance after surgical stress, and inadequate caloric intake	Catabolic response to stress of surgery Inability to tolerate oral feedings during first few postoperative days due to decreased GI motility, anorexia, nausea, and general discomfort Failure of health care providers to administer sufficient calories via the parenteral route	Weight loss of approximately ¼ to ½ lb/d in adult (provided fluids are not abnormally retained) Perhaps a decrease in serum albumin, transferrin, and retinol binding protein levels (although delivery of a large volume of blood products or the long half-life of certain secretory proteins can interfere with correct interpretation)

ADH, antidiuretic hormone; GI, gastrointestinal.
(From Metheny, N.M. [2000]. *Fluid and electrolyte balance* [4th ed., p. 308]. Philadelphia: Lippincott Williams & Wilkins.)

TABLE 7–6   The Burn Patient Receiving Parenteral Fluid Therapy

	Objectives/Mechanisms	Intervention
First 48 hours	Maintain fluid volume relative to loss and third spacing.	Ensure venous access; administer fluids consistent with clinical condition and physician's orders.
Intravascular to interstitial shift	Treat volume depletion.	Administer albumin as ordered to correct third-space shifts; maintain fluid status and IV access.
Shock	Re-establish inadequate tissue perfusion. Deliver oxygen to metabolically active cells.	Replace water, electrolytes, and protein (from skin). In a patient with a 50% burn, edema, may exceed total plasma volume of patient.
Dehydration	Water and electrolyte loss are less than protein loss.	Determine replacement needs and administer fluids adequate to restore perfusion.
	Osmotic pressure draws fluid from undamaged tissues.	Administer colloids to draw fluid in from other compartments, thus increasing vascular volume.
Hypovolemia	Exudate from burned area, water (as vapor), and blood loss occur.	Ensure adequate venous access to provide fluid volume.
Decreased urine output	Ensure that kidneys are working before administration of potassium replacement. Antidiuretic hormone exceeds water reabsorption by kidneys.	Replace blood volume and maintain kidney output. Monitor intake and output to ensure elimination of wastes.
Potassium excess	Hyperkalemia; cells release potassium, and decreased renal flow obstructs normal excretion of potassium.	Initiate fluid replacement with albumin, dextran, Hetastarch.
Sodium deficit	Due to edema and loss of exudate	Administer nonelectrolyte solution to replace insensible losses.
Metabolic acidosis	Due to accumulation of fixed acids released from tissue	Administer only enough fluid to maintain blood volume/urine output.
Second to third day	Shift from interstitial fluid to plasma.	Reduce parenteral fluids accordingly; excess urinary output is evidence of need to decrease fluid therapy.
	Avoid circulatory overload.	Maintain fluid volume and monitor patient for hypophosphatemia.

TABLE 7–7   Rule of Nines for Estimating Burned Body Area in Adults

Body Parts	Percentage of Body
Head and neck	9
Anterior trunk	18
Each arm	9
Posterior trunk	18
Genitalia	1
Each leg	18

ASSESSMENT

Ongoing assessment of the patient is needed to tailor fluid replacement to individual patient needs. Monitoring parameters include urine volume, sensorium, vital signs, and central venous pressure.

Urine output is the best indicator of adequate fluid resuscitation. Adult output should be 30 to 50 mL/hour. Lack of urine output or a substantial decrease in volume may be attributed to inadequate fluid replacement, gastric dilation, or renal failure. Daily weights are a helpful tool for monitoring the burned patient. A weight gain of 15% to 20% may indicate fluid retention. Adequacy of tissue perfusion is measured by assessing the patient's sensorium. Sensorium should remain normal with appropriate fluid replacement unless other factors, such as head injury, are present.

SAFE PRACTICE ALERT Vital signs should be monitored hourly in the burned patient.

Blood pressure should remain at near normal values with consideration given to the patient's baseline pressure. Temperature may be elevated and tachycardia may be present. Rate and character of respirations should be evaluated. Peripheral pulses and capillary refill times should be monitored. Vasoconstriction of unburned skin is a compensatory response to help preserve normal blood flow in the hours immediately after a severe burn. Hence, unburned skin may be cool to the touch and appear pale at first.

Central venous and arterial pressure monitoring may be used to evaluate the effects of fluid replacement. Signs of inadequate fluid replacement are decreased urine output, thirst, restlessness and disorientation, hypotension, and increased pulse rate. Circulatory overload may be suspected with an elevated central venous pressure reading (15 to 20 cm H_2O), shortness of breath, and moist crackles.

The Diabetic Patient

Diabetic acidosis is an endocrine disorder causing complex fluid and electrolyte disturbances. It occurs when a lack of insulin prevents the metabolism of glucose, and essential calories are provided instead by the catabolism of the patient's own fat and protein. Acidosis results from the accumulation of acid by-products. Understanding the physiologic changes in diabetic acidosis aids the nurse in detecting early imbalances and the subsequent treatment.

PHYSIOLOGIC CHANGES IN DIABETIC ACIDOSIS

Lack of insulin prevents cellular metabolism of glucose and its conversion into glycogen. Glucose accumulates in the bloodstream (hyperglycemia). When the blood glucose level rises >180 mg/100 mL, glucose spills over into the urine (**glycosuria**). The kidneys require 10 to 20 mL water to excrete 1 g glucose; water excretion increases (polyuria).

The body's fat and protein are used to provide necessary calories for energy. Ketone bodies, metabolic by-products, reduce plasma bicarbonate, and acidosis occurs.

FLUID AND ELECTROLYTE DISTURBANCES

Dehydration results from excessive fluid and electrolyte losses. Cellular fluid deficit occurs when water is drawn from the cells by the hyperosmolality of the blood. Extracellular fluid deficit occurs when

- Glycosuria increases the urinary output.
- Ketone bodies raise the load on the kidneys and increase the water to excrete them.
- Vomiting causes loss of fluid and electrolytes.
- Oral intake falls because of the patient's condition.
- Hyperventilation is induced by the acidotic state.

Ketosis

Ketosis is the excessive production of ketone bodies in the bloodstream. Ketone bodies are the end products of oxidation of fatty acids. Ketosis occurs when a lack of insulin results in excessive fatty acids being converted by the liver to ketones and the decreased utilization of ketones by the peripheral tissues. Electrolytes and ketone bodies, retained in high serum concentration, increase the acidosis; the increase in the number of hydrogen ions, from the retention of ketone bodies, may drop the blood pH to 7.25 and lower. The bicarbonate anions decrease to compensate for the increase in ketone anions and may drop the bicarbonate level to 12 mEq/L or less.

Hyperglycemic Hyperosmolar Nonketotic Coma

Hyperglycemic hyperosmolar nonketotic coma (HHNC) is a syndrome that may develop in the middle-aged or elderly type 2 diabetic patient. The condition is often associated with the stress of cardiovascular disease, infection, or pharmacologic treatment with steroids or diuretics. It is also precipitated by too-rapid infusion of parenteral nutrition fluid. Blood glucose levels may reach 4,000 mg/dL but without the ketosis of diabetic ketoacidosis. Fluid volume deficit is profound and may lead to death. Underlying factors contributing to development of diabetic ketoacidosis or HHNC are found in Table 7–8. Signs and symptoms of diabetic acidosis are summarized in Box 7–1.

PARENTERAL THERAPY

Insulin is given to metabolize the excess glucose and combat diabetic acidosis. Because absorption is quickest by the bloodstream, insulin is administered IV. When

TABLE 7–8   Factors Contributing to Development of DKA or HHNC in Susceptible Persons

DKA	HHNC
Infections, illness	Chronic renal disease
Physiologic stresses (e.g., trauma, surgery, myocardial infarction, dehydration, pregnancy)	Chronic cardiovascular disease
	Acute illness, infection
Psychologic/emotional stress	Surgery burns, trauma
Omission/reduction of insulin	Hyperalimentation, tube feedings
Failure of insulin delivery system (pump)	Peritoneal dialysis
Excess alcohol intake	Mannitol therapy
	Pharmacologic agents
	Chlorpromazine
	Cimetidine
	Diazoxide
	Diuretics (thiazide, thiazide-related, and loop diuretics)
	Glucocorticoids and immunosuppressive agents
	L-Asparaginase
	Phenytoin
	Propranolol

DKA, diabetic ketoacidosis; HHNC, hyperglycemic hyperosmolar nonketotic coma.
(From Metheny, N.M. [2000]. *Fluid and electrolyte balance* [4th ed., p. 335]. Philadelphia: Lippincott Williams & Wilkins.)

given subcutaneously or intramuscularly, the slower rate of absorption of insulin may be further decreased by peripheral vascular collapse in the presence of shock. The dose of insulin, when administered by continuous infusion, is usually 4 to 8 U/hour. Many types of infusion pumps are available to ensure accurate and continuous administration of medications.

Parenteral fluids are administered to increase the blood volume and restore kidney function. Early treatment of the hypotonic patient usually consists of the administration of 0.9% sodium chloride solution to replace sodium and chloride losses and to expand the blood volume. Later, hypotonic fluids with sodium chloride may be used. Bicarbonate replacement may be necessary in severe acidosis.

Potassium administration is contraindicated in the early treatment of diabetic acidosis. During the later stages (10 to 24 hours after treatment), the plasma potassium level falls; improved renal function increases potassium excretion and, in anabolic states, as the glucose is converted into glycogen, a sudden shift of potassium from extracellular fluid to intracellular fluid further lowers the plasma potassium level. If the patient is hydrated, potassium should be administered when the plasma potassium concentration falls.

A severe potassium deficit may occur if symptoms are not recognized and early treatment begun. Symptoms include weak grip, irregular pulse, weak picking at the bedclothes, shallow respiration, and abdominal distention.

BOX 7–1   Signs and Symptoms of Diabetic Ketoacidosis

Infusion nurses need to become familiar with the signs and symptoms that characterize diabetic acidosis. By recognizing impending diabetic acidosis, early treatment may be initiated and complications prevented.

Hyperglycemia—When a lack of insulin prevents glucose metabolism, glucose accumulates in the bloodstream.

Glycosuria—When the accumulation of glucose exceeds the renal tolerance, glucose spills over into the urine.

Polyuria—Osmotic diuresis occurs when the heavy load of nonmetabolized glucose and the metabolic end products increase the osmolality of the blood. In turn, the increased renal solute load requires more fluid for excretion.

Thirst—Cellular dehydration, arising from the osmotic effect produced by hyperglycemia, prompts thirst.

Weakness and fatigue—The body's inability to use glucose and a potassium deficit lead to weakness and fatigue.

Flushed face—Flushing results from the acid condition.

Rapid, deep breathing—The body's defense against acidosis, expiration of large amounts of carbon dioxide reduces carbonic acid and increases the pH of the blood.

Acetone breath—Increased accumulation of acetone bodies results in acetone-scented breath.

Nausea and vomiting—Distention resulting from atony of gastric muscles causes nausea and vomiting.

Weight loss—An excess loss of fluid (1 L body water equals 2.2 lb, or 1 kg, body weight) and a lack of glucose metabolism contribute to weight loss.

Low blood pressure—Severe fluid deficit leads to low blood pressure.

Oliguria—Decreased renal blood flow that results from a severe deficit in fluid volume produces oliguria.

References and Selected Readings

Asterisks indicate references cited in text.

*Adelman, R.D., & Solhung, M.J. (1996). Pathophysiology of body fluids and fluid therapy. In: R.E. Behrman, R.M. Kliegman, & A.M. Arvin (Eds.). *Nelson textbook of pediatrics* (15th ed., pp. 185–222). Philadelphia: W.B. Saunders.

*Baxter Healthcare. (1999). *Clinical guide to infusion therapy: Water and electrolytes.* S. Weinstein (Ed.).

Foley, M. (1998). *Lippincott's need-to-know nursing reference facts* (pp. 107–148). Philadelphia: Lippincott-Raven.

*Klotz, R. (1998). The effects of infusion solutions on fluid and electrolyte balance. *Journal of Infusion Nursing, 21,* 20–24.

*Metheny, N.M. (2000). Fluid and electrolyte balance (4th ed.). Philadelphia: Lippincott Williams & Wilkins.

*Terry, J., et al. (1995). *Infusion therapy: Clinical principles and practice* (pp. 111–115). Philadelphia: W.B. Saunders.

Review Questions

1. Which of the following contributes to respiratory alkalosis?
   A. Inhalation of excess carbon dioxide
   B. Shallow breathing
   C. Depletion of carbon monoxide
   D. Increased oxygenation

2. Symptoms associated with respiratory alkalosis include all of the following *except:*
   A. Tetany
   B. Unconsciousness
   C. Convulsions
   D. Lethargy

3. Respiratory acidosis is associated with all of the following *except:*

   A. Diabetes

   B. Emphysema

   C. Asthma

   D. Pneumonia

4. Kidney function controls which of the following?

   A. Bicarbonate concentration

   B. Sodium exchange

   C. Intracellular potassium

   D. Acidity

5. Symptoms associated with metabolic alkalosis include:

   A. Muscular hyperactivity

   B. Tetany

   C. Depressed respirations

   D. Increased respirations

6. Metabolic acidosis is associated with a deficit of:

   A. Bicarbonate ion

   B. Carbon dioxide

   C. Sodium

   D. Chloride

7. Symptoms of metabolic acidosis include which of the following?

   A. Stupor and shortness of breath

   B. Weakness and unconsciousness

   C. A plasma pH below 7.35

   D. Plasma bicarbonate concentration below 24 mEq/L

8. Regulating mechanisms that maintain the constancy of body fluid volume, electrolyte composition, and osmolality are functions of which of the following?

   A. Renocardiovascular system

   B. Endocrine system

   C. Respiratory system

   D. Kidneys

9. Normal intake of 2,500 mL from all sources is estimated to deliver a loss of approximately how many milliliters in breath and perspiration?

   A. 1,000 mL

   B. 1,400 mL

   C. 1,500 mL

   D. 1,800 mL

10. Which of the following is the major electrolyte of the intracellular compartment?

    A. Calcium

    B. Potassium

    C. Sodium

    D. Bicarbonate

CHAPTER 8

Principles of Parenteral Fluid Administration

KEY TERMS

Acidifying Infusions
Alkalizing Fluid
Dehydration
Hemolysis
Hexoses
Hydrating Fluids
Hyperinsulinism

Hypertonic
Hypodermoclysis
Hypotonic
Isotonic
Osmolality
Turgor
Water Intoxication

Parenteral Fluids

To help enhance patient outcomes, a knowledge of parenteral fluids is essential when delivering infusion therapy. This is particularly important because rapid and critical changes in fluid and electrolyte balance may be caused by infusates.

Until the 1930s, intravenous (IV) fluids consisted of dextrose and saline solutions. Little was known about electrolyte therapy (see Chap. 1). Today, however, more than 200 types of commercially prepared fluids are available. The great increase in their use leads to a more common occurrence of fluid and electrolyte disturbances. Moreover, with the increased administration of fluids in alternative care settings, nurses must know the chemical composition and the physical effects of the infusions they administer.

> **LEGAL ISSUES:** Fluid Injections
>
> Nurses have a legal and professional responsibility to know the:
>
> - Normal amount of any IV infusion they administer
> - Desired and untoward effects of any IV infusion
> - Type of fluid, the amount, and the rate of flow, determined only after the physician has carefully assessed the patient's clinical condition

Intravenous Infusion

Today, methods of infusion have changed dramatically, and small-volume parenteral *fluids* may be administered as a secondary infusate or in a volume-controlled reservoir for electronic drug delivery.

An infusion is usually regarded as an amount of fluid >100 mL designated to be infused parenterally because the volume must be administered over a long period. However, when medications are administered as a *piggyback* (secondary to and delivered with the initial infusion) small-volume (50 to 100 mL) parenteral infusion, a shorter period (usually 30 to 60 minutes) may be required, whereas volumes of 150 to 200 mL may require >1 hour. Today, methodologies have changed to be consistent with the clinical needs of patients, and alternate delivery systems are readily available (see Chaps. 11 and 12).

Intravenous fluids are mistakenly referred to as *IV solutions*. The term *solution* is defined in the *United States Pharmacopeia* (USP) as a liquid preparation that contains one or more soluble chemical substances usually dissolved in water. Solutions are distinguished from injections, for example, because they are not intended for administration by infusion or injection (USP, 1999). Moreover, methods of preparation may vary widely. The USP refers to parenteral fluids as injections, and methods of preparation must follow standards for injection.

Official Requirements of Intravenous Fluids

Intravenous injections must meet the tests, standards, and all specifications of the USP applicable to injections. This includes quantitative and qualitative assays of infusions, including tests for pyrogens and sterility.

PARTICULATE MATTER

Each fluid container must be carefully examined to detect cracks. The fluid must be examined for cloudiness or particles. The final responsibility falls on the pharmacist and the nurse who administers the fluid. Tests to detect particulate matter, and standards for an acceptable limit of particles, have been established by the USP. A large-volume injection for single-dose infusion meets the requirements of the test if it contains not more than 50 particles per milliliter that are ≥ 10.0 μm, and not more than 5 particles per milliliter that are ≥ 25.0 m in effective linear dimension.

pH VALUE

The pH indicates hydrogen ion concentration or free acid activity in solution. All IV fluids must meet the pH requirements set forth by the USP. Most of these requirements call for a fluid that is slightly acid, usually ranging in pH from 3.5 to 6.2. Dextrose requires a slightly acid pH to yield a stable fluid. Heat sterilization, used for all commercial fluids, contributes to the acidity. It is important to know the pH of the commonly used IV fluids because it may affect the stability of an added drug and cause the drug to deteriorate. The acidity of dextrose fluids has been criticized for its corrosive effect on veins.

TONICITY

Parenteral fluids are classified according to the tonicity of the fluid in relation to normal blood plasma. The osmolality of blood plasma is 290 mOsm/L. Fluid that approximates 290 mOsm/L is considered isotonic. IV fluids with an osmolality significantly >290 mOsm (+50 mOsm) are considered **hypertonic,** whereas those with an osmolality significantly <290 mOsm (−50 mOsm) are **hypotonic.**

Parenteral fluids usually range from approximately one-half isotonic (0.45% sodium chloride) to 5 to 10 times **isotonic** (25% to 50% dextrose). The tonicity of the fluid infused into the circulation affects fluid and electrolyte metabolism and may result in disastrous clinical disturbances (see Table 8–1 for more information on the effects of isotonic, hypertonic, and hypotonic fluids).

Knowing the osmolality of the infusion and the physical effect it produces alerts the nurse to potential fluid and electrolyte imbalances. The choice of veins used for an infusion is affected by the tonicity of the fluid; hyperosmolar fluids, for example, must be infused through veins that carry a large blood volume to dilute the fluid and prevent trauma to the vessel.

The tonicity of the fluid also affects the rate at which it can be infused. Hypertonic dextrose infused rapidly may result in diuresis and dehydration.

Because of the direct and effective role osmolality plays in IV therapy, the nurse involved in administering IV fluids needs to be familiar with various terms and calculations. For instance, the *osmotic pressure* is proportional to the total number of particles in the fluid. The *milliosmole* (mOsm) is the unit that measures the particles or the osmotic pressure. By converting milliequivalents to milliosmoles, an approximate osmolality may be determined. A quick method for approximating the tonicity of IV injections follows.

TABLE 8–1 Results of Infusion of Fluids With Different Tonicities

Tonicity	Effect
Hypertonic fluid	Increases osmotic pressure of plasma Draws fluid from the cells
Hypotonic fluid	Lowers the osmotic pressure of plasma Causes fluid to invade the cell
Isotonic fluid	Increases extracellular volume

Fluids Containing Univalent Electrolytes

Each milliequivalent is approximately equal to a milliosmole because univalent electrolytes, when ionized, carry one charge per particle. An injection of normal saline (0.9% sodium chloride) contains 154 mEq sodium and 154 mEq chloride per liter of fluid, making a total of 308 mEq/L, or approximately 308 mOsm/L.

Fluids Containing Divalent Electrolytes

Because each particle carries two charges when ionized, the milliequivalents per liter of fluid or the number of electrical charges per liter when divided by the charge per ion (2) gives the approximate number of particles or milliosmoles per liter. As an example, when 20 mEq magnesium sulfate is introduced into a liter of fluid, each ionized particle carries two charges. By dividing 20 mEq or 20 charges by 2, an approximate 10 particles or 10 mOsm/L is reached for each component, or 20 mOsm/L total.

The osmolality of electrolytes in solution may be accurately computed but involves using the atomic weight and the concentration of the given electrolytes in milligrams per liter. The methods for accurately computing the osmolality of an electrolyte, such as potassium (K), in solution follow:

$$\frac{\text{milligrams of electrolyte/L}}{(\text{Atomic weight})\,(\text{valance})} = \text{milliosmoles/L}$$

Example: 35 mg K/L

$$\frac{35}{35 \times 1} = 0.5 \text{ mOsm/L}$$

Example: 40 mg K/L

$$\frac{40}{40 \times 2} = 1 \text{ mOsm/L}$$

Kinds and Composition of Fluids

Various kinds of fluids are used for parenteral injections. These fluids are composed of dextrose in water, sodium chloride in water, sodium bicarbonate, ammonium chloride, and other substances.

Dextrose in Water

When glucose is part of parenteral injections, it is usually referred to as *dextrose*, a designation by the USP for glucose of requisite purity. Dextrose is available in concentrations of 2.5%, 5%, 10%, 20%, and 50% in water. To determine the osmolality or the caloric value of a dextrose fluid, the nurse needs to know the total number of grams or milligrams per liter. Because 1 mL water weighs 1 g, and 1 mL is 1% of 100 mL, milliliters, grams, and percentages can be used interchangeably when calculating solution strength. Thus, dextrose 5% in water equals 5 g dextrose in 100 mL, or 50 g dextrose in 1 L. The metabolic effects of dextrose are listed in Box 8–1.

BOX 8–1   Metabolic Effects of Dextrose

- Provides calories for essential energy
- Improves hepatic function because glucose is converted into glycogen by the liver
- Spares body protein (prevents unnecessary breakdown of protein tissue)
- Prevents ketosis or excretion of organic acid (which may occur when fat is burned by the body without an adequate supply of glucose)
- Stored intracellularly in the liver as glycogen, causes the shift of potassium from the extracellular to the intracellular fluid compartment (*Note: This effect is desired as treatment for hyperkalemia. It is achieved by infusing dextrose and insulin.*)

CALORIES

Hexoses (glucose or dextrose and fructose) do not yield 4 calories per gram, as do dietary carbohydrates (e.g., starches). Each gram of hydrous or anhydrous dextrose provides approximately 3.4 or 3.85 calories, respectively. One liter of 5% glucose infusion yields 170 calories; 1 liter of 10% glucose yields 340 calories (American Association of Healthcare Pharmacists [ASHP], 1998; see Chap. 16 for more information).

TONICITY OF DEXTROSE 5% IN WATER

Dextrose 5% in water is considered an isotonic fluid because its tonicity approximates that of normal blood plasma, or 290 mOsm/L. Because dextrose is a nonelectrolyte and the total number of particles in solution does not depend on ionization, the osmolality of dextrose fluids is determined differently from that of electrolyte fluids. One millimole (one formula weight in milligrams) of dextrose represents 1 mOsm (unit of osmotic pressure). One millimole of monohydrated glucose is 198 mg, and 1 liter of dextrose 5% in water contains 50,000 mg. Thus:

$$\frac{50,000 \text{ mg}}{198} = 252 \text{ mOsm/L}$$

pH VALUE

The USP requirement for the pH of dextrose fluids is 3.5 to 6.5. This broad range may at times contribute to an incompatibility in one bottle of dextrose and not in another when an additive is involved (see Chap. 16).

INDICATIONS FOR USE

Dextrose fluids are used for patients with dehydration, hyponatremia, and hyperkalemia. They are also vehicles for drug delivery and nutrition.

Dehydration

In cases of **dehydration,** dextrose 2.5% in water and dextrose 5% in water provide immediate hydration for medical as well as surgical patients. Dextrose 5% in water is considered isotonic only in the bottle. Once infused into the vascular system, the dextrose is rapidly metabolized, leaving water. The water decreases the osmotic pressure of the blood plasma and invades the cells, providing immediately available water to dehydrated tissues.

Hypernatremia

If the patient is not in circulatory difficulty with extracellular expansion, dextrose 5% in water may be administered to decrease the concentration of sodium.

Medication Administration

Many of the drugs for IV therapy are added to infusions of dextrose 5% in water.

Nutrition

Concentrations of dextrose 20% and 50% in conjunction with electrolytes provide long-term nutrition. Insulin is frequently added to prevent overtaxing the islet tissue of the pancreas.

 SAFE PRACTICE ALERT Because the kidneys do not store potassium, prolonged fluid therapy with electrolyte-free fluids may result in **hypokalemia**. This happens when cells are anabolized by the metabolism of glucose and potassium shifts from the extracellular to the intracellular fluid. Conversely, when renal function is impaired, IV potassium should be used cautiously. Remain alert for signs of **hyperkalemia**. If such signs develop, notify the physician and be prepared to replace fluid *components* with more appropriate electrolytes.

Hyperkalemia

Infusions of dextrose in high concentration with insulin cause anabolism (buildup of body cells), which results in a shift of potassium from the extracellular to the intracellular compartment, thereby lowering the serum potassium concentration.

DANGERS OF USE

Among abnormalities resulting from infusion of dextrose are dehydration, hypokalemia, hyperinsulinism, and water intoxication.

Dehydration

Osmotic diuresis occurs when dextrose is infused at a rate faster than the patient's ability to metabolize it. A heavy load of nonmetabolized glucose increases the osmolality of the blood and acts as a diuretic; the increased solute load requires more fluid for excretion. A normal, healthy person with a urine specific gravity of 1.029 to 1.032 requires 15 mL water to excrete 1 g solute, whereas people with poor kidney function or low concentrating ability of the kidneys require much more water to excrete the same amount of solute (Metheny, 2003).

Hyperinsulinism

A rapid infusion of hypertonic carbohydrate solutes may result in **hyperinsulinism**. In response to a rise in blood glucose level, extra insulin pours from the beta cells of the pancreatic islets in an attempt to metabolize the infused carbohydrate. Terminating the infusion may leave excess insulin in the body, resulting in symptoms such as nervousness, sweating, and weakness caused by the severe hypoglycemia that may be induced. Typically, after infusion of hypertonic dextrose, a small amount of isotonic dextrose is administered to cover the excess insulin (Metheny, 2003).

Water Intoxication

An imbalance resulting from an increase in the volume of the extracellular fluid from water alone is known as **water intoxication**. Prolonged infusions of isotonic or hypotonic dextrose in water may cause this condition, which is compounded by stress and leads to inappropriate release of antidiuretic hormone (ADH) and fluid retention. The average adult can metabolize water at a rate of approximately 35 to 40 mL/kg/day, and the kidney can safely metabolize only approximately 2,500 to 3,000 mL/day in an average patient receiving IV therapy (Metheny, 2003). Under stress, the patient's ability to metabolize water decreases (Box 8–2).

ADMINISTRATION

Isotonic dextrose may be administered through a peripheral vein. Hyperosmolar fluids, such as dextrose 50% in water, should be infused into the superior vena cava through central venous access. Hypertonic dextrose administered through a peripheral vein with small blood volume may traumatize the vein and cause thrombophlebitis. Infiltration can result in tissue necrosis.

Sodium-free dextrose injections should not be administered by **hypodermoclysis** (direct administration into subcutaneous tissue to enhance hydration). Dextrose fluids, by attracting body electrolytes in the pooled area of infusions, may cause peripheral circulatory collapse and anuria in sodium-depleted patients.

Electrolyte-free dextrose injections should not be used in conjunction with blood infusions. Dextrose mixed with blood causes **hemolysis** of the red blood cells.

The amount of water required for hydration depends on the clinical condition and the needs of the patient. The average adult patient requires 1,500 to 2,500 mL

BOX 8–2   Potential Consequences of Infusing Specific Fluids

- **Cellular dehydration** may result from excessive infusions of hypertonic fluids.
- **Water intoxication** results when hypotonic fluid is infused beyond the patient's tolerance for water.
- **Circulatory overload** can result from isotonic fluid administration.

water each day. In patients with prolonged fever, however, the water requirement depends on the degree of temperature elevation. For example, the 24-hour fluid requirement for a patient with a body temperature between 101°F and 103°F increases by at least 500 mL; the fluid requirement for a prolonged temperature above 103°F increases by at least 1,000 mL.

The rate of administration depends on the patient's condition and the purpose of therapy. When the infusion is used to supply calories, the rate must be slow enough to allow complete metabolism of the glucose (0.5 g/kg/hour in normal adults). The maximum rate usually should not exceed 0.8 g/kg/hour (ASHP, 1998). When the infusion is used to produce diuresis, the rate must be fast enough to prevent complete metabolism of the dextrose, thereby increasing the osmolality of the extracellular fluid.

Isotonic Sodium Chloride Infusions

Sodium chloride injection (0.9%), USP (normal saline), contains 308 mOsm/L (sodium, 154 mEq/L; chloride, 154 mEq/L). It has a pH between 4.5 and 7.0 and is usually supplied in volumes of 1,000, 500, 250, and 100 mL. The term *normal* (or *physiologic*) is misleading because the chloride in normal saline is 154 mEq/L, compared with the normal plasma chloride value of 103 mEq/L, whereas the sodium is 154 mEq/L, or approximately 9% higher than the normal plasma value of 140 mEq/L. Because normal saline lacks the other electrolytes present in plasma, the isotonicity of the fluid depends on the sodium and chloride ions, resulting in a higher concentration of these ions (ASHP, 1998).

INDICATIONS FOR USE

Normal sodium chloride injection is indicated for the following:

- Extracellular fluid replacement when chloride loss is relatively greater than or equal to sodium loss.
- Treatment of metabolic alkalosis in the presence of fluid loss; the increase in chloride ions provided by the infusion causes a compensatory decrease in the number of bicarbonate ions.
- Sodium depletion. When there is an extracellular fluid volume deficit accompanying the sodium deficit, an isotonic solution of sodium chloride is used to correct the deficit (Metheny, 2003).
- Initiation and termination of blood transfusions. When 0.9% sodium chloride is used to precede a blood transfusion, the hemolysis of red blood cells, which occurs with dextrose in water, is avoided.

 SAFE PRACTICE ALERT Sodium chloride 0.9% solution (normal saline) provides more sodium and chloride than the patient needs. Marked electrolyte imbalances have resulted from the almost exclusive use of normal saline. Hypernatremia, acidosis, and circulatory overload may result when normal saline is administered in excess of the patient's tolerance.

DANGERS OF USE

An adult's dietary requirement for sodium is approximately 90 to 250 mEq/day, with a minimum requirement of 15 mEq and a maximum tolerance of 400 mEq (ASHP, 1998). When 3 L 0.9% sodium chloride or dextrose 5% in 0.9% sodium chloride is administered, the patient receives 462 mEq sodium (154 mEq/L), a level that exceeds normal tolerance.

Hypernatremia

Infusion of saline during a period of sodium retention—for example, during stress—can result in hypernatremia. The danger of hypernatremia increases in the elderly, in patients with severe dehydration, and in patients with chronic glomerulonephritis; these patients require more water to excrete the salt than do patients with normal renal function. Isotonic saline does not provide water, but requires most of its volume for the excretion of salt.

Acidosis

One liter of 0.9% sodium chloride solution contains one-third more chloride than is present in the extracellular fluid. When infused in large quantities, the excess chloride ions cause a loss of bicarbonate ions and result in acidosis.

Hypokalemia

Infusion of saline increases potassium excretion and at the same time expands the volume of extracellular fluid, further decreasing the concentration of the extracellular potassium ion.

Circulatory Overload

Continuous infusions of isotonic fluids expand the extracellular compartment and lead to circulatory overload.

REQUIREMENTS

In an average adult, the daily requirements of sodium chloride are met by infusing 1 L of 0.9% sodium chloride or 1 to 2 L of 4.5% sodium chloride, but the dosage depends on the patient's age, weight, clinical condition, and fluid, electrolyte, and acid–base status (ASHP, 1998).

Dextrose 5% in 0.9% Sodium Chloride

Dextrose 5% in 0.9% sodium chloride (normal or isotonic saline solution), which contains 252 mOsm dextrose (chloride, 154 mEq/L; sodium, 154 mEq/L), has a pH of 3.5 to 6.0 and is available in volumes of 1,000, 500, 250, and 150 mL. When normal saline is infused, the addition of 100 g dextrose prevents both the formation of ketone bodies and the increased demand for water the ketone bodies impose for renal excretion. The dextrose prevents catabolism and, consequently, loss of potassium and intracellular water.

INDICATIONS FOR USE

Isotonic saline with dextrose injection is indicated for the following:

- Temporary treatment of circulatory insufficiency and shock caused by hypovolemia in the immediate absence of a plasma expander
- Early treatment along with plasma or albumin for replacement of loss caused by burns
- Early treatment of acute adrenocortical insufficiency

DANGERS OF USE

The hazards are the same as those for normal saline injection (see preceding section).

Dextrose 10% in 0.9% Sodium Chloride

Dextrose 10% in 0.9% sodium chloride contains 504 mOsm/L dextrose (sodium, 154 mEq/L; chloride, 154 mEq/L), has a pH of 3.5 to 6.0, and is usually supplied in volumes of 1,000 and 500 mL.

INDICATIONS FOR USE

This fluid is used as a nutrient and an electrolyte (sodium and chloride) replenisher.

ADMINISTRATION

Dextrose 10% in 0.9% sodium chloride, because of its hypertonicity, must be administered IV, preferably through a wide vein to dilute the fluid and reduce the risk of trauma to the vessel. Close observation and precautions are necessary to prevent infiltration and damage to the tissues.

Hypertonic Sodium Chloride Infusions

These infusions include 3% sodium chloride (sodium, 513 mEq/L; chloride, 513 mEq/L) and 5% sodium chloride (sodium, 850 mEq/L; chloride, 850 mEq/L).

INDICATIONS FOR USE

Infusion of hypertonic sodium is indicated for

- Severe dilutional hyponatremia (water intoxication). Hypertonic sodium chloride, on infusion, increases the osmotic pressure of the extracellular fluid, drawing water from the cells for excretion by the kidneys.
- Severe sodium depletion. Infusions of hypertonic saline replenish sodium stores. An estimate of the sodium deficit can be made by taking the difference between the normal sodium concentration and the patient's current sodium concentration and multiplying the difference by 60% of the body weight in kilograms; sodium depletion is based on total body water, and not on extracellular fluid.

ADMINISTRATION

Hypertonic sodium chloride injection must be administered with great caution to prevent pulmonary edema. Cautions include frequent re-evaluation of the patient's clinical and electrolyte status during administration. A 3% or 5% solution of sodium chloride is used to correct the deficit, providing the fluid volume is normal or excessive; the amount of sodium administered depends on the sodium deficit in the plasma (Metheny, 2003).

Hypertonic saline solutions should be infused slowly (e.g., 200 mL over a minimum of 4 hours), and the patient should be observed constantly. The fluid must be infused with great care taken to prevent infiltration and trauma to the tissues. Box 8–3 summarizes the important nursing considerations in the administration of hypertonic saline infusion.

Hypotonic Sodium Chloride in Water

One-half hypotonic saline (0.45% saline containing sodium, 77 mEq/L, and chloride, 77 mEq/L) is used as an electrolyte replenisher. When there is a question regarding the amount of saline fluid required, hypotonic saline is preferred over isotonic saline. In general, 0.45% sodium chloride is preferable to 0.9% sodium chloride.

Hydrating Fluids

Because fluids consisting of dextrose with hypotonic saline provide more water than is required for excretion of salt, they are useful as **hydrating fluids.** These fluids

---

BOX 8–3 Nursing Considerations for Administering Hypertonic (3% and 5%) Saline Solution

- Check the serum sodium level before administering the solution and frequently thereafter.
- These solutions are dangerous and should be used only in critical situations in which the serum sodium level is very low (ie, <110 mEq/L) and the patient exhibits neurologic signs.
- Administer the solution only in intensive care settings where the patient can be closely monitored. Watch for signs of pulmonary edema and worsening of neurologic signs. Use with great caution in patients with congestive heart failure or renal failure.
- Only small volumes are needed (e.g., 5 or 6 mL/kg body weight of 5% sodium chloride) to elevate the serum sodium level by 10 mEq/L. For example, elevating the serum sodium level of a 70-kg patient from 110 to 120 mEq/L requires approximately 350 to 420 mL.
- The serum sodium should not rise more rapidly than 2 mEq/L/hour unless the clinical state of the patient indicates the need for more rapid treatment.
- The fluid can be administered with an electronic infusion device. The device should be monitored closely because no instrument is foolproof.
- Therapy aims to elevate the serum sodium level enough to alleviate neurologic signs—not to raise the serum sodium level to normal quickly. Recommendations include raising the serum concentration no higher than 125 mEq/L with hypertonic saline. The health care provider may prescribe furosemide to promote water loss and prevent pulmonary edema. Urine should be saved because renal sodium and potassium losses may need to be measured to allow for replacement.

include dextrose 2.5% in 0.45% saline (dextrose, 126 mOsm/L, with sodium, 77 mEq/L, and chloride, 77 mEq/L), dextrose 5% in 0.45% saline (dextrose, 252 mOsm/L, with sodium, 77 mEq/L, and chloride, 77 mEq/L), and dextrose 5% in 0.2% saline (dextrose, 252 mOsm/L, with sodium, 34.2 mEq/L, and chloride, 34.2 mEq/L).

INDICATIONS FOR USE

Commonly called *initial hydrating fluids*, hypotonic saline dextrose infusions are indicated as follows:

- To assess the status of the kidneys before electrolyte replacement and maintenance is initiated
- To provide hydration for medical and surgical patients
- To promote diuresis in dehydrated patients

ADMINISTRATION

To assess the status of the kidneys, the fluid is administered at the rate of 8 mL/m^2 body surface area (BSA) per minute for 45 minutes. The restoration of urine flow shows that the kidneys have begun to function. The hydrating fluid then may be replaced by more specifically needed electrolytes. If after 45 minutes the urine flow is not restored, the rate of infusion is reduced to 2 mL/m^2 BSA per minute for another hour. If this does not produce diuresis, renal impairment is assumed (Metheny, 2003).

Initial hydrating fluids must be used cautiously in edematous patients with cardiac, renal, or hepatic disease. Once good renal function is obtained, appropriate electrolytes should be administered to prevent hypokalemia.

Hypotonic Multiple-Electrolyte Fluids

Hypotonic multiple-electrolyte fluids are patterned after the type devised by Butler and colleagues at Massachusetts General Hospital, who were the first to emphasize that basic water and electrolyte requirements are proportionate to the BSA. Butler-type fluids are one third to one half as concentrated as plasma. They provide fluid to meet the patient's fluid volume requirement. In so doing, they provide cellular and extracellular electrolytes in quantities balanced between the minimal needs and the maximal tolerance of the patient. These fluids, because of their hypotonicity, provide water for urinary elimination and metabolic needs and take advantage of the body's homeostatic mechanisms to retain the electrolytes and reject those not needed, thereby maintaining water and electrolyte balance.

Hypotonic fluids should contain 5% dextrose for its protein-sparing and antiketogenic effect. The dextrose increases the tonicity of the fluid in the container, but once infused, the dextrose is metabolized, leaving the water and salt. Whether the patient has received too much or too little water depends on the tonicity of the electrolyte and not the osmotic effect of dextrose.

A balanced solution of hypotonic electrolytes is ideal for routine maintenance. Of the various modifications of the Butler-type fluids, those containing 75 mEq total cations per liter are used for older infants, children, and adults.

ADMINISTRATION

A useful formula for maintenance water requirements, based on studies by Crawford, Butler, and Talbot, is the following: maintenance water equals 1,600 mL/m^2 BSA per day. For obese or edematous patients, this should be calculated on ideal weight rather than actual weight. The water requirement must be patterned after the condition of the patient.

When infection, trauma involving the brain, or stress lead to inappropriate release of ADH, maintenance requirements are less. Excessive fluid losses through urine, stool, expired air, and so forth, require increased water. The rate of infusion is usually 3 mL/m^2 BSA per minute.

DANGERS OF USE: WATER INTOXICATION

The patient's tolerance limits for water can be exceeded. Care should be exercised in maintaining the prescribed flow rate and in ensuring that the patient receives the prescribed volume of fluid. Water intoxication is more likely to occur when inappropriate release of ADH, in response to stress, causes water retention. These patients should be carefully watched to detect any early signs of an imbalance so that a change in therapy can be initiated before the condition becomes precarious. Weighing the patient is the best way to monitor the status of water balance. Daily weights are extremely important in following the state of hydration in extremely ill patients.

Isotonic Multiple-Electrolyte Fluids

Many types of commercial replacement fluids are available. When severe vomiting, diarrhea, or diuresis results in a heavy loss of water and electrolytes, replacement therapy is necessary. Balanced fluids of isotonic electrolytes with an ionic composition similar to plasma are used.

Rapid initial replacement is seldom necessary. However, if a severely dehydrated patient shows signs of impaired circulation and renal function and it is necessary to restore the patient's blood pressure quickly, 30 mL/kg of an isotonic fluid may be provided in the first 1 or 2 hours.

Fluid overload must be prevented. Central venous pressure monitoring is especially helpful in elderly patients and in those with renal or cardiovascular disorders.

Extracellular replacement can usually be assumed to be complete after 48 hours of replacement therapy unless proved otherwise by clinical or laboratory evidence. To continue replacement fluids after deficits have been corrected may result in sodium excess, leading to pulmonary edema or heart failure. Patients receiving replacement therapy should be observed closely to detect any signs of circulatory overload.

Gastric replacement fluids provide the usual electrolytes lost by vomiting or gastric suction. They contain ammonium ions, which are metabolized in the liver to hydrogen ions and urea, replacing the hydrogen ion lost in gastric juices. They are useful in metabolic alkalosis caused by excessive ingestion of sodium bicarbonate. The usual adult dose is 500 to 2,000 mL, and the rate should be consistent with the patient's clinical condition but not >500 mL/hour.

Gastric replacement fluids are contraindicated in patients with hepatic insufficiency or renal failure. They require the same precautions as any fluid containing potassium and should be avoided in patients with renal damage or Addison's disease. Also, the low pH causes incompatibilities with many additives.

Lactated Ringer's injection is considered safe in certain conditions. Because the electrolyte concentration closely resembles that of the extracellular fluid, it may be used to replace fluid loss from burns and fluid lost as bile and diarrhea. Lactated Ringer's injection has been useful in mild acidosis, the lactate ion being metabolized in the liver to bicarbonate.

> ⚠ **SAFE PRACTICE ALERT** Three liters of lactated Ringer's injection contain approximately 390 mEq sodium, which can quickly elevate the sodium level in a patient who is not sodium deficient. Lactated Ringer's injection is contraindicated in severe metabolic acidosis or alkalosis and in liver disease or anoxic states that influence lactate metabolism.

Alkalizing Fluids

When anesthesia or disorders, such as dehydration, shock, liver disease, starvation, and diabetes, cause a patient to retain chlorides, ketone bodies, or organic salts, or when a patient loses excessive bicarbonate, metabolic acidosis occurs. Treatment consists of infusing an appropriate **alkalizing fluid.** These fluids include one-sixth molar isotonic sodium lactate (1.9%, with sodium, 167 mEq/L, and lactate ions, 167 mEq/L, and a pH of 6.0 to 7.3), one-sixth molar sodium bicarbonate injection, USP (1.5%, with sodium, 178 mEq/L, and bicarbonate, 178 mEq/L, and a pH of 7.0 to 8.0), and hypertonic sodium bicarbonate injection (7.5% or 5%).

One-Sixth Molar Sodium Lactate

The lactate ion must be oxidized in the body to carbon dioxide before it can effect acid–base balance; the complete conversion of sodium lactate to bicarbonate requires approximately 1 to 2 hours.

INDICATIONS FOR USE

One-sixth molar sodium lactate is used when acidosis results from a sodium deficiency in such disorders as vomiting, starvation, uncontrolled diabetes mellitus, acute infection, and renal failure (ASHP, 1998).

DANGERS OF USE

Because oxidation is necessary to increase the bicarbonate concentration, sodium lactate is not used for patients experiencing oxygen lack, as in shock or congenital heart disease with persistent cyanosis. It is also contraindicated in liver disease because the lactate ions are improperly metabolized.

ADMINISTRATION

The usual dose is 1 L of a one-sixth molar solution, but the dosage depends on the patient's condition and the serum sodium level. One-sixth molar infusion may be administered by venoclysis or hypodermoclysis and usually at a rate not greater than 300 mL/hour (ASHP, 1998). The patient should be observed closely for any evidence of alkalosis.

Sodium Bicarbonate Injection

Sodium bicarbonate injection, USP (1.5%, with sodium, 178 mEq/L, and bicarbonate, 178 mEq/L) is an isotonic fluid that provides bicarbonate ions for conditions of excess depletion.

INDICATIONS FOR USE

Sodium bicarbonate injection is used for severe hyperpnea early in the treatment of severe acidosis until the signs of dyspnea and hyperpnea subside. The bicarbonate ion is released in the form of carbon dioxide through the lungs, leaving an excess of sodium cation behind to exert its electrolyte effect (Terry, 2001).

Recommendations and practice related to pharmacologic management of cardiopulmonary resuscitation suggest a cautious use of sodium bicarbonate to manage acidosis (Metheny, 2000).

ADMINISTRATION

The usual dose is 500 mL in a 1.5% solution. The dosage depends on the patient's weight, condition, and carbon dioxide content. If the isotonic infusion is not available, it may be made by adding two 50-mL ampules containing 3.75 g each of sodium bicarbonate to 400 mL hypotonic saline.

The fluid should be infused slowly IV. Rapid injection may induce cellular acidity and death.

The patient should be watched for signs of hypocalcemic tetany, and calcium supplement should be administered if required; calcium does not ionize well in an alkaline medium. Extravasation of hypertonic sodium bicarbonate injections must be avoided (ASHP, 1998). Bicarbonate therapy should cease when the pH reaches 7.2.

Acidifying Infusions

Normal saline (0.9% sodium chloride injection, USP) is not usually listed among the **acidifying infusions.** However, because metabolic alkalosis is a condition associated with excess bicarbonate and loss of chloride, isotonic saline provides conservative treatment. When the chloride ions are infused, the bicarbonate decreases in compensation and the alkalosis is relieved.

Ammonium chloride, the usual acidifying agent, is available as isotonic 0.9% ammonium chloride injection (ammonium, 167 mEq/L; chloride, 167 mEq/L) and hypertonic 2.14% ammonium chloride injection (ammonium, 400 mEq/L; chloride,

400 mEq/L). The pH range is 4.0 to 6.0. Both concentrations are supplied in 1-L bottles.

INDICATIONS FOR USE

Ammonium chloride is used as an acidifying infusion in severe metabolic alkalosis caused by loss of gastric secretions, pyloric stenosis, or other causes. Ammonium ions are converted by the liver to hydrogen ions and to ammonia, which is excreted as urea.

ADMINISTRATION

The 2.14% ammonium chloride is usually used in the treatment of the adult patient; 0.9% ammonium chloride is used for children.

   The dosage depends on the condition of the patient and on an accurate chemical picture, including plasma carbon dioxide–combining power. Ammonium chloride must be infused at a very slow rate to enable the liver to metabolize the ammonium ions, not to exceed 5 mL/minute in adults. Rapid injection can result in toxic effects, causing irregular breathing, bradycardia, and twitching (ASHP, 1998). See Table 8–2 for more information on contents of fluids.

> △ **SAFE PRACTICE ALERT** Because its acidifying effect depends on the liver for conversion, ammonium chloride must not be administered to patients with severe hepatic disease or renal failure. It is contraindicated in any condition in which the patient has a high ammonium level.

Evaluation of Water and Electrolyte Balance

A rational approach is necessary if the patient is to receive safe and successful IV therapy. In the past, the nurse's technical responsibility in maintaining the infusion and patent venous access were emphasized. With the current increase in the use of IV therapy, however, clinical disturbances in fluid and electrolyte metabolism are more common.

   Changes in the patient's status can occur quickly and in the absence of the physician. Today, the nurse's responsibility consists of monitoring the fluid and electrolyte status of the patient as well as the progress of the infusion. Greater emphasis must be placed on the causes and effects of fluid and electrolyte abnormalities so that these imbalances may be anticipated and recognized before they become disastrous.

Monitoring Parameters

The nurse should be familiar with the parameters used in evaluating fluid and electrolyte imbalances and in supplying fluid and electrolyte requirements.

TABLE 8–2   Contents of Selected Water and Electrolyte Solutions

Solution	Cautions and Considerations

Dextrose 5% in water (D_5W):
  No electrolytes
  50 g of dextrose
	Supplies approximately 170 cal/L and free water to aid in renal excretion of solutes
	Should not be used in excessive volumes in patients with increased antidiuretic hormone activity or to replace fluids in hypovolemic patients

0.9% NaCl (isotonic saline):
  Na^+ 154 mEq/L
  Cl^- 154 mEq/L
	Isotonic fluid commonly used to expand the extracellular fluid in presence of hypovolemia
	Because of relatively high chloride content, can be used to treat mild metabolic alkalosis

0.45% NaCl (½-strength saline):
  Na^+ 77 mEq/L
  Cl^- 77 mEq/L
	A hypotonic solution that provides N^+, Cl^-, and free water; Na^+ and Cl^- provided in fluid allows kidneys to select and retain needed amounts
	Free water desirable as aid to kidneys in elimination of solutes

0.33% NaCl (⅓-strength saline):
  Na^+ 56 mEq/L
  Cl^- 56 mEq/L
	A hypotonic solution that provides Na^+, Cl^-, and free water
	Often used to treat hypernatremia (because this solution contains a small amount of N^+, it dilutes the plasma sodium while not allowing it to drop too rapidly)

3% NaCl:
  Na^+ 513 mEq/L
  Cl^- 513 mEq/L
	Grossly hypertonic solutions used only to treat severe hyponatremia
	See Box 8–3 summary of important nursing considerations in administration.

5% NaCl:
  Na^+ 855 mEq/L
  Cl^- 855 mEq/L
	Dangerous solutions

Lactated Ringer's solution:
  Na^+ 130 mEq/L
  K^+ 4 mEq/L
  Ca^{2+} 3 mEq/L
  Cl^- 109 mEq/L
	A roughly isotonic solution that contains multiple electrolytes in approximately the same concentrations as found in plasma (note that this solution is lacking in Mg and PO_4)
	Used in the treatment of hypovolemia, burns, and fluid lost as bile or diarrhea

Lactate (metabolized to bicarbonate) 28 mEq/L	Useful in treating mild metabolic acidosis

Sodium lactate solution, ⅙ M:
  N^+ 167 mEq/L
  Cl^- 167 mEq/L
	A roughly isotonic solution used to correct severe metabolic acidosis (lactate is metabolized to bicarbonate in 1–2 h by the liver)
	Not used in patients with liver disease (lactate cannot be converted to bicarbonate in such patients); also not used in patients with oxygen lack (unable adequately to convert lactate to bicarbonate)

Sodium bicarbonate, 5%:
  Na^+ 595 mEq/L
  Cl^- 595 mEq/L
	A very hypertonic solution used to correct severe metabolic acidosis
	Should be cautiously administered at a slow rate, using EID
	Should be administered only with extreme caution to salt-retaining patients (e.g., those with cardiac, renal, or liver damage)

Ammonium chloride, 2.14%:	Acidifying solution used to correct severe metabolic alkalosis Because of high ammonium content, must be administered cautiously in those with compromised hepatic function

Potassium chloride, 0.15%:
  K^+ 20 mEq/L
  Cl^- 20 mEq/L
	Premixed potassium chloride solution

Potassium chloride, 0.30%:
  K^+ 40 mEq/L
  Cl^- 40 mEq/L
	Premixed potassium chloride solution

CENTRAL VENOUS PRESSURE

Central venous pressure monitoring provides a simple, accurate, and valuable guide in detecting changes in blood volume and assessing fluid requirements. It is particularly valuable in assessing the ability of the heart to tolerate the infusion. Many erroneous conclusions are drawn from false values recorded when the infusion line is not properly responsive to right atrial pressures.

Normal venous pressure indicates an adequate circulatory blood volume; elevated venous pressure may mean an increase in circulatory volume and right heart pressure, with the possibility of circulatory overload. It may also indicate other problems such as a pulmonary embolus, myocardial infarction, or lack of digitalis. Determination of the hematocrit value supplements clinical information.

A low venous pressure, too low to measure, indicates that the patient has probably lost fluid or blood. The nurse must not overlook the fact that fluid loss can result from drug-induced vasodilation or improper administration of IV fluids. If rapid infusion of dextrose exceeds the patient's tolerance, massive diuresis with dehydration and diminished circulatory volume may occur. The decreased venous blood return into the right atrium is reflected by a decrease in the central venous pressure.

PULSE

The pulse quality and rate provide valuable clinical information for assessing fluid and electrolyte changes in the patient. A high pulse pressure, bounding and not easily obliterated by pressure, indicates a high cardiac output caused by circulatory overload. A regular pulse, easily obliterated by pressure, indicates low cardiac output resulting from a lowered blood volume.

A bounding, easily obliterated pressure signifies a drop in blood pressure with a wide pulse pressure, indicative of impending circulatory collapse. As the patient's condition deteriorates, the pulse becomes rapid, weak, thready, and easily obliterated, signifying circulatory collapse.

HAND VEINS

Examination of the hand veins provides a means of evaluating the plasma volume. The hand veins usually empty in 3 to 5 seconds when the hand is elevated and fill in the same length of time when the hand is lowered to a dependent position. Peripheral vein filling takes longer than 3 to 5 seconds in patients with sodium depletion and extracellular dehydration.

Slow emptying of the hand veins indicates overhydration and excessive blood volume; slow filling indicates a low blood volume and often precedes hypotension. Hand veins that become engorged and clearly visible indicate an increase in plasma volume secondary to an interstitial-to-vascular fluid shift or an increase in extracellular fluid volume (Metheny, 2000). A rapid guide for fluid assessment is found in Table 8–3.

NECK VEINS

Changes in fluid volume are reflected by changes in neck vein filling, provided the patient is not in heart failure. In the supine position, the patient's external jugular

TABLE 8–3   Rapid Fluid Imbalance Assessment Guide

Assessment Focus	Fluid Volume Excess (Hypervolemia)	Fluid Volume Deficit (Hypovolemia)
Cardiovascular system	Bounding pulse Elevated pulse rate Jugular distention Overdistended hand veins	Decreased blood pressure Decreased pulse rate Flat neck veins Narrow pulse pressure Slow hand vein filling
Integumentary system	Warm, moist skin Sternal fingerprinting	Decreased turgor over sternum/forehead Lowered skin temperature
Neurologic system	—	Altered orientation: confusion
Respiratory system	Moist crackles Respiratory rate >20/min Dyspnea Pulmonary edema	Clear lungs
Eyes	Periorbital edema	Dry conjunctiva Sunken eyes Decreased tearing
Lips	—	Dry and cracked
Mouth	—	Dry mucous membranes
Tongue	—	Dry, leathery texture Longitudinal furrows
Weight	Mild: 2% above normal Moderate: 5% above normal Severe: >8% above normal	Mild: <2% below normal Moderate: 5% below normal Severe: >8% below normal

veins fill to the anterior border of the sternocleidomastoid muscle. Flat neck veins in the supine position indicate a decreased plasma volume.

WEIGHT

A sudden gain or loss in weight is a significant sign of a change in the fluid volume. A change in the volume of body fluid can be computed by weighing the patient daily at the same time of day, on the same scales, with the same amount of clothing. A loss or gain of 1 kg body weight reflects a loss or gain of 1 L body fluid. A rapid 2% loss of total body weight indicates mild fluid volume deficit, and a rapid loss of 8% or more represents severe fluid volume deficit. Conversely, weight gain occurs when total fluid intake exceeds total fluid output. A rapid 2% gain of total body weight indicates mild fluid volume excess; a 5% gain represents a moderate fluid volume excess; and 8% or greater indicates a severe fluid volume excess.

THIRST

Thirst is an important symptom denoting a deficit in body fluid or, more specifically, cellular dehydration. This type of dehydration occurs when the extracellular fluid becomes hypertonic, either as a result of water deprivation or the infusion of hypertonic saline. The increase in osmotic pressure causes fluid to be drawn from the cells, resulting in cellular dehydration, the stimulus to thirst. Normally, thirst governs the need for water but, in certain conditions, the lack of thirst may accompany dehydration. This is especially true in the aged, in whom thirst is not urgent. These patients may lose their thirst and as a result become severely dehydrated before the condition is recognized. In the severely burned patient, the great thirst experienced may lead to ingestion of excess water and to a serious sodium deficit.

INTAKE AND OUTPUT

Water intake and output should be carefully measured and recorded. Hourly urine output measurements may be particularly important. A urine output of 200 mL/hour indicates that too much water is being infused too rapidly. By regulating the urine output between 30 and 50 mL/hour, the patient receives at least enough fluid for the kidneys to work efficiently.

A decreased urinary output accompanies a decreased blood volume; changes in the arterial pressure and pressure in the glomeruli result in the oliguria or anuria of profound shock. The increase in urinary output accompanying an increase in blood volume is primarily caused by changes in arterial pressure and pressure in the glomeruli. Output should include urine, vomitus, diarrhea, drainage from fistulas, and drainage from suction apparatus.

SKIN TURGOR

Observing changes in skin **turgor** (elasticity) and texture is helpful in assessing the state of water balance. To test skin turgor, the skin is pinched over the sternum, inner aspect of the thigh, or forehead in the adult or the medial aspects of the thigh or abdomen in the child, and then released; in the normal person, the pinched skin returns to its original position. Skin that remains in a raised position for several seconds indicates a deficit in fluid volume.

TONGUE TURGOR

A dry, leathery tongue may indicate a fluid volume deficit or mouth breathing. To differentiate between the two, the mucous membrane may be checked for moisture by running the finger between the gums and the cheek; dryness indicates a fluid volume deficit.

Normally, the tongue has one longitudinal furrow. In the patient with fluid volume deficit, additional longitudinal furrows are present and the tongue is smaller because of the fluid loss. Not significantly affected by age, the tongue is a good parameter to measure in all age groups.

EDEMA

Edema reflects an increase in the extracellular fluid volume outside the circulating intravascular compartment. It depends on an imbalance or a disturbance in the exchange of water and electrolytes between the patient and the environment or the exchange of water and electrolytes between the compartments of the body. The fluid and electrolyte exchange between the body compartments may be affected by an alteration in the circulatory system, the lymphatic system, or the concentration of albumin in the serum; water and electrolytes escape from the circulation faster than they enter, and edema ensues.

Edema may be generalized, as in congestive failure; localized, as with ascites; or peripheral. By detecting edema early, a clinical imbalance may be corrected before the patient's condition deteriorates. Early peripheral edema may be detected by fingerprinting, a procedure in which the finger is rolled over the bony prominence of the sternum or tibia. As edema increases, pitting edema occurs and may be detected by pressure of the fingers on the subcutaneous tissue. Figure 8–1 shows the degrees of edema.

In generalized edema, such as that seen in cardiac failure, total extracellular water volume as well as interstitial edema increase. Symptoms such as venous engorgement, restlessness, dyspnea, cyanosis, and pulmonary rales indicate generalized edema.

Laboratory Values

Laboratory values, when used to supplement clinical observations, aid in forming diagnostic and therapeutic guidelines. Electrolyte studies (serum sodium, potassium, chloride, bicarbonate, and pH) performed daily are important in assessing the fluid and electrolyte status of the patient receiving IV fluids. In patients with massive electrolyte losses, such studies may be required two or three times a day. Blood cell count and hematocrit determinations are helpful in detecting hemoconcentration or hemodilution; *hemoconcentration* reflects a diminished plasma volume caused by dehydration, and *hemodilution*, an increased volume from overtreatment with water.

Measurement of serum protein with the albumin/globulin ratio helps in detecting a change in fluid volume; large quantities of rapidly administered parenteral fluid dilute and decrease the serum protein concentration. This determination is helpful when used to supplement clinical observation—otherwise, it may be misleading and interpreted as showing actual depletion. A decrease in serum protein

FIGURE 8–1.   Edema scale. Severity of edema is ranked on a scale of +1 to +4, with +1 being barely perceptible and +4 being visible and remarkable.

reduces the osmotic pressure of the extracellular compartment, causing some edema and loss of plasma volume. Blood urea nitrogen should be measured frequently to evaluate kidney function, an important parameter in treating fluid and electrolyte imbalances.

Clinical Disturbances of Water and Electrolyte Metabolism

Most of the common clinical disturbances in water and electrolyte balance result from changes in the volume of total body water or in one or more of the fluid compartments of the body. Clinical disturbances in water and electrolyte metabolism have been classified into six types: isotonic, hypertonic, and hypotonic expansion and isotonic, hypertonic, and hypotonic contraction. These are discussed in the following sections.

Isotonic Expansion

Isotonic expansion (circulatory overload) occurs when fluids of the same tonicity as plasma are infused into the vascular circulation. Because fluids isotonic to plasma do not affect the osmolality, water does not flow from the extracellular to the intracellular compartment. The extracellular compartment expands in proportion to the fluid infused and is the only compartment affected. The increase in the volume of fluid dilutes the concentration of hemoglobin and lowers the hematocrit and total protein levels, but the serum sodium level remains the same.

Isotonic expansion is a critical complication of IV therapy. Patients who receive isotonic fluids around the clock are at particular risk and should be observed closely for early signs of circulatory overload. Sodium chloride (0.9%) or fluids containing balanced isotonic multiple electrolytes are used for pre-existing or continuing fluid and electrolyte losses and are not the ideal fluids for maintenance therapy. The electrolyte isotonicity of these fluids causes expansion of the extracellular compartment and does not provide the extra water that balanced hypotonic fluids provide for the kidney to retain or secrete as needed. The early postoperative or posttrauma patient is susceptible to this critical complication. The increased endocrine response to stress during the first 2 to 5 days after surgery results in retention of sodium chloride and water. When a patient under stress is receiving isotonic infusions, the nurse must anticipate and watch for signs of circulatory overload.

Elderly patients receiving isotonic fluids must be carefully monitored because they have a lower tolerance for fluids and electrolytes. Because they are also likely to have some degree of cardiac and renal impairment, the ability of the kidneys to eliminate fluid is likely to be diminished. The status of these patients can change quickly. In the patient who has had a craniotomy, large-volume isotonic infusions can increase the intracranial pressure and prove detrimental.

Patients who are potential candidates for isotonic expansion must be watched carefully and turned frequently to prevent fluid from settling in the lungs. Pulmonary edema can result from the cardiac and pulmonary side effects of IV therapy. The apices of the lungs, which are high, tend to be fairly dry, but the bases of the lungs, posteriorly and inferiorly, can be fairly wet (Metheny, 2003). As a result, hypostatic pneumonia secondary to gravity may develop.

MANIFESTATIONS

The nurse who monitors IV infusions must be familiar with the early clinical manifestations that accompany isotonic expansion to recognize and prevent its development; mild pulmonary edema progressing to severe pulmonary edema is a late stage that must be prevented. Early clinical manifestations include (a) weight gain; (b) increased fluid intake over output; (c) high pulse pressure; (d) increase in central venous pressure; (e) peripheral hand vein emptying time; (f) peripheral edema; and (g) hoarseness. If IV therapy is allowed to continue, isotonic expansion becomes more apparent and dangerous, with easily recognized signs: cyanosis, dyspnea, coughing, and neck vein engorgement. Laboratory characteristics include a drop in the hematocrit value and reduced concentrations of hemoglobin and total protein.

TREATMENT

Treatment for circulatory overload when detected early is relatively simple and consists of withholding all fluids until excess water and electrolytes have been eliminated by the body. After the condition is rectified, hypotonic maintenance fluids provide the patient with fluid and a minimum daily requirement of electrolytes. The hypotonicity of the fluid allows the kidneys to maintain the needed amount and selectively retain or excrete the excess.

Isotonic Contraction

Isotonic contraction occurs when there is loss of fluid and electrolytes isotonic to the extracellular fluid, such as whole blood or large volumes of fluid from diarrhea or vomiting. The extracellular compartment contracts. Because the fluid lost is isotonic, the osmolality of the extracellular compartment remains unchanged and no movement of water occurs between the compartments; only the extracellular volume is affected.

MANIFESTATIONS

Because of the loss of fluid, the hematocrit level and the concentrations of hemoglobin and total protein are increased. The serum sodium concentration does not change. Clinical manifestations include:

- Weight loss
- Negative fluid balance (a decrease in urinary output but a greater output than total fluid intake)
- Regular pulse rate, easily obliterated by pressure, and, as the patient's condition deteriorates, becoming weak and thready
- Possible increase in peripheral hand vein filling time above the normal 3 to 5 seconds when the hand is moved from an elevated to a dependent position

TREATMENT

Treatment consists of replacing the fluid loss with isotonic fluids containing balanced electrolytes.

Hypertonic Expansion

Hypertonic expansion occurs when the volume of body water is increased by the IV infusion of hypertonic saline. Sodium chloride 3% or 5% is used to replace a massive sodium loss or remove excess accumulation of body fluids, but, if the infusion is administered rapidly, hypertonic expansion can result. The saline increases the osmotic pressure of the extracellular compartment, causing water to be drawn from the intracellular compartment until both compartments are isosmotic. The volume of the extracellular compartment increases and that of the intracellular compartment decreases. The osmolality of the extracellular fluid is higher than before the infusion but lower than the high level after the infusion because of the increased extracellular fluid volume (ASHP, 1998).

Caution must be used in the IV administration of hypertonic saline fluid. Circulatory overload with hypernatremia can occur. An understanding of the reason for the infusion, the condition of the patient, the proper rate of administration, and the signs and symptoms of hypertonic expansion provides a basis for sound IV practice.

MANIFESTATIONS

Clinical manifestations include a gain in body weight dependent on the volume infused. A small volume (500 mL) does not contribute to a significant weight gain (Metheny, 2003).

An increased sodium load results in a decreased rate of water excretion; however, the abrupt increase in plasma volume may cause an increase in the rate of water excretion as the body attempts to excrete the excess salt and water. The degree of thirst depends on the hypertonicity of the plasma and consequently the amount of cellular dehydration.

Peripheral hand vein emptying time may be increased beyond the normal 5 seconds when the hand is elevated, but depends on the degree of expansion of the extracellular compartment. A bounding pulse is significant in detecting hypertonic expansion. The serum sodium concentration is increased. The hematocrit level and the concentrations of hemoglobin and total serum protein are decreased as a result of the expanded fluid volume in the extracellular compartment.

TREATMENT

Treatment consists of stopping the infusion to allow the kidneys to eliminate the overload of salt and water. If no cardiovascular side effects are noted, dextrose 5% in water may be infused slowly to reduce the tonicity of the extracellular fluid and replace body water.

Hypertonic Contraction

Hypertonic contraction (hypertonic dehydration) occurs when water is lost without a corresponding loss of salt. This condition occurs in patients who are unable to take sufficient fluid for a prolonged period or in patients with excess insensible water loss through the lungs and skin.

In elderly patients, hypertonic dehydration is a common clinical disturbance; they frequently experience a decrease in the thirst stimuli in response to hypertonicity of body fluids, and adequate intake of fluid is not met. In the unconscious or incontinent patient, frequency and excess urination may go undetected or may be interpreted as a sign of good renal function. A loss of tubular ability to concentrate urine in the aged results in a large urinary volume when an increased solute load is presented to the patient (Metheny, 2000).

Elderly patients also have a diminished response to ADH. Large amounts of dilute urine may be lost, resulting in hypertonic dehydration (see Chap. 22). To prevent fluid imbalance, the nurse must recognize that individuals differ widely in the water they require; patients whose kidneys do not concentrate urine well require more water than those whose kidneys do concentrate urine well.

The daily fluid requirement must be met. In hypertonic contraction, the loss of water from the extracellular compartment results in an increase in the osmolality, causing water to flow from the cells to the extracellular compartment. Dehydration occurs as water leaves the cellular compartment to replace the plasma volume.

Both the intracellular and the extracellular compartments are affected by the water loss; there is a decrease in volume and an increase in osmolality in both compartments. In contrast, in isotonic contraction, only the extracellular compartment is affected and the contraction is more serious. Because signs of hypertonic contraction are not obvious in the early stages, the nurse must anticipate such an imbalance and be alert to any changes.

MANIFESTATIONS

Clinically, thirst is an early and reliable sign of hypertonic contraction, but it may be absent in the elderly, complicating early recognition of this imbalance. Weight loss occurs. Negative fluid balance (output greater than intake) is present. Hourly output measurements show a decrease in the rate of excretion of water.

The pulse has a normal quality and is regular in the early stages of hypertonic contraction. The hand vein filling time may be within the normal limits; cellular fluid has partly replenished the plasma.

Irritability, restlessness, and possibly confusion may be present. Skin turgor diminishes and is a sign of dehydration in the later stages. A dry mouth with a furrowed tongue indicates dehydration. Laboratory studies show an increase in serum sodium concentration, hematocrit level, hemoglobin concentration, and total serum protein concentration.

TREATMENT

Treatment consists of hydrating the patient by administering a balanced hypotonic fluid such as the Butler-type fluids: 2,400 mL/m^2 BSA per day for moderate pre-existing deficit and 3,000 mL/m² BSA per day for severe pre-existing deficit. The usual rate for IV administration is 3 mL/m² BSA. A therapeutic test for functional renal depression may be necessary before infusing water and electrolytes for maintenance.

Hypotonic Expansion

Hypotonic expansion (water intoxication, dilutional hyponatremia) occurs when the increase in the volume of body fluids is caused by water alone. Water expands the extracellular compartment, causing a decrease in the concentration. Water then diffuses into the cells until both compartments are isosmotic. Both the extracellular and the intracellular compartments are affected; the volume is increased and the concentration is decreased.

The serum sodium concentration and the hematocrit, hemoglobin, and total serum protein levels are reduced. Hypotonic expansion occurs in patients who are receiving large quantities of electrolyte-free water to replace excessive fluid and electrolytes lost from gastric suction, vomiting, diarrhea or diuresis, or insensibly through the skin.

Patients receiving continuous infusion of dextrose 5% in water are particularly susceptible to water intoxication. This fluid contains 252 mOsm dextrose per liter, making it an isotonic fluid in the container. Once introduced into the circulation, the dextrose is quickly metabolized, leaving the water free to dilute and expand the extracellular compartment. With the decreased osmolality of the extracellular fluid, water diffuses into the cells and hypotonic expansion occurs. The patient's tolerance to water can be exceeded by infusion of excess amounts of hypotonic fluids. The kidneys of the normal adult can metabolize water in amounts of 35 to 45 mL/kg/day, but the kidneys of the average patient can metabolize only 2,500 to 3,000 mL/day; above these volumes, abnormal accumulation of water occurs (Metheny, 2003).

Hypotonic expansion is more likely to occur during the early postoperative period, when retention of water is affected by the response to stress, particularly in the elderly patient, in whom the response to stress is compounded by impairment in renal function. Small amounts of adjusted hypotonic saline (sodium, 90 mEq/L; chloride, 60 mEq/L; and lactate, 30 mEq/L) may be used in the early postoperative management of the aged.

MANIFESTATIONS

When acute onset of behavioral changes, such as confusion, apathy, and disorientation, occurs in the elderly postoperative patient, overhydration should be suspected.

Central nervous system disturbances such as weakness, muscle twitching, and convulsions are seen, as are headaches, nausea, and vomiting. Fluid intake is increased over fluid output. Weight gain is always present.

Blood pressure usually is normal but may be elevated. Peripheral hand veins are usually full, and hand emptying time is increased beyond the normal 5 seconds when the hand is elevated from a dependent position. The pulse may be regular and not easily obliterated when pressure is applied.

TREATMENT

Treatment consists of withholding all fluids until the excess water is excreted. In severe hyponatremia, it may be necessary to administer small quantities of hypertonic saline to increase the osmotic pressure and the flow of water from the cells to the extracellular compartment for excretion by the kidneys. Hypertonic saline must be used cautiously and must not be administered to patients with congestive heart failure.

Hypotonic Contraction

Hypotonic contraction (hypotonic dehydration) occurs when fluids containing relatively more salt than water are lost from the body. This loss results in a decrease in the effective osmolality of the extracellular compartment. Water is drawn into the cells until osmotic equilibrium is established. Because of the invasion of water, the intracellular compartment is expanded and the extracellular compartment is contracted. This imbalance may result from the loss of salt from any one of several sources: urine of patients receiving diuretics, fistula drainage, severe burns, vomitus, and sweat. The elderly are affected by the loss of small quantities of sodium.

MANIFESTATIONS

Clinical manifestations include weight loss; negative fluid balance; pulse rate that is increased, weak or thready, and easily obliterated; increased hand filling time; and decreased skin turgor. Laboratory studies show a decrease in serum sodium concentration and an increase in hematocrit, hemoglobin, and total serum protein levels.

TREATMENT

Treatment of hypotonic contraction consists of replacing the fluids and electrolytes that have been lost. Because other electrolytes are usually lost along with the sodium loss, a balanced electrolyte fluid may be administered.

References and Selected Readings

Asterisks indicate references cited in text.

*American Society of Healthcare Pharmacists [ASHP]. (1998). Bethesda, MD: American Hospital Formulary Service, 1486, 1490, 1514–1517, 1527–1529.

Carpenito, L.J. (1995). *Nursing diagnosis applied to clinical practice* (6th ed., pp. 120–127). Philadelphia: J.B. Lippincott.

*Terry, J. (2001). Fluids and electrolytes. In: J. Terry, L. Baranowski, & C. Hedrick (Eds.). *Intravenous therapy:*

Clinical principles and practice (p. 120). Philadelphia: W.B. Saunders.

*Metheny, N.M. (2000). *Fluid and electrolyte balance* (5th ed.). Philadelphia: Lippincott Williams & Wilkins.

United States Pharmacopeia [USP]. (1999). (26th ed., pp. 803, 1027). Easton, PA: Mack Publishing.

Review Questions

Note: Questions below may have more than one right answer.

1. Which of the following IV dextrose fluids is considered isotonic?
   A. 2.5%
   B. 5%
   C. 0%
   D. 20%

2. A teaching plan for a patient diagnosed with hypermagnesemia should include:
   A. Preventing injury due to hypotension or weakness
   B. Availability of an antacid to prevent gastric acidity or reflux
   C. Preventing constipation by routine laxative administration
   D. Restricting fluid intake

3. Edema is the result of excess fluid in which of the following areas?
   A. Interstitial space
   B. Intracellular space
   C. Intrathecal space
   D. Intravascular space

4. One-sixth molar sodium lactate may be infused by which of the following methods?
   A. IV push
   B. Hypodermoclysis
   C. Venoclysis
   D. Syringe pump

5. The electrolyte concentration of lactated Ringer's injection closely resembles that of:
   A. Extracellular fluid
   B. Intracellular fluid
   C. Pericardium
   D. Intravascular compartment

6. Which of the following is true of high pulse pressure?
   A. Indicates high cardiac output
   B. Indicates reduced cardiac output
   C. Indicates impending circulatory collapse
   D. Indicates low cardiac output

7. Hypotonic expansion may also be known as which of the following:
   A. Dilutional hyponatremia
   B. Water intoxication
   C. A only
   D. A and B

8. Slow filling of the hand veins indicates which of the following?
   A. Excessive blood volume
   B. Low blood volume
   C. Increased plasma volume
   D. Increased extracellular fluid volume

9. Gastric replacement fluids are contraindicated in patients with:
   A. Renal failure
   B. Hepatic insufficiency
   C. Increased pulse pressure
   D. Isotonic expansion

10. Which of the following is not true of hypertonic fluid?
    A. Lowers osmotic pressure of plasma
    B. Causes fluid to invade the cell
    C. Increases extracellular volume
    D. Draws fluid from the cells

CHAPTER
9

Complications and Interventions

KEY TERMS

Air Embolism

Catheter Embolism

Cellular Toxicity

Débridement

Ecchymosis

Edema

Extravasation

Hematoma

Infiltration

Ischemia

Necrosis

Phlebothrombosis

Reflex Sympathetic Dystrophy
  (RSD)

Root Cause Analysis

Sentinel Events

Speed Shock

Thrombogenicity

Thrombophlebitis

Thrombosis

Understanding Complications

As many as 90% of all hospitalized patients in the United States receive some form of infusion therapy, and the number of patients in the alternative care settings continues to proliferate. Although most infusion therapy is administered without problems, complications, ranging from minor to more serious, do occur. Such complications increase hospital rate of stay, length of therapy, and nursing responsibilities, and may put the patient at risk for additional problems. Fortunately, most of these complications are preventable. A comprehensive knowledge of the inherent risks and measures to prevent their occurrence may eliminate many of the hazards associated with infusion therapy (Perdue, 2001). The IV nurse needs to recognize complications and respond with appropriate nursing interventions to ensure quality of care. Complications are varied and may be local or systemic. Local complications occur frequently, but are rarely serious. Systemic complications, although rarer, are serious and frequently life threatening. They require immediate recognition and medical attention. **Sentinel events**, as defined by the Joint Commission on Accreditation of Healthcare Organizations (JCAHO), are unexpected occurrences involving death or serious physical or psychologic injury, or the risk thereof. This chapter addresses the full range of complications as well as sentinel events and appropriate nursing interventions.

Local Complications

Local complications are those seen at or near the catheter insertion site as a result of trauma to the vessel wall or as a result of mechanical failure. In general, they are easily corrected and are associated with no serious problems when appropriate interventions are initiated (Perdue & Dugger, 2004). Occasionally, local complications are not recognized until considerable damage occurs, making early recognition of complications a key factor in infusion therapy. Early recognition may prevent the following:

- Extensive **edema** that deprives the patient of urgently needed fluid and medications
- **Necrosis** (localized death of tissue)
- **Thrombophlebitis** with the subsequent danger of embolism

Local complications that are mechanical in nature are generally resolved by correction of the mechanical failure, such as adjusting a tourniquet, insertion site, cannula, container, tubing, or patient position. Local complications may also occur as the result of trauma to the wall of the vein. Among the common local complications are ecchymosis or hematoma, infiltration, extravasation, phlebitis, postinfusion phlebitis, thrombosis, thrombophlebitis, and phlebothrombosis.

Ecchymosis/Hematoma

Ecchymosis denotes the infiltration of blood into the tissues; **hematoma** usually refers to uncontrolled bleeding at a venipuncture site, generally creating a hard, painful lump. Both are commonly associated with venipunctures that are performed by unskilled professionals or on those patients who have a tendency to bruise easily. Ecchymosis and hematomas often occur when multiple entries are made into a vein, or when attempts are made into veins that are not easily palpated. These injuries limit veins for future use (Perdue, 2001).

> **SAFE PRACTICE ALERT** If ecchymosis occurs during venipuncture, the cannula should be removed and light pressure should be applied. These areas may take days to weeks to disappear. If hematoma occurs during a venipuncture attempt, the cannula is immediately removed, direct pressure is applied to the area, catheter integrity is assessed, and the extremity is elevated until bleeding has stopped. A dry, sterile dressing is applied to the site and the area is monitored for signs of breakthrough bleeding. Ice may be applied and the area is observed for circulatory, neurologic, and motor function. (Perdue, 2001).

Infiltration

Dislodgment of the catheter with consequent **infiltration** of fluid is common and frequently is considered of minor significance. With the increasing numbers of irritating solutions and the frequency with which potent drugs are infused in IV solutions, serious problems may occur when the fluid invades the surrounding tissues. Hypertonic, acid, and alkaline fluids are contraindicated for hypodermoclysis and are not intended for other than venous infusions. If they are allowed to infiltrate, necrosis may occur.

If necrosis is avoided, edema may nevertheless

- Deprive the patient of fluid and drug absorption at the rate essential for successful therapy
- Limit veins available for venipuncture, complicating therapy
- Predispose the patient to infection

> **SAFE PRACTICE ALERT** To confirm an infiltration, apply a tourniquet proximal to the injection site tightly enough to restrict the venous flow. If the infusion continues regardless of this venous obstruction, extravasation is evident.

Extravasation

Extravasation can easily be recognized by increasing edema at the site of the infusion. Comparing the infusion area with the identical area in the opposite extremity can help the nurse identify swelling.

In many cases, the edema is allowed to increase to great proportions because of the misconception that backflow of blood into the adapter is significant proof that the infusion is entering the vein. This is not a reliable method for detecting possible infiltration because the point of the IV catheter may puncture the posterior wall of the vein, leaving the greater portion of the bevel in the lumen of the vein. Blood return is obtained on negative pressure, but if the infusion is allowed to continue, fluid seeps into the tissues at the point of the catheter, thereby increasing the edema (see Chap. 8).

Occasionally, a blood return is not obtained on negative pressure. This may occur when the needle occludes the lumen of a small vein, obstructing the flow of blood. Evidence of backflow should not be the sole criterion for confirming extravasation.

Drugs that contribute to necrosis that results from extravasation are most often osmotically active or **ischemia** inducing, or they cause direct **cellular toxicity.** Mechanical compression in the infiltrated tissue can increase the extent of damage, as can infection of the resulting wound. If only superficial tissue loss occurs and the area remains free of infection, **débridement** yields a clean bed capable of granulation. If deep structures are involved, however, spontaneous wound healing may be averted, resulting in the need for wide excision, debridement, and grafting or amputation to restore tissue integrity.

Phlebitis

Phlebitis, or inflammation of the intima of the vein, is a commonly reported complication of infusion therapy. The inflammatory process occurs as a result of irritation to the endothelial cells of the vein intima, creating a rough cell wall where platelets readily adhere. Phlebitis is characterized by pain and tenderness along the course of the vein, erythema, and inflammatory swelling with a feeling of warmth at the site (Perdue, 2001). Phlebitis may be mechanical, chemical, or bacterial. See Box 9–1, Factors Contributing to Venous Inflammation, and Box 9–2, Phlebitis Rating Scale.

Mechanical phlebitis is associated with cannula placement; cannulas placed in areas of flexion may result in mechanical phlebitis. As the extremity is mobilized, the cannula may irritate the vein intima, causing injury and resultant phlebitis. The cannula should closely approximate the lumen of the vessel to avoid mechanical phlebitis. Proper taping and securement is also essential.

> **SAFE PRACTICE ALERT** To evaluate a mechanical phlebitis, check the tourniquet, site, cannula, solution container, tubing, and involved extremity.

Bacterial phlebitis is an inflammation of the vein intima associated with a bacterial infection. The condition may be serious and predispose the patient to systemic complications addressed later in this chapter. See Box 9–1. Handwashing is the

---

BOX 9–1   Factors Contributing to Venous Inflammation

Inflammation of the vein can occur from any foreign body and is mediated by the following:

- Duration of the infusion
- Composition of the solution
- Site of the infusion
- Venipuncture technique
- Method used

BOX 9–2   Phlebitis Rating Scale

	0	1+	2+	3+
Edema	No	Possible	Possible	Yes
Erythema (with or without pain)	No	Yes	Yes	Yes
Streak formation	No	No	Yes	Yes
Palpable cord	No	No	No	Yes

---

single most important procedure for preventing nosocomial infections, and aseptic technique is essential in the preparation and care of venipuncture sites (APIC, 1998).

Chemical phlebitis is associated with a response of the vein intima to chemicals producing inflammation. The inflammatory response is created by the administration of solutions or medications or as a result of certain cannula materials. We know that the normal blood pH is 7.35 to 7.45 and is slightly alkaline. The normal pH for solutions is 7.0, which is neutral. The pH of dextrose solutions ranges from 3.5 to 6.5 (Perdue, 2001). Acidity is needed to prevent caramelization of the dextrose during sterilization and to maintain the stability of the solution during storage. Solutions and medications with a high pH or osmolality predispose the vein intima to irritation (Perdue, 2001). The more acidic an IV admixture, the greater the risk. In addition, additives such as potassium chloride, vancomycin hydrochloride, and many antineoplastic agents can contribute to chemical phlebitis. Refer to Thrombophlebitis later in this chapter.

 SAFE PRACTICE ALERT   Chemical phlebitis may be caused by irritating medications or solutions, medications improperly diluted or administered too rapidly, particulate matter, cannula material, or extended dwell time.

Post-Infusion Phlebitis

Post-infusion phlebitis refers to inflammation of the vein that usually presents within 48 to 96 hours of cannula removal. Factors contributing to the development of post-infusion phlebitis include the following: poor cannula insertion technique, a debilitated patient, poor vein condition, hypertonic or acidic solutions, ineffective filtration, placement of a large-gauge cannula in a small vessel, and failure to change tubings, dressing, infection site caps, and cannulas consistent with the Infusion Nursing Standards of Practice. (Perdue, 2001; INS, 2005). Measures for preventing post-infusion phlebitis are provided in Box 9–3.

BOX 9–3   Standard Precautions

Use Standard Precautions, or the equivalent, for the care of all patients, *Category IB**

A. Handwashing

(1) Wash hands after touching blood, body fluids, secretions, excretions, and contaminated items, whether or not gloves are worn. Wash hands immediately after gloves are removed, between patient contacts, and when otherwise indicated to avoid transfer of micro-organisms to other patients or environments. It may be necessary to wash hands between tasks and procedures on the same patient to prevent cross-contamination of different body sites. *Category IB*
(2) Use a plain (nonantimicrobial) soap for routine hand washing. *Category IB*
(3) Use an antimicrobial agent or a waterless antiseptic agent for specific circumstances (e.g., control of outbreaks or hyperendemic infections), as defined by the infection control program. *Category IB*. (See Contact Precautions for additional recommendations on using antimicrobial and antiseptic agents.)

B. Gloves
Wear gloves (clean, nonsterile gloves are adequate) when touching blood, body fluids, secretions, excretions, and contaminated items. Put on clean gloves just before touching mucous membranes and nonintact skin. Change gloves between tasks and procedures on the same patient after contact with material that may contain a high concentration of micro-organisms. Remove gloves promptly after use, before touching noncontaminated items and environmental surfaces, and before going to another patient, and wash hands immediately to avoid transfer of micro-organisms to other patients or environments. *Category IB*

C. Mask, Eye Protection, Face Shield
Wear a mask and eye protection or a face shield to protect mucous membranes of the eyes, nose, and mouth during procedures and patient-care activities that are likely to generate splashes or sprays of blood, body fluids, secretions, and excretions. *Category IB*

D. Gown
Wear a gown (a clean, nonsterile gown is adequate) to protect skin and to prevent soiling of clothing during procedures and patient-care activities that are likely to generate splashes or sprays of blood, body fluids, secretions, or excretions. Select a gown that is appropriate for the activity and amount of fluid likely to be encountered. Remove a soiled gown as promptly as possible, and wash hands to avoid transfer of micro-organisms to other patients or environments. *Category IB*

E. Patient-Care Equipment
Handle used patient-care equipment soiled with blood, body fluids, secretions, and excretions in a manner that prevents skin and mucous membrane exposures, contamination of clothing, and transfer of micro-organisms to other patients and environments. Ensure that reusable equipment is not used for the care of another patient until it has been cleaned and reprocessed appropriately. Ensure that single-use items are discarded properly. *Category IB*

F. Environmental Control
Ensure that the hospital has adequate procedures for the routine care, cleaning, and disinfection of environment surfaces, beds, bedrails, bedside equipment, and other frequently touched surfaces, and ensure that these procedures are being followed. *Category IB*

G. Linen
Handle, transport, and process used linen soiled with blood, body fluids, secretions, and excretions in a manner that prevents skin and mucous membrane exposures and contamination of clothing, and that avoids transfer of micro-organisms to other patients and environments. *Category IB*

(Continued)

BOX 9–3   **Standard Precautions**   *(Continued)*

H. Occupational Health and Bloodborne Pathogens

(1) Take care to prevent injuries when using needles, scalpels, and other sharp instruments or devices; when handling sharp instruments after procedures; when cleaning used instruments; and when disposing of used needles. Never recap used needles, or otherwise manipulate them using both hands, or use any other technique that involves directing the point of a needle toward any part of the body; rather, use either a one-handed scoop technique or mechanical device designed for holding the needle sheath. Do not remove used needles from disposable syringes by hand, and do not bend, break, or otherwise manipulate used needles by hand. Place used disposable syringes and needles, scalpel blades, and other sharp items in appropriate puncture-resistant containers, which are located as close as practical to the area in which the items were used and place reusable syringes and needles in a puncture-resistant container for transport to the processing area. *Category IB*

(2) Use mouthpieces, resuscitation bags, or other ventilator devices as an alternative to mouth-to-mouth resuscitation methods in areas where the need for resuscitation is predictable. *Category IB*

I. Patient Placement

Place a patient who contaminates the environment or who does not (or cannot be expected to) assist in maintaining appropriate hygiene or environmental control in a private room. If a private room is not available, consult with infection control professionals regarding patient placement or other alternatives. *Category IB*

---

*Category IB. Strongly recommended for all hospitals and reviewed as effective by experts in the field and a consensus of HICPAC based on strong rationale and suggestive evidence, even though definitive scientific studies have not been done.

From Guideline for isolation precautions in hospitals developed by the Centers for Disease Control and Prevention and the Hospital Infection Control Practices Advisory Committee (HICPAC), January 1996.

Thrombosis

Any injury that roughens the endothelial cells of the venous wall allows platelets to adhere and a thrombus to form (Fig. 9–1). Because the point of the IV catheter traumatizes the wall of the vein where it touches, a thrombus or thrombi form on the vein and at the tip of the catheter. The result of local thrombi obstructing the circulation of blood is **thrombosis**. Thrombi not only obstruct circulation, they also form an excellent trap for bacteria, whether the bacteria are carried by the bloodstream from an infection in a remote part of the body or enter the body through a subcutaneous orifice.

Thrombosis of the deep veins (axillary, subclavian, innominate, internal jugular, and superior vena cava) and subsequent risk of infection occur when catheters are placed in the venous system. The device that poses the greatest risk of iatrogenic bloodstream infection is the central venous catheter (CVC) in its numerous forms (Centers for Disease Control and Prevention [CDC], 2001). The reported incidence is difficult to determine, but studies indicate a variation from 0.02% to 13%. These studies included patients with peripherally inserted central catheters, implanted venous access ports, and CVCs (Bennett & Brachman, 1998; Table 9–1; see Chapter 14).

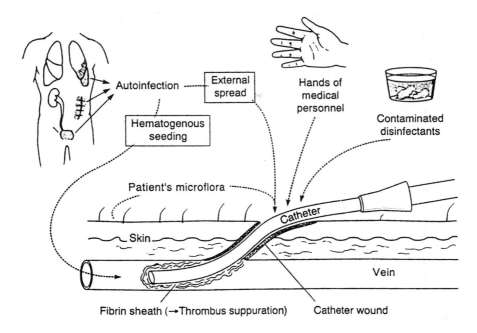

FIGURE 9–1. Sources of vascular catheter-related infection.

Thrombophlebitis

Thrombophlebitis denotes a twofold injury—thrombosis plus inflammation. The development of thrombophlebitis is easily recognized. Classic symptoms of tenderness, erythema, and swelling are seen the longer a catheter remains in place. A painful inflammation develops along the length of the vein. If the infusion is allowed to continue, the thrombosis progressively obstructs the circulation and the vein becomes hard, tortuous, tender, and painful. Early detection may prevent an obstructive thrombophlebitis that can slow and eventually stop the infusion. This condition, which is painful, may persist indefinitely, incapacitating the patient and limiting available veins for future therapy.

CONTRIBUTING FACTORS

Any irritation involving the wall of the vein predisposes the patient to thrombophlebitis. *Duration of the infusion* is a significant factor in the development of thrombophlebitis. As the duration increases, so do the incidence and degree of inflammation.

The *composition of the solution* may play a role. Venous irritation and inflammation may result from the infusion of hypertonic glucose solutions, certain drug additives, or solutions with a pH significantly different from that of the plasma. Dextrose solutions are irritating to the vein. The *United States Pharmacopeia* (USP) specifications for pH of dextrose solutions range from 3.5 to 6.5; acidity is necessary to prevent caramelization of the dextrose during autoclaving and to preserve the stability

TABLE 9–1   Approximate Risks of Bloodstream Infection Associated With Various Types of Devices for Intravascular Access*

Type of Device	Representative Rate	Representative Range
Short-term temporary access[a]		
Peripheral IV cannulas		
Winged steel needles	<0.2	0–1
Peripheral IV catheters		
Percutaneously inserted	0.2	0–1
Cutdown	6	0–1
Midline catheters	0.7	0.7–0.8
Arterial catheters	1	—
Central venous catheters		
All-purpose, multilumen	3	1–7
Pulmonary artery	1	0–5
Hemodialysis	10	3–18
Long-term indefinite access[b]		
Peripherally inserted, central venous catheters	0.20	—
Cuffed central catheters	0.20	0.10–0.53
Subcutaneous central venous ports	0.04	0.00–0.10

IV, intravenous.
*Based on data from recently published, prospective studies.
[a]Number of bloodstream infections per 100 devices.
[b]Number of bloodstream infections per 100 device-days.
(Reproduced with permission from Bennett, J.V., & Brachman, P.S. [1998]. *Hospital infections* [4th ed., p. 696]. Philadelphia: Lippincott Williams & Wilkins.)

of the solution during storage. Studies show a significant reduction in thrombophlebitis when buffered glucose solution have been infused. Neut, a sodium bicarbonate 1% solution, may be added to increase the pH of acid IV solutions. This additive, however, poses a problem of incompatibility when added to solutions containing drugs. The greatest number of incompatibilities may be produced by changes in pH (Bennett & Brachman, 1998). As an example, tetracycline hydrochloride, with a pH of 2.5 to 3.0, is unstable in an alkaline environment.

The *infusion site* can be a factor contributing to thrombophlebitis. The veins in areas over joint flexion undergo injury when motion of the catheter irritates the venous wall. The veins in the lower extremities are especially susceptible to trauma, which may be enhanced by stagnant blood in varicosities and stasis in peripheral venous circulation.

> ⚠️ **SAFE PRACTICE ALERT** When used for infusing an irritating solution, small veins are subject to inflammation.

The *infusion catheter* may occlude the entire lumen of the vein, obstructing the flow of circulating blood; the solution then flows undiluted, irritating the wall of the vein.

Venipuncture technique can mean the difference between a successful infusion and the complication of thrombophlebitis. Only minimal trauma results from a skillfully executed venipuncture, whereas a carelessly performed venipuncture may seriously traumatize the venous wall. Phlebitis associated with sepsis may be related to the technique of the clinician. Infection is always a risk if sterile technique is not zealously observed. Thorough cleansing of the skin is important in preventing infections. Maintenance of asepsis is essential during long-term therapy, particularly in the use of the through-the-needle catheter (Bennett & Brachman, 1998).

Infusion methods for parenteral solutions may foster septic thrombophlebitis. This complication is most often associated with the through-the-needle catheter. The catheter threaded through the needle remains sterile and does not come in contact with the skin, but provides a large subcutaneous orifice facilitating entry of bacteria around the catheter and seepage of fluid.

The over-the-needle catheter is not without fault because it comes in direct contact with the skin before being introduced into the vein. However, the tight fit through the skin may bar further bacterial entry. (Box 9–1 summarizes contributing factors.)

TREATMENT

Most cases of superficial thrombophlebitis respond to prompt removal of the IV catheter and local application of heat, although the affected vein may remain firm for several months.

A sterile inflammation usually develops from a chemical or mechanical irritation. When the inflammation is the result of sepsis, however, the condition is much more serious and carries with it the potential danger of septicemia and acute bacterial endocarditis. Additional treatment measures are required, possibly including excision of the infected vein. The wound is then left to heal secondarily. Antibiotic therapy then begins and continues for 7 to 10 days.

An additional complication is embolism when thrombosis occurs. The more pronounced the inflammation and the more intense the pain, the more organized the thrombus is likely to become. Embolism is less likely to occur from the well-attached clot of thrombophlebitis than from phlebothrombosis.

PREVENTIVE MEASURES

In performing venipunctures, the nurse exercises every caution to avoid injuring the wall of the vein needlessly. Multiple punctures, through-and-through punctures, and damage to the posterior wall of the vein with the point of the catheter can lead to thrombosis. The nurse can minimize the risk of phlebitis by implementing these measures:

- Refrain from using veins in the lower extremities.
- Select veins with ample blood volume when infusing irritating substances.
- Avoid veins in areas over joint flexion and use an arm board if the vein must be located in an area of flexion.
- Anchor the catheter securely to prevent motion, which may loosen the catheter.

To prevent septic phlebitis, thorough preparation of the skin, together with aseptic technique and maintenance of asepsis during infusion, is imperative. Periodic inspection of the injection site will detect developing complications before serious damage occurs.

Complaints of a painful infusion make it necessary to differentiate between early phlebitis and venospasm from an irritating solution. In the case of venospasm, slowing the infusion and applying heat to the vein dilates the vessel and increases the blood flow, thereby diluting the solution and relieving the pain. After a hypertonic solution infusion, infusion with an isotonic fluid flushes the vein of irritating substances.

If inflammation accompanies the pain, a change in the injection site should be considered. Continuing the infusion leads to progressive trauma and limits available veins. Adherence to time limits for removal of the catheter reduces the incidence of phlebitis (Infusion Nurses Society [INS], 2005). (Box 9–2 ranks the severity of phlebitis.)

During removal of the infusion catheter, care must be taken to prevent injury to the wall of the vein; the catheter should be removed at an angle nearly flush with the skin. Pressure should be applied for a reasonable length of time to prevent extravasation of blood.

Phlebothrombosis

Phlebothrombosis denotes thrombosis and usually indicates that the inflammation is relatively inconspicuous. It is thought to give rise to embolism because the thrombus is poorly attached to the wall of the vein. Both thrombophlebitis and phlebothrombosis have a degree of inflammation and are associated with potential embolism. Factors that promote thrombosis are summarized in Table 9–2.

Systemic Complications

Serious, even life-threatening systemic complications range from septicemia to embolism to shock and infection. These complications need to be prevented or identified as soon as possible and treatment interventions begun.

Septicemia

Septicemia is caused by invasion of the bloodstream by micro-organisms or their by-products, including bacteria, fungi, mycobacteria, and rarely, viruses. Clinical

TABLE 9–2   Genesis of Thrombosis

Type	Clinical Manifestation	Contributing Factors
Fibrin sheath thrombosis	Inability to aspirate blood; catheter occlusion	Thrombogenic catheter material
Vascular mural thrombosis	Vein obstruction; classic symptoms of thrombosis	Difficult insertions; multiple attempts at venipuncture; sustained contact of the catheter with the venous wall

manifestations of septicemia include chills, fever, general malaise, and headache. See Chapter 14.

CONTRIBUTING FACTORS

Certain predisposing factors put the infusion therapy patient at risk:

- Age younger than 1 year or older than 60 years
- Granulocytopenia
- Immunocompromised state
- Loss of skin integrity
- Distant infection that might contribute to hematogenous seeding.

Also contributing to the development of septicemia are catheter-related factors, such as the size of the catheter, number of lumens, function and use of the catheter, catheter material, bacterial adherence, and **thrombogenicity.**

TREATMENT

Supportive therapy for the patient with septicemia includes fluid replacement, blood pressure maintenance, oxygenation, cardiac output maintenance, nutritional support, and preservation of acid–base balance. Ancillary treatments involve administration of steroids, naloxone, and endotoxin vaccination.

PREVENTIVE MEASURES

Because intravascular systems should be considered potential portals for infection, prevention programs support the use of 0.2-μm air-eliminating, bacterial-retentive filters. In addition, good hand-washing techniques, line care protocols, and adherence to the INS Standards of Practice for monitoring, maintenance of infusion, tubing changes, and catheter care all contribute to an environment that does not readily support development of septicemia in patients receiving infusion therapies (see Chapters. 4 and 10).

Pulmonary Embolism

Pulmonary embolism occurs when a substance, usually a blood clot, dislodges and floats freely, propelled by the venous circulation to the right side of the heart and into the pulmonary artery (Metheny, 2000). Emboli may obstruct the main pulmonary artery or the arteries to the lobes, occluding arterial apertures at major bifurcations (INS, 2005). Obstruction of the main artery then results in circulatory and cardiac disturbances. Recurrent small emboli may eventually result in pulmonary hypertension and right heart failure (Metheny, 2000). See Chapter 14.

Precautions for preventing this serious complication include the following:

- Filter infusions of blood or plasma through an adequate filter to remove any particulates that could promote small emboli formation.

- Do not perform venipuncture in the veins of the lower extremities. These veins are particularly susceptible to trauma that predisposes the patient to thrombophlebitis. Although superficial veins rarely seem to be the source of emboli (INS, 2005), a thrombus may extend into the deep veins, resulting in a potentially viable clot; superficial and deep veins unite freely in the lower extremities.
- Avoid applying positive pressure to relieve clot formation.

> **SAFE PRACTICE ALERT** Avoid irrigating a plugged catheter. Doing so may embolize small catheter thrombi, some of which are infected.

- Check for patency of the lumen of the catheter by kinking the infusion tubing approximately 8 inches from the catheter. Then kink and release the tubing between the catheter and the pinched tubing. If the tubing becomes hard and meets with resistance, obstruction is evident. The catheter should be removed and the infusion reinstated.
- Take special precautions with drug additives. Reconstituted drugs must be completely dissolved before being added to parenteral solutions because it is the inherent nature of red blood cells to adhere to particles, adding to the danger of clot formation.
- Examine fluids to detect particulate matter.

Air Embolism

Although **air embolism** is a significant possible complication with air-dependent containers, it is more frequently associated with central venous lines. There is a potential risk for air embolism to result from the insertion of a CVC, inadequate sealing of the tract before disconnecting a CVC, disconnection of central lines, and bypassing the pump housing of an electronic volumetric pump with an IV piggyback connection. Smart pump technology has eliminated some of the potential for error. See Chapters 11 and 14.

> **SAFE PRACTICE ALERT** A fatal embolism may occur when small bubbles accumulate dangerously and form tenacious bubbles that block the pulmonary capillaries. Recognition of the circumstances that contribute to this hazard and measures taken to prevent its occurrence are imperative for safe fluid therapy.

Symptoms associated with air embolism arising from sudden vascular collapse include cyanosis, drop in blood pressure, weak, rapid pulse, rise in venous pressure, and loss of consciousness.

⚠ **SAFE PRACTICE ALERT** If air embolism occurs, the source of air entry must be immediately rectified. The patient should be turned on the left side with his or her head down. This causes the air to rise in the right atrium, preventing it from entering the pulmonary artery. Oxygen is then administered and the physician notified.

CONTRIBUTING FACTORS: GRAVITY INFUSIONS

If a vented container is allowed to run dry, air enters the tubing and the fluid level drops to the proximity of the patient's chest. The pressure exerted by the blood on the walls of the veins controls the level to which the air drops in the tubing. A negative pressure in the vein may allow air to enter the bloodstream. Negative pressure occurs when the extremity receiving the infusion is elevated above the heart (Metheny, 2000).

Infusions flowing through a CVC carry an even greater risk of air embolism when the container empties than infusions flowing through a peripheral vein. Because the central venous pressure is lower than the peripheral venous pressure, a negative pressure that could suck air into the circulation is more likely. The nurse therefore needs to take precautions while changing the administration set of a central venous infusion. See Chapter 14.

Running solutions simultaneously is a key factor. One empty vented container becomes the source of air for the flowing solution. This happens because the atmospheric pressure is greater in the open tubing to the empty container than below the partially restricted clamp on the infusion side. Recurrent small air bubbles are constantly aspirated into the flowing solution and on into the venous system. The introduction of air may be prevented by running one solution at a time. Vigilance is imperative if vented solutions are prescribed to run simultaneously. The tubing must be clamped off completely before the solution container is allowed to empty (Bennett & Brachman, 1998).

This principle is also involved in the piggyback setup for secondary infusions. The potential danger of air embolism exists whenever solutions from two vented sets run simultaneously through a common catheter. Again, advanced technologies have minimized the use of piggyback setups.

All connections of an infusion set must be tight. Any faulty opening or defective hole in the set allows air to be emitted into the flowing solution. If a stopcock is used, the outlets not in use must be completely shut off.

The regulating clamp on the infusion set should be located no higher than the patient's chest. Because the pressure exerted by the blood on the venous wall normally raises a column of water from 4 to 11 cm above the heart, a restricting clamp placed above this point results in a negative pressure in the tubing. If great enough, the pressure can suck air into the flowing solution should a loose connection or a faulty opening exist between the clamp and the catheter (Bennett & Brachman, 1998). The lower the clamp, the greater the chance of defects occurring above the clamp, where positive pressure can force the solution to leak out (Bennett & Brachman, 1998).

KEY INTERVENTIONS: Removing Air When Changing the IV Administration Set

If the fluid container on a continuous infusion should empty, fresh fluid will force trapped air into the circulation and air embolus may result. To help ensure that air does not enter the patient's system during an IV administration, take the following precautions:

1. Immediately before and during the time that the catheter will be open to the air, assist the patient to lie flat and supine in bed and perform the Valsalva maneuver (forced expiration with the mouth closed).
2. To remove the air from the administration set, first place a hemostat (clamp) close to the infusion catheter.
3. Hang the fresh solution container.
4. With an antiseptic agent, clean the section of the tubing proximal to the hemostat and below the air level in the tubing.
5. Insert a sterile needle to allow the air to escape.
6. *Unclamp the hemostat* and readjust flow.

A. When the infusate container runs dry during simultaneous infusion of fluids through a Y-type administration set, pressure below the partially constricted clamp is lower than the atmospheric pressure, allowing air from the empty container (atmospheric) to enter the infusion. **B.** Without an automatic shutoff valve on a secondary infusion piggybacked through the injection site of a primary IV set, air from the empty infusate container will enter the patient's circulation.

The Y-type infusion set used with vented containers is a less obvious source of air embolism but one by which unknown quantities of air can be drawn into the bloodstream.

An infusion set long enough to drop below the extremity gives added protection against air being drawn into the vein should the infusion bottle empty. Inlying pressure chambers on administration sets should be kept filled at all times. Manual compression of an empty chamber forces air into the bloodstream.

Catheter Embolism

Catheter embolism may occur during the insertion of a through-the-needle catheter if part of the catheter breaks off, which may happen if the proper procedure is not strictly followed. The catheter should never be pulled back through the needle. If it becomes necessary to remove the catheter, the entire unit should be removed and a new catheter inserted. Catheter embolism may also occur during the insertion of an over-the-needle catheter if the needle is either partially or totally withdrawn and then reinserted. If the catheter shears off into circulation, fluoroscopic cardiac catheterization may be necessary to visualize and remove the embolus. See Chapter 14.

Pulmonary Edema

Overloading the circulation is hazardous to any patient, but especially to elderly patients and to patients with impaired renal and cardiac function. Infusing fluids too rapidly increases the venous pressure, with the possibility of consequences such as cardiac dilation and pulmonary edema (see Chapters 14 and 22).

Signs and symptoms, such as venous dilation with engorged neck veins, increased blood pressure, and a rise in venous pressure, should alert the nurse to the danger of pulmonary edema. Rapid respiration and shortness of breath may occur.

TREATMENT

With signs of circulatory overload, the infusion should be slowed to a minimal rate and the physician notified. Raising the patient to a sitting position may facilitate breathing.

PREVENTIVE MEASURES

Several preventative measures may reduce the likelihood of pulmonary edema:

- Maintain infusions at the prescribed flow rate.
- Avoid applying positive pressure using the pressure-chamber administration sets to infuse solutions. If the patient requires fluids so rapidly that positive pressure is required, infusion then becomes the physician's responsibility.
- Use of a controlled-volume infusion set often provides additional protection. These sets control the volume from 10 to 150 mL and prevent large quantities of fluid from being accidentally infused. See Chapter 11.
- Discard solutions not infused within the 24-hour period prescribed. Do not infuse them with the following day's fluids. Fluids administered in excess of the quantity ordered can overtax the homeostatic controls, thereby increasing the danger of pulmonary edema.

Speed Shock

Speed shock is the systemic reaction that occurs when a substance foreign to the body is rapidly introduced into the circulation. Caution must be observed in administering IV push injections. Rapid injection permits medication to concentrate in the plasma and reach toxic proportions. The toxin may then flood the organs that are rich in blood, such as the heart and brain. As a result, syncope, shock, and cardiac arrest may occur (Metheny, 2000).

Some precautionary measures can minimize the potential danger of speed shock. Using a pediatric-type infusion set to reduce the size of the drops of infusate provides greater accuracy and thereby reduces the risks attendant on rapid administration. These sets are valuable when solutions containing potent drugs must be maintained at a minimal rate of flow. Electronic flow control devices may be used to control the rate of infusion, with the nurse who initiates the infusion making sure that the solution is flowing freely before adjusting the rate. The nurse also needs to keep in mind that movement of a catheter in which the aperture is partially obstructed by the wall of the vein can cause an increase in the flow, contributing to the danger of speed shock.

Allergic Reactions

An allergic reaction is a response to the medication or infusate to which the patient is sensitive. Such reactions may occur from the passive transfer of sensitivity to the patient from a blood donor, or sensitivities to substances normally present in the blood, as seen in transfusion reactions. See Chapter 17.

SAFE PRACTICE ALERT If an allergic reaction is suspected, the infusion should be stopped immediately, the tubing and solution container changed, and the vein kept open to permit treatment of possible anaphylactic shock. Notify the physician and initiate appropriate interventions as ordered.

Intravascular Infection

Intravascular infection is related to many factors, such as the intravascular device (catheter/cannula), contaminated solution or other substances, and bloodborne pathogens, among others.

Intravascular device–related bloodstream infections are perhaps the least frequently recognized nosocomial infection (Bennett & Brachman, 1998). Catheter-related infections are those that originate from the catheter material itself or from migration of organisms through the open skin along the catheter (Table 9–1). Solution-related infections are those that result from contamination of IV solutions, either in the manufacturing process or in use.

SOURCES OF INFECTION

Bacteria responsible for IV-associated infection come from three main sources: air, skin, and blood. Micro-organisms (flora and fauna) characteristic of a given location are referred to accordingly, hence the terms *skin flora*, *intestinal flora*, and so on. Table 9–3 identifies microbial pathogens associated with infusion-related septicemia (Bennet & Brachman, 1998).

Air

The number of microbes per cubic foot of air varies depending on the particular area involved. Where infection is present, bacteria escape in bodily discharges, contaminating

TABLE 9–3   Microorganisms Most Frequently Encountered in Various Forms of Intravascular Line–related Infection

Source	Pathogens
Catheter-related	
Peripheral IV catheter	Coagulase-negative staphylococci*
	Staphylococcus aureus
	Candida spp.*
Central venous catheters	Coagulase-negative staphylococci
	S. aureus
	Candida spp.
	Corynebacterium spp. (especially JK-1)
	Klebsiella and *Enterobacter* spp.
	Mycobacterium spp.
	Trichophyton beigelii
	Fusarium spp.
	*Malassezia furfur**
Contaminated IV infusate	Tribe Klebsiella
	Enterobacter cloacae
	Enterobacter agglomerans
	Serratia marcescens
	Klebsiella spp.
	Burkholderia cepacia
	Burkholderia acidovorans, Burkholderia pickettii
	Stenotrophomonas maltophilia
	Citrobacter freundii
	Flavobacterium, spp.
	Candida tropicalis
Contaminated blood products	*E. cloacae*
	S. marcescens
	Ochrobactrum anthropi
	Flavobacterium spp.
	Burkholderia spp.
	Yersinia spp.
	Salmonella spp.

IV, intravenous.
*Also seen with peripheral IV catheters in association with the administration of lipid emulsion for parenteral nutritional support.
(Reproduced with permission from Bennett, J.V., & Brachman, P.S. [1998]. Hospital infections [4th ed., p. 698]. Philadelphia: Lippincott Williams & Wilkins.)

clothing, bedding, and dressings. Activity, such as making a bed, sends bacteria flying into the air on particles of lint, pus, and dried epithelium (Bennett & Brachman, 1998). Increased activity raises the number of airborne particles and provides an environment that interferes with aseptic technique and potentially contributes to contamination. Airborne micro-organisms may be plentiful in patient areas and utility rooms. These contaminants find easy access to unprotected IV fluids.

Skin

The skin is the source of bacteria mainly responsible for IV-associated infection. The bacteria found on the skin are referred to as resident or transient. Resident bacteria are those normally present, and they are relatively constant in a given individual. They adhere tightly to the skin and usually include *Staphylococcus albus* as well as diphtheroids and *Bacillus* species (Bennett & Brachman, 1998). Because not all bacteria are removed by scrubbing, meticulous care must be observed to avoid touching sterile equipment.

> **SAFE PRACTICE ALERT** Quaternary ammonium compounds such as aqueous benzalkonium chloride are inactivated by organic debris. Therefore, they are ineffective against gram-negative organisms and should not be used for skin disinfection.

The transient bacteria are responsible for infection carried from one person to another. Touch contamination is a potential hazard of infection because hospital personnel move about frequently, touching patients and objects. Frequent hand washing is imperative.

The patient's skin is fertile soil for bacterial growth. Some estimates indicate that a minimum of 10,000 organisms are present per square centimeter of normal skin (Parras et al., 1994). A square centimeter is equal to 0.155 square inches. Organisms such as gram-positive *Staphylococcus epidermidis*, *Staphylococcus aureus*, gram-negative bacilli (especially *Klebsiella*, *Enterobacter*, and *Serratia*), and enterococci are ubiquitous on the skin of hospitalized patients (Bennett & Brachman, 1998).

Blood

Like the skin, the blood may harbor potentially dangerous micro-organisms. Therefore, care must be taken to prevent bacterial or other contamination from blood spills when drawing blood samples and performing venipunctures. Refer to Chapter 17 for a discussion of bloodborne pathogens; also see Box 9–3 for a summary of standard precautions for preventing infections, particularly bloodborne infections.

SURVIVABILITY OF BACTERIA AND OTHER CONTAMINANTS

Infection depends on the ability of bacteria to survive and proliferate. The factors that influence their survival are the specific organisms present, the number of such organisms, the resistance of the host, and the environmental conditions (Pearson, 1996).

Specific Organisms

Bacteria are referred to as pathogenic or nonpathogenic. Pathogenic bacteria are capable of producing disease. All bacteria should be considered pathogenic because current data show that bacteria previously considered nonpathogenic may produce infection. In one study, *Serratia* species were implicated in 35% of cases of gram-negative septicemia resulting from IV therapy (Bennett & Brachman, 1998).

Bacteria are classified as gram-positive and gram-negative. In recent years, gram-negative bacteria have replaced gram-positive bacteria as the leading cause of death from septicemia (Pearson, 1996; INS, 2005). The single most important reason for the intensity of the problem is probably the increased use of antibiotics that are highly effective against gram-positive organisms but only selectively effective against gram-negative organisms. With the competitive inhibition of gram-positive bacteria eliminated, the more resistant gram-negative organisms have proliferated in the hospital environment (Metheny, 2000; Smith, 1998).

Number of Organisms

The number of contaminants present influences the probability of an infection arising. The power of bacteria to proliferate must not be underestimated. It is simply not true that small amounts of bacteria from touch contamination are harmless. Contamination of IV fluids and bottles with even a few organisms is extremely dangerous because some fungi and many bacteria can proliferate at room temperature in a variety of IV solutions to more than 105 organisms/mL within 24 hours (Bennett & Brachman, 1998).

Host Resistance

The resistance of the host influences the development and course of infection, particularly septicemia. Underlying conditions such as diabetes mellitus, chronic uremia, cirrhosis, cancer, and leukemia may adversely affect the patient's capacity to resist infection. Treatment with immunosuppressive drugs, corticosteroids, anticancer agents, and extensive radiation therapy may depress immunologic response and permit the invasion of infection. Therapy may mask infection so that serious infection remains unrecognized until autopsy.

Environmental Conditions

Environmental conditions that affect the survival and propagation of bacteria in IV fluids are the pH, temperature, and the presence of essential nutrients in the infusion.

Some organisms grow rapidly in a neutral solution and are less likely to grow in an acid medium. Buffering of acidic dextrose solutions has been recommended for preventing phlebitis, although the neutral environment provided by the buffer may enhance the survival and proliferation of bacteria.

The temperature of the fluid may affect the ability of bacteria to multiply. At room temperature, strains of *Enterobacter cloacae, Enterobacter agglomerans*, and other members of the tribe Klebsiella proliferate rapidly in commercial solutions of 5% dextrose in water.

Total parenteral nutrition fluids should be used as soon as possible after preparation. When they must be stored temporarily, they should be refrigerated at 4°C. At this temperature, growth of *Candida albicans* is suppressed (Bennett & Brachman, 1998).

Certain nutrients must be present to support bacterial growth. Blood and crystalloid solutions provide nutrients that broaden the spectrum of pathogens capable of proliferation. Maki and associates stated that the administration of blood or reflux of blood into the infusion system may provide sufficient nutrients to broaden this spectrum (Alhimyary, Fernandez, & Picard, 1996). Accordingly, the American Association of Blood Banks requires blood to be stored at a constant controlled refrigeration of 1°C to 6°C (see Chap. 17).

Saline fluids are likely to contain enough biologically available carbon, nitrogen, sulfur, phosphate, and traces of other material to support, under favorable conditions, the survival and multiplication of any gram-negative bacillus introduced to as many as 1 million organisms per milliliter.

CONTRIBUTORS TO CONTAMINATION AND INFECTION

Extrinsic contamination and other factors that contribute to infection range from faulty handling of fluids to faulty devices and techniques.

Faulty Handling and Flawed Procedures

Containers of parenteral fluid are accepted as being sterile and nonpyrogenic on arrival from the manufacturer. The potential risk of contamination occurring in transit or in use is frequently overlooked by hospital personnel. However, through faulty handling or carelessness, glass containers may become cracked or damaged and plastic bags punctured. Bacteria and fungi may penetrate a hairline crack in an IV container, even though the crack is so fine that fluid does not leak from the container.

Besides providing carbon and energy, IV solutions of dextrose include the extra nutrients needed to support the growth of 10 million organisms per milliliter of fluid. If the fluid is not examined closely, its opalescence may be overlooked, and subsequent infusion of a few hundred milliliters of such contaminated fluid results in deep shock or possibly death.

The nurse is responsible for examining containers of fluid before their use. They should be inspected against a light and dark background for cracks, defects, turbidity, and particulates. Plastic containers should be squeezed to detect any puncture hole. Accidental puncture may occur without being evident and provide a port for entry for micro-organisms (Bennett & Brachman, 1998). Any container with a crack or defect must be regarded as potentially contaminated and unusable. Similarly, any glass container lacking a vacuum when opened should not be used.

Unsterile Conditions

When a 1-L glass container is opened, approximately 100 mL of air rushes in to fill the vacuum. In areas with a high concentration of airborne particles, contamination of unprotected fluids is a potential risk. The sterile environment of a laminar flow hood prevents this problem.

Outdated Solutions

The longer the container is in use, the greater the proliferation of bacteria and the greater the risk of infection should contamination inadvertently occur. The risk of infusing outdated fluids can be avoided by adhering to special limits, supported by a strong monitoring policy. Every container should be labeled with the time it is opened. The guidelines of the CDC and INS Standards of Practice should be followed, in addition to adhering to the guidelines developed by the Hospital Infection Control Advisory Committee (Bennett & Brachman, 1998; CDC, 1998).

Improperly Prepared Admixtures

Allowing untrained hospital personnel to add drugs to IV containers contributes to the potential for contamination. This risk is reduced when admixtures are prepared under laminar flow hoods by skilled personnel adhering to strict aseptic technique in accord with a pharmacy additive program.

Nurses and physicians who have to prepare admixtures in an emergency, and other personnel involved in the preparation and administration of IV drugs, should receive special training in the preparation of admixtures and the handling of IV fluids and equipment. Adherence to strict aseptic methods is vital. It must be emphasized that touch contamination is the primary source of infection. Although laminar flow hoods prevent airborne contamination, they do not ensure sterility when a break in aseptic technique occurs (see Chap. 18).

Manipulation of Equipment

Infusion fluids can be inadvertently contaminated by faulty techniques in manipulating the equipment. In open systems, in which fluids are not protected by air filters, the simple procedure of hanging the container may be taken for granted and the risk of contamination overlooked.

When an administration set is inserted into the container and the container is inverted, the fluid tends to leak out the vent onto the unsterile surface of the container. Regurgitation of the contaminated fluid into the container occurs when the container vents. Instructions in the use of the equipment often go unread and unheeded. Squeezing the drip chamber of the administration set before inserting it into the container and releasing it when the container is inverted prevents regurgitation of fluid and minimizes the risk of contamination.

Exposure of Injection Ports and Stopcocks

Meticulous aseptic technique must be observed in using injection ports because they are a potential source of contamination when used to piggyback infusions. The injection port location, at the distal end of the tubing, exposes it to patient excreta and drainage, which enhance the growth of micro-organisms.

The injection port must be scrubbed at least 1 minute with an accepted antiseptic, such as 70% isopropyl alcohol. Scrubbing the injection cap for 30 seconds with an antimicrobial (e.g., povidone–iodine) fluid provides good protection.

Today's use of needleless systems has minimized the risk associated with connecting a needle to an injection port. However, when a needle must be used, it should be firmly engaged up to the hub in the injection site and securely taped to prevent any in-and-out motion of the needle from introducing bacteria into the infusion (see Chaps. 11 and 12).

Similarly, three-way stopcocks are potential mechanisms of bacterial transmission because their ports, unprotected by sterile coverings, are open to moisture and other contaminants. Connected to CVCs and arterial lines, they are still used in some settings for drawing blood samples. Accordingly, aseptic practices are vital in preventing bacteria from being introduced into the IV line. Attaching a sterile catheter plug when the stopcock is added and changing the devices after each use reduce the risk of contamination. Whenever fluid leakage is discovered at injection sites, connections, or vents, the IV set should be replaced.

Catheter Insertion

Within 24 to 48 hours after a plastic catheter is inserted into a vessel, a loosely constructed fibrin sheath develops around the intravascular portion of the device, forming a nidus within which micro-organisms can multiply. The nidus shields them to an extent from host defenses and antibiotics. The thrombus or thrombi generated by the catheter material may play a role in systemic infection.

INFECTION PREVENTION

Catheter care and antibiotic lock technique are two interventions used to prevent catheter-related infection. Additional preventive measures involve careful adherence to policies and procedures based on INS standards with respect to rotating the infusion site and limiting the time that the catheter dwells in the vessel (in-dwell time). This may reduce the inherent problems of catheter-associated infection, even though most device-related septicemias are actually caused by the patient's own skin flora or by micro-organisms transmitted from the hands of the health care professional.

Antibiotic Lock Technique

The antibiotic lock technique has been used to reduce the potential for CVC-related infection in the immunocompromised patient (Table 9–3). Vancomycin, amphotericin B, and fluconazole have all been successfully used as flush solutions. A small amount of concentrated antibiotic or antifungal agent is instilled in the catheter, and the distal portion of the catheter is capped.

Skin Preparation

Microbes on the hands of health care personnel contribute to hospital-associated infection. Too often, breaks in sterile technique occur from failure to wash the hands before changing containers or administration sets or preparing admixtures. Besides the usual skin flora, antibiotic-resistant gram-negative organisms frequently contaminate the hands of hospital personnel.

To maintain asepsis, the CDC recommends that the hands be thoroughly washed before insertion of CVCs. Furthermore, guidelines support the use of sterile gloves.

In a study made of 118 patients receiving IV therapy through an indwelling polyvinyl catheter, 53 catheters were found to be contaminated with bacteria; in 28 of these, the organisms were comparable with those cultured from the skin of the patient before the skin was cleaned with iodine.

Frequently, the question arises of whether to shave the insertion site. The need to remove hair is not substantiated by scientific evidence. Antiseptics used to clean the skin also clean the hair. Moreover, shaving may produce microabrasions, which can enhance the proliferation of bacteria.

Alcohol 70% is typically used to prepare the skin site for venipuncture. Studies show that ethyl alcohol, 70% by weight, is an effective germicide for the skin when applied with friction for 1 minute, and INS standards support its use. It is as effective as 12 minutes of scrubbing and reduces the bacterial count by 75%. Because a minimum of 10,000 organisms/cm^2 is present on normal skin, the count is reduced to 2,500. Too frequently, alcohol use consists of a quick wipe, which fails to reduce the bacterial count significantly (INS, 2005).

Iodine and iodine-containing disinfectants are still the most reliable agents for preparing the skin for venipuncture because they provide bactericidal, fungicidal, and sporicidal activity. Because of occasional patient allergy to iodine, the possibility of sensitivity should be investigated before its use. Tincture of iodine (2% iodine in 70% alcohol) is inexpensive and well tolerated. The solution should be liberally applied, allowed to dry for at least 30 seconds, and washed off with 70% alcohol. Both agents should be applied with friction, working from the center of the field to periphery. Iodophor preparations, when used for patients with sensitive skin, should not be washed off because the sustained release of free iodine may be necessary for germicidal action. Iodophor preparations require a 30-second contact time.

Equipment Preparation

The tourniquet itself may be a source of cross-infection and contamination owing to its potential for reuse from patient to patient. Using an IV start kit with a disposable tourniquet minimizes the problem. However, if reusable tourniquets are consistent with clinical practice, the tourniquet should be disinfected frequently.

Once the venipuncture is completed and the catheter is in the lumen of the vein, the catheter must be securely anchored. To-and-fro motion of the catheter in the puncture wound may irritate the intima of the vein and introduce cutaneous bacteria.

Thought should be given next to the possible contamination of the adhesive tape used to secure the catheter. Because rolls of tape last indefinitely, they may harbor contaminants; they are transported from room to room, placed on patients' beds and tables, and frequently roll to the floor. Furthermore, before venipuncture, strips of tape often are torn off the roll and placed in convenient locations on the bed, table, and uniform. These facts should be kept in mind. Adhesive tape should not be applied over the puncture wound. The puncture wound must be considered an open wound, and asepsis must be maintained.

Access Device and Site Care

The CDC recommends using a topical antibiotic or antiseptic ointment at the IV site after catheter insertion. The wound should be protected by a sterile, occlusive dressing. Dressing changes should be consistent with INS standards. The same applies to catheter site rotations. Frequent observations should be made for signs of malfunction of the catheter, infiltration, and phlebitis characterized by erythema, induration, or tenderness (Bennett & Brachman, 1998). Such signs require immediate removal of the catheter.

RESEARCH ISSUES: Central Venous Catheters (Refer to Chapter 14)

Krzywda, E. (1999). Predisposing factors, prevention, and management of central venous catheter occlusions. *Journal of Intravenous Nursing, 22*(6S), 14–16.
The author addressed current research on and clinical practices associated with central venous catheter occlusion. The summary demonstrated the effect of interruption of care on therapy, catheter replacement, limitations in vascular access, and other serious sequelae associated with thrombotic complications. The primary approach should be one of prevention.
Hadaway, L.C. (1998). Major thrombotic and nonthrombotic complications: Loss of patency. *Journal of Intravenous Nursing, 21*(5S), 143–160.
    In this study, the author demonstrated that maintaining catheter function depends on both catheter and vessel patency.

Besides monitoring for signs of catheter malfunction, the nurse needs to monitor the condition of the catheter. Contamination may result from a break in aseptic technique, from contaminated fluid or administration set, from bacterial invasion of the puncture wound, or from clinically undetected bacteremia arising from an infection in a remote area of the body, such as a tracheostomy, the urinary tract, or a surgical wound. The clot around or in the catheter serves as an excellent trap for circulatory micro-organisms and as a source of nutrients for bacterial proliferation (Alhimyary, Fernandez, and Picard, 1996; Bennett & Brachman, 1998; Parras et al., 1994). See the accompanying CVC research display for more information.

CONFIRMATION OF INFECTION

Intravenous-associated sepsis is not always accompanied by phlebitis. Symptoms of infection consist of chills and fever, gastric complaints, headache, hyperventilation, and shock. Should infection develop from an unknown source in a patient receiving IV therapy, the IV system should be suspected and the entire system, including the catheter, removed. The catheter and the infusion fluid should then be cultured. See Procedure 9–1 for a step-by-step approach to culturing the catheter.

All containers of fluid previously administered to the patient should be suspected and, if possible, retained and cultured. All information and identification, including the lot number of the suspected fluid, should be recorded on the culture requisition and the patient's chart. The U.S. Food and Drug Administration, the CDC, and the local health authorities should be notified if contamination during manufacturing is suspected; fluids bearing implicated lot numbers should be stored for investigation. See Procedure 9–1 for more information.

Cultures and Culture Profiles

Culture results identify micro-organisms in suspected IV infections. Before removing a catheter for culture, the surrounding skin should be cleaned with 70% isopropyl alcohol and allowed to air dry. If purulent drainage is present, a specimen of the drainage should be obtained before the skin is cleaned.

PROCEDURE 9.1
Step-by-Step Approach to Culturing the Catheter

Equipment

Alcohol

Sterile scissors

Culture medium and labels

Action	Rationale
1. Cleanse the skin around the catheter site with alcohol and allow the alcohol to air dry	1. Allowing the alcohol to air dry maintains a clean field.
2. Maintaining asepsis, remove the catheter.	2. Maintaining asepsis avoids contamination.
3. Snip 1 cm of the catheter tip into the culture medium.	3. Tip is immediately exposed to the medium.
4. Label and send the culture medium to the laboratory in accord with institutional policies and procedures.	4. Proper transit ensures accuracy of results.

When line sepsis is suspected, three blood culture specimens should be drawn, ideally from separate venipuncture sites. Deep candidal sepsis (systemic candidiasis) is often associated with negative culture results. It is common practice in a number of clinical settings, such as intensive care units, to develop a culture profile for the patient with suspected sepsis and routinely to culture the blood of patients receiving multiple infusion therapies. Quantitative blood cultures, using pour plates, are an excellent tool for diagnosing catheter-related infection.

Semiquantitative Technique for Culturing Catheters

In the presence of purulent drainage, before removing a catheter, the nurse cleans the skin around the insertion site with an alcohol-impregnated pad to reduce contaminating skin flora and to remove any residual antibiotic ointment. After the clean area dries, the nurse withdraws the catheter, taking care to avoid contact with the surrounding skin. If pus can be expressed from the catheter wound, it is prepared for Gram's staining and culture separately. For short indwelling catheters, the entire length of the catheter is cut from the skin–catheter junction (Fig. 9–2) using sterile scissors. With longer catheters, a 2-inch segment that includes the tip and the intracutaneous segment is cultured. Segments are

FIGURE 9–2. Segments of vascular catheters cultured semiquantitatively. (Reprinted with permission of D.G. Maki and Little, Brown & Co. © 1986.)

cultured as soon as possible after removal and within 2 hours. In the laboratory, the segment is rolled back and forth across the surface of a 100-mm 5% blood agar plate four times. Plates are then incubated aerobically at 37°C for at least 72 hours. This technique has outstanding sensitivity and specificity in diagnosing catheter-related infections. Box 9–4 lists criteria for defining a nosocomial bacteremia as catheter-related.

BOX 9–4   Criteria for Defining a Nosocomial Bacteria Catheter-Related Infection

- Isolation of the same species in significant numbers on semiquantitative culture of the catheter and from blood cultures obtained by separate venipunctures with negative culture of infusate
- Clinical and microbiologic data disclosing no other apparent source of septicemia
- Clinical features consistent with bloodstream infection

KEY INTERVENTIONS: Culturing the Infusion Fluid

The following procedure should be used for culturing the infusion fluid:

1. Aseptically withdraw 20 mL of fluid from the IV line: Use 1 mL to prepare a pour plate; use the remaining fluid to inoculate two blood culture containers.
2. To the remaining IV fluid in the container, add an equal volume of brain–heart infusion broth enriched with 0.5% beef extract. Inoculate at 37°C. This is a more sensitive culture for detecting low-level contamination.

Additional Hazards: Particulates

Particulate matter comprises the mobile, undissolved substances unintentionally present in parenteral fluids. Such foreign matter may consist of rubber, glass, cotton fibers, drug particles, molds, metal, or paper fibers.

The pulmonary vascular bed acts as a filter for infused particles. Particles introduced into the vein travel to the right atrium of the heart, through the tricuspid valve, and into the right ventricle. From there they are pumped into the pulmonary artery and on through branches of arteries that decrease in size until the particles are trapped in the massive capillary bed of the lungs, where the capillaries measure 7 to 12 μm in diameter.

Five μm, the size of an erythrocyte suspended in fluid, has been suggested as the largest allowable size for a particle in the pulmonary capillary bed. Particles >5 μm are recognized as potentially dangerous because they are likely to become lodged. Particles as large as 300 μm can pass through an 18-gauge catheter, and much larger particles may pass through an indwelling catheter with a larger lumen. Table 9–4 lists particle size comparisons.

If the occlusion of a small arteriole inhibits oxygenation or normal metabolic activities, cellular damage or tissue death may result. Where there is ample collateral circulation, the occlusion would have no appreciable biologic effect. However, a particle that is not biologically inert may incite an inflammatory reaction, a neoplastic response, or an antigenic, sensitizing response.

Particles may gain access to the systemic circulation, where occlusion of a small arteriole in the brain, kidney, or eye can be serious, for the following reasons:

- The pulmonary vascular bed cannot filter out all particles. Prinzmetal and associates demonstrated that glass beads up to 390 μm may pass through the pulmonary capillary bed and reach the systemic circulation (Parras et al., 1994; Pearson, 1996).
- Large arteriovenous shunts exist in the human lung. Particles may bypass the pulmonary capillary bed and enter the systemic circulation, where a systemic occlusion could be serious.

TABLE 9–4   Particle Size Comparisons

Micrometers		Inch
175	=	0.007
150	=	0.006
125	=	0.005
100	=	0.004
75	=	0.003
50	=	0.002
25	=	0.001

Note: One micrometer equals 40 millionths of an inch (approx.). A human hair is approximately 125 μm in thickness. Bacteria range in size from 0.3 to 0.5 μm. We cannot see a particle or hole smaller than 20 μm. A hole 25 μm in diameter in a HEPA filter is more than 75 times larger than the contaminants and bacteria passing through.

- Particles >5 μm may reach the systemic circulation by way of interarterial injection or infusion.

Sources of Particulates

The USP sets the acceptable limit of particles for single-dose infusion at not more than 50 particles/mL that are ≥10.0 μm and not more than 5 particles/mL that are ≥25.0 μm in effective linear dimension (see Chap. 11).

Over the years, manufacturers have made great efforts to produce high-quality products, but these efforts may be negated by manipulating the products before their infusion.

MEDICATION ADDITIVES

Drugs constitute a major source of particulate matter. Improper technique in preparing drugs may result in the formation of insoluble particles. Use of an IV additive service precludes the need to mix drugs on the nursing unit (see Chap. 18).

GLASS AMPULES

Glass ampules have been responsible for the injection of thousands of glass particles into the circulation. Turco and Davis, in a classic study prompted by the frequency of high-dose administration of furosemide, showed that a dose of 400 mg, which at that time required the breaking of 20 ampules, could add 1,085 glass particles >5 μm to the injection. A dose of 600 mg, requiring 30 ampules, could result in 2,387 particles >5 μm.

ANTIBIOTIC INJECTABLES

Particulate contamination of bulk-filled antibiotics may be 2 to 10 times greater than that of stable antibiotic solutions and lyophilized antibiotics. Filtration is impossible because packaging by the sterile bulk-fill method involves extracting and processing the antibiotic in sterile bulk powder form and then aseptically placing the bulk antibiotic into dry, presterilized vials.

In the lyophilized and the stable liquid packaging processes, the particulate matter can be terminally removed by filtration directly into pre-sterilized vials. Most antibiotics are packed by the bulk-fill method, however.

Particulate matter in IV injections may be responsible for much of the phlebitis that so often occurs with the infusion of these drugs. Studies demonstrate the major pathologic conditions caused by particulate matter are direct blockage of vessels; platelet agglutination leading to formation of emboli; local inflammation caused by impaction of particles; and antigenic reactions with subsequent allergic consequence.

Reducing the Particulate Level

Because particulate matter infused through IV fluids may produce pathologic changes that can have an adverse effect on critically ill patients, every effort must be made to reduce the particulate count in IV injections. In general, nurses and physicians have been unaware of the potential dangers that exist and have unknowingly added to the contamination. To promote awareness, official agencies have developed standards for an acceptable particulate limit in IV fluids, and industry has provided the health care profession with filters to limit direct access of particulates, bacteria, fungi, and other contaminants to the bloodstream.

FILTERS

A filter aspiration needle specially designed to remove particulate matter from IV medications is available. With this device attached to a syringe, the medication is drawn from the vial or glass ampule and the particles are filtered out. The filter needle must then be discarded to prevent the particles trapped on the filter from being injected when the medication is added to the IV fluid.

FINAL FILTERS

The National Coordinating Committee on Large Volume Parenterals has recommended the inline filter that is both particulate and microbe retentive for patients receiving hyperalimentation and patients who are immunodeficient or immunocompromised. The particulate-retentive IV filter is usually recommended for patients receiving IV infusions when the fluid contains many additives or when drugs requiring constitution are known to include many particulates.

   The INS policy advocates the routine use of 0.2-μm air-eliminating filters in delivering routine IV therapy because these filters remove particulates, bacteria, and air, and some remove endotoxins as well (INS, 2003, 2005).

   Filters are manufactured in a variety of forms, sizes, and materials. Some block the passage of air under normal pressure when wet. Used with electronic infusion devices, they play an important role in preventing air from being pumped into the bloodstream should the fluid container empty.

   A knowledge of filter characteristics, use, and proper handling is important for patient safety. Faulty handling can result in occlusion of the filter, with the patient not receiving prescribed fluids. In addition, the infusion may need to be discontinued and venipuncture repeated to insert a new line. Moreover, a ruptured filter may go undetected and introduce filter fragments, bacteria, and possibly air into the IV system. A thorough discussion of IV filtration and its benefits is provided in Chapter 11.

Ongoing Monitoring and Precautions

The practice setting in which care is delivered has no relevance to the level of diligence needed to provide high-quality infusion therapy. This theory is based on the fact that the patient is accustomed to the flora in his or her own environment. In any clinical environment, principles of asepsis must be adhered to in an effort to minimize the risk of IV catheter-related infection and to ensure a high level of IV patient care (see Chaps. 22 and 23).

Extensive guidelines for monitoring infusion therapy and preventing catheter-related infection have been published (CDC, 1998). Preventive measures described throughout this chapter should be adhered to. In addition, any device intended for vascular access must be thought of in fundamental terms as a direct conduit between the external world and the patient's bloodstream (CDC, 1998; INS, 2000 and 2005).

Inappropriate catheter care and lack of monitoring and nursing interventions may contribute to catheter-related infections. The use of specialty IV teams to ensure a high level of aseptic technique during and after catheter insertion has been associated with substantially lower rates of catheter-related infection (Hadaway, 1998; Krzywda, 1999).

Sentinel Events

We know that a sentinel event refers to an unexpected occurrence involving death or serious physical or psychologic injury, or the risk thereof. Serious injury specifically includes loss of limb or function. The phrase "or the risk thereof" includes any process variation for which a recurrence would carry a significant chance of a serious adverse outcome. Such events are called "sentinel" because they signal the need for immediate investigation and response (JCAHO, 2000; see Box 9–5).

BOX 9–5   Sentinel Event Policy

Goals of the Policy

The goals of the policy are fourfold:

- To have a positive impact in improving patient care
- To focus the attention of an organization that has experienced a sentinel event on understanding the causes that underlie that event and on making changes in the organization's systems and processes to reduce the probability of such an event in the future
- To increase the general knowledge about sentinel events, their causes, and strategies for prevention
- To maintain the confidence of the public in the accreditation process

Components of the Policy

The policy has the following components:

- Standards relating to sentinel events
- Reviewable sentinel events
- Sentinel event database

Standards Relating to Sentinel Events

- Leadership chapter
- Improving performance

Adapted from http://www.aracnet.com/~oahhs/issues/jcaho/sentnl12.htm

ROOT CAUSE ANALYSIS

Root cause analysis is a process for identifying the basic or causal factors that underlie variation in performance, including the occurrence or possible occurrence of a sentinel event. A root cause analysis focuses primarily on systems and processes, not individual performance. It progresses from special causes in clinical processes to common causes in organizational processes and identifies potential improvements in processes or systems that would tend to decrease the likelihood of such events in the future, or determines, after analysis, that no such improvement opportunities exist. (JCAHO, 2000). Refer to Chapter 2.

Previously, if a surveyor identified a sentinel event in the course of conducting an on-site survey, he or she would review the root cause analysis on site, often affecting the flow and focus of the survey and introducing a potential variation in the root cause analysis review process. Currently, if during the course of a survey, a reviewer identifies a potentially reviewable sentinel event that has not previously been reported to the JCAHO, he or she will take the following steps:

- Inform the chief executive officer (CEO) that the event has been identified
- Inform the CEO that the event will be reported to the Joint Commission for further review and follow-up under the provisions of the Sentinel Event Policy

During the on-site survey, the surveyor(s) will assess the organization's compliance with sentinel event–related standards in the following ways:

- Review the organization's process for responding to a sentinel event
- Interview the organization's leaders and staff about their expectations and responsibilities for identifying, reporting, and responding to sentinel events
- Ask for and review an example of a root cause analysis that has been conducted in the past year to assess the adequacy of the organization's process for responding to a sentinel event. Additional examples may be reviewed if needed to more fully assess the organization's understanding of, and ability to conduct, root cause analyses. In selecting an example, the organization may choose a closed case or a "near miss" to demonstrate its process for responding to a sentinel event (JCAHO, 2004).

REFLEX SYMPATHETIC DYSTROPHY

Reflex sympathetic dystrophy (RSD) is a condition of burning pain, stiffness, swelling, and discoloration of the hand (Fig. 9–3). RSD includes other medical diagnoses such as causalgia, Sudeck's atrophy, and shoulder-hand syndrome. RSD occurs from a disturbance in the sympathetic (unconscious) nervous system that controls the blood flow and sweat glands in the hand and arm. When the nervous system becomes overactive, burning pain is felt and swelling and warmth are left in the affected arm. If not treated, RSD can cause stiffness and loss of use of the affected part of the arm.

In some cases, the cause of RSD is unknown. Often an injury can cause RSD, or the symptoms may appear after a surgery or sometimes insertion of an IV cannula.

FIGURE 9–3. On the right, the swollen, painful hand of early RSD with reddened joints.

(Weinstein, 2005). Other causes include pressure on a nerve, infection, cancer, neck disorders, stroke, or heart attack. These conditions can cause pain, which sets off the sympathetic reflex causing RSD symptoms. Nerve injuries may change the way the nerve impulses are sent, causing a "short circuit" (Fig. 9–4).

Signs and Symptoms

The pain associated with reflex sympathetic dystrophy is often described as burning. Swelling can cause painful joints and stiffness. RSD has three stages:

1. Stage I (acute) may last up to 3 months. During this stage the symptoms include pain and swelling, increased warmth in the affected part/limb, and excessive sweating. There may be faster-than-normal nail and hair growth and joint pain during movement of the affected area.
2. Stage II (dystrophic) can last 3 to 12 months. Swelling is more constant, skin wrinkles disappear, skin temperature becomes cooler, and fingernails become brittle. The pain is more widespread, stiffness increases, and the affected area becomes sensitive to touch.
3. Stage III (atrophic) occurs from 1 year on. The skin of the affected area is now pale, dry, tightly stretched, and shiny. The area is stiff, pain may decrease, and there is less hope of getting motion back.

Diagnosis

The diagnosis usually is made when at least three of the following symptoms are present: pain and tenderness, signs of changed blood flow (either increased or decreased), swelling with joint stiffness, or skin changes.

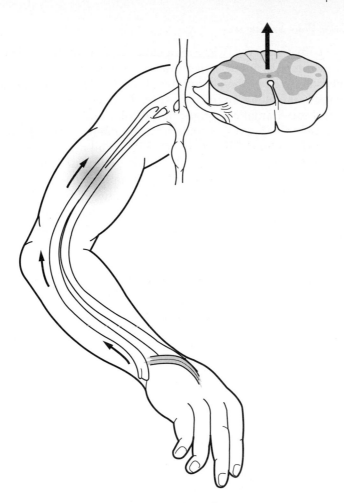

FIGURE 9–4.   This illustration shows how a nerve injury may cause a "short circuit" in the nervous system, resulting in sympathetic overactivity in the hand with burning pain, swelling, and increased sweating.

Treatment

Early diagnosis and treatment are important. Three forms of treatment may be combined: medication, physical therapy, and surgery. Medication taken by mouth can help decrease the symptoms. To reduce symptoms and provide long-term relief, local anesthetics may be injected into a nerve bundle at the base of the neck (stellate ganglion block). In some cases, a tourniquet is applied to the arm and medication can be injected into a vein along with an anesthetic. A hand surgeon may recommend therapy by a hand, occupational, or physical therapist, or by a physiatrist. Therapy is important to regain function and reduce discomfort caused by RSD. Successful treatment depends on the patient's full and active effort in therapy (AAOS, 2004).

COMPLEX REGIONAL PAIN SYNDROME

Complex regional pain syndrome (CRPS) is a chronic pain condition. The key symptom of CRPS is continuous, intense pain out of proportion to the severity of the injury, which gets worse rather than better over time. CRPS most often affects one of the arms, legs, hands, or feet. Often the pain spreads to include the entire arm or leg. Typical features include dramatic changes in the color and temperature of the skin over the affected limb or body part, accompanied by intense burning pain, skin sensitivity, sweating, and swelling. The cause of CRPS is unknown, but a proliferation of infusion-related injury cases cause one to suspect IV-related injuries (Weinstein, 2005). In some cases the sympathetic nervous system plays an important role in sustaining the pain. Another theory is that CRPS is caused by a triggering of the immune response, which leads to the characteristic inflammatory symptoms of redness, warmth, and swelling in the affected area.

Often the pain spreads to include the entire arm or leg, even though the initiating injury might have been only to a finger or toe. Pain can sometimes even travel to the opposite extremity. It may be heightened by emotional stress.

References and Selected Readings

Asterisks indicate references cited in text.

*Alhimyary, A., Fernandez, C., Picard, M., et al. (1996). Safety and efficacy of total parenteral nutrition delivered via a peripherally inserted central venous catheter. *Nutrition in Clinical Practice, 11,* 199–203.

*Association for Practitioners in Infection Control (1998). Your most powerful defense against infections. http://www.guideline.gov/summary/summary.aspx?ss=14&doc_id=2226&string=. Accessed August 1, 2005.

American Academy of Orthopedic Surgeons (2004). http://orthoinfo.aaos.org/brochure/thr_report.cfm?Thread_ID=50&topcategory=Hand. Accessed March 2, 2005.

*Bennett, J.V., & Brachman, P.S. (1998). *Hospital infections* (4th ed., pp. 689–723). Philadelphia: Lippincott Williams & Wilkins.

*Centers for Disease Control and Prevention. (2001). *Guidelines for prevention of intravascular infection.* Atlanta, GA: Author.

Gura, K.M. (2004) Incidence and nature of epidemic nosocomial infections. *Journal of Infusion Nursing, 27*(3) 175–178.

*Hadaway, L.C. (1998). Major thrombotic and nonthrombotic complications: Loss of patency. *Journal of Intravenous Nursing, 21*(5S), 143–160.

http://www.ninds.nih.gov/disorders/reflex_sympathetic_dystrophy/detail_reflex_sympathetic_dystrophy.htm. Accessed March 1, 2005.

*Infusion Nurses Society (2005) Policies and procedures for infusion nursing. 28(Suppl. 1).

*Infusion Nurses Society (2005) Revised infusion nursing standards of practice; in preparation. *Journal of Infusion Nursing,* (Suppl.).

*Infusion Nurses Society (2000) Revised standards of practice. *Journal of Infusion Nursing.* 23(Suppl. 1).

*Infusion Nurses Society (2000) Revised standards of practice. *Journal of Infusion Nursing.* 28(Suppl. 1).

Intravenous Nurses Society. (1998). Revised intravenous nursing standards of practice. *Journal of Intravenous Nursing, 21*(Suppl. 1).

*Joint Commission on Accreditation of Healthcare Organizations (2000). http://www.aracnet.com/~oahhs/issues/jcaho/sentnl12.htm. Accessed March 1, 2005.

* Joint Commission on Accreditation of Healthcare Organizations (2004) http://www.jcrinc.com/subscribers/perspectives.asp?durki=8423&site=10&return=7728. Accessed March 15, 2005.

*Krzywda, E. (1999). Predisposing factors, prevention and management of central venous catheter occlusions. *Journal of Intravenous Nursing, 22*(6S), 14–16.

*Metheny, N.M. (2000). *Fluid and electrolyte balance* (5th ed.). Philadelphia: Lippincott Williams & Wilkins.

*Parras, F., Ena, J., Bouza, E., et al. (1994). Impact of an educational program for the prevention of colonization of intravascular catheters. *Hospital Epidemiology and Infection Control, 15,* 335–337.

*Pearson, M.L. (1996). The Hospital Infection Control Advisory Committee: Guideline for prevention of intravascular-device-related infections. *Hospital Epidemiology and Infection Control, 17,* 438–473.

*Perdue, M.B. (2001). Intravenous complications. In: J. Hankins, R.A. Waldman-Lonsway, C. Hedrick, & M. Perdue (Eds.). *Infusion therapy in clinical practice* (2nd ed., pp. 418, 423–424, 427). Philadelphia: W.B. Saunders.

*Smith, J.P. (1998). Thrombotic complications in intravenous access. *Journal of Intravenous Nursing, 21*(2), 96–98.

*Weinstein, S.M (2005). Reflex sympathetic dystrophy: Cause and effect of infusion-related complications. Submitted to *Journal of Infusion Nursing.* Dec 2005.

Review Questions

Questions below may have more than one right answer.

1. Gram-negative organisms include all of the following *except:*
   A. *Staphylococcus aureus*
   B. *Pseudomonas aeruginosa*
   C. *Klebsiella*
   D. *Escherichia coli*

2. Which of the following micro-organisms is *not* associated with IV infusate contamination?
   A. *Coccidioides immitis*
   B. *Enterobacter cloacae*
   C. *Klebsiella pneumoniae*
   D. *Serratia marcescens*

3. A diagnosis of reflex sympathetic dystrophy may include all of the following *except:*
   A. Sudeck's atrophy
   B. Causalgia
   C. Finger-hand compression
   D. Shoulder-hand syndrome

4. In the event of a suspected air embolism, the appropriate nursing intervention is to
   A. Turn patient on left side, head down
   B. Turn patient on right side, head down
   C. Turn patient on left side, head raised
   D. Turn patient on right side, head raised

5. Which of the following is *not* a sign of impending pulmonary edema?
   A. Venous dilation
   B. Increased blood pressure
   C. Engorged neck veins
   D. Slow, shallow respirations

6. To minimize the danger of speed shock, it is necessary to
   A. Control volume
   B. Avoid free flow
   C. Catch up all solutions
   D. Use positive pressure

7. Classic symptoms of air embolism include all of the following *except*
   A. Cyanosis
   B. Dyspnea
   C. Churning over precordium
   D. Increase in pulse pressure

8. The recommended method of culture for purulent drainage is
   A. Agar
   B. Broth culture
   C. Semiqualitative
   D. Semiquantitative

9. Factors influencing the survival of bacteria include all of the following *except:*
   A. Number and type of organisms present
   B. Environmental conditions
   C. Resistance of the host
   D. Use of filtration

10. Clinical manifestations of septicemia include which of the following?
    A. Chills and fever
    B. Chills and fever, headache, and general malaise
    C. General malaise only
    D. Fever and headache only

CHAPTER 10

Evidence-Based Infusion Practice

KEY TERMS

Clinical Decision Making
Documentation
Evidence-Based Practice
Informatics

Outcomes
Performance Criteria
Research
Variable

Evidence-Based Nursing

Current trends in nursing reflect a continuing emphasis on evidence-based practice. **Evidence-based practice** is nursing activity that incorporates the findings of pertinent, valid, and reliable research studies into nursing care and process. Evidence-based practice calls for a nurse to select and review appropriate **research** studies from the health-related literature and apply relevant findings to patient care. Appropriate selections include studies that warrant immediate attention by nurses who are attempting to keep pace with important advances in the profession. Some specific purposes of evidence-based nursing are presented in Box 10–1. Infusion (IV) nurses, in particular, are constantly challenged to keep up with the rapidly growing and changing information base in their area of practice. In addition to knowing where to obtain the information (Box 10–2), nurses must evaluate the quality of the material.

Evidence-based leadership in nursing makes each experience count. Evidence-based practice pools the wide array of skill sets that each participant brings to the health care setting and influences decisions related to patient care. Essential compo-

---

BOX 10–1   Purposes of Evidence-Based Nursing

- To identify, using predefined criteria, the best quantitative and qualitative original and review studies on quality assurance; continuing professional development; and, especially, the meaning, cause, course, diagnosis, prevention, treatment, or economics of health problems managed by nurses
- To summarize these studies in structured abstracts that describe their objectives, methods, results, and evidence-based conclusions in a reproducible and accurate fashion
- To provide brief, highly expert commentary on the context of each study, its methods, and clinical applications that its findings warrant
- To disseminate the summaries in a timely manner to nurses

Based on Banks, N. (1999). Positive outcome after looped peripherally inserted central catheter malposition. *Journal of Intravenous Nursing, 22*(1), 14–17.

---

nents for the creation of evidence-based practice (EBP) include institutional support, strong clinical leadership, availability of resources, and feedback on outcomes. (Newell-Stokes, 2004). Evidence-based model comparisons are presented in Box 10-3.

Evidence-Based Practice and Outcomes

Evidence-based nursing integrates the best evidence from research findings with clinical expertise, patient preferences, and existing resources to form decision-making tools about the health care of individual patients (DiCenso, Cullum, & Ciliska, 1998a, 1998b). The quality of information that nurses demand and how effectively they evaluate and use it for **clinical decision making** influences patient **outcomes** and, ultimately, the role of nurses in the health care delivery system.

Nurses comprise the greatest number of health care professionals in the largest area of practice in the most settings. In the past few decades, clinical research has

---

BOX 10–2   Sources of Information

- Textbooks
- Journals
- Bibliographic databases
- Sources of distilled and consolidated information (some of the critical appraisal work has already been done for the reader and only a distillation of the best studies is presented), such as the journal *Evidence-Based Nursing*
- Internet sites

    www.urmc.rochester.edu/hslt/miner/resources/evidence-based/index.cfm (clinical experts respond to patient queries)
    http://www.hsl.unc.edu (references and sources related to evidence-based practice)

BOX 10–3   Evidence-Based Model Comparisons

Rosswum	Stetler	Titler
Assess need for practice change	Phase I: preparation External versus internal factors	Problem-focused triggers Knowledge-focused triggers/process: new research or literature
Link problem with interventions/ outcomes • Use standardized classification system • Select outcomes		
Synthesize • Review literature • Rate strength • Benefit versus risk • Feasibility	Phase II: validation • Use tables and group reviews • Rate strength Phase III: comparative evaluation and decision making • Fit and feasibility • Look at current practice • Review substantiating evidence • Decide to adopt, adapt, reject	Assemble and critique research. Determine if there is a sufficient research base. Pilot if sufficient research. Look at other evidence or research if research insufficient.
Design practice change protocol or procedure	Phase IV: translation and application Operational implementation • Instrumental use • Cognitive use • Symbolic use Pilot if "consider for use"	Determine if change is appropriate for adoption.
Implement (pilot), evaluate: Decide to adopt, adapt, not to use Integrate into practice and maintain	Evaluation: • Formal • Informal	Evaluation: Analyze structure, process, and outcome.

From Newell-Stokes, G. (2004). *Journal of Infusion Nursing, 27*(6), p. 385.

proliferated in nursing-related health services and in **informatics** (the use of computer-based searches). The application of these research findings to practice is great. However, it requires an investment of attention, methods, and resources to achieve the best outcomes for a specific patient population.

Applicable Research Evidence

An example of an IV therapy-related research study with findings that are applicable to nursing practice may be found in the article, "Fewer Patients Dislodged Peripheral Intravenous Catheters with Transparent Dressings than with Gauze Dressings." This original work by Tripepi-Bova, Woods, and Loach appeared in the *American Journal of Critical Care* in 1997. Diane Palmer, lecturer at the School of Nursing, the University of Hull (United Kingdom), commented on the original manuscript, noting that the study evaluates the effectiveness of two frequently used dressings in a randomized, controlled trial. The authors measured adhesive properties, reduction in peripheral vein thrombophlebitis, dislodgment by patients, and infiltration. To ensure standardization of insertion and dressing techniques, nurses attended mandatory training sessions, received written instructions, and had access to diagrams. Patients were monitored until the IV catheter for that specific insertion site was discontinued (Tripepi-Bova, Woods, & Loach, 1997).

When recommending changes in procedure or policy, or both, based on others' studies, the nurse must also consider the local practice and published standards, such as the Intravenous Nurses Society (INS) *Standards of Practice*. A serious-minded review of published studies such as that of Tripepi-Bova and colleagues could be beneficial to clinicians evaluating the feasibility of specific dressing materials (INS, 1998, 2005).

Nurses know that patients benefit from the care that nurses provide. But how can that effectiveness be verified? Alvin Tarlov and colleagues in 1989 took into account the specific outcomes that gauge the effectiveness of nursing care (Kelly, 1994; Tarlov, 1989), including the patient's health status, quality of life, knowledge, and ability to function and manage symptoms. A more recent study documented significant relationships between nursing and patient outcomes, including mortality and patient satisfaction (Scott, Sochalski, & Aiken, 1999).

By measuring patient outcomes, nurses can respond to two pivotal questions: Do our patients benefit from our care? And if so, how? A focus on outcomes may help nurses survive an unstable job market, evaluate the efficacy of IV teams, and ensure that the nursing perspective regarding outcome management is represented.

Outcomes are the consequences of a treatment or intervention. Indicators are valid and reliable measures related to performance. *Outcome indicators*, or measures, gauge how patients are affected by their nursing care; for example, is the rate of nosocomial infections down? Is the incidence of IV-related infections lower? *Process indicators*, such as pressure ulcers, evaluate the nature and amount of care that nurses provide. *Structure indicators* assess the organization and delivery of nursing care from a standpoint of staffing. Indicators are commonly reviewed to evaluate patient status in relation to outcomes—for example, the ability to bear weight is an indicator used to evaluate ambulation. (Other terms associated with outcomes, research, and evidence-based practice are given in Box 10–4.)

BOX 10–4   Terms Used in Evidence-Based Practice

Case control—(Dawson-Saunders, 1997): An observational study beginning with patients who have had the health problem and with control subjects who do not have the health problem; looks backward to identify possible causal factors

Cohort—A group of people with a common characteristic or set of characteristics

Constant comparison—(Crombie, 1996): A procedure in qualitative research wherein newly collected data are compared in an ongoing fashion with data obtained earlier to refine theoretically relevant categories

Data saturation—(Crombie, 1996): Process of collecting data in a qualitative research study without generating new themes

Double-blind study—A research design in which neither subject nor researcher knows to which group or study methods the various subjects are assigned

Effectiveness—Extent to which an intervention does more good than harm for participants who receive the intervention under usual conditions; answers the question *does it work*?

Random effects model—(Polit & Hungler, 1995): Provides a summary estimate of the magnitude of effect in meta-analysis; takes into account both within-study and between-study variance and gives a wider confidence interval to the estimate than a fixed-effects model if there is significant between-study variation

Relative risk—Risk of adverse effects resulting from treatment as opposed to risks attendant to non-treatment

---

Evidence-Based Practice and Performance Improvement

Across the health care arena, organizations are developing national quality initiatives (Table 10–1). One such organization is ECRI (Plymouth Meeting, PA), a firm that tests medical devices and develops guidelines and test programs. Formerly known as Emergency Care and Research Institute, ECRI has developed a comprehensive guide to quality practice using the principles of evidence-based disease management. Disease management is an approach to patient care that coordinates medical resources for patients across the entire health care delivery system.

In 2004, the Agency for Health Care Policy and Research (AHCPR) restructured its popular clinical practice guideline and technology assessment programs. AHCPR's Evidence-Based Practice Program now sponsors the development of technology assessments and evidence reports by 12 designated evidence-based practice centers. The new initiative includes the development of a National Guideline Clearinghouse (NGC) that will be a comprehensive database. ECRI has been chosen to create the database, abstract existing guidelines, compare guidelines on similar topics, and establish the NGC Web site. For each guideline, ECRI will produce:

- A standardized summary about the guideline and its development
- A comparison of guidelines covering similar topic areas, listing the major interventions addressed and the areas of agreement and disagreement
- The full text of guidelines or links to the full text

TABLE 10–1   National Quality Indicators

Organization	Initiative	Description
Joint Commission on the Accreditation of Hospitals and Healthcare Organizations (JCAHO)	ORYX	Integrates use of outcomes and performance measures
National Committee for Quality Assurance (NCQA)	Health Plan Employer Data and Information Set (HEDIS)	Targets effectiveness of care, access and availability, patient satisfaction, costs
American Nurses Association (ANA)	Nursing Report Card	Provides indicators and measurement tools for evaluating quality of nursing care in acute care settings
Health Care Financing Administration (HCFA)	OASIS (Outcome and Assessment Information Set)	Provides assessment questions used to collect clinical, financial and administrative data in home health care
Foundation for Accountability	Foundation for Accountability	Improves information available to consumers when they are choosing health plan, provider, hospital, treatment

Measurements: Performance Criteria and Research Studies

Measurement in nursing may be traced to Florence Nightingale, who used mortality statistics as a quality-of-care measure for British soldiers during the Crimean War. The ORYX initiative of the Joint Commission on the Accreditation of Healthcare Organizations (JCAHO) integrates patient outcomes and other performance measures into the accreditation process. "Oryx" is from the Latin word for gazelle. The long-range goal of this program is to establish a data-driven continuous survey and accreditation process to complement the standards-based assessment. Although accreditation is still based on standards, trends in data and in an organization's response to its data are being used as part of JCAHO's overall assessment as the performance measures database expands (JCAHO, 2004).

The INS *Standards of Practice* were developed as a framework for establishing infusion policies and procedures in all practice settings and for defining **performance criteria** for nurses responsible for administering infusion therapy. In the 2005 edition, the standards define the criteria relative to nursing accountability in the delivery of infusion therapies. They provide a framework for nurses to evaluate patient outcomes. They also provide a tool for evaluating the quality of patient care and the competency of the nurse delivering infusion therapy (INS, 1998, 2000, 2005).

Whereas performance may be measured by established standards, health and other focuses can be measured in many different ways. The various measurable aspects of health are known as **variables.** In a treatment study, such as one by Banks (1999), in which the author demonstrated positive outcomes after looped, peripher-

(text continues on p. 197)

TABLE 10–2   Summary of Documented PICC Malpositions and Methods of Resolution

Source	Location of Malposition	Incidence of Malposition	Technique Used for Resolution	Successful Outcomes	Unsuccessful Outcomes
Frey	Curled in subclavian vein	2 of 269 insertions	Infusions with an infusion pump		
	"Figure 8" in basilic vein	1 of 269 insertions	None cited	Used for 6 weeks	
	Looped in basilic vein	1 of 269 insertions	None cited	Used for 3 weeks	
	"Several other" PICCS looped back on themselves in the upper arm during insertion	Unknown	Removed		Classified as unsuccessful inserts
James et al.	Right basilic insertions: subclavian, axillary, jugular or right atrium	42 malpositions (34%) on first insertion	CXRs obtained with guidewire in place		
	Right cephalic insertions: subclavian, axillary, right atrium, or peripheral vein (1)		Removing guidewire and allowing tip to fall into SVC or partially withdrawing wire and readvancing catheter	11 of 42 lines (26%) successfully repositioned	11 of 42 in subclavian or axillary position (26%) could not be repositioned using any of these techniques
	Left basilic insertions: other locations (not specified)				
	Right cephalic insertions: other locations (not specified)		Rapid saline flush with patient in semi-Fowler's position	2 of 42 lines (4%) successfully repositioned	Unsuccessful in 3 of 42 lines (7%)
LaRue	May–Dec. 1992: unable to thread catheter past subclavian-jugular-innominate junction	14 of 100 attempts (14%)	Turning patient's head more severely in chin-to-shoulder position (toward insertion side), vigorous flush technique or changing arm position	1 out of 14 attempts at repositioning was successful (1%) using one or more of these techniques	13 of 14 attempts at repositioning were unsuccessful (93%) using one or more of these techniques

	Dec.–Oct.1993: change in insertion technique (7 cm withdrawal of guidewire after half of line inserted)	99 of 100 lines (99%) successfully placed		Successful SVC placement
	Jugular placement	1 of 100 lines (1%)	Withdrawn and reinserted with new technique	
LaFortune	Malpositioned tip in 26% of patients: looped or coiled in branches or tributaries off the axillary vein	6 of 11 malpositions 5 of 11 malpositions	Readvancing catheter after withdrawing catheter 2–6 cm and performing one or more of the following actions: Withdrawal of catheter 2–6 cm Hyperextension of arm Rotation of arm Traction applied to wrist Having patient open and close fist Relaxation and distraction	7 of 11 lines repositioned after one or two attempts One patient needed repositioning under fluoroscopy	One line in an 8-year-old child was removed after one attempt at repositioning was unsuccessful
Lum and Soski	Internal jugular vein	20 of 62 (32.2%)	Patient positioning	8 of 10 cases (80%)	
	Axillary vein	22 of 62 (35.5%)	Guidewire exchange	9 of 13 cases (69%)	
	Opposite innominate vein	7 of 62 (11.3%)	Rapid flushing	22 of 40 cases (55%)	
	Subclavian vein	4 of 62 (6.5%)	Partial withdrawal	17 of 18 cases (94%)	
	Right atrium	6 of 62 (9.7%)	Removal		
	Innominate vein	1 of 62 (1.6%)		22 of 22 cases (100%)	
	Basilic vein	1 of 62 (1.6%)			
	Unknown vein	1 of 62 (1.6%)			

(Continued)

TABLE 10–2 **Summary of Documented PICC Malpositions and Methods of Resolution** *(Continued)*

Source	Location of Malposition	Incidence of Malposition	Technique Used for Resolution	Successful Outcomes	Unsuccessful Outcomes
Abi-Nader	Primary malposition (tip site not specified)	5 of 92 insertions (5%)	Line removed and reinserted	100% effective	
	Tip located in heart	14 of 92 insertions (15%)	Pulled back to correct position using CXR	Effective	
	Curled in axillary vein	1 of 92 insertions (1%)	Line left in place, second PICC line inserted in a different vein	Second PICC line found to have straightened out the first line on second CXR	
Alhimyary et al.	Coiling or malposition (site of tip not specified)	7 of 135 insertions (5%)	3 PICC lines removed and reinserted		
			3 PICC lines removed and replaced with subclavian catheters		
			1 PICC line successfully repositioned; technique not specified		
Ng et al.	Cephalad to internal jugular vein	27 of 963 insertions (2.8%)	Resolution techniques not discussed		
	Right atrium or right ventricle	13 of 963 insertions (1.3%)			
	Looped in subclavian or axillary vein	16 of 963 insertions (1.6%)			

CXR, chest x-ray; PICC, peripherally inserted central catheter; SVC, superior vena cava.

ally inserted central catheter (PICC) malposition, the intervention (independent variable) was the noninvasive approach. The outcomes (dependent variables) were central tip placement of the catheter and prevention of additional costs and potential discomfort for the patient. Banks summarized documented PICC malpositions and resolutions (Table 10–2).

Evaluation of the Evidence

In reviewing the literature, the professional nurse is urged to determine whether the study and its methods and measures are reliable and valid. *Reliability* refers to the degree to which a measure gives the same result two or more times under similar circumstances. *Validity* is the ability of a measurement tool to measure accurately what it is intended to measure. Criterion-related validity requires comparing a given measure with a gold standard, such as the INS *Standards of Practice* (see Chap. 4).

Thus, readers of research reports should consider the types of measures used, the reliability and validity of the measures, and methods used in measuring the outcomes. Examples of published findings specific to infusion therapy may be found in the accompanying research display, Noteworthy Research Relevant to Infusion Therapy.

 RESEARCH ISSUES: Noteworthy Research Relevant to Infusion Therapy

Treatment
Clark, A., Carr, D., & Loyd, G. (1998). The influence of epidural analgesia on cesarean delivery rates: A randomized, prospective clinical trial. *American Journal of Obstetrics and Gynecology*, *179*, 1527–1533.
Heyland, D.K., MacDonald, S., & Keefe, L. (1998). Total parenteral nutrition in the critically ill patient: A meta-analysis. *Journal of the American Medical Association, 280*, 2013–2019.
Kupensky, D.T. (1998). Applying current research to influence clinical practice: Use of midline catheters. *Journal of Intravenous Nursing, 21*, 271–279.

Prognosis
Massicotte, M.P., Dix, D., & Monagle, P., on behalf of the Canadian Childhood Thrombophilia Program. (1998). Central venous catheter related-thrombosis in children: Analysis of the Canadian Registry of Venous Thromboembolic Complications. *Journal of Pediatrics, 133*, 770–776.
Mazzola, J.R., Schott-Baer, D., & Addy, L. (1999). Clinical factors associated with the development of phlebitis after insertion of a peripherally inserted central catheter. *Journal of Intravenous Nursing, 22*, 36–41.

Outcome
Goodwin, M.L., & Carlton, I. (1993). The peripherally inserted central catheter: A retrospective look at three years of insertions. *Journal of Intravenous Nursing, 16*, 92–103.
Pauley, S.Y., Vallande, N.C., & Riley, E.N. (1993). Catheter-related colonization associated with percutaneous inserted central catheters. *Journal of Intravenous Nursing, 16*, 50–54.

Competency-Based Programs and Documentation

The IV nurse specialist, through study, supervised practice, and validation of competency, acquires knowledge and develops skills necessary for the practice of IV nursing. Such a nurse is competent to practice.

Competency-based orientation programs are designed to orient the IV nurse who is new to an institution to the practices, policies, and procedures of that institution or agency. Such a program benefits the institution or agency as well as the patient (Weinstein, 2000). And such a program must be standardized but individualized, quality based but cost effective (Weinstein, 2000).

Orientation or institutional competencies are derived from standards of accrediting organizations, such as JCAHO, and the standards of practice of specialty nursing organizations. JCAHO, for example, requires **documentation** of competence not only at orientation but on an ongoing basis. State health departments also require documentation of clinical competence. Competency programs incorporate self-assessment tools, orientation curriculum, skills checklists, and in-house education, which includes simulated practice, written and didactic examination, and program evaluation. Adult learning principles, as described by Knowles, are an integral component of the program (Case, 1996).

Documentation is essential as a legal record of care provided, a communication tool for other health care professionals, and a determinant of eligibility for reimbursement. Detailed, accurate, adequate documentation prevents reinvention of the wheel (or duplication of effort and services) by saving time, ensures that the patient masters skill sets, and protects the health care provider or the institution. Tools used to document care include nursing care plans (see Chap. 4), flow sheets, progress notes, periodic updates developed by home care providers, and discharge summaries (Rankin & Stallings, 1996).

Documentation should include the intervention performed, the patient's response to the intervention, and the subsequent outcomes. Sentinel or adverse events should also be documented consistent with institutional policy. By providing an accurate record of the care delivered and by structuring that care on evidence-based nursing practice and published standards, the nurse who is responsible for providing IV care ensures safe practice.

References and Selected Readings

Asterisks indicate references cited in text.

Alhimyary, A., Fernandez, C., & Picard, M. (1996). Safety and efficacy of total parenteral nutrition. *Nutrition in Clinical Practice, 11,* 199–203.

*Banks, N. (1999). Positive outcome after looped peripherally inserted central catheter malposition. *Journal of Intravenous Nursing, 22*(1), 14–17.

*Case, B. (1996). Breathing air into adult learning. *Journal of Continuing Education in Nursing, 27*(4), 148–158.

Connor, V.W. (1999). Patient confidentiality in the electronic age. *Journal of Intravenous Nursing, 22,* 199–200.

*Crombie, I.K. (1996). *The pocket guide to critical appraisal: A handbook for healthcare professionals* (p. 47). London: BMJ Publishing Group.

Dawson-Saunders, B., & Trapp, R.G. (1997). *Basic and clinical biostatistics.* Norwalk, CT: Appleton & Lange.

*DiCenso, A., Cullum, N., & Ciliska, D. (1998a). *Evidence-based nursing* (p. 66). Kent, United Kingdom: RCN Publishing.

*DiCenso, A., Cullum, N., & Ciliska, D. (1998b). Implementing evidence-based nursing: Some misconceptions. *Evidence-Based Nursing,* 38–40.

Evidence-Based Nursing user's guide. (2004). *Evidence-Based Nursing, 7*(1) 4–8.

Frey, A.M. (1995). Pediatric peripherally inserted catheter program report. *Journal of Intravenous Nursing, 18,* 280–291.

Hagland, M. (1998). The gap: HIPAA and secure information technology. *Health Management Technology, 19*, 24–30.

*Intravenous Nurses Society. (1998). Revised intravenous nursing standards of practice. *Journal of Intravenous Nursing, 21*, 19, 25, 516.

*Infusion Nurses Society (2000). Revised standards of practice. *Journal of Infusion Nursing. 23*(Suppl. 1).

*Infusion Nurses Society (2005). Revised standards of practice. *Journal of Infusion Nursing. 28*(Suppl. 1).

*Infusion Nurses Society (2005). Revised infusion nursing standards of practice. *Journal of Infusion Nursing.*

James, L., Bledsoe, L, Hadaway, L.C. (1993). A retrospective look at tip location and complications of peripherally inserted catheter lines. *Journal of Intravenous Nursing, 16*, 104–109.

*Joint Commission on Accreditation of Healthcare Organizations (JCAHO). (2004). ORYX: The next evolution in accreditation. [On-line]. Available: http://www.jacho.org/perfmeas/oryx_qa.html.0

*Kelly, K.C. (1994). The Medical Outcomes Study: A nursing perspective. *Journal of Professional Nursing, 10*, 209–216.

LaRue, G.D. (1995). Improving central placement rates of peripherally inserted catheters. *Journal of Intravenous Nursing, 18*, 24–27.

*Newell-Stokes, G. (2004). Applying evidence-based practice: A place to start. *Journal of Infusion Nursing, 27*(6), 381–385.

Ouriel, K., Veith, F.J., & Sasahara, A.A. (1998). A comparison of recombinant urokinase with vascular surgery as initial treatment for acute arterial occlusion of the legs. *New England Journal of Medicine, 338*, 1105–1111.

*Polit, D.E., & Hungler, B.P. (1995). *Nursing research: Principles and methods* (p. 22). Philadelphia: Lippincott-Raven.

*Rankin, S.H., & Stallings, K.D. (1996). *Patient education issues, principle, practices*. (3rd ed., pp. 122, 162–164, 183–187). Philadelphia: Lippincott-Raven.

*Scott, J.G., Sochalski, J., & Aiken, L. (1999). Review of magnet hospitals research. *Journal of Nursing Administration, 29*(1) 9–18.

*Tarlov, A.R., Ware, J.E. Jr., Greenfield, S. et al. (1989). The Medical Outcomes Study: An application of methods for monitoring the results of medical care. *Journal of the American Medical Association, 262*, 925–930.

*Tripepi-Bova, K.A., Woods, K.D., & Loach, M.C. (1997). A comparison of transparent polyurethane and dry gauze dressings for peripheral IV catheter sites: Rates of phlebitis, infiltration, and dislodgment by patients. *American Journal of Critical Care, 6*, 377–381.

*Weinstein, S.M. (2000). Certification and credentialing to ensure competency-based practice. *Journal of Intravenous Nursing, 23*, 1, 21–28.

Review Questions

Note: Questions below may have more than one right answer.

1. Outcomes can best be described as which of the following?
   A. Use of protocols to render health care
   B. Ability to provide consistent care in all regions of the country
   C. End results of treatment or intervention
   D. Use of less invasive and less costly procedures

2. Measurable aspects of health are known as:
   A. Regional practices
   B. Variables
   C. Standards
   D. AHA requirements

3. Quality of care was originally measured by which of the following?
   A. Mortality rate
   B. Length of stay
   C. Functional ability
   D. Cost of service

4. Which of the following is *not* an example of a useful outcome indicator to measure quality of nursing care?
   A. Functional status
   B. Patient satisfaction
   C. Patient discomfort
   D. Health insurance plan

5. Measurement issues reviewed when perusing the literature include which of the following?
   A. Reliability
   B. Validity
   C. Length
   D. Bias

6. Patient outcomes are influenced by which of the following?
   A. Quality of information
   B. How information is used in clinical decision making
   C. a only
   D. a and b

7. Tools used to document care include which of the following?
   A. Nursing care plans
   B. Flow sheets
   C. Progress notes
   D. Discharge summaries

8. Reliability refers to:
   A. Validity of the measurements
   B. Degree to which the same results are achieved two or more times
   C. Degree to which results are achieved under same circumstances
   D. Determining what is important to measure

9. Data saturation refers to:
   A. Process of collecting data in qualitative research study
   B. Extent to which intervention does more harm than good
   C. Observational study of patients with similar health problems
   D. Comparison of new data with earlier data

10. Treatment-related research in the area of evidence-based nursing includes that by which of the following authors?
    A. Goodwin
    B. Heyland
    C. Mazzola
    D. Pauley

UNIT 3

Clinical Decision
Making

CHAPTER 11

Infusion Equipment and Safety

KEY TERMS

Absorption	Hypovolemia
Bubble point	Latex
Calibrated	Linear
Controller	Needleless
Differential Pressure	Osmolality
Elastomeric	Point of Care
Electronic Infusion Devices	Pressure Pump
Free Flow	Psi
Gravity	Ramping
Hemorepellant	Resealable Injection Site
Hydrophilic	Smart Technology
Hydrophobic	Systems Approach
Hydrostatic	Wetted

Physical Principles of Equipment Use

As technology has continued to keep pace with advances in medical science, the delivery of patient care has improved and more sophisticated devices and innovative equipment have become available for administering infusion therapy. However, no matter how sophisticated and reliable or easy to use infusion devices and accessories are, the infusion (IV) nurse first needs a solid understanding of the physical principles that govern flow and other facets of infusion therapy.

Hadaway Associates offers an online course to teach staff patient assessment, planning, implementation, and evaluation of outcomes. Peripheral IV Therapy in Adults is ready for use and meets the needs of registered nurses and licensed vocational nurses new to infusion therapy. The course is based on the familiar nursing process and guides the learner through all aspects of safely delivering infusion therapy through peripheral veins using short peripheral catheters. The course features access 24 hours a day and 7 days a week consistent with varied schedules, interactive anatomy graphics, and numerous other photographs of equipment and supplies used in IV therapy. See Figure 11-1 for sample pages from the course. On successful completion, the learner will receive a certificate for 1.8 contact hours.

Flow Dynamics

Pressure, a principle of physics underlying infusion therapy, is the force that overcomes the natural resistance to flow created by infusion equipment, such as the IV administration set, in-line filters, and narrow-gauge needles, and by venous or arterial back pressure. Fortunately, the human body readily adapts to changes in pressure, which enables clinicians to deliver IV therapy safely.

PRESSURE

Pressure in the arterial system ranges from 80 mm Hg in the aorta to a low of 5 to 10 mm Hg in the venous return system. Intravenous pressure is created by the weight of a column of fluid in the catheter tubing—the weight is due to gravity—and we refer to it as **hydrostatic** pressure. Fluid always flows from an area of higher pressure to one of lower pressure. For a fluid to infuse by gravity, it is necessary to create a pressure only slightly more than normal, or 40 mm Hg in a peripheral line.

A number of resistance factors may interfere with or inhibit fluid flow. These factors include the patient's vascular pressure, internal diameter of the tubing, in-line filters, viscosity of the fluid, narrow-gauge needles, and the length of the tubing. Resistance to flow is determined by the smallest component in the IV system; this is usually the catheter. An example of equipment that incorporates principles of pressure for delivery of precise amounts of drugs and fluids is the electronic infusion device (EID), which is discussed later in this chapter (see section on Electronic Infusion Devices).

GRAVITY

Gravity is the physical force that propels the flow of the infusate, although this flow also depends on head pressure. Roller clamps and screw clamps used to adjust and maintain rates of flow on gravity infusions vary considerably in their efficiency and accuracy. Rate minders or flow-control mechanisms may also be used to regulate and adjust flow. When a rate minder is added to an IV administration set, the desired flow rate may be preset. Levels of accuracy vary with the type of device used.

Introduction

The safe delivery of intravenous therapy requires knowledge of vascular anatomy, physiology of blood flow, rapidly changing technology, infection control principles, and potential complications. Skills required include patient assessment, venipuncture, choosing appropriate equipment, and correct interventions for complications. Increasing patient acuity, demanding nursing workloads, and the expanding complexity of therapy increase the risk of IV-related complications.

Your basic nursing education may have provided very limited exposure to the underlying principles and practices for safe IV therapy practice. Or, you may have never worked in a situation where you were expected to deliver IV therapy.

Next >

Components of the Set

The spike contains a sharp point for piercing the seal on the bag or bottle.

Push the spike straight into the port on a plastic bag to avoid accidental puncture of the side of the bag contaminating the tubing and the fluid.

The drip chamber allows fluid to flow from the container into the tubing. The size of the tube extending into the chamber determines the drop factor or the number of drops required to deliver 1 milliliter of fluid.

Each manufacturer has a different size tube:

- Abbott delivers 15 drops per ml
- Baxter delivers 10 drops per ml
- McGaw delivers 15 drops per ml
- Microdrip set for all brands delivers 60 drops per ml

Spike

< Prev   Next >

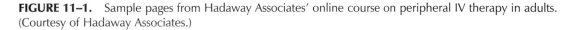

FIGURE 11–1.   Sample pages from Hadaway Associates' online course on peripheral IV therapy in adults. (Courtesy of Hadaway Associates.)

FIGURE 11–1. (Continued)

Factors such as venous spasm, venous pressure changes, patient movement, manipulations of the clamp, and bent or kinked tubing may cause variations in the flow rate. To monitor consistency of the flow rate, preprinted or self-made time tapes may be attached to the IV container. The time tape should be attached to the container and hourly increments marked on the tape or strip, beginning with the time the infusion began (Fig. 11–2).

FLOW

To determine the flow rate intelligently, the nurse must have a knowledge of parenteral solutions, their effect, and the rate of administration. The nurse must also understand other factors that influence the speed of the infusion. These factors include the patient's body surface area (BSA), condition, age, and tolerance to the infusion. The composition of the fluid is also a factor in the rate of administration.

Body Surface Area

The BSA is proportionate to many essential physiologic processes (organ size, blood volume, respiration, and heat loss) and, therefore, to total metabolic activity. Knowing the BSA helps the nurse determine fluid and electrolyte amounts and compute infusion rates. The larger the person, the more fluid and nutrients are required and the faster they can be used. The usual infusion rate is 3 mL/m^2 BSA/minute (see nomograms in Fig. 11–3). This rate applies to maintenance and replacement fluids. However, the speed must be adjusted carefully to each individual.

Patient's Clinical Condition and Age

Because the heart and kidneys play a vital role in using infused solutions, the cardiac and renal status of the patient affect the desired rate of administration. Blood volume may expand when rapidly infused fluids overtax an impaired heart and when renal damage causes retention of fluid. Patients with **hypovolemia** must receive plasma and blood rapidly, but the desired rate of the infusion should be specified by the physician. Vital signs must be carefully observed and the speed of the infusion decreased as the blood pressure rises. For specific parameters regarding the influence that age has on the rate of administration, refer to Chapters 21 and 22.

Patient's Tolerance

Tolerance to fluids varies among individuals and influences the rate of infusion. A 5% infusion of alcohol has been administered at the rate of 200 to 300 mL/hour to sedate without intoxicating an average adult. However, when such a fluid is to be administered, the rate must be titrated to the individual and prescribed by the physician. The infusion should be checked frequently to maintain the required rate of flow. Because of certain factors, the rate is subject to change.

Composition of Solution

The composition of the fluid may affect the rate of flow. When the solution is used as a vehicle for administering drugs, the speed of the infusion depends on the drug and the desired clinical effect. Because of its deleterious effect on the heart when infused

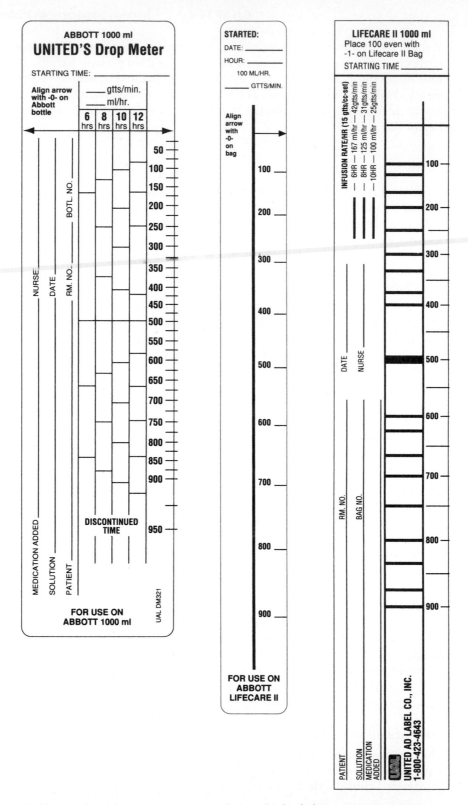

FIGURE 11–2. Time tapes. (Courtesy of United Ad Label Co., Inc., Brea, CA.)

FIGURE 11–3. A nomogram.

at a rapid rate, potassium should be administered with caution. Approximately 20 to 40 mEq potassium in a liter of fluid infused over an 8-hour period is an average rate for administering potassium parenterally.

Concentration of solutions must be considered because the flow rate may alter the desired effect. When dextrose is administered for caloric benefits, it is infused at a rate that ensures complete utilization. Dextrose has been administered at a maximum rate of 0.5 g/kg body weight/hour without producing glycosuria in a normal person. At this rate, it would take approximately 1.5 hours to administer 1 L of 5% dextrose to a person weighing 70 kg, or twice as long for 1 L of 10% dextrose. This maximum rate is faster than usual and is not customarily used except in an emergency.

When a diuretic effect is desired, a more rapid infusion is necessary. If the fluid is too rapidly infused for complete metabolism, the glucose accumulates in the bloodstream, increases the **osmolality,** and acts as a diuretic.

When oliguria or anuria occurs, the status of the kidneys must be determined before fluids containing potassium can be administered. Urinary suppression may be caused by a blood volume deficit or kidney damage. An initial hydrating fluid, to test kidney function, is usually administered at a rate of 8 mL/m² BSA/minute for 45 minutes. If urine does not flow, the rate is slowed to approximately 2 mL/m² BSA/minute for another hour. If urine output does not occur after this period, kidney damage is likely to be present (Methony, 2000). For more information, refer to Chapters 7 and 8.

Height of the Infusion Container

Intravenous fluids are propelled by gravity. Any change in gravity induced by raising or lowering the infusion container, relative to the patient's position, alters the rate of flow. When patients receiving infusions are ambulatory or transported to ancillary departments, the containers should be retained at the same height or the speed of the infusion should be readjusted to maintain the prescribed rate of flow.

Clot in the Catheter

Any temporary stoppage of the infusion, such as a delay in hanging subsequent fluids, may cause a clot to form in the lumen of the catheter, partially or completely obstructing it. Clot formation may also occur when an increase in venous pressure in the extremity receiving the infusion forces blood back into the catheter. This results from restriction of the venous circulation. In arm infusion sites, this is most commonly caused by the blood pressure cuff on the infusion arm; restraints placed on or above the infusion catheter; and the patient lying on the arm receiving the infusion.

Change in Catheter Position

A change in the catheter's position may push the bevel of the catheter against or away from the wall of the vein. Special precautions should be taken to prevent speed shock or vascular overload by making sure that the fluid flows freely before adjusting the rate.

Other Changes

Stimulation of vasoconstrictors from any infusion of cold blood or irritating fluid may cause venous spasm, impeding the rate of flow. A warm pack placed on the vein proximal to the infusion catheter offsets spasms. Any injury, such as phlebitis or thrombosis, that reduces the lumen of the vein decreases the flow of the fluid. In addition, a clogged air vent in the administration set used with air-dependent containers causes the infusion to stop.

If the nurse has any question as to the rate of administration, the physician should be consulted. This applies particularly to IV administration of drugs in fluid.

The rates should also be established for patients receiving two or more infusions simultaneously. Any change in the rate from that normally used should be prescribed by the attending physician.

Computation of Administration Rate

When determining drops per minute, the nurse rounds the drop rate to a whole number. The milliliters per hour also are rounded to a whole number when gravity infusion sets are being used. Flow rate calculations require the following base of information: amount of fluid to be infused, duration of the administration, and drop factor of the set to be used.

Calculating the appropriate infusion rate is easy. The nurse must first know the drop factor of the set that is being used; then he or she can set up a fraction showing the volume of infusate over the number of minutes in which the volume should be infused. For example, if the patient is to receive 100 mL of fluid within 1 hour, the fraction would be

$$\frac{100 \text{ mL}}{60 \text{ minutes}}$$

The fraction is multiplied by the drop factor to determine the number of drops per minute to be infused, using this simple equation:

$$\text{Drops per minute} = \frac{\text{total mL}}{\text{total minutes}} \times \text{drop factor}$$

If 1,000 mL of fluid is ordered over an 8-hour period, the equation is modified as follows:

$$\text{Flow rate} = \frac{1,000 \text{ mL}}{8 \text{ hours}} = 125 \text{ mL/hour}$$

For microdrip or pediatric systems, the equation is:

$$\text{mL/hour} = \text{drop factor}$$

A simple, computer-generated table is presented in Figure 11-4.

Safety Principles and Selection of Equipment

General IV equipment includes IV catheters and accessories; air-venting, microbe-retentive filters; administration sets; and EIDs. A working knowledge of the selection and use of these devices is vital for the nurse who must provide IV therapy and

FIGURE 11–4.   Program for calculating flow rates. (IV drip calculator, courtesy of Globalrph, www.globalrph.com)

ensure the patient's safety and comfort. Although purchasing decisions are increasingly being made with a group purchasing contract in mind, nurses should be involved in selecting IV equipment as members of a product evaluation committee, equipment task force, or safety committee. The concept of safety will always have a profound impact on practice. Worker safety, in particular, is a top priority for health care institutions today (Pugliese, 2004). Protecting health care workers from injury is essential, especially in infusion therapy, where injuries resulting from sharp objects and devices—referred to as *sharps injuries*—are more prevalent than in other areas of nursing practice. Sharps injuries are related not only to needles but also to any sharp objects and devices that have the potential to cause harm by exposing the nurse or others to the blood and body fluid of patients. Box 11–1 lists examples of these objects.

BOX 11–1   Sharps Used in IV Practice

Disposable syringes with needles
Medication cartridge syringes
Needles (injection, vascular access, anesthetic, IV)
Suture needles
Intravascular catheters
Lancets
Scalpels
Razors
Surgical instruments
Glass vacuum blood tubes
Glass capillary tubes or pipettes
Glass medication vials or ampules
Glass IV bottles

Safety Devices and Programs

Many IV nurses find that gathering information concerning the availability and use of safety devices in an institution or agency is helpful in implementing safety programs. Data on injuries may be gathered from local sources and from the more than 70 health care facilities participating in Exposure Prevention Information Network (EPINet) and the International Health Care Worker Safety Center (Ippolito, Puro, & Petrosillo, 1997; Tereskerz, Bentley, Coyner, & Jagger, 1996; Tokars et al., 1993). See the appendices for information on EPINet and needlestick tracking information.

INSTITUTE OF MEDICINE AND OTHER SAFETY REPORTS

The 1999 Institute of Medicine (IOM) Report estimated that medical errors kill approximately 44,000 to 98,000 people annually. A 2004 report by Health Grades, Inc., evaluated 37 million patient records and estimated that 195,000 people in the United States died in 2000, 2001, and 2002 as a result of potentially avoidable medical errors (Patient Safety Press). A potential adverse drug reaction (PADE) is a medication error that has the potential to cause harm, but actually does not do so, either because of circumstances, chance, or because someone corrects and intercepts the error before it reaches the patient.

A companion to the Institute of Medicine Report is *Keeping Patients Safe: Transforming the Work Environment of Nurses*. This report identifies solutions to problems in hospital, nursing home, and other health care organization work environments that threaten patient safety through their effect on nursing care. The report's findings and recommendations address the related issues of management practices, workforce capability, work design, and organizational safety culture. Actions needed from the federal and state governments and from coalitions of parties involved in shaping the work environments of nurses also are specified.

Because of the high-risk nature of intravenous medications, the potential for harm is greatly enhanced over oral medications. A **systems approach** to medical safety is needed to ensure positive outcomes related to patient care.

> **RESEARCH ISSUES:** OSF Healthcare's Journey in Patient Safety
>
> Whittington, J., Cohen, H. (2004). OSF Healthcare's journey in patient safety. *Quality Management in Health Care, 13*(1), 53–59.
>
> This article describes OSF Healthcare's recent journey in patient safety. It discusses the involvement of its 6 hospitals in collaboration with each other and the Institute for Healthcare Improvement. OSF focused on a strategy for decreasing adverse drug events (ADEs). They worked on impacting 4 major areas: safety culture, high-risk medication, dispensing of medication, and medication reconciliation. By doing this, OSF decreased its rate of ADEs per 1000 units of medication administered from 3.84 to 1.39 over the course of 20 months.

System Approach to Safety

Following the IOM's landmark study, the literature has been replete with articles addressing patient safety related to medication administration. Examples of situations that require vigilance to avoid medication errors are listed in Table 11–1 (Hughes & Ortiz, 2005). Common barriers to safe medication administration are divided into five categories and presented in Table 11–2 (Burke, 2005). Public awareness has pushed this effort forward, and a mandate for reform has involved clinicians, researchers, manufacturers, pharmacists, and biomedical engineers in an effort to manage the challenge and develop a system approach to safety. This includes the advent of smart technology that can assist in averting infusion errors at the point of care, thus creating an additional layer of safety for patients (Wilson, 2004).

The role of **smart technology** is to recall whatever rules apply, i.e., dosing limits and clinical advisories for a particular clinical area, by incorporating the rules within the software. See Smart Technologies later in this chapter.

Infusion Safety

Manufacturers such as BD and others have met our demands for safer technology by providing equipment to meet our clinical needs and to enhance patient outcomes. See Figures 11-5, 11-6, and 11-7 for detailed information on how these products are used in the clinical setting. Key features of B-D's Vacutainer Push Button Collection Set are included in Box 11-2 as an example of the types of features available.

SAFETY ASSESSMENT

Safety assessment should include the number of sharps-related injuries and the type of devices involved. Data from studies on human immunodeficiency virus (HIV) seroconversion after needlestick injuries show that injuries caused by large-gauge, hollow-bore needles directly inserted into a vein or artery are associated with a high risk of inadvertent intramuscular or subcutaneous injection (Cardo, Culver, & Ciesielski, 1997). Because they are hollow, blood-filled needles, IV introducer needles, and phlebotomy devices pose a significant risk for transmitting bloodborne infection

TABLE 11–1   Examples of Situations Requiring Vigilance to Avoid Errors

Inadequate patient information	Unknown allergies Unknown medications
Inability to monitor	Vital signs/lab values prior to dosing
Compromised health	Failure to recognize significance of lab values
Number of medications	Multiple meds/frequency of dosing
Unfamiliarity with medication	Knowledge deficit
Monitoring effect of treatment	Lack of follow-up
Administration errors	Rapid administration
Route of administration	Lack of a therapeutic dose when changing route of administration
Drugs in need of manipulation	Inaccurate dosing when splitting, crushing, or suspending a medication
Calculations needed	Miscalculation of drug for dose/weight
Handwritten prescriptions	Incomplete information Incorrect dosage form/strength Illegible Decimal errors Nonstandard terminology
Pediatrics	Wrong dose/route/frequency Incorrect calculations Neonatal administration Dosing errors
Elderly patients	Multiple drugs Compromised health status Multiple care providers Sensitivity to medications
Women	Pregnancy Lactation

(Adapted from Bates, D.W., Leape, L.L., & Petrycki, S. [1993]. Incidence and preventability of adverse drug events in hospitalized adults. *Journal of General Internal Medicine, 8*[6]:289–294.)

(Tereskerz et al., 1996; see Chap. 17). The global focus on safety devices continues to proliferate. Smart infusion systems are available that can avert high-risk errors and provide previously unavailable data for continuous quality improvement efforts.

NEEDLELESS SYSTEMS

In a study by the Centers for Disease Control and Prevention (CDC), 89% of occupational exposures to HIV were caused by percutaneous injuries; most were needlesticks (CDC, 1998). In today's practice arena, the **needleless** system has nearly revolutionized infusion therapy. In general, the product consists of a blunt-tipped plastic insertion device and an injection port that opens to reduce the incidence of accidental needlestick injuries and to promote safety in infusion practice. Again, diverse systems are available to meet clinical needs in many settings.

TABLE 11–2   Common Barriers to Safe Medication Administration

Research
• Outcomes not easily adapted to practice
• Lack of recognition of impact and limitations of technology
• Lack of funding

Education
• Knowledge deficit
• Insufficient clinical practice
• Lack of training on-site

Policy
• Lack of nurse involvement
• Lack of standardization
• Practice/policy implications

Practice
• Lack of best practices
• Lack of standardization
• Lack of focus on safety
• Excessive non-nursing responsibilities
• Inadequate/inaccurate reporting
• Technology and practice failures

Administration
• Lack of administrative support for safety initiatives
• Integration challenges
• Lack of nursing involvement at all levels
• Inadequate allocation of financial resources

(Adapted from Burke, K.G. [2005]. The state of the science on safe medication administration symposium. http://www.nursingcenter.com. *American Journal of Nursing, 105*[Suppl.], 4–9.)

BOX 11–2   B-D Vacutainer Push Button Collection Set: Key Features

• Intended for blood collection and short-term infusion
• Facilitates the prevention of accidental needlestick injury
• Ease-of-use reduces training time while improving activation compliance
• Easily activated without patient discomfort
• Ideal for use in high-risk environment
• Latex-free
• Flash visualization confirms venous access prior to collection of specimen
• Blood flashback is seen clearly through the translucent body
• One-handed safety activation also allows attention to the patient and venipuncture site

Courtesy and © of Becton, Dickinson and Company.

• Holding both colored shields, twist and remove white shield	• Screw on holder (if using Pronto™, hold white tab while screwing in needle)	• Rotate safety shield back

• Twist and pull needle shield straight off	• Perform venipuncture	• Firmly push forward on the safety shield, lock into place and inspect

Things to Remember:
- Handle all biologic samples and blood collection sharps (lancets, needles, luer adapters and blood collection sets) according to the policies and procedures of your facility
- Obtain appropriate medical attention in the event of any exposure to biologic samples (for example, through a puncture injury) since they may transmit viral hepatitis, HIV (AIDS) or other infectious diseases
- Utilize any built-in needle protector if the blood collection device provides one
- BD does not recommend reshielding used needles, but the policies and procedures of your facility may differ and must always be followed
- Discard BD Vacutainer Brand Eclipse Blood Collection Needle in the nearest sharps collector. Follow your institution's policy for safe disposal of all medical waste

FIGURE 11–5. Vacutainer Eclipse blood collection needle, economical needle-based safety device for injection in a variety of sizes. (Adapted from BD Vacutainer Eclipse Blood Collection Needle Quick Reference Card. Courtesy and © of Becton, Dickinson and Company.)

PERIPHERAL VASCULAR ACCESS DEVICES

Innovations in catheter technology have produced catheters to meet the patient's every need, from routine peripheral infusion to the most sophisticated therapy. Catheters vary in gauge, length, design, and composition. Their composition may be polyvinylchloride (PVC), polyurethane, or silicone. Thin-walled catheters promote increased flow rates, which allow smaller catheters to be used. Most catheters are radiopaque or contain a stripe of radiopaque material to enable radiographic visualization.

Some products have wings, which confer all the advantages of a small-vein needle for insertion and taping. In these devices, the adapter of the IV set connection is located a few inches from the catheter, which provides ease and smoother technique

1

To use the BD Vacutainer®
Push Button Blood Collection Set,
peel off the paper backing and
remove the device. Avoid contact
with the activation button during
the removal of the device.

2a

With thumb and index finger,
grasp the wings together and
access vein using standard needle
insertion technique.

OR

2b

If preferred by your institution,
the body of the device can be held,
instead of the wings, during
insertion.

3

Proper access to the vein will
be indicated by the presence of
"flash" directly behind and below
the button.

4a

The device is designed to be
activated while the needle is still
in the patient's vein. Following the
collection procedure, and while the
needle is still in the vein, push the
button to retract the needle into the
body of the device.

4b

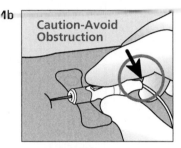

To ensure complete and immediate
retraction of device, make sure to
keep fingers and hands away from
the end of the blood collection set
during retraction. Do not impede
retraction.

4c

Apply pressure to the venipuncture
site in accordance with your facility's
protocol.

5

Confirm that the needle is in the
shielded position prior to disposal.

6

Discard the entire shielded blood
collection set and holder into an
approved sharps disposal container.

FIGURE 11–6.   BD Vacutainer push-button blood collection/in-vein needle activation. (Adapted from BD
Vacutainer Push Button Blood Collection Set InService Poster. Courtesy and © of Becton, Dickinson and Company.)

Aspiration

Draw up medication in accordance with established protocol.

Injection

Administer medication in accordance with established protocols, making sure that all medication has been dispensed.

Activation can occur either inside or outside* the patient.

Activation

Push plunger rod to activate the safety mechanism. Depress until you sense two "clicks."

If Activation is performed before needle is withdrawn from patient, do not advance needle while depressing plunger rod.

* If Activation is performed after needle is withdrawn from patient, minimal splatter may occur. When activating the device outside of the patient, hold the device downward at arm's length, and activate while pointing away from self and others. Keep device within sight at all times to avoid accidental needlestick injury.

Retraction

The needle will disappear into the syringe and the plunger will be recessed into the barrel when activation is complete. There is no exposure to the used needle. Immediately discard into an approved sharps container.

Things to Remember:

• BD Integra Needle and Syringe are not a standard luer connection.

• After pressurizing the medication vial, do not continue to press the plunger rod past the point of resistance, as this may cause premature activation.

FIGURE 11–7. BD Integra 3-mL syringe, a low-waste space syringe with detachable retracting needle. (Adapted from BD Integra 3 mL Syringe Quick Reference Card. Courtesy and © of Becton, Dickinson and Company.)

when changing sets, thereby reducing the potential for mechanical phlebitis and contamination. Such catheters are available with injection sites as an integral part of the catheter; the mixing of drugs or blood components with primary parenteral fluid is reduced to a minimum (0.4 mL), minimizing the potential for incompatibilities.

Product Selection and Evaluation Criteria

A multidisciplinary health care team that includes front-line health care workers should be involved in selecting safety products. Other potential team members include infection control, safety, quality improvement, occupational health, materials management, medical staff, emergency/trauma, surgical, anesthesia, diagnostic radiology, home care, critical care, and laboratory staff. The IV specialist must be included in the team that assesses products used in infusion therapy.

In determining the criteria for selecting IV safety devices, design and performance should be considered. Consideration should be given also to latex-free components of a device that may have prolonged contact with a patient, such as an IV catheter (U.S. Food and Drug Administration [FDA], 1996). The suggested FDA criteria are given in Box 11–3.

An evaluation survey instrument may also be developed to measure accurately staff opinion during product evaluation. An example of forms used by the Training for the Development of Innovative Control Technology Project convened by Dr. June Fisher of the University of California at San Francisco is given in Figure 11–8 (Pugliese, 2004).

BOX 11–3   U.S. Food and Drug Administration Suggested Criteria for Selecting a Safety Device

- Device provides a barrier between the hands and the needle following use.
- Device allows or requires worker's hands to remain behind the needle at all times.
- Safety constitutes an integral part of the device, is not an accessory.
- Safety features are effective before disassembly and remain in effect after disposal.
- Device should be simple and easy to use, requiring little or no training.

Adapted from U.S. Food and Drug Administration. (1995). Supplementary guidance on the content of premarket notification (510K) submission for medical devices with sharps injury prevention features (draft). Rockville, MD: General Hospital Device Branch, Pilot Device Evaluation Division, Office of Device Evaluation.

Date:_____ Department:_____ Occupation:_____

Product Evaluated:_____ Number of times used:_____

Please circle the most appropriate answer for each question. A rating of one (1) indicates the highest level of agreement with the statement, five (5) the lowest. Not applicable (N/A) may be used if the question does not apply to this product.

agree...........disagree

1. The safety feature can be activated using a one-handed technique.	1	2	3	4	5	N/A
2. The safety feature does not interfere with normal use of this product.	1	2	3	4	5	N/A
3. Use of this product requires you to use the safety feature.	1	2	3	4	5	N/A
4. This device does not require more time to use than a nonsafety device.	1	2	3	4	5	N/A
5. The safety feature works well with a wide variety of hand sizes.	1	2	3	4	5	N/A
6. The device allows for rapid visualization of flashback in the catheter or chamber.	1	2	3	4	5	N/A
7. Use of this product does not increase the number of sticks to the patient.	1	2	3	4	5	N/A
8. The product stops the flow of blood after the needle is removed from the catheter (or after the butterfly is inserted) and just prior to line connections or hep-lock capping.	1	2	3	4	5	N/A
9. A clear and unmistakable change (either audible or visible) occurs when the safety feature is activated.	1	2	3	4	5	N/A
10. The safety feature operates reliably.	1	2	3	4	5	N/A
11. The exposed sharp is blunted or covered after use and prior to disposal.	1	2	3	4	5	N/A
12. The product does not need extensive training to be operated correctly.	1	2	3	4	5	N/A

FIGURE 11–8. An infusion device's safety feature evaluation form. (From the American Hospital Association).

INFUSION CATHETERS

Most IV catheters consist of a flexible, nonthrombogenic tubing that remains within the lumen of the vessel, negating many of the formerly routine complications associated with IV therapy (see Chap. 9). The gold standard is the over-the-needle catheter (ONC). Once the venipuncture is made, the catheter is slipped off the needle into the vein and the steel needle removed. The use of obturators, which are inserted into the catheter to maintain patency for intermittent infusion, is infrequent today.

Catheters are made of diverse materials; for many years, PVC was used almost exclusively. Ideally, to reduce the risk of thrombus formation on the catheter, the catheter should be made of a **hemorepellant** material, such as silicone. Catheters should be radiopaque for detection by imaging equipment in the event the catheter is severed and lost in the circulation (INS, 1998, 2000, 2005). Some formations of polyurethane, such as Vialon, have an ultrasmooth microsurface, an exclusive lubrication process, and the ability to soften up to 70% while in the vessel. This biomaterial decreases the chance of irritation to the vessel wall, thereby reducing the potential or mechanical phlebitis. These catheter characteristics allow for ease of insertion, kink resistance, and reduced risk of phlebitis and infiltration, and also translate into optimum dwell times (Gaukroger, Robert, & Manners, 1988; Maki & Ringer, 1991; McKee, Shell, Warren, & Campbell, 1989; Stanley, Meister, & Fuschuber, 1992).

STEEL NEEDLES

The type of steel needle used for infusion therapy is the winged infusion device, or small-vein needle. The gauge of the needle refers to both the inside and the outside diameters of the lumen—the smaller the gauge, the larger the lumen. Steel needles are typically thin walled. Because the wall of the needle is thinner than that of the standard needle, a larger lumen is obtained for the same external diameter, offering the advantage of enhanced flow rates. Today, steel needles are most commonly used for sampling venous blood.

Factors to be considered in selecting a steel needle are length of bevel, gauge, and length of the needle. A short bevel reduces the risk of trauma to the endothelial wall, infiltration from a puncture to the posterior wall, and hematoma or extravasation occurring when the steel needle enters the vein. When a steel needle with a long bevel is inserted into the vessel, blood may leak into the tissues before the entire bevel is in the lumen of the vein.

Whenever possible, the gauge of the needle should be appreciably smaller than the lumen of the vein to be entered; when the gauge of the needle approaches the size of the vein, trauma may occur. When a large needle occludes the flow of blood, irritating fluids flowing through the vein with no dilution of blood may cause chemical phlebitis. Mechanical phlebitis may result from motion and pressure exerted by the needle on the endothelial wall of the vein.

When large amounts of fluid are required, a needle of adequate size must be used; a small lumen interferes with the flow of fluid. The flow of blood varies inversely as the fourth power of the radius of the lumen of the needle. Thus, a needle with an internal radius of 1 mm that delivers 1 mL of blood with a fixed pressure on the plunger or in the infusion bottle delivers only $\frac{1}{16}$ of a milliliter when the radius is

TABLE 11–3   Peripheral Venous Access Devices and Their Use

Device	Description	Advantages	Disadvantages
Catheter	ONC catheter Variety of sizes and lengths Radiopaque	Easily inserted	Short-term use; site should be rotated consistent with institutional policy
Midline catheter	A mid-catheter device usually placed in either the basilic or cephalic vein	ONC: Aquavene elastomeric polymer expands two gauge sizes and up to 1 inch in length when hydrated; longer indwell time	Inherent risk of puncturing and shearing the catheter during insertion
PICC catheter	20 to 24 inches long and used for long term access in patients with poor central access and those at risk for complications from central insertion	Reduced incidence of complications; may be placed by physician or nurse[a]; diversity of size ranges and manufacturers; may be inserted using guidewire, stylet, or introducer	Care must be taken when threading the catheter through the introducer needle not to withdraw or pull the catheter back through the needle (avoid shearing); may occlude smaller peripheral vessels
Winged infusion needle	Steel needle or flexible catheter with fixed extension set	Easily inserted and secured with wings; extension set ensures access	

ONC, over-the-needle catheter; PICC, peripherally inserted central catheter.
[a]Consistent with state Nurse Practice Act.

reduced to 0.5 mm. A large needle is also required with fluids of high viscosity. The rate of flow of the fluid decreases in proportion to the viscosity of the fluid.

The flow of the fluid varies inversely with the length of the needle shaft. If the length of the needle is increased, other conditions being equal, the volume flowing is reduced. Use of a short needle for infusions reduces the risk of infiltration. Because a short needle affords more play than a long needle, more motion is needed to puncture the vessel wall.

Making a wise choice of a catheter for an infusion is a relatively straightforward process. Although the number and types of lines have increased dramatically, several factors remain considerations in all choices (Table 11–3). In addition, a number of safety devices are available to facilitate delivery of peripheral infusion therapy.

Winged Infusion Needles

The winged infusion device or small-vein needle is similar to the steel cannula, with the hub replaced with two flexible wings. Originally designed for pediatric and geri-

FIGURE 11–9. Winged infusion needle.

atric use, it has been used in prolonged therapy for all ages. Two types of small-vein needles are available, one with a short length of plastic tubing and a permanently attached **resealable injection site,** the other with a variable length of plastic tubing permanently attached to a female Luer adapter that accommodates an administration set. The small-vein needle with the resealable injection site allows the intermittent administration of medications or fluids. Variations of the winged infusion needle are available for short-term infusion use. A dilute solution of heparinized saline or saline solution maintains patency of the needle when it is not in use. Winged infusion needles also enhance safety and protection (Fig. 11–9).

Needle Shields

Manufacturers have incorporated safety needle shields into their respective designs. Shields or sheath covers help to prevent inadvertent needlesticks. Needle-Pro (Smith Industries Medical Systems) and Safety Tip are examples of these products (Fig. 11–10).

Midline Catheters

The introduction of the midline catheter provided an alternative to central line catheter placement for prolonged IV access. The materials that midline catheters are made of are significant safety features. For instance, polytetrafluoroethylene (Teflon) is less thrombogenic and less inflammatory than polyurethane or PVC. Vialon is nonhemolytic and free of plasticizers. It is slick after immersion in fluid and softens after insertion, minimizing vein trauma and clot induction. Aquavene has also been used; it is an elastomeric hydrogel that softens and expands when hydrated (in contact with aqueous fluids, such as blood). Advantages of using the product include reduction of peripheral IV restarts, elimination of the need for central IV lines with their associated complications, and ease of midline insertion (see Chap. 12). The complete softening and expansion process takes approximately 90 minutes. This product permits long-term placement when venous access is limited or when therapy is prescribed for a specific time. The product is considered a peripheral venous catheter according to INS standards. Professionals are encouraged to develop policies and procedures relevant to indwell time and consistent with INS standards and institutional guidelines (INS, 1998, 2000, 2005).

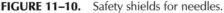

FIGURE 11–10.   Safety shields for needles.

FLUID CONTAINERS

Sterile glass containers first became available in 1929. Although currently used much less frequently, glass remains the container of choice for those fluids that, because of their characteristics, may not be administered in plastic containers. For example, nitroglycerin can be absorbed into plastic containers and tubing, and lipid emulsions can absorb certain plastics from the container into the fluid.

Glass Containers

At manufacture, glass IV containers are sealed under vacuum and therefore must be vented when delivered to the patient. The air vent on the administration set (typically as part of the piercing pin) should have an air filter to prevent the ingress of microbes as the fluid is vented. If a nonvented administration set is used with a glass container, the fluid will not flow. Air must displace the fluid in the container for flow to occur.

Medications should be added to glass containers through the rubber stopper. Glass is also an absolute barrier to gases such as carbon dioxide and oxygen. Some drugs such as lipids and bicarbonate are not stable in current plastic containers because of gas diffusion.

Plastic Containers

Baxter Healthcare (Deerfield, IL) was the first manufacturer to develop plastic containers for parenteral fluids. Plastic containers are easily transported, minimize the risk of damage to the container, and are easily disposed of. Air venting is not required because the container collapses as the fluid is delivered. This in turn reduces the risk of air embolism and airborne contamination. Because plastic containers do not have stoppers or bushings, the risk of coring and particulate matter is eliminated. Plastic IV containers range in size from 25 to 1,000 mL for IV infusion.

Syringes and Safety Syringes

A syringe may be a fluid container, especially when used with an infusion device that accommodates syringe delivery. Delivery of fluid or medication from a syringe is well suited to patient care areas in which small volumes of medication or fluid are required. The limiting feature of the syringe is its volume capacity (see Chap. 21). Using standard syringes, delivery times vary from 15 to 60 minutes with an accuracy rate of ±15%.

The development of safety syringes has contributed greatly to practice. Several manufacturers provide safety syringes with needle guards to protect the health care worker and patient (Fig. 11–11).

DRUG DELIVERY SYSTEMS

Three of six IV drug delivery systems were rated superior by a national panel of clinicians (Consensus Development Conference, September 27 and 28, 1999). The systems were manufacturer-prepared IV delivery systems, point-of-care–activated IV delivery systems, and pharmacy-based IV admixture programs. IV push, volume-control chambers, and syringe pumps were ranked lower by the panel of experts. The use of these systems varies within a given institution and in specific clinical circumstances; for example, in a medical emergency, IV push may be preferred (CDC, 1998; Occupational Safety and Health Administration, 1998; Tereskerz et al., 1996).

Manufacturer-Prepared Systems

Manufacturer-prepared fluids have revolutionized practice because increasing numbers of medications are marketed in this way. Premixed fluids are prepared under sterile conditions in the designated diluent and container with specific instructions for use. Easily transported and stable, manufacturer-prepared fluids have changed the way in which home care is delivered (see Chap. 23).

Point-of-Care System

A use-activated **(point-of-care)** container is compartmentalized, with premeasured drug in one compartment and the required fluid in another compartment. To activate the container for infusion, the nurse must remove or dislodge a diaphragm or seal between the compartments. This simplifies drug delivery by allowing the drug and the fluid to mix. It also eliminates the need for separate drug and diluent vials and yields an appropriate admixture for delivery.

Pharmacy-Based Infusion Admixture

Although many medications come in a prefilled container for IV piggyback administration, some medications must be added to fluid before administration. Methods for adding medications to fluid containers vary with each system, and new safety parameters have been added to currently available devices. The plastic bag contains

• To assemble, hold needle and syringe by flanges (wings) and twist needle until firmly seated

• During aspiration, press index finger against flanges to prevent sleeve movement

• After injection, grasp sleeve firmly and twist flanges to loosen the sleeve

• Fully retract needle into sleeve until it locks in the protected position
• When the Safe Lock Indicator green band fully covers the red band and an audible click is heard, the sleeve is locked into position

Things to Remember:

• Aseptic technique and proper skin preparation of the site are essential
• Discard Safety-Lok Syringe in the nearest sharps collector. Follow your institution's policy for safe disposal of all medical waste.

FIGURE 11–11. B-D Safety-Lok Syringe, the original shielding safety hypodermic needle requiring two-handed activation. (Adapted from BD Safety-Lok Syringe Quick Reference Card. Courtesy and © of Becton, Dickinson and Company.)

a resealable medication port through which the medication is injected, although some products permit needleless access to the container.

When medications are added to the plastic containers during an infusion, care must be taken to ensure that the clamp on the administration set is closed and the flow interrupted before the medication is added. This prevents inadvertent administration of an undiluted and potentially toxic dose of medication that has not been fully diluted in the IV container. Medications and fluids should always be mixed thoroughly before administration, regardless of the system used. Most drug delivery systems use universal piercing pins. Use of such products eliminates the need to remove an existing air vent from the piercing pin.

INFUSION ADMINISTRATION SETS

An important factor in the administration set is the rate of flow the given set is gauged to produce. Commercial sets vary, delivering anywhere from 10 to 15 drops/mL, depending on the nature of the fluid. The nurse must be aware of the drop factor to set the rate of flow correctly. Increased fluid viscosity may slow the rate of infusion, but does not affect the drop factor.

Most conventional sets use the roller clamp or slide clamp for controlling the flow rate. Fluid temperature, room temperature, height of the fluid container, and the patient's catheter size all affect flow rate. The nurse should recheck the infusion rate regularly to ensure that the prescribed flow rate is maintained.

Alternatives to the roller clamp are available from a number of manufacturers; they can save nurses valuable time and are helpful in maintaining the rate of infusion. One device has a flow-metering system that essentially eliminates changes in flow rate. The metering device consists of an adjustable dam. The dam is usually added to a standard administration set and can be removed if desired. The rate can be set and is maintained as long as the head height of the fluid container remains constant. This minimizes the risk of runaway infusions and free flow, which can occur if the roller clamp fully opens accidentally.

Specialty-Use Sets

Non-PVC IV administration sets are available for gravity and volumetric EIDs. Nitroglycerin and other drugs can be administered without altering the dosage of the drug through **absorption** into the walls of PVC tubing. Fat emulsion leaches plasticizers from the PVC tubing; these specialty sets may have non-PVC layers in fluid contact or use plasticizers that do not leach as easily.

In many cases, the flow must be maintained at a minimal rate. One method is to reduce the drop size by using a microdrip set. These sets deliver 60 drops/mL. At the rate of 60 drops/minute, it would take 1 hour to infuse 60 mL. A variety of commercial sets are available for alternate or simultaneous infusion of two fluids. Some sets contain a filter (Fig. 11–12).

Positive-pressure sets are designed to increase the rate of infusion and are an asset when rapid replacement of fluid becomes necessary. When used with the collapsible plastic fluid container, the danger of air embolism is minimal because as the bag collapses, the risk of air in the system is reduced. In contrast to the collapsible

FIGURE 11–12. **A.** Air-eliminating properties of an IV filter. **B.** Hydrophilic/hydrophobic membrane properties of an IV filter. **C.** Optimal IV filter for add-on or in-line use. (Courtesy of Abbott Laboratories, Abbott Park, IL.)

plastic container, glass containers must be vented to allow the fluid to flow, and air is thus present in the system. As the last portion of fluid from the glass container is delivered to the patient, the air under pressure may rapidly enter the vein before the clamp can be applied, resulting in an embolus. The nurse should never apply positive pressure to infuse fluids.

Check Valve Sets

Check valve sets were traditionally used to administer secondary medications as a piggyback into the injection site located below the valve. The valve automatically shut off the main-line infusion while the admixture was running and automatically allowed the main infusion to start when the medication had run in. Variations of this set are available for use with electronic flow control devices (EIDs), which enable the user to back-prime the small-volume container (piggyback) with primary fluid (see section on Electronic Infusion Devices).

Volume-Controlled Sets

Accuracy in controlling the volume of IV fluids has always been facilitated by using a volume-controlled set. Used less frequently today because of the plethora of EIDs available on the market and market pricing of those devices, the volume-controlled set still maintains a place in the clinical setting. Sets contain vented, **calibrated** burette chambers that control the volume from 100 to 150 mL. The burette chamber of some sets contains a rubber float that prevents air from entering the tubing once the infusion is completed (see Fig. 11-13).

Some calibrated burette chambers contain a microporous filter to block the passage of air when the chamber empties. Refilling these chambers requires a specific procedure. The word *OSCAR* is a memory helper to recall the procedure:

O—Open clamp,
S—squeeze drip chamber and hold,
C—close clamp close to drip chamber,
A—and
R—release drip chamber.

FIGURE 11–13. Volume-controlled infusion set. (Courtesy of Abbott Laboratories, Abbott Park, IL.)

Electronic Infusion Device–Specific Sets

Some administration sets are made specifically for use with EIDs. These sets also come in a number of configurations. Such sets and their respective electronic delivery systems ensure safe delivery of infusion therapy to patients of all ages in a variety of clinical settings. By extracting fluid from the IV container and ejecting it at predetermined intervals through the administration set, the EID delivers the appropriate preset amount of diluent.

FINAL INFUSION FILTERS

Filters prevent passage of undesirable substances into the vascular system (Fig. 11–14).

Particulate filters of 1 or 5 μm are recommended when IV medications are being prepared. A bacteria-retentive filter of approximately 0.2 μm is recommended for the

FIGURE 11–14. Primary Venoset with IVEX-2 integral filter.

routine delivery of IV therapies. The time of change should ideally coincide with the changing of the administration set (see Chap. 4).

Filters come in diverse configurations, including add-on and integral units. Add-on filters should be securely connected to the administration set and treated as a part of that set. Integral filters are attached by the manufacturer to the administration set. To achieve final filtration, the filter should be located as close to the catheter site as possible.

The industry standard is a membrane filter. Membrane filters are screen-type filters with uniformly sized pores that provide an absolute rating. A 0.2-μm screen-type filter retains on the flat surface membrane all particles larger than 0.2 μm. A 0.2-μm filter is considered an absolute, bacteria-retentive, air-eliminating filter and decreases the complications of infection and the potential for air embolism.

The *United States Pharmacopeia* (1999) has established an acceptable limit of particles for single-dose infusion as not more than 50 particles/mL that are ≥10.0 μm and not more than 5 particles/mL that are ≥25.0 μm in effective linear dimension.

Effect of Pressure and Air on Filters

At a certain pressure, all filters allow air to pass from one side of the **wetted** hydrophilic membrane to the other. This pressure value is called the **bubble point** of that particular membrane. Distinguishing features that affect the bubble point are the different filter materials (e.g., hydrophobic, hydrophilic,), depth, screen, different wetting (**hydrophilic**)or nonwetting (**hydrophobic**) characteristics, and the test liquid. Water or saline solution, for example, is the test liquid of choice when testing hydrophilic membranes for IV filters because fluids that are administered IV are primarily water. Water is inexpensive, can be filtered easily for control of particulates and micro-organisms, and is readily available. There are other advantages to using water as a bubble point test fluid. Water tests the wetting characteristics of hydrophilic membrane filters. To define this point further, an explanation of bubble point tests in relation to membranes is required.

Bubble Point Tests

Bubble point testing is particularly important in IV therapy because it is crucial that the filter in the IV line prevent air from passing through it at low pressures, such as those used in IV therapy.

Testing involves encapsulation of the membrane in an integral housing. Two different types of bubble point tests may be performed, open bubble and closed bubble point, depending on downstream flow and the ability to see the membrane (Fig. 11–15). An open bubble point test can be performed only if the direction of normal flow is such that the bubbles produced can be seen as they form. This means that the housing of the filter must be transparent and the downstream side of the membrane can be observed. This test is performed by first flowing the test liquid through the device at low pressures until it is wetted out. Usually, this pressure is the same as that used in administering fluid by gravity feed pressures (36 to 39 inches of water). Then, after the membrane is wetted out, air pressure is applied as before. The bubble point

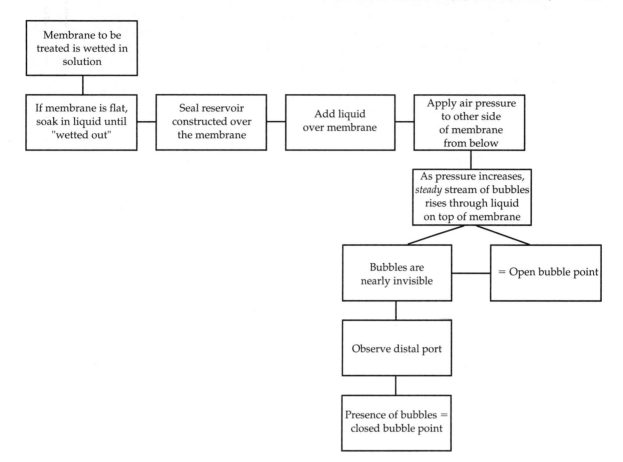

FIGURE 11–15.   Bubble point tests. An open bubble point test can be performed only if the direction of normal flow permits bubbles to form.

has been reached when a steady stream of bubbles is seen on the downstream side of the membrane.

A closed bubble point test must be performed when the downstream side of the membrane cannot be visualized. Closed bubble points result in slightly higher values than open bubble points because the air pressure during the test is steadily increasing and it takes more time for the air bubbles to escape through the distal port. If the pressure is increased slowly, the test is more accurate.

Testing of IV membranes and filter devices with water is significant. Most hydrophilic membranes incorporate either external (applied after they are made) or internal (in the base formula) wetting agents to render them more wettable with water. It is particularly important in IV therapy because it is critical that the membrane should wet properly so that air does not pass the membrane at low pressures.

The 0.2-μm air-venting filters automatically vent air through a nonwettable (hydrophobic) membrane and permit uniform high gravity flow rates through large, wettable (hydrophilic) membranes. They prevent an air block, which could ultimately result in a plugged catheter.

Filters are also rated according to the pounds per square inch **(psi)** of pressure they withstand, an important consideration in selecting the proper filter. The filter should withstand the pressure exerted by the infusion pump or rupture may occur. If the psi rating of the housing is less than that of the membrane, excess force will break the housing, leaving the filter intact.

Optimal filters should (a) automatically vent air; (b) retain bacteria, fungi, and endotoxins; (c) not bind drugs; (d) allow high gravity flow rates; and (e) be able to withstand the pressure exerted by the infusion pump. The pressure rating of the housing, when less than that of the filter membrane, may provide added protection.

INFUSION ACCESSORIES

A plethora of accessories, such as injection caps, loops, latex ports, and needleless systems, is available today (Fig. 11–16). Most include safety features. The injection port or catheter cap may be used to adapt any indwelling device to an intermittent infusion device. Available either as an individual unit or incorporated into the design of an ONC or winged infusion set, injection ports have simplified the administration of intermittent therapies using needleless systems.

A   B

FIGURE 11–16. Among the many accessory items for IV therapy are **(A)** loops and **(B)** injection ports.

Intermittent infusion devices may also be called *heparin locks*, *INTS*, or *PRN adapters* because heparin or saline is routinely instilled into the cap and its housing to maintain patency. Most health care organizations routinely instill saline rather than dilute heparin in such devices.

LATEX DEVICES AND SENSITIVITY

Shortly after the turn of the century, **latex** sensitivity remains a challenge for health care workers and patients alike, with powdered latex gloves being the most common latex equipment to exacerbate allergies. In addition, many of the clinical supplies used to deliver IV fluids and fluids are made of latex.

The various types of latex reactions include irritant or contact dermatitis, allergic contact-type IV hypersensitivity, and type I hypersensitivity. Allergic reactions are potentially avoidable for both the patient and clinicians. The nurse delivering IV therapy should be cognizant of the prevalence, symptoms, risk factors, diagnosis, and treatment of latex allergy (Beezhold et al., 1996; Gritter, 1999; National Institute for Occupational Safety and Health [NIOSH], 1997; Warshaw, 1998).

Standard precautions mandate that health care providers wear gloves for prolonged periods of patient care. Latex is a natural rubber product derived from the sap of the commercial rubber tree *Hevea brasiliensis*. The latex fluid is composed of carbohydrates, lipids, phospholipids, and *cis*-1,4 polyisoprene. Latex is a complex protein by-product of the rubber tree containing more than 28 antigenic peptide proteins and contributing to allergic reactions in people with hypersensitivity latex allergy (Table 11–4).

Exposure can occur through cutaneous, mucosal, parenteral, or aerosol routes. Parenteral exposure includes medications injected through latex IV injection sites or drawn through rubber stoppers of vials. Powder released into the air during the removal of a powdered latex glove may precipitate respiratory distress. Latex proteins may remain airborne for as long as 5 to 12 hours (Beezhold et al. 1996; Warshaw, 1998). Diagnosis is confirmed by detailed history, including risk factors and suspected reactions. Physical examination may reveal a lack of symptoms. A skin prick test is a reliable indicator of an antigen allergy. Radioallergosorbent testing (RAST) is an in vitro test for IgE antibodies to a specific antigen. The results of RAST may be inconclusive, however. Use, challenge, or patch tests may be performed, along with

TABLE 11–4 Type I Reactions to Latex

System Affected	Clinical Manifestation
Cardiovascular	Hypotension, sinus tachycardia, arrhythmias, cardiac arrest
Gastrointestinal	Nausea, vomiting, diarrhea, abdominal cramping
Respiratory	Bronchospasm, shortness of breath, cyanosis, laryngeal edema, wheezing, respiratory arrest
Cutaneous	Flushing, urticaria, pruritus, rash
Systemic	Faintness, generalized edema

BOX 11–4   Web Site Sources of Information: Latex Sensitivity

- Education for Latex Allergy/Support Team and Information Coalition (ELASTIC)
  http://www.ncbi.nlm.nih.gov/entrez/query.fcgi?cmd=Retrieve&db=PubMed&list_uids=9216304&dopt=Citation
- Latex Allergy Links
  http://www.ncbi.nlm.nih.gov/entrez/query.fcgi?cmd=Retrieve&db=pubmed&list_uids=10893510&dopt=Citation
- National Institute for Occupational Safety and Health (NIOSH)
  www.cdc.gov/niosh/homepage.html

---

intradermal testing, basophil histamine release, and inhalation tests. Prevention is achieved by providing a latex-free environment. NIOSH recommends that if latex gloves are worn, they should be the low-antigen type and powderless (Warshaw, 1998). For more information, see Box 11–4.

ELECTRONIC INFUSION DEVICES AND SMART TECHNOLOGIES

Complex infusions of medications are administered using **electronic infusion devices** (EIDs) that, although designed to be easy to use, have been associated with serious programming errors that can result in overdosing or underdosing. Earlier versions of EIDs are now being replaced by smart computerized devices with comprehensive drug libraries, dosing limits, and best-practice guidelines that are prescriptive and restrictive. Each hospital develops its own complete data set, including drug names, concentrations, dosing units, and dose limits, and loads the devices with this information. Some smart pumps include additional features such as drug information and weight, rate, and volume limits specific to the clinical area in which they are used. These devices add to a new level of safety in IV administration that was previously impossible. (Vanderveen, 2005).

The INS Standards of Practice address regulation of flow (see Chap. 4). Electronic infusion devices should be used when warranted by the patient's age and condition, setting, and prescribed therapy. The nursing professional is responsible and accountable for the use of EIDs. Use of EIDs, their deployment, selection criteria, and classifications should be outlined in institutional policy and procedure manuals. The nurse's knowledge base concerning EIDs should include, at the minimum, indications for use, mechanical operation, safe use and troubleshooting techniques, and the psi rating.

The psi rating is important because **differential pressure** is often a component of such devices. With a range of two or three levels, such equipment may sense a change in pressure, usually 5 psi over baseline, and some devices monitor and read out (display) line pressure. *Operating* or *line pressure* is the pressure generated by a pump that causes fluid to flow at a predetermined rate. *Maximum occlusion pressure* is the limit to operating pressure at which an occlusion alarm is triggered. Needle pressure is the same as venous pressure. During an infusion, pressure at the tip of the catheter is only slightly greater than the pressure in the vein or artery, regardless of the output pressure of the pump. The pressure at the needle tip needs to be slightly higher than vascular pressure for fluid to flow. An understanding of pressure and the psi rating is essential to safe use of EIDs, filters, and other components of the IV system.

EIDs are invaluable in neonatal, pediatric, and adult intensive care units, where critical infusions of small volumes of fluid or doses of high-potency drugs are required. These devices have increased the level of safety in parenteral therapy. Today, the risk of air embolism is reduced by alarm systems and by the automatic interruption of the infusion when a container empties. A controlled rate of flow reduces the risk of circulatory overload.

The devices have saved valuable nursing time; uniform control of fluid eliminates the need to count drops and continually adjust flow rates. Plugging of the catheter, which occurs when blood backs into the catheter because of an increase in venous pressure from coughing, crying, or straining, is eliminated. The pressure generated by the EID pump may exceed the maximum venous pressure.

SAFE PRACTICE ALERT   Strengths and Weaknesses of Medication Technology

Technology	Strengths	Weaknesses
Automated dispenser	Patient-specific Requires secure access Includes R.Ph. review Specifies dose/amount	Restocking errors User input errors
Electronic medication Administration/recording	Bar coding Drugs/nurse badges Patient ID scanning	Transcription errors Scanning errors
Computerized infusion devices	Drug library Dose limits Alarms in place	Input errors (missing decimal points, etc.)

Adapted from Nicholas, P.K., Agius, C.R. (2005). Toward safer IV medication administration. *American Journal of Nursing, 105*(Suppl.), 25–30.

Ambulatory Infusion Devices

Self-care is an important component of current health care delivery systems. The development of compact, battery-driven EIDs has simplified care in diverse ambulatory clinical settings, including home care.

External Infusion Pumps

The size, weight, and portability of the unit are important considerations in choosing a system. An active patient must be comfortable wearing the lightest pump possible; a sedentary patient may prefer the advantages of a larger device. Accessories and loading procedures vary with the manufacturer and the product selected. Infusion capacity may dictate the choice of the system. Pump-specific sets may be required, such as with the patient receiving nutritional support or pain medication. Integral safety features include:

- Occlusion alarm
- Low-volume safety alarm
- Low-battery alarm

Competition in this exciting area of growth has stimulated many new companies to enter the electronic infusion market, resulting in greater availability of more sophisticated products for the professional IV nurse.

Elastomeric Balloon Devices

An **elastomeric** device is made of a soft, rubberized material capable of inflating to a predetermined volume. The balloon deflates at a rate determined by the diameter of the restricting outlet located in the preattached tubing or in the neck of the container. The size of the tunnel controls the passage of fluid. The balloon, safely encapsulated inside a rigid, transparent container, becomes the reservoir for fluid. The shape of this device is manufacturer specific, and it may be round, disk shaped, or cylindrical. A tamper-proof port for injecting medication into the balloon is attached. Typically, the capacity is 50 to 100 mL and the devices are for one-time use only.

Spring-Coil Piston Syringes

The volume of a spring-coil piston syringe ranges from 30 to 60 mL, and a spring powers the plunger in the absence of manual pressure. Like the elastomeric balloon, this device has limited applications and is for one-time use only. The syringe is filled by withdrawing the piston and overextending the spring. As the spring regains its shape, it forces the piston down, expelling its contents.

Spring-Coil Container

This container combines the principles of the spring-coil piston syringe in a multiuse and small-volume container. An overextended spring in an enclosed space between two disks seeks to recover its original shape, pulling the top and bottom together and forcing the fluid contents out of the restricting orifice. Handy and convenient for the ambulatory patient, the spring-coil container is ideal for home use.

Therapy-Specific Devices

EIDs are finding increasing use in keep-open arterial lines and infusion of drugs, blood, and viscous fluids such as parenteral nutrition fluids. Advances in technology have provided us with more sophisticated devices. Many types and models are available. In general, pumps are devices that generate flow under positive pressure. Such devices may be peristaltic, syringe, or pulsatile. **Controllers** are devices that generate flow by gravity and are capable of either drop counting or volumetric delivery.

Controllers

Controllers do not exert positive pressure greater than the head height of the infusion container, which is usually 2 psi. The controller is used to monitor the infusion for accuracy, to sound an alarm if flow is interrupted, and to provide even, consistent delivery of fluid. A controller uses drop-sensor technology. Manufacturers have developed variations on this theme, specific to patient populations and clinical needs.

Pumps

A diversity of pump products is available, including syringe, positive-pressure, and volumetric devices.

Syringe Pumps   Many manufacturers have met the demand for syringe infusion systems. Syringe pumps are calibrated in milliliters per hour, are used with standard disposable syringes, and provide smooth and precise delivery of low volumes of fluid to specific patient populations. A variety of new products on the market may be configured to suit special clinical situations, with options such as auto bolus reduction to minimize the possibility of administering an accidental bolus of drug, preset upper bolus rates, maintenance notification, and downloading capability between instruments.

Positive-Pressure Infusion Pumps   A positive-pressure device overcomes vascular resistance, tubing compromises such as excessive length, and the normal physical limitations that cause an IV to function improperly.

Pressure exerted by the unit is expressed in pounds per square inch (psi) or millimeters of mercury (mm Hg). One psi and 50 mm Hg exert the same amount of pressure. The psi rating of an EID is important because it may affect the type of filter being used or the ability of the unit to infuse fluids through arterial lines. The pressure exerted should not exceed the pressure the filter can withstand because otherwise a rupture may occur; when the pump is used for arterial infusion, the pressure must be high enough to overcome arterial pressure. Positive **pressure pumps** are used in most clinical settings.

Volumetric Infusion Pumps   With the volumetric pump, the unit calculates the volume delivered by measuring the volume displaced in a reservoir that is a component of the disposable administration set. The mechanism of action may be piston generated or **linear**.

Computer-Generated Technology

The computer has become the focal point of the IV drug delivery system. Electronic flow is now the norm rather than the exception. EIDs today are available in diverse sizes and technologies for a broad range of purposes. Accompanying these computerized systems is a whole new lexicon of terms with which the nurse must become familiar to use the equipment safely and properly. For example, commonly heard terms include *tapering* or **ramping**, which describe the progressive increase or decrease of infusion rate. Another common term is **free flow**. Free-flow alarms may be life saving if the administration set has no intrinsic valves or reservoirs that require motion of the pumping mechanism to propel the fluid. Many pumps incorporate free-flow alarms that are capable of detecting open flow of fluid to the patient. Others have internal clamps or devices that lock into place when tubing is removed from the pump, preventing free flow of fluid to the patient. Other safety features are available on a number of products.

Compared with a smart pump, an IV medication safety system offers a technology platform that can provide harm- and dose-error reduction software across multiple types of infusion devices. This type of system integrates infusion and patient monitoring modules using a common user interface. It may even be networked with a hospital's information technology system, providing immediate access to data and accelerating best practice and process improvements. (Vanderveen, 2004)

Equipment Safety and Use

ECRI (Plymouth Meeting, PA), an independent, nonprofit agency that tests equipment for safety and effectiveness and continually designs new criteria for evaluation of equipment, is dedicated to improving the safety, efficacy, and cost effectiveness of health care technology, facilities, and procedures. Among the products assessed are EIDs from various manufacturers. The organization develops strict evaluation criteria aimed at helping care providers in the clinical setting perform with a high degree of safety and accuracy.

In relation to EIDs and infusion therapy, evaluation criteria are wide ranging to meet the needs of nursing staff in today's complex health care setting. The impact of downsizing and the integration of health care organizations has affected staffing patterns nationwide; therefore, nurses must be familiar with the literature and with the device to be used. They must take all precautions to ensure safe, efficient operation. One constant remains, however. The EID should never be used as a substitute for high-quality care and patient monitoring (see Chaps. 2 through 4).

Product Selection and Evaluation

Selection of equipment is a complex task. Hospitalized patients now receive a multitude of therapies through their vascular systems. The type of device used to initiate flow depends on the complexity of care, the range of required flow, pressure, the insertion site, and the delivery rate.

Product selection should be a serious consideration and should be based on needs assessed in the clinical setting. The ability to deliver a specified dose in μg/kg/minute, μg/kg/hour, mg/kg/minute, or mg/kg/hour by entering the appropriate concentration, patient weight, bolus amount, and mass units is a feature often required in the critical care setting. Demands for features such as bolus capabilities, syringe size sensing, and delivery in body weight, mass, continuous, or volume-over-time modes have challenged today's manufacturers to produce ever more advanced products.

Decision-Making Process

The product evaluation committee is usually involved in the selection of EIDs in the clinical setting. This focus should carry into the alternative care setting as well, so that the EIDs chosen clearly meet the patients' clinical and therapeutic needs while fulfilling a real function as accessories to high-quality IV nursing care. When selection is made by a group purchasing contract, nursing input is vital to the selection process.

Patient Selection and Education

Patients should be carefully evaluated for their ability to comprehend and perform self-care procedures, especially when EIDs are to be used. The patient should be taught how to wear the pump, how to operate and care for the equipment (pump and line as well), and what troubleshooting steps to take in case of technical problems (see Chap. 23).

References and Selected Readings

Asterisks indicate references cited in text.

Barnsteiner, J.H. (2005). Medication reconciliation: Transfer of medication information across settings—keeping it free from error. *Journal of Infusion Nursing, 28*(Suppl.), 31–36.

*Bates, D.W., Leape, L.L., & Petrycki, S. (1993). Incidence and preventability of adverse drug events in hospitalized adults. *Journal of General Internal Medicine, 8*(6):289–294.

*Beezhold, D.H., Sussman, G.L., Liss, G.M., et al. (1996). Latex allergy can induce clinical reactions to specific foods. *Clinical and Experimental Allergy, 26,* 416–422.

Blum, D.Y. (1995). Untoward events associated with use of midterm IV devices. *Journal of Intravenous Nursing, 18,* 116–119.

*Burke, K.G. (2005). The state of the science on safe medication administration symposium. http://www.nursingcenter.com. *American Journal of Nursing, 105*(Suppl.), 4–9.

*Cardo, D.M., Culver, D.H., & Ciesielski, C.A. (1997). A case-control study of HIV seroconversion in health care workers after percutaneous exposures. *New England Journal of Medicine, 177,* 1485–1490.

*Centers for Disease Control and Prevention (1998). Guidelines for prevention of intravascular infection. Atlanta, GA: Author.

Chiarello, L.A. (1995). Selection of needlestick prevention devices: A conceptual framework for approaching product evaluation. *American Journal of Infection Control, 23,* 386–395.

ECRI (1999). Needlestick prevention devices. *Health Devices, 28*(10), 381–407.

*Gaukroger, P.B., Robert, J.G., Manners, T.A. (1988). Infusion thrombophlebitis: A prospective comparison of 645 Vialon and Teflon cannulae in anaesthetic and postoperative use. *Anaesthesia and Intensive Care. 16,* 265–271

Goetz, A.N., Miller, J., Wagener, M.M., & Muder, R.R. (1998). Complications related to intravenous midline catheter usage. *Journal of Intravenous Nursing, 21,* 76–79.

*Gritter, M. (1999). Latex allergy: Prevention is the key. *Journal of Intravenous Nursing, 22,* 281–285.

Hanchett, M., & Kung, L. (1999). Do needleless intravenous systems increase the risk of infection? *Journal of Intravenous Nursing, 22,* 117–119.

Hatcher, I. Sullivan, M. Hutchinson, J. et al. (2004). An intravenous medication safety system: Preventing high-risk medication errors at the point of care. *Journal of Nursing Administration, 34*(10), 437–439.

*Hughes, R.G., Ortiz, E. (2005). Medication errors. *Journal of Infusion Nursing, 28*(Suppl.), 14–23.

*Infusion Nurses Society. (2005). Draft document. Revised Standards of Practice.

*Institute of Medicine. (1999). *To err is human: Building a safer health system.* Washington, DC. National Academy Press.

Institute for Safe Medication Administration. (2004). ISMP list of high alert medications. Available at: www.ismp.org/MSAarticles/highalert.htm. Accessed August 15, 2005.

International Health Care Worker Safety Center (1997). Uniform needlestick and sharp-object injury report. *Advances in Exposure Prevention, 3*(2), 15–16.

*Intravenous Nurses Society. (1998). Revised intravenous nursing standards of practice. *Journal of Intravenous Nursing, 21*(Suppl. 1), 41–45, 46, 50.

*Ippolito, G., Puro, V., & Petrosillo, N. (1997). *Prevention, management and chemoprophylaxis of occupational exposure to HIV* (p. 12). Charlottesville, VA: International Health Care Worker Safety Center, University of Virginia.

Luebke, M.A., Arduino, M.J., & Duda, T.E. (1998). Comparison of microbial properties of a needleless and a conventional needle-based intravenous access system. *American Journal of Infection Control, 26,* 431–436.

*Maki, D.G., Ringer, M. (1991). Risk factors for infusion-related phlebitis with small peripheral venous catheters: A randomized controlled trial. *Annals of Internal Medicine, 114,* 845–854.

*McKee, J.M., Shell, J.A., Warren, T.A., Campbell, V.P. (1989). Complications of intravenous therapy: A randomized prospective study—Vialon vs. Teflon. *Journal of Intravenous Nursing, 12*(5), 288–295.

*Metheny, N.M. (2000). *Fluid and electrolyte balance* (4th ed.). Philadelphia: Lippincott Williams & Wilkins.

Morimoto, T., Gandhi, T.K., Seger, A.C., et al. (2004). Adverse drug events and medication errors: Detection and classification systems. *Quality & Safety in Health Care, 13,* 306–314.

*National Institute for Occupational Safety and Health. (1997). *NIOSH alert: Preventing allergic reactions to natural rubber latex in the workplace* (Publication 97-135). Washington, DC: Author.

National Symposium on Patient Safety (1999). Consensus Development Conference. Washington, DC.

*Nicholas, P.K., Agius, C.R. (2005). Toward safer IV medication administration. *Journal of Infusion Nursing, 28*(Suppl.), 25–30.

*Occupational Safety and Health Administration. (1998). Occupational Safety and Health Administration docket no. H370A: Occupational exposure to bloodborne pathogens; request for information. *Federal Register, 63*(174), 48250–48252.

*Patient Safety Press. http://www.medicalnewstoday.com/medicalnews.php?newsid=11856. Accessed January 4, 2006.

*Pugliese, G. (2004). *Sharps injuries.* Chicago: American Hospital Publishing.

Schneider, P.J. (Ed.). (2004). Addressing harm with high-risk drug administration. *Hospitals & Health Networks, 78*(Suppl), 18–20.

*Stanley, M.D., Meister, E., Fuschuber, K. (1992). Infiltration during intravenous therapy in neonates: Comparison of Teflon and Vialon catheters. *Journal of the Southern Medical Association; 85*(9), 883–886.

*Tereskerz, P.M., Bentley, M., Coyner, B.J., & Jagger, J. (1996). Percutaneous injuries in health care workers. *Advances in Exposure Prevention, 2*(5), 1–3.

*Tokars, J.I., Marcus, R., Culver, D.H., Schable, C.A., McKibben, P.S., Bandea, C.I., Bell, D.M. (1993). Surveillance of HIV infection and zidovudine use among health-care workers after occupational exposure to HIV-infected blood. *Annals of Internal Medicine, 118*, 913–919.

United States Pharmacopeia [USP]. (1999). (26th ed., pp. 803, 1027). Easton, PA: Mack Publishing.

*U.S. Food and Drug Administration. (1996). Latex containing devices; user labeling; proposed rules. *Federal Register, 61*, 32618–32621.

U.S. Public Health Service. (1998). Guidelines for the management of healthcare worker exposures to HIV and recommendations for post-exposure prophylaxis. *Morbidity and Mortality Weekly Report Reports and Recommendations, 47* (RR-7).

*Vanderveen, T. (2004). Variability in IV Therapy: A 65-hospital analysis of IV best practices. In: Schneider, P.J. (Ed.). Infusion safety: Addressing harm with high-risk drug administration. *Hosp Health Networks 78* (Suppl.), 18–20.

*Vanderveen, T. (2005) How IV safety systems have prevented medication errors. *Journal of Infusion Nursing, 28*(Suppl.), 40–41.

*Warshaw, E.M. (1998). Latex allergy. *Journal of the American Academy of Dermatology, 38*, 1–24.

*Whittington, J., Cohen, H. (2004). OSF Healthcare's journey in patient safety. *Quality Management in Health Care, 13*(1), 53–59.

*Wilson, K., Sullivan, M. (2004). Preventing medication errors with smart infusion technology. *American Journal of Health-System Pharmacy, 61*(2), 177–183.

Review Questions

Note: Questions below may have more than one right answer.

1. Which of the following factors should be considered in selecting IV equipment?

   A. Latex-free components

   B. Safety design

   C. Performance

   D. All of the above

2. The porosity rating of an inline IV filter is what size in micrometers (μm)?

   A. 0.2

   B. 0.5

   C. 1.0

   D. 1.2

3. Which of the following statements is true concerning syringe delivery of medication?

   A. The limiting feature in adult patients is volume.

   B. It is a fluid container when used with a syringe-loaded EID.

   C. A only

   D. A and B

4. Preferred IV drug delivery systems include which of the following?

   A. Manufacturer-prepared

   B. Point-of-care–activated

   C. Pharmacy-based admixture

   D. Volume-control chambers

5. Which of the following statements is true concerning hypovolemic patients?

    A. Plasma and blood must be delivered rapidly.

    B. Plasma and blood must be delivered slowly.

    C. Rate of infusion decreases with increased blood pressure.

    D. Rate of infusion increases with changes in blood pressure.

6. An initial hydrating fluid to test kidney function is administered at 8 mL/m^2/minute over how many minutes?

    A. 10

    B. 30

    C. 45

    D. 60

7. Latex fluid is composed of which of the following?

    A. Carbohydrates

    B. Lipids and phospholipids

    C. A only

    D. A and B

8. Which of the following systems may reduce the incidence of needlestick injuries?

    A. Needleless

    B. Filters

    C. Luer locks

    D. Universal connectors

9. Examples of sharps involved in IV practice include which of the following?

    A. Lancets

    B. Needles

    C. V catheters

    D. B and C

10. Type I latex reactions manifested by the respiratory system include which of the following?

    A. Angioedema, respiratory arrest

    B. Shortness of breath

    C. Cyanosis and wheezing

    D. Laryngeal edema, wheezing

CHAPTER 12

Peripheral Infusion Therapy Techniques

KEY TERMS

Arteriospasm

Arteriovenous Fistula

Axillary Dissection

Fear Cascade

Sympathetic Reaction

Syncope

Vasovagal Reaction

Approach to Preparation

How the nurse approaches the patient about to receive IV therapy may have a direct bearing on that patient's response to treatment. Because an undesirable response can affect the patient's ability to accept treatment, the nurse's manner and attitude are significant factors.

Although routine for the nurse, IV therapy may be a new and frightening experience for any patient unfamiliar with the procedure. Various factors enter into the patient's perception of IV therapy, including accounts in the mass media, rumors related to errors or fatalities, or simple miscommunications. The nurse who provides a careful explanation of the procedure does much to alleviate fear and ensure patient compliance. Considerations in preparing the patient for the procedure may be found in Box 12–1.

Clinical Conditions

The critically ill patient is particularly susceptible to fears, which can sometimes become exaggerated, triggering an undesirable autonomic nervous system response

---

BOX 12–1   Considerations in Preparing the Patient for IV Therapy

- Patient's clinical condition
- Type of therapy ordered
- Duration of treatment
- Patient's experience level and IV history
- Other treatment modalities
- Vascular assessment

---

known as the **vasovagal reaction,** which may manifest itself as **syncope.** In many cases, the nurse can prevent the vasovagal response and consequent syncope by appearing confident and reassuring the patient.

It is desirable to prevent syncope to avoid the **sympathetic reaction** that may follow and result in vasoconstriction. The peripheral collapse attendant to vasoconstriction then limits the supply of available veins, which complicates venipuncture. Repeated attempts at venipuncture can result in an experience so traumatic as to affect the further course of IV therapy. Only a skilled clinician should perform a venipuncture on an anxious patient who has limited access and difficult veins. (See Chaps. 21 and 22 for special considerations for special populations.)

Exaggerated reactions to fear may trigger the **fear cascade** (Fig. 12–1). This result not only makes therapy difficult, but may constitute a real threat to the patient, particularly one with severe cardiac disease.

Type of Therapy Prescribed

The type of therapy ordered often dictates the plan of care. The ambulatory surgical patient has decidedly different educational needs than the critically ill patient with multiple IV accesses. If the patient will be involved in self-care and self-administration of IV medications and solutions, the approach must encourage and support the patient's independence and confidence. Plans for promoting self-care and independence should begin at the time of admission to the hospital or with the patient's first encounter with the IV service.

Duration of Therapy

A prolonged course of therapy requires multiple solutions, which makes preservation of the veins essential. Performing the venipuncture distally with each subsequent puncture proximal to the previous one and alternating arms contributes to venous preservation.

The patient's comfort also needs to be considered when solutions are required over an extended period. For instance, performing venipunctures on veins located on the dorsal surface of the extremities provides more freedom and comfort for the patient.

FIGURE 12–1.   The fear cascade.

Patient's Experience and IV History

Prior experience with IV therapy, good or bad, affects the patient's acceptance of treatment. If venipuncture by an experienced clinician has been a positive experience for the patient, he or she may feel more comfortable and relaxed. If the patient's history includes complications associated with IV therapy, venipuncture may be difficult.

Other Treatment Modalities

Use of multiple clinical modalities (ie, nutritional support, antibiotics, and transfusions) has a significant effect on preparations for IV therapy. In such cases, the clinician may consider using a multilumen catheter so that administration of subsequent medications can be timed to avoid interference with the line providing nutrition or the line providing transfusion therapy. Other concerns include non-IV therapies. For example, if the patient is also undergoing physical or occupational therapy, the nurse may find it difficult to use the hand veins for an IV line because such placement makes maintaining secure, dry connections and a tightly sealed dressing difficult.

Vascular Assessment

Initially, the nurse makes a vascular assessment. If findings confirm that limited vascular access precludes successful venipuncture and long-term treatment, consideration should be given to the proposed course of therapy and use of alternative access devices, such as a midline or peripherally inserted central catheter (PICC). Then, after ensuring the patient's privacy and comfort, the nurse implements various procedures, including hand washing, making sure to avoid an **arteriovenous fistula** or graft inserted for dialysis (because catheterization of a graft or fistula is determined by institutional policy), and avoiding the dependent extremity of a patient who has had a mastectomy or cerebral vascular accident. See Chapters 13 and 14.

Considerations for Vein Selection

The selection of the vein may be a deciding factor in the success of the infusion and the preservation of veins for subsequent treatment (Table 12–1). The most prominent vein is not necessarily the most suitable for venipuncture. Prominence may result from a sclerosed condition, which occludes the lumen and interferes with the flow of solution, or the prominent vein may be located in an area impractical for infusion purposes. Scrutiny of the veins in both arms is desirable before a choice is made. The prime factors to be considered in selecting a vein are

- Suitable location
- Condition of the vein
- Purpose of the infusion
- Duration of therapy

Location

Most superficial veins are accessible for venipuncture (Fig. 12–2), but some of these veins, because of their location, are not practical. For example, the antecubital veins are a poor choice for routine therapy because they are located over an area of joint flexion where any motion could dislodge the IV catheter and cause infiltration or result in mechanical phlebitis. If these large veins are impaired or damaged, phlebothrombosis may occur, which can limit access to the many available hand veins. The antecubital veins offer excellent sources for withdrawing blood and may be used many times without damage to the vein, provided good technique and sharp needles are used. However, one infusion of long duration may traumatize the vein, limiting

TABLE 12–1   Site Selection: Superficial Veins of the Arm

Vein	Location	Device	Considerations
Cephalic	Radial aspect of lower arm along radial bone of forearm	18- to 22-gauge cannula; usually ONC	Large vein, easily accessed Start distal and work upward Good for infusing blood or chemically irritating drugs
Basilic	Ulnar aspect of lower arm along the ulnar bone	18- to 22-gauge ONC	Difficult to access Large vein, easily palpated Stabilize during venipuncture
Accessory cephalic	Branches off cephalic vein along radial bone	18- to 22-gauge ONC	Medium–large vein, easily stabilized Valves at cephalic junction may inhibit catheterization Short length may require short (1-inch) catheter
Upper cephalic	Radial aspect of upper arm above elbow	16- to 20-gauge ONC	Difficult to visualize Good site for confused patients
Median antebrachial	Extends up front of forearm from median antecubital	18- to 22-gauge ONC	Nerve endings preclude cannulation Infiltration may occur
Median basilic	Ulnar aspect of forearm	18- to 22-gauge ONC	Appropriate site
Median cubital	Radial aspect of forearm	18- to 22-gauge ONC	Appropriate site
Antecubital fossa	Bend of elbow	Any size; may be used for midline or peripherally inserted central catheter insertion	Best for emergency interventions

ONC, over-the-needle catheter.

the availability of vessels that most readily provide ample quantities of blood when needed. Because of the proximity of the arteries to the veins in the antecubital fossa, special care must be taken to prevent intra-arterial injection when medications are introduced.

Aberrant arteries in the antecubital area are present in 1 of 10 people. When a patient complains of severe pain in the hand or arm on infusion, an **arteriospasm** caused by an intra-arterial injection is to be suspected, and the infusion must be stopped immediately.

Surgery often dictates which extremity can be used. Veins should be avoided in the arm on the same side as an **axillary dissection,** as in radical mastectomy, because the circulation may be impaired, affecting the flow of the infusion and increasing edema. When the patient is turned sideways during the operation, the upper arm is used for the IV infusion; increased venous pressure in the lower arm may interfere with free flow of the solution.

FIGURE 12–2. IV placement chart. (Courtesy of Becton Dickinson Vascular Access, Sandy, UT.)

Use of the veins in the lower extremities usually depends on a physician order because of the danger of pulmonary embolism caused by a thrombus extending into the deep veins. Complications may also arise from the stagnant blood in varicosities, which makes them susceptible to trauma. In addition, pooling of infused medications in stagnant blood can cause untoward reactions when drug concentrations reach toxic levels in circulating blood.

Guidelines from the Centers for Disease Control and Prevention (CDC) strongly recommend using upper-extremity veins in adult patients, or if necessary, subclavian and jugular sites (CDC, 2000). Guidelines of the Infusion Nurses Society (INS) support that premise (INS, 1998, 2000, 2005).

Condition of the Vein

Frequently, the dorsal metacarpal veins provide points of entry that should be used first to preserve the proximal veins for further therapy. The use of these veins depends on their condition. In some elderly patients, the dorsal metacarpal veins may be a poor choice; blood extravasation occurs more readily in small, thin veins, and it may be difficult to secure the catheter adequately because of thin skin and lack of supportive tissue. At times, these veins do not dilate sufficiently to allow for successful venipuncture; when hypovolemia occurs, the peripheral veins collapse more quickly than do larger, more proximal ones.

Palpation of the vein is an important step in determining the condition of the vein and in differentiating it from a pulsating artery. A thrombosed vein may be detected by its lack of resilience; its hard, cordlike feeling; and by the ease with which it rolls. Use of such traumatized veins results in repeated attempts at venipuncture, pain, and undue stress.

Occasionally, when thrombosis from multiple infusions interferes with the flow of solution and limits available veins, the venipuncture may be performed with the catheter inserted in the direction of the distal end. Lack of valves in these small peripheral veins permits rerouting of the solution and bypassing of the involved vein.

Often, large veins may be detected by palpation and offer advantages over the smaller but more readily discernible veins. Because of the small blood volume, the more superficial veins may not be easily palpated and may not make a satisfactory choice for venipuncture.

Continual use by the nurse of the same fingers for palpation increases their sensitivity. The thumb should never be used because it is not as sensitive as the fingers; also, a pulse may be detected in the nurse's thumb, and this may be confused with an aberrant artery.

Although not apparent, edema may conceal an available vein; application of finger pressure for a few seconds may help to disperse the fluid and define the vein.

Purpose of the Infusion

The purpose of the infusion dictates the rate of flow and the solution to be infused—two factors that inherently affect the selection of the vein. When large quantities of fluid are to be rapidly infused, or when positive pressure is indicated, a large vein must be used. When fluids with a high viscosity, such as packed red blood cells, are required, a vein with an adequate volume of flow is necessary to ensure flow of the solution.

Large veins are used when hypertonic solutions or solutions containing irritating drugs are to be infused. Such solutions traumatize small veins; the supply of blood in these veins is not sufficient to dilute the infused fluid. Large vessels provide better hemodilution of the drug or solution, thereby minimizing the potential for developing phlebitis.

Venous Distention

Special care must be taken to distend the vein adequately. To achieve this, a soft, preferably latex-free, tourniquet is applied with enough pressure to impede venous flow while maintaining arterial flow. If the radial pulse cannot be felt, the tourniquet is too tight.

To fill the veins to capacity, apply pressure until radial pulsation ceases and then release pressure until pulsation begins. A blood pressure cuff may be used; inflate the cuff and then release it until the pressure drops to just below the diastolic pressure.

The tourniquet is applied to the midforearm if the selected vein is in the dorsum of the hand. If the selected vein is in the forearm, the tourniquet is applied to the upper arm.

Very little pressure is applied when performing venipuncture on patients with sclerosed veins. If the pressure is too great or the tourniquet is left on for an extended time, the vein becomes hard and tortuous, causing added difficulty when the catheter is introduced. For some sclerosed veins, a tourniquet is unnecessary and only makes the phlebotomy more difficult (see considerations for the geriatric patient in Chap. 22).

If pressure exerted by the tourniquet does not fill the veins sufficiently, the patient may be asked to open and close his or her fist. This action of the muscles forces the blood into the veins, causing them to distend considerably more. A light tapping usually fills the vein. It may be helpful, before applying the tourniquet, to lower the extremity below the heart level to increase the blood supply to the veins. On occasions when these methods are inadequate to fill the vein sufficiently, application of heat helps. To be effective, the heat must be applied to the entire extremity for 10 to 20 minutes and must be retained until the venipuncture is performed (see Table 12–1).

Considerations Before Beginning the Infusion

Selecting the Device

Many diverse infusion devices are available; particular consideration should be given to the use of safety equipment. See Chapter 11 for an extensive discussion of safety devices for IV access.

Ensuring Secure and Optimal Environment

Proper lighting is very important and should not be overlooked. A few extra seconds spent in obtaining adequate light may actually save time and free the patient from unnecessary venipunctures. The ideal light is either ample daylight or a spotlight that does not shine directly on the vein, but leaves enough shadow for clearly defining the vessel.

Checking Solution and Container

Careful inspection is necessary to ensure that the fluid is clear and free of particulates and the container intact—with no cracks in the glass bottle or holes in the plastic bag. The label must be checked to verify that the correct solution is being used and that the container is not outdated. The nurse also needs to check the time and the date the container was opened. After 24 hours, the fluid is outdated and should not be used (see Chap. 4). Hang time is determined in institutional policy.

Attaching Administration Set to Fluid Container

The nurse attaches the IV administration set to the solution container by closing the roller clamp to equalize pressure, squeezing the drip chamber, and inserting the set into the container with a thrust, not a twisting motion. The drip chamber is released, causing the air vent to function immediately and the drip chamber to fill on suspension of the container. This prevents the fluid from leaking through the air vent and clears the infusion set of air, thereby preventing bubbles from entering the tubing. In systems that do not require air venting—plastic and semirigid containers—squeezing the drip chamber before insertion avoids the subsequent introduction of air into the container.

Establishing Height of the Fluid Container

The nurse suspends the fluid container approximately 3 feet above the injection site. The pressure from this height is adequate to ensure a maximum flow rate. The greater the height of the container, the greater the force with which the fluid flows into the vein should the flow-control clamp release, and the greater the risk of speed shock.

Ensuring Privacy and Comfort

The nurse may ask visitors to leave the room during the procedure and close bedside curtains if the patient has a roommate. The patient should be in a comfortable position with the arm on a flat surface. If necessary, a strip of tape can be used to secure the arm to an arm board to prevent an uncooperative or disoriented patient from jerking the arm during catheter insertion.

If the area selected for venipuncture is hairy, clipping the hair permits better cleansing of the skin and makes removal of the catheter less painful when the infusion is terminated. Shaving is not recommended, consistent with INS standards (INS, 1998, 2000). Products such as Skin-Prep decrease bacterial flora and may be considered for use before venipuncture.

Applying Anesthetic Products

Eutectic mixture of local anesthetics (EMLA; Astra Pharmaceuticals, Westborough, MA) is a cream mixture of two local anesthetics (lidocaine 2.5% and prilocaine 2.5%). If appropriate, EMLA may be applied to the skin under an occlusive dressing. The release of lidocaine and prilocaine into the epidermal and dermal layers of the skin provides anesthesia. The two agents stabilize neuronal membranes by inhibiting the conduction of impulses (Astra Pharmaceuticals, 1997). Use of the product is contraindicated in patients with a known history of sensitivity to local amide anesthetics (Procedure 12–1).

Between 1 and 2 mg of topical nitroglycerin (Nitro-Bid; Hoechst Marion Roussel, Kansas City, MO) may also be applied. Studies indicate that this product distends the veins without the need for tapping, pumping the hand, or clenching the

PROCEDURE 12.1
Applying EMLA Cream

Equipment

Antiseptic skin cleanser

Sterile wipes or sponges

EMLA cream

Occlusive dressing

Action	*Rationale*
1. Cleanse skin with antiseptic.	1. Prevents risk of infection
2. Apply 2.5 g EMLA cream thickly at intended site.	2. Ensures covering entire dermal at surface
3. Place an occlusive dressing over the EMLA cream and smooth edges of the dressing. Keep dressing in place until it is time for venipuncture.	3. Ensures occlusion
4. Record application time.	4. Ensures appropriate absorption time and documentation of procedure

fist. Alternatively, some professionals advocate administering intradermal lidocaine before venipuncture. This is done with 0.1 to 0.2 mL of 1% lidocaine and a tuberculin syringe. Lidocaine may, however, expose the patient to allergic reaction, anaphylaxis, inadvertent injection of the drug into the vascular system, and obliteration of the vein.

Considerations for Venipuncture Procedure

Variations in direct and indirect methods are described in Table 12–2. The injection site should be scrubbed with an antiseptic that remains in contact with the skin for at least 30 seconds before venipuncture. An appropriate single-dose antiseptic agent should be used. Avoid aqueous benzalkonium-like compounds or hexachlorophene. Recommended agents include chlorhexidine, 10% povidone-iodine, alcohol, or 2% tincture of iodine. If the vein has sustained a through puncture (evidenced by a developing hematoma) and the venipuncture is unsuccessful, the catheter should be immediately removed and pressure applied to the site.

TABLE 12–2   Comparing Approaches to Venipuncture

Direct (One Step)	Indirect (Two Complete Motions)
Nurse thrusts catheter through skin and into vein with quick motion.	Nurse inserts catheter through skin below the point where vein is visible but above the vein.
Catheter enters directly over the vein.	This approach depresses the vein, obscuring its position.
Direct technique is not suitable for small veins because of potential for hematoma formation.	The catheter is adjacent to the vein, but has not penetrated the vessel wall. Gently locate the vein, decrease catheter angle, and enter the vessel.

 SAFE PRACTICE ALERT Allow antiseptic agent to air dry. If using povidone-iodine as the primary antiseptic agent, do not apply alcohol, as it will negate povidone-iodine's antimicrobial effect. If using alcohol as a single agent, apply for a minimum of 30 seconds. If using tincture of iodine, allow it to dry, then remove with alcohol and allow it to dry.

 SAFE PRACTICE ALERT Never reapply a tourniquet to the extremity immediately after a venipuncture; a hematoma will occur, limiting veins and providing an excellent culture medium for bacteria.

Anchoring the Device

Once the catheter is in place, the nurse needs to make sure it stays securely in place and safe from dislodgment. This involves a special taping technique.

TAPING

Using half-inch-wide tape over the hub of the catheter, the nurse anchors the device flush with the skin. No elevation of the hub is necessary because this would only increase the risk of puncturing through the vein (known as a *through puncture*) with the point of the introducer needle.

After placing a half-inch strip of tape—adhesive up—under the hub of the catheter, the nurse folds one end of the strip tightly and diagonally over the catheter and repeats the motion with the other end crossing the first end. This secures the catheter firmly and prevents any sideways movement. Tape should not be placed directly over the injection site.

LOOPING THE TUBING

After the device is secured by tape, the IV tubing is looped to relieve tension and secured with tape independent of the catheter tape. This prevents dislodging the catheter by an accidental pull on the tubing.

KEY INTERVENTIONS: A Step-by-Step Approach to Basic Venipuncture

1. To ensure sterility of field, wash hands and put on gloves before applying tourniquet.
2. Select appropriate site that will best enhance venous distention.
3. Prepare skin according to recommendations consistent with INS Standards of Practice.
4. Establish minimum rate of flow. To do this, adjust clamp. Then kink infusion tubing between third and fourth fingers of the dominant hand. (When the kinked tubing is released, the minimum rate of flow prevents the rapid fluid or drug infusion that has the potential to induce speed shock. (*Note: the tubing may also be kinked by placing it through the slots on the roller clamp.*)
5. Hold patient's hand or arm with other hand using your thumb to keep skin taut. This helps to anchor the vein and prevent rolling.
6. Align steel introducer needle with the vein, approximately one-half inch from entry site. Keeping the needle in bevel-up position facilitates venipuncture and is atraumatic. (*Note: In some cases, the bevel-down approach may be used in small veins to avoid extravasation. Then readjustment may be made before releasing the tourniquet to prevent puncturing the vein and producing a hematoma.*)
7. To ensure simultaneous entry through skin and tissue, insert the needle at a 45° angle.
8. Relocate vein and decrease angle slightly to minimize trauma.
9. Then, slowly (with a downward motion) pick up the vein. Doing this levels the introducer needle and catheter almost flush with the skin.
10. Watch for a flashback of blood, which may indicate successful entry. Also anticipate both a sense of increased resistance when the catheter meets the wall of the vein and a snap felt at the loss of resistance as the catheter enters the vein.
11. Release tourniquet, remove introducer needle, and activate the needleless cover (see Chap. 11 for information concerning safety devices). The catheter may then be advanced manually or with infusing fluid.
12. Release pressure exerted by little finger (Step 4).
13. Connect administration set to hub and release kinked tubing to initiate flow.
14. Check injection site for swelling.

DRESSING AND DOCUMENTING

An occlusive dressing is applied over the catheter entrance site to allow for routine, standardized inspection. The type, gauge, insertion date, and nurse's initials are written on tape near the dressing and documented in the clinical record. Variations in taping are shown in Figure 12–3.

Other Securement Devices

Other securement devices may also be used. A number of manufacturers provide these products to meet ongoing needs for quality infusion care.

ARM BOARDS

An arm board may be helpful for immobilizing the extremity when undue motion can result in infiltration or phlebitis. It is a valuable aid in restraining the arm when infusions

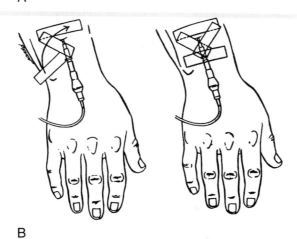

FIGURE 12–3. Variations in taping. **(A)** Chevron taping technique. **(B)** Taping variations for over-the-needle catheters.

are initiated on uncooperative, disoriented, or elderly patients or children, or when the catheter is inserted on the dorsum of the hand or in an area of joint flexion.

When the metacarpal veins are used, the fingers should be immobilized to prevent any movement of the catheter that could result in phlebitis. This complication results from failure to recognize that the hand has both transverse and longitudinal arches and that if the knuckle joints (metacarpophalangeal) are immobilized in a straight position, they develop motion-preventing contracture. Patients who are receiving long-term therapy and who have edema or muscular weakness are particularly vulnerable. Intensive physical therapy, splinting, and even surgery may be required to restore mobility.

To preserve maximal function, the hand should be immobilized in a functional position on the arm board. If a plastic arm board is used, the nurse can cover it with absorbent paper or a bandage to prevent the arm from perspiring and sticking to the board. Any tape placed on the catheter must be independent of the board so that a motion of the arm on the board does not cause a pull on the catheter. If the arm must be restrained, the restraint is secured to the board, not to the patient's arm above the puncture area. Such restraint might act as a tourniquet, causing a backflow of blood into the catheter and resulting in clotting and obstruction of the flow. Arm board design has changed dramatically, and many manufacturers now provide sophisticated devices aimed at ensuring patient comfort.

⚠ SAFE PRACTICE ALERT The function of the hand may be endangered and even permanently impaired by the widespread practice of flattening the hand on an arm board during infusion therapy.

DRESSINGS

Consistent with INS Standards of Practice, an occlusive dressing should be applied over the infusion site. The occlusive dressing may be gauze or tape, or a transparent, semipermeable membrane dressing. Follow manufacturer's recommendations for the use of all transparent dressings (Fig. 12–4).

Infusion sites should be labeled with type of catheter (Fig. 12–5), length and size, date, time, and initials of the person who initiated the infusion. Many labels are available to facilitate this practice (Fig. 12–6).

FIGURE 12–4.   Using a dressing such as the Tegaderm IV transparent dressing allows the IV nurse to see the injection site without removing the dressing. (Courtesy of 3M, Minneapolis, MN.)

FIGURE 12–5. Labeling of the venipuncture site consistent with INS standards. (Courtesy of United Ad Label Co., Inc., Brea, CA.)

IV Dressing Changed
Date _____ Initial _____
Catheter size _____
Next change due _____

IV246 Fl. Pink

Intrathecal Catheter No IV Access	Intrathecal Catheter No IV Access

IV247 Fl. Green

HEPARIN LOCK
Device _____ Size: _____
Inserted: Date _____ Time: _____
Init _____

IV214 Fl. Yellow

CAUTION Epidural Catheter No IV Access	CAUTION Epidural Catheter No IV Access

IV248 Fl. Red

DATE:
TIME:
GAUGE:
NAME:

IV251 White

P.I.C.C. Peripherally Inserted Central Catheter	P.I.C.C. Peripherally Inserted Central Catheter

IV249 Fl. Yellow

HEPARIN FLUSH _____ UNITS

IV111 Fl. Red

SALINE FLUSH

IV110 Fl. Green

WRAP AROUND IV TUBING	IV TUBING CHANGED Date _____ Hr. _____ By _____

IV407 Fl. Orange

FIGURE 12–6. Variety of labels used to identify catheter sites, types, dressings, and other products and procedures.

Describe relevant anatomy/physiology	Meets expectations	Needs education
Skin	☐	☐
Layers of vein	☐	☐
Venous and arterial system	☐	☐
Determine appropriate placement of device		
Length and duration of therapy	☐	☐
Age and clinical condition	☐	☐
Verbalizes factors influencing selection	☐	☐
Verifies physician order		
Type, rate, volume to be delivered	☐	☐
Isotonic, hypertonic, hypotonic	☐	☐
Rate and volume	☐	☐
Inspects integrity of equipment		
Fluid container	☐	☐
Administration set	☐	☐
Infusion device, accessories	☐	☐
Performs successful venipuncture (initial attempt)		
One attempt per device (success rate >85%)	☐	☐
Implements Standards of Practice		
Occlusive dressing application	☐	☐
Ongoing monitoring	☐	☐
Site rotation	☐	☐
Set changes	☐	☐

FIGURE 12–7. Performance checklist for IV therapy.

Techniques associated with infusion therapy remain consistent throughout the clinical settings in which care is delivered. Adherence to institutional guidelines and Standards of Practice ensures good-quality outcomes. Figure 12–7 provides a performance checklist.

RESEARCH ISSUES: Advantages of Securement Devices

Sheppard, K., LeDesma, M., Morris, N., & O'Connor, K. (1999). A prospective study of two intravenous catheter securement techniques in a skilled nursing facility. *Journal of Intravenous Nursing, 22*(3), 151–153.

In this prospective, controlled study in a skilled nursing facility, the authors determined IV dwell times and outcomes associated with a securement device. The device resulted in significantly longer average catheter dwell times (3.95 days vs. 2.45 days) and significantly fewer local complications (65 vs. 155). The securement device also reduced clinical time in managing vascular access by 13.5 minutes.

References and Selected Readings

Asterisks indicate references cited in text.

American Association of Blood Banks. (2003). *Technical manual* (13th ed., pp. 378, 456–458). Arlington, VA: Author.

*Astra Pharmaceuticals. (1997). Product literature. Westborough, MA: Author.

Banks, N. (1999). Positive outcome after looped peripherally inserted central catheter malposition. *Journal of Intravenous Nursing, 22*(1), 14–18.

*Centers for Disease Control and Prevention. (2000). *Guidelines for prevention of intravascular infection.* Atlanta, GA: Author.

*Intravenous Nurses Society. (1998). Revised intravenous nursing standards of practice. *Journal of Intravenous Nursing, 21*(Suppl. 1), S53–58.

*Infusion Nurses Society. (2005). Draft revised Standards of Practice.

Lopez, V., Molassiotis, A., Chan, W.-K., Ng, F., & Wong, E. (2004) An intervention study to evaluate nursing management of peripheral intravascular devices. *Journal of Infusion Nursing, 27*(5),322–344.

Mazzola, J.R., Schott-Baer, D., & Addy, L. (1999). Clinical factors associated with the development of phlebitis after insertion of a peripherally inserted central catheter. *Journal of Intravenous Nursing, 22*(1), 36–39.

Metheny, N.M. (2000). *Fluid and electrolyte balance* (5th ed.). Philadelphia: Lippincott Williams & Wilkins.

Pierce, C., & Baker, J.J. (2004). A nursing process model: Quantifying infusion therapy resource consumption. *Journal of Infusion Nursing, 27*(4), 232–234.

*Sheppard, K., Ledesma, M., Morris, N., & O'Connor, K. (1999). A prospective study of two intravenous catheter securement techniques in a skilled nursing facility. *Journal of Intravenous Nursing, 22*(3), 151–153.

3M Corporation. (1999). Product literature. Minneapolis, MN.

Review Questions

Note: Questions below may have more than one right answer.

1. The term *vasovagal reaction* refers to an autonomic nervous system response to:

   A. Stress

   B. Fluid resuscitation

   C. Sudden hydration

   D. Circulatory overload

2. Appropriate actions for the nurse to take if a patient's veins do not become prominent after application of a tourniquet include all of the following *except:*

   A. Asking the patient to pump his or her hand

   B. Placing the extremity in a dependent position

   C. Tapping the vein gently

   D. Tightening the tourniquet to restrict arterial flow

3. Which of the following is true concerning the height of the fluid container?

   A. Place 36 inches above the injection site

   B. Place 48 inches above the injection site

   C. The greater the height, the lower the force

   D. The lower the height, the greater the force

4. Which of the following veins should be assessed first to preserve veins for future use?

   A. Dorsal metacarpal

   B. Cephalic

   C. Basilic

   D. Digital

5. The dorsal metacarpal veins may be a poor choice in which of the following patients?

   A. Elderly

   B. Home care

   C. Diabetic

   D. Renal patient

6. A thrombosed vein may be detected by which of the following factors:

   A. Resilience

   B. Soft, pliable feel

   C. Cord-like feel

   D. Lack of resilience

7. Application of digital pressure applied to disperse fluid denotes presence of which of the following?

   A. Circulatory collapse

   B. Edema

   C. Hypertension

   D. All of the above

8. EMLA cream is a mixture of which of the following anesthetic agents?

   A. Lidocaine, Novocain, and prilocaine

   B. Novocain and lidocaine

   C. Prilocaine and Novocain

   D. Lidocaine and prilocaine

9. Before venipuncture, the injection site should be scrubbed with an antiseptic that is allowed to remain in contact with the skin for:

    A. 15 seconds

    B. 30 seconds

    C. 45 seconds

    D. 60 seconds

10. Dislodging of the catheter by an accidental pull may be a result of which of the following procedures?

    A. Looping the tubing

    B. Taping catheter flush with the skin

    C. Placing tape over the injection site

    D. All of the above

CHAPTER 13

Short Peripheral Access

KEY TERMS

Catheter Patency
Hypodermoclysis
Peripheral

Phlebotomy
Negative Fluid Displacement

Short Peripheral Catheters

Short peripherally placed catheters have long been the standard of care for short-term peripheral use and remain so today. The term *short peripheral catheter* denotes a product that is <3 inches long, although typically a 1-inch catheter is placed.

Insertion Techniques

Whether performing a basic IV insertion procedure or varying the procedure in accordance with the patient's condition or equipment available, the IV nurse's competence in performing peripheral IV therapy should be assessed periodically. Of course, the competent IV nursing professional should be able successfully to perform the procedure using aseptic technique. See Chapter 12.

Variations in insertion techniques are common and may depend on devices available (catheter products are covered completely in Chap. 11). This section addresses particular insertion techniques for some products. An ongoing challenge, particularly for the less experienced nurse, is identifying available veins for venipuncture. The

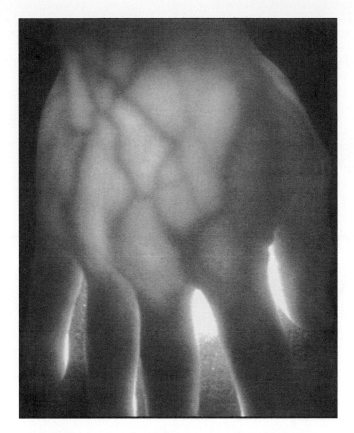

FIGURE 13–1.   Transhand illumination with IRIS Vascular Viewer. (Courtesy of InfraRed Imaging Systems, Inc.)

IRIS Vascular Viewer answers these clinical needs by providing direct, real-time visualization of vascular structures (Fig. 13–1). The inadequacies of current vascular access practices significantly compromise patient care and contribute to rising health care costs. Multiple access attempts and outright failures delay patient treatment, frustrate health care professionals, and increase the likelihood of downstream complications and expense (Fig. 13–2).

Closed Catheter Systems

Closed catheter systems, such as that offered by BD (Nexiva), offer greater insertion success, increased protection against blood exposure and accidental needlestick injuries, simplified processes, and enhanced patient safety and satisfaction (BD, 2005). Because the device is preassembled, there are fewer components involved and a reduced risk of in-use contamination. With a closed Luer access port, the nurse can ensure needleless administration of fluid and medication, in addition to venous sampling. The system is totally closed to contamination (BD, 2005), which has certainly facilitated safe practice. See Chapter 9 and Fig. 13–3.

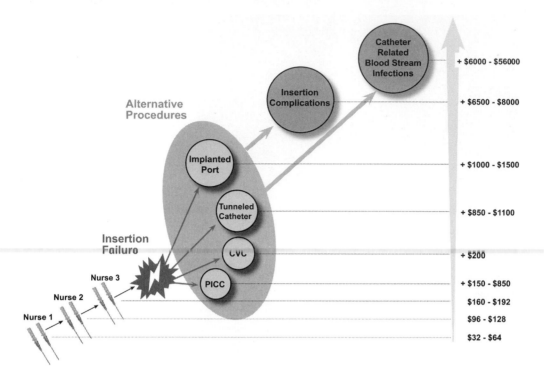

FIGURE 13–2.   For patients with indication for IV therapy, failure to place IVs can result in delayed therapy treatment, increased costs, and the prospect of complications. (Courtesy of InfraRed Imaging Systems, Inc.)

RyMed has developed the first needle-free IV connector designed to prevent **negative fluid displacement**, which causes the retrograde of the patient's blood within the catheter lumen. This is a variation on the typical needle-free injection port system aimed at minimizing error and ensuring safety. InVision-Plus is focused on minimizing the two most critical catheter management issues of the day: intraluminal thrombotic catheter occlusions and intraluminal catheter-related bloodstream infections. For example, an important key to reducing thrombotic catheter occlusions, particularly for intraluminal occlusions, is to prevent the retrograde flow of blood into the catheter lumen. See Boxes 13–1 and 13–2 and Fig. 13–4 concerning negative displacement.

A similar concern is the possibility of touch contamination (see Chap. 9). Again, RyMed has found a way to minimize the potential for touch contamination of the

---

BOX 13–1   Neutral Fluid Displacement: Ease of Use Advantages

- Eliminates the need for positive-pressure technique
- Eliminates the need for clamping and ends the confusion on whether or not to clamp during the connection to or disconnection from the IV connector system

Before Insertion

After Insertion

Shielded Needle

FIGURE 13–3.   Nexiva Closed Catheter System. (Courtesy and © of Becton, Dickinson and Company.)

catheter hub or vascular access device during initial setup or during the replacement of their InVision-Plus (Fig. 13–5). Figures 13–6 and 13–7 show further InVision details.

Maintaining **catheter patency** is critical to successful IV therapy outcomes. Many catheters are left indwelling for extended periods, often up to several years. During flushing procedures, at the time of syringe disconnection from the injection cap/port, blood can be drawn back into the catheter lumen. This can lead to catheter occlusion and disruption of therapy.

Clinicians have used a variety of methods known as positive-pressure flushing techniques over the years. In the last decade, needleless access injection systems have

---

BOX 13–2   Neutral Fluid Displacement: Flushing Advantages

- Flush using normal saline only or with heparin and saline
- Eliminates potential risk of heparin-induced thrombocytopenia (HIT)
- Potential cost savings to health care facility by elimination of heparin
- Improves the overall simplicity and ease of use

FIGURE 13–4.   Negative displacement. (Courtesy of RyMed Technologies, Inc.)

been introduced into infusion therapy process to offer the health care worker protection from accidental needlesticks. Although these devices have protected the health care worker, they have made ineffective some of the positive-pressure flushing techniques that nurses previously relied on. As a result, the incidence of catheter occlusion has increased. In the mid-1990s, several new devices were brought to the market with designs focused on overcoming this complication. These devices, known as positive-displacement needleless access caps/ports, have been shown to reduce the incidence of catheter occlusion (Table 13–1).

Insertion of the Over-the-Needle Catheter

To insert the over-the-needle catheter, the nurse puts on gloves, applies a tourniquet above the injection site, selects the vein, and prepares the injection site according to authorized recommendations. If palpation of the vein is necessary, the nurse prepares

FIGURE 13–5. InVision touch-free package and handling. (Courtesy of RyMed Technologies, Inc.)

FIGURE 13–6. InVision Long. (Courtesy of RyMed Technologies, Inc.)

FIGURE 13–7. Cutaway view of the InVision. (Courtesy of RyMed Technologies, Inc.)

TABLE 13–1   Positive Displacement

Practice	Product	Comments
Applying pressure to the syringe plunger on needle withdrawal from the injection cap/port		This technique was very effective when using small-bore needles to flush through a rubber injection cap, not as effective with large-bore plastic cannula, and not effective with Luer-activated valves.
Withdrawing flush syringe/needle from the injection cap/port during the infusion of the last 1 mL of flush solution		Not effective with needleless Luer-activated valves.
Engaging the clamp on the catheter or extension set prior to syringe disconnection from the injection cap/port		This requires the presence of an extension set and clamp, and it is effective only as long as the clamp is left engaged.
	Positive-displacement Luer access valve products	These products consist of a reservoir that empties into the catheter lumen on disconnection of the syringe. The displacement volume is variable depending on the product and may not be adequate to overcome the volume of reflux.
Syringes designed to reduce syringe-induced reflux		BD Medical offers a specially designed syringe (BD PosiFlush), which reduces the impact of rebound as the plunger bottoms out into the syringe barrel.

the fingertip in the same manner. Without touching the proposed insertion site, the nurse performs the venipuncture in the usual manner and proceeds as follows:

1. Once the needle has punctured the venous wall, introduce the needle ½ inch farther to ensure entry of the catheter into the lumen of the vein.
2. Hold the needle in place and slowly slide the catheter hub until the desired length is in the vein. If the venipuncture is unsuccessful, do not reinsert the needle into the catheter. To do so can sever the catheter.
3. Remove the needle by holding the catheter hub in place. To minimize leakage of blood while removing the needle and connecting the infusion set, apply pressure on the vein beyond the catheter with the little finger.
4. Attach the IV administration set, which has been previously cleared of air, and regulate the flow rate. A number of accessories are available to facilitate the process (Figs. 13-4 through 13-7).
5. Consider applying a topical antiseptic iodophor ointment, or a broad-spectrum antiseptic ointment for patients sensitive to iodine.
6. Tape the catheter securely to prevent motion that could contribute to phlebitis. However, avoid taping over the injection site. Then cover the site with a sterile gauze sponge or transparent, semipermeable dressing.
7. Loop the tubing and tape independent of the catheter to prevent an accidental pull from withdrawing the catheter.
8. Initial the tape close to the dressing and indicate the length, gauge, and type of catheter and the date of insertion. Document the procedure in the clinical record.
9. Remove gloves and wash hands.

Insertion of the Midline Catheter

Midline catheters were introduced in the 1950s and have undergone several transitions. Improvements in the early midline facilitated placement via a split-away plastic introducer. Currently, the design is 7 to 8 inches long and composed of polyurethane or silicone. The catheter may be placed in the basilic, cephalic, or median cubital veins of the upper arm or antecutital area, with the tip residing in the cephalic or basilic vein in the upper portion of the arm. The midline catheter is designed for peripheral infusion of general IV solutions and medications and for venous sampling. Indications for midline IV therapy include administration of antibiotics, hydration, pain medication, peripheral nutrition solutions of 12.5% or less final glucose concentration, and selected antineoplastic agents (excluding vesicants, which the Oncology Nursing Society recommends be infused through a central line). See Chapter 14.

The procedure should be performed using sterile technique, and only by experienced nurses with excellent IV insertion skills, and then only after careful consideration of the possible risks, including thrombosis, phlebitis, air embolism, infection, vascular perforation, bleeding, and catheter transection (see Chap. 11).

As with any venipuncture, adequate assessment of the patient and the venous status is essential to ensure success. The basilic vein is the vein of choice for longer-line IV insertions because of its larger size, straighter course, and adequate hemodilution capability.

Before insertion, the clinician should carefully select the vessel site and aseptically prepare it consistent with institutional policy and recommended INS Standards of Practice, then establish a sterile field and apply gloves. Again, the technique is specific

BOX 13–3   Procedure for Midline Catheter Insertion

1. Gather equipment and supplies.
2. Explain the procedure to the patient, including rationale for use.
3. Assist the patient in obtaining a comfortable supine position.
4. Extend the patient's arm, supporting it with a rolled towel.
5. Abduct the arm at a 45-degree angle.
6. Prepare the work area.
7. Position protective covering under the extremity.
8. Place the tourniquet on the mid-upper arm for vein assessment.
9. Clip the hair 8-10 inches from around the antecubital fossa.
10. Apply sterile gloves.
11. Flush the catheter with 0.9% sodium chloride solution.
12. Cleanse insertion area three times with alcohol swabsticks, starting at the insertion site (refer to Chap. 9).
13. Remove and discard gloves.
14. Apply tourniquet.
15. Apply new gloves.
16. Drape arm with fenestrated drape or sterile towels, leaving an opening for the venipuncture.
17. Perform venipuncture using manufacturer's recommended techniques.
18. Slowly advance catheter to desired initial length, intermittently flushing with 0.9% sodium chloride and alternating blood withdrawal to determine placement/return.
19. Continue to follow manufacturer's recommendations for the use of their product, consistent with INS Standards of Practice.
20. Remove tourniquet.
21. Attach administration set or cap and initiate infusion slowly while observing upper arm for swelling.
22. Secure consistent with institutional policy and established Standards of Practice.

Adapted from Perucca, R. (2001). Obtaining vascular access. In: Hankins, J. *Infusion therapy in clinical practice* (2nd ed., p. 382). Philadelphia: W.B. Saunders.

to the manufacturer's recommendations for the use of its product. Box 13–3 provides guidance for inserting a midline catheter.

Midline catheters came under scrutiny during the mid-1990s owing to adverse events related to anaphylaxis and phlebitis. The Landmark catheter (MenloCare, Menlo Park, CA), was removed from the market in 1997.

Those products currently being used are uncoated and inserted in the same manner as a PICC. See Chapter 14.

RESEARCH ISSUES: Financial Feasibility of Midline Catheters

Thomson, S. (1993). IV therapy: A financial feasibility study. *Nursing Management, 24,* 68A–G.

Thomson published a financial study comparing the use of midline catheters with use of multiple short peripheral catheters. The operational cost of placing a peripheral catheter was $24.06, which was confirmed by other studies (Kokotis K., Santolucito J.). In Thomson's study, the need for catheter rotation every 72 hours was eliminated, which resulted in nursing time and equipment cost savings.

Peripherally Inserted Central Catheter Placement

The INS has developed an extensive PICC Education Module for use by nurse instructors. The module contains a narrative outline and 179 slides to ensure consistency in the content of PICC presentations. The information in the module is based on INS Standards of Practice. Sample pretests and post-tests with answer sheets, a PICC insertion data collection form, competency/skills checklist, and a student syllabus are included. PICC placement is covered extensively in Chapter 14.

RESEARCH ISSUES: Advantages of Securement Devices

Sheppard, K., LeDesma, M., Morris, N., O'Connor, K. (1999). A prospective study of two intravenous catheter securement techniques in a skilled nursing facility. *Journal of Intravenous Nursing, 22*(3), 151–153.

In this prospective, controlled study in a skilled nursing facility, the authors determined IV dwell times and outcomes associated with a securement device. The device resulted in significantly longer average catheter dwell times (3.95 days vs. 2.45 days), and significantly fewer local complications (65 vs. 155). The securement device also reduced clinical time in managing vascular access by 13.5 minutes.

Hypodermoclysis

The IV nursing professional should be familiar with the term *hypodermoclysis* and its clinical applications, which are used more often now. When performing a hypodermoclysis, the subcutaneous route is used as a vehicle for absorption of IV isotonic hydration fluids. Fluid selection is tantamount to success, and solutions containing sodium chloride, with or without glucose, are most commonly used. Electrolyte solutions, including Ringer's solution, lactated Ringer's solution, and Normosol R may also be used. Additives are used to enhance absorption within the tissues (Walsh, 2005). Two new products are Amphadase (Amphastar Pharmaceuticals, Inc., Cucamonga, CA) and Vitrase (ISTA Pharmaceuticals, Irvine, CA). Wydase, previously used, is off of the market.

A clysis needle, resembling the standard winged infusion needle, is entered into the lateral aspect of the patient's thigh and the infusion is initiated. Standard skin preparation consistent with INS Standards of Practice should be followed before the procedure and for removal of the needles at the completion of the clysis. Some manufacturers provide therapy-specific clysis administration sets, such as the Aqua-C Hydration System from Norfolk Medical (Skokie, IL). The use of a specially prepared set may decrease the possibility of mistaking the subcutaneous infusion for an intravenous line (Walsh, 2005). In lieu of such a set, a standardized 78-inch administration set may be used.

Phlebotomy

The professional IV nurse performs phlebotomy in many institutions. The **phlebotomy**, a bleeding of between 400 and 500 mL blood, is performed for transfusion purposes, as well as therapeutically for acute pulmonary congestion, polycythemia vera, hemochromatosis, and porphyria cutanea tarda.

Phlebotomy for Transfusion Purposes

ROUTINE DONATION

When phlebotomy is performed for routine bank blood, donor selection is based on the medical history and the physical examination (weight, temperature, pulse, blood pressure, and hemoglobin). The procedure is performed according to the standards of the American Association of Blood Banks (AABB; AABB, 2003).

AUTOTRANSFUSION

Autotransfusion is used to return the patient's own blood to the circulation. The phlebotomy may be performed either by blood bank procedure or non–blood bank procedure.

When the phlebotomy is performed in the blood bank, the usual blood bank procedure is followed. The blood can be stored at 4°C or the red blood cells can be frozen.

When the bleeding is performed outside the blood bank, the same technique (according to the standards of the AABB) is used. However, the donor criteria can be modified. For example, people with a history of cancer cannot make a routine donation but may donate for themselves. Blood, which is suitable only for the donor, must be labeled with the donor's name and hospital number or Social Security number. The donated blood is then segregated from other donor bloods. The ABO type is confirmed just before transfusion.

An important fact to bear in mind is the possibility of sepsis. Clinically undetected bacteremia may exist in the patient with a catheter, a tracheostomy, or a disease process.

Phlebotomy for Therapeutic Purposes

The therapeutic phlebotomy is performed to remove blood from and promote the health of the donor. The practice requires a written order by the physician specifying the date, the amount of blood to be drawn, the frequency for performing the procedure, and the hemoglobin or hematocrit value at which the patient's blood should be drawn. If the patient's physician approves and if the label conspicuously indicates the patient's diagnosis and that the blood was drawn therapeutically, the blood may be used for transfusion (see Chap. 17).

RELIEF OF ACUTE PULMONARY CONGESTION

An inpatient phlebotomy may be performed to reduce venous pressure and relieve the workload on the heart of a patient with acute pulmonary edema resulting from cardiac failure or overtransfusion. Overtransfusion is much less likely to occur today because central venous pressure monitoring provides a valuable guide for fluid administration. Also, effective drugs are available to increase cardiac output and lower the central venous pressure.

Polycythemia Vera

Although a therapeutic phlebotomy for polycythemia vera can be an inpatient or outpatient procedure, it is most frequently performed on a hospitalized patient in an effort to obtain a remission of the disease, which is characterized by a striking increase in the number of circulating red blood cells. Either alone or in combination with radioactive phosphorus (^{32}P), phlebotomy reduces the red blood cell mass, lowers the blood volume, reduces blood viscosity, and improves circulatory efficiency. The number of and interval between phlebotomies should be specified by the physician and the hematocrit value determined after the blood donation.

> **SAFE PRACTICE ALERT** Because the patient with acute pulmonary congestion is critically ill, the phlebotomy should probably be done by or in the presence of the patient's physician.

Hemochromatosis

Excessive body stores of iron characterize hemochromatosis. The phlebotomy is usually an outpatient procedure performed to reduce the total body iron concentration. Because patients with hemochromatosis usually have a hematocrit value in the normal range, periodic checks on the hematocrit value are desirable.

Porphyria Cutanea Tarda

How outpatient phlebotomy acts to relieve the skin lesions of porphyria cutanea tarda is not clear. These patients may have a normal hematocrit reading; thus, they are likely to undergo phlebotomy too often.

Donor Phlebotomy Procedure

To allay apprehension and avoid a vasovagal reaction, the nurse should explain the procedure and reassure the patient before proceeding as follows.

Patient Preparation

> **SAFE PRACTICE ALERT** Verifying the patient's identity is a safety imperative.

1. Identify the patient. Match the donor with the record and the order for the phlebotomy.
2. Make sure that identically numbered labels are applied to the donor record, the blood collection container, and the test tubes for donor blood samples. In addition, make sure that the processing tubes are correctly numbered and kept with the container during the blood collection. Consult institutional policy for prep solutions.
3. Prepare the donor's arm to provide an aseptic site for venipuncture. This protects both the blood donor and the blood recipient. In preparing the area,

always start at the venipuncture site and move outward in concentric spirals for at least 1½ inches. Use only sterile materials and instruments.
4. Put on gloves. Then, using a 15% aqueous (not alcoholic) soap or detergent solution, scrub the donor's arm vigorously for at least 30 seconds with gauze or 60 seconds with cotton balls.
5. Apply 10% acetone in 70% isopropyl alcohol to remove the soap. Let the site dry.
6. Apply tincture of iodine (3% in 70% ethyl alcohol) to the site and allow it to dry.
7. Use 10% acetone in 70% isopropyl alcohol to remove the iodine; again allow the site to dry.
8. Place dry sterile gauze over the site until ready to perform the venipuncture.

An alternative procedure is as follows:

1. Put on gloves.
2. Use 0.7% aqueous scrub solution of iodophor compound (povidone–iodine or poloxamer–iodine complex). Scrub the area for 30 seconds. Remove the foam; it is not necessary to dry the arm.
3. Prepare the site with iodophor complex solution (eg, 10% povidone–iodine); allow to stand 30 seconds. The solution need not be removed.
4. Place a dry, sterile gauze sponge over the site until ready to perform the venipuncture. Do not repalpate vein.

COLLECTION OF BLOOD

The following procedure for collecting blood using a plastic bag is reproduced from the AABB's *Technical Manual* (AABB, 2003). This procedure may be modified when the blood is to be discarded.

1. Inspect bag for any defects. Apply pressure to check for leaks. The anticoagulant solution must be clear.
2. Position bag carefully, making sure it is below the level of the donor's arm.
   • If a balance system is used, ensure counterbalance is level and adjusted for the amount of blood to be drawn. Unless metal clips and a hand sealer are used, make a very loose overhand knot in tubing. Hang the bag and route tubing through the pinch clamp.
   • If a balance system is not used, be sure there is some way to monitor the volume of blood drawn.
   • If a vacuum-assist device is used, follow the manufacturer's instructions.
3. Reapply tourniquet or blood pressure cuff. Have donor open and close hand until previously selected vein is again prominent.
4. Uncover sterile needle and do venipuncture immediately. A clean, skillful venipuncture is essential for collection of a full, clot-free unit. Tape the tubing to hold needle in place and cover site with sterile gauze.
5. Open the temporary closure between the interior of bag and tubing, if present.
6. Have donor open and close hand, squeezing a rubber ball or other resilient object slowly every 10 to 12 seconds during collection. Keep donor under observation throughout phlebotomy. The donor should never be left unattended during or immediately after donation.

7. Mix blood and anticoagulant gently and periodically (approximately every 30 seconds) during collection. Mixing may be done by hand, by placing bag on a mechanical agitator, or by using a rocking vacuum-assist device.

8. Ensure blood flow remains fairly brisk so that coagulation activity is not triggered. Rigid time limits are not warranted if there is continuous agitation, although units requiring more than 8 minutes to draw may not be suitable for preparation of platelet concentrates, fresh frozen plasma, or cryoprecipitate.

9. Monitor volume of blood being drawn. If a balance or vacuum-assist device is used, blood flow stops after the proper amount has been collected. One milliliter of blood weighs 1.053 g, the minimum allowable specific gravity for female donors. A convenient figure to use is 1.06 g; a unit containing 405 to 495 mL should weigh 430 to 525 g plus the weight of the container with its anticoagulant.

10. Clamp tubing temporarily using a hemostat. Collect blood-processing sample by a method that precludes contamination of the donor unit. This may be accomplished in several ways:
    - If the blood collection bag contains an in-line needle, make an additional seal with hemostat, metal clip, hand sealer, or tight knot made from a previously prepared loose knot just distal to the in-line needle. Open the connector by separating needles. Insert proximal needle into processing test tube, remove hemostat, allow tube to fill, and reclamp tubing. Carefully reattach slide connector. Donor needle is now ready for removal.
    - If the blood collection bag contains an in-line processing tube, ensure that the processing tube or pouch is full when the collection is complete and the original clamp is placed near the donor needle. The entire assembly may now be removed from donor.
    - If a straight-tubing assembly set is used, there are two alternative procedures. In the first method, remove the needle from donor's arm as soon as tubing is clamped. Take bag and assembly to the sealer area or collect the processing tube at the donor chair by placing a hemostat close to where donor tubing enters the bag, leaving the tubing full of blood. Remove clamp next to donor needle, empty contents of donor tubing into processing test tube, reapply clamp or permanently seal next to donor needle, remove hemostat next to donor bag, and allow donor tubing to refill with blood, well mixed, from donor bag.

        In the second method, place two hemostats or temporary seals on tubing. Cut tubing between the seals, put the cut end of tubing into the processing test tube, remove proximal hemostat, allow tube to fill, and reclamp tubing.

11. Deflate and remove tourniquet. Remove needle from arm. Apply pressure over gauze and have donor raise arm (elbow straight) and hold gauze firmly over phlebotomy site with the other hand.

12. Discard needle assembly into rigid container designed to prevent accidental injury to and contamination of personnel.

13. Strip donor tubing as completely as possible into the bag, starting at seal. Work quickly to avoid allowing the blood to clot in the tubing. Invert bag

several times to mix thoroughly, then allow tubing to refill with anticoagu-
lated blood from the bag. Repeat this procedure once.

14. Seal the tubing left attached to the bags into segments on which the segment
number is clearly and completely readable. Knots, metal clips, or a dielectric
sealer may be used to make segments suitable for cross-matching. It must be
possible to separate segments from the container without breaking sterility
of the container.

15. Reinspect container for defects.

16. Recheck numbers on container, processing tubes, and donation record. Be
sure the expiration date of the unit is on the container label.

KEY INTERVENTIONS: Suggested Therapeutic Phlebotomy Procedure

In therapeutic phlebotomies, collected blood must be discarded. The procedure itself is not
adequate for recipient protection. Equipment needed includes a phlebotomy pack, a counterbalance stand or small spring scale, blood pressure cuff or tourniquet, tincture of iodine (3%
in 70% ethyl alcohol) or iodophor complex solution (10% povidone–iodine), 10% acetone in
70% isopropyl alcohol for use with tincture of iodine, and sterile sponges.
The nurse then proceeds as follows:

1. Put on gloves.
2. Select the most suitable vein. Apply a tourniquet or a blood pressure cuff inflated to 50
to 60 mm Hg. Have the patient open and close his or her fist to make the vein more
prominent, if necessary. Remove the tourniquet.
3. Prepare the venipuncture site with cleansing solution applied to sterile gauze sponges.
Always start at the puncture site and move out in concentric spirals.
4. Apply tincture of iodine; allow to dry. Question patient before applying; some patients
may be allergic to iodine.
5. Apply 10% acetone in 70% isopropyl alcohol to remove iodine. Allow to dry. Iodophor
complex (10% povidone–iodine) may be substituted for iodine. It does not cause skin
reactions even in iodine-sensitive people. Do not wash off iodophor complex. Cover
the site with dry, sterile gauze to prevent contamination until the phlebotomy is begun.
6. Begin blood collection by suspending bag from donor scale as far below donor's arm
as possible.
7. If counterbalance scales are used, adjust the balance for amount of blood to be drawn.
8. Make loose overhand knot in donor tube near needle.
9. Apply tourniquet (do not impair arterial circulation).
10. Do not touch or repalpate vein.
11. Perform phlebotomy.
12. Tape needle in place and cover with sterile sponge.
13. Pinch bead into bag from junction of donor tube and bag to open lumen and allow
blood to flow.
14. Instruct patient to open and close fist slowly.
15. Collect blood until bag falls on scale. If spring scales are used, collect until prescribed
amount has been withdrawn.
16. Pull knot tight.
17. Release tourniquet, withdraw needle, and apply pressure with gauze pad until bleeding has stopped. Do not flex arm. The arm may be elevated while applying pressure.
18. Dispose of blood and equipment as directed by hospital procedure.
19. Record procedure in clinical record.

17. Place blood at appropriate temperature. Unless platelets are to be removed, whole blood should be placed at 1°C to 6°C immediately after collection. If platelets are to be harvested, blood should not be chilled, but should be maintained at room temperature (approximately 20°C to 24°C) until platelets are separated. Platelets should be separated within 6 hours after collection of the unit of whole blood.

TREATMENT OF ADVERSE DONOR REACTIONS

Stop the phlebotomy at the first sign of reaction and call the physician. If the donor faints:

- Elevate the donor's feet above head level.
- Loosen tight clothing.
- Ascertain that the donor has an adequate airway.
- Apply cold compresses to forehead and back of neck.
- Check and record blood pressure, pulse, and respiration periodically.

If the donor experiences nausea and vomiting, instruct the donor to breathe slowly. If the patient exhibits muscular twitching or tetanic spasms of hands or face, assist him or her to rebreathe into a paper bag. Do not give oxygen.

If the donor has convulsions (rare), call for assistance. Then, prevent injury by turning the donor on the left side. For more serious reactions or if the donor does not respond, call for medical assistance.

Record the nature and treatment of all reactions on the donor's record. Include opinion as to the future use of the donor for blood donations.

Techniques associated with infusion therapy remain consistent throughout the clinical settings in which care is delivered. Adherence to institutional guidelines and Standards of Practice ensures good-quality outcomes.

References and Selected Readings

Asterisks indicate references cited in text.

*American Association of Blood Banks. (2003). *Technical manual* (14th ed., pp. 378, 470–478). Arlington, VA: Author.

Banks, N. (1999). Positive outcome after looped peripherally inserted central catheter malposition. *Journal of Intravenous Nursing, 22*(1), 14–18.

*BD Corporation. (2005). Product literature. Sandy, UT.

Dasgupta, M., Binns, M.A., & Rochon, P.A. (2000). Subcutaneous fluid infusion in a long-term care setting. JAGS; 48(7) 795-799.

*InfraRed Imaging Systems (2005). Product literature. Columbus, OH.

*Infusion Nurses Society (2000). Revised standards of practice. *Journal of Infusion Nursing. 23*(Suppl 1).

*Infusion Nurses Society (2005). Revised standards of practice. *Journal of Infusion Nursing. 28*(Suppl 1).

*Infusion Nurses Society. (2005). Draft of revised Standards of Practice.

*Intravenous Nurses Society. (1998). Revised intravenous nursing standards of practice. *Journal of Intravenous Nursing, 21*(Suppl. 1), S53–58.

Mazzola, J.R., Schott-Baer, D., & Addy, L. (1999). Clinical factors associated with the development of phlebitis after insertion of a peripherally inserted central catheter. *Journal of Intravenous Nursing, 22*(1), 36–39.

Metheny, N.M. (2000). *Fluid and electrolyte balance* (4th ed.). Philadelphia: Lippincott Williams & Wilkins.

*RyMed Corporation. (2004). Product literature.

Sassoon, M., Shvartzman, P. (2001). Hypodermoclysis: An alternative infusion technique. *American Family Physician, 64*(9), 1575–1578.

*Sheppard, K., LeDesma, M., Morris, N., & O'Connor, K. (1999). A prospective study of two intravenous catheter securement techniques in a skilled nursing facility. *Journal of Intravenous Nursing, 22*(3), 151–153.

*Thomson, S. (1993). IV therapy: A financial feasibility study. *Nursing Management, 24,* 68A–G.

3M Corporation. (1999). Product literature. Minneapolis, MN.

*Walsh, G. (2005). Hypodermoclysis: An alternate method for rehydration in long-term care. *Journal of Infusion Nursing, 28*(2), 123–129.

Review Questions

Note: Questions below may have more than one right answer.

1. Which of the following is true of small peripheral catheter insertion?
   A. Techniques vary.
   B. Standards of practice should be followed.
   C. An infusion specialist is skilled to insert.
   D. All of the above

2. Which of the following is correct about closed catheter systems?
   A. They offer flexibility.
   B. They detract from safety.
   C. They cannot be used for venous sampling.
   D. They replaced needle-free systems.

3. Which of the following is true of midline catheters?
   A. They were introduced in the 1970s.
   B. They were recalled in 1975.
   C. They are composed of polyurethane or silicone.
   D. They cannot be placed in the antecubital fossa.

4. Hypodermoclysis refers to which of the following?
   A. Intravenous insertion
   B. Infusion of Wydase
   C. Subcutaneous absorption of isotonic hydration fluids
   D. Subcutaneous absorption of hypertonic hydration fluids

5. A clysis needle is placed in which of the following areas?
   A. Lateral aspect of the thigh
   B. Dorsal aspect of the thigh
   C. Lateral aspect of the forearm
   D. Dorsal aspect of the forearm

6. In lieu of a specific clysis administration set, which of the following may be used?
   A. In-line filter set
   B. 78-inch administration set
   C. 30-inch administration set
   D. Central line

7. Blood obtained through phlebotomy may be stored at which of the following temperatures?
   A. 4°C
   B. 7°C
   C. 10°C
   D. 12°C

8. Polycythemia vera is characterized by which of the following?
   A. Decreased RBCs
   B. Increased RBCs
   C. Decreased eosinophils
   D. Increased eosinophils

9. Hemochromatosis refers to which of the following?
   A. Decreased iron stores
   B. Increased iron stores
   C. Decreased cholesterol
   D. Increased triglycerides

10. Which of the following is true of blood obtained through therapeutic phlebotomy?
    A. It may be transfused.
    B. It should be stored at 4°C.
    C. It must be discarded.
    D. It does not require HIV testing.

CHAPTER 14

Central Venous Access

KEY TERMS

Basilic Vein
Brachiocephalic Vein
Central Venous Catheter
Central Venous Pressure
Cephalic Vein
Elastomeric Hydrogel
External Jugular Vein

Pinch-Off Syndrome
Polyurethane
Silicone
Subclavian Vein
Superior Vena Cava
Thrombolytic
Valsalva Maneuver

Central Venous Access

Definition

A **central venous catheter,** commonly referred to as a *central line,* is the catheter threaded into the central vasculature. The central venous catheter (CVC) tip is placed in the superior vena cava at the junction of the right atrium. Central venous access permits administration of fluids, blood components, medications, and nutritional solutions, and also facilitates hemodynamic monitoring. Knowledge of the vascular system is essential for providing care to the patient with a central venous catheter. Vessels involved include the cephalic, basilic, axillary, jugular, subclavian, and brachiocephalic veins as well as the superior vena cava (Fig. 14–1).

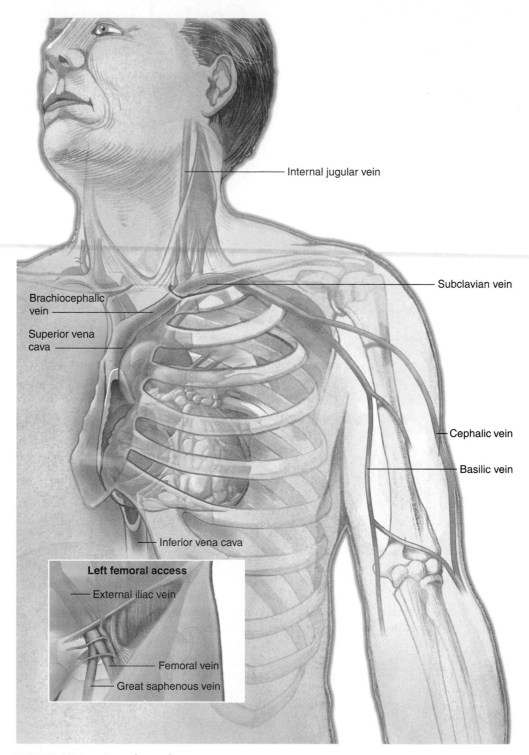

FIGURE 14–1.   Central vascular structures.

Vascular Structures Used for Central Venous Access

CEPHALIC VEIN

The **cephalic vein** ascends along the outer border of the biceps muscle to the upper third of the arm. It passes in the space between the pectoralis major and deltoid muscles. It terminates in the axillary vein, with a descending curve, just below the clavicle. The cephalic vein is occasionally connected with the external jugular or subclavian vein by a branch that passes from it upward in front of the clavicle.

BASILIC VEIN

The **basilic vein** is larger than the cephalic. It passes upward in a smooth path along the inner side of the biceps muscle and terminates in the axillary vein.

AXILLARY VEIN

The **axillary vein** starts upward as a continuation of the basilic vein, increasing in size as it ascends. It receives the cephalic vein and terminates immediately beneath the clavicle, at the outer border of the first rib, at which point it becomes the subclavian vein.

EXTERNAL JUGULAR VEIN

The **external jugular vein** is easily recognized on the side of the neck. It follows a descending inward path to join the subclavian vein above the middle of the clavicle.

INTERNAL JUGULAR VEIN

The **internal jugular vein** descends first behind and then to the outer side of the internal and common carotid arteries. The carotid plexus is situated on the outer side of the internal carotid artery. The internal jugular vein joins the subclavian vein at the root of the neck. At the angle of junction, the left subclavian receives the thoracic duct, whereas the right subclavian receives the right lymphatic duct.

SUBCLAVIAN VEIN

The **subclavian vein,** a continuation of the axillary vein, extends from the outer edge of the first rib to the inner end of the clavicle, where it unites with the internal jugular to form the innominate vein. Valves are present in the venous system until approximately 1 inch before the formation of the innominate vein.

RIGHT AND LEFT BRACHIOCEPHALIC VEINS

Each of the two veins is formed by the union of the right or left internal jugular vein and the corresponding subclavian vein. The **right brachiocephalic vein** is approximately 1 inch long. It passes almost vertically downward and joins the **left brachiocephalic vein** just below the cartilage of the first rib. The left brachiocephalic vein is approximately 2.5 inches long and larger than the right. It passes from left to right across the upper front chest in a downward slant. These vessels join to form the superior vena cava.

SUPERIOR VENA CAVA

The **superior vena cava** receives all blood from the upper half of the body. It is composed of a short trunk 2.5 to 3 inches long. It begins below the first rib close to the sternum on the right side, descends vertically slightly to the right, and empties into the right atrium of the heart.

Advantages, Disadvantages, and Indications for Central Venous Access

The main advantage of a CVC is immediate access to the central circulatory system. Rapid administration and dilution of large volumes of fluids are possible because the catheter tip is in a large vessel. Additionally, rapid dilution reduces the risk of phlebitis and venous sclerosis. Other advantages of CVCs include longer dwell times of weeks to years, depending on the type; appropriateness for all types of therapies and multiple incompatible solutions via multilumen catheters; insertion at the bedside or in ambulatory care without general anesthesia; and access for central venous pressure monitoring. Disadvantages include the need for physician placement of the catheter except for peripherally inserted central catheters (PICCs), increased risk of infection without tunneling or a cuff, and the invasiveness of the procedure (Camp-Sorrell, 2004).

CVCs are used for multiple purposes. Nontunneled CVCs are used in emergency situations for treating shock with massive fluid replacements and in surgery for rapid administration of fluids. They may be placed for administration of parenteral nutrition, frequent and long-term blood transfusions, long-term fluid replacement or medications, and administration of irritant, vesicant, or highly concentrated drugs. Frequent blood sampling is less painful using a CVC.

Overview of CVC Types, Materials, and Properties

There are five main types of CVCs, as seen in Box 14–1. Their dwell time ranges from days to years or indefinitely until a complication becomes evident. Improvements in catheter materials and properties, safety features, and device options have made this an ever-evolving field of technology. It is important for nurses to know the principles of central vascular access and understand the needs of an individual patient to recommend the most appropriate device and interventions.

Catheter Materials

The ideal central venous catheter would be composed of a material that inhibits thrombus formation, inserts easily, and is biocompatible and radiopaque.

BOX 14–1   Overview of Central Venous Access Devices

Nontunneled Central Venous Catheter (CVC)	Large-bore catheter inserted percutaneously into central vascular structures; used for short-term (days to weeks) therapy.
Peripherally Inserted Central Catheter (PICC)	Very-small-gauge catheter inserted percutaneously into an upper extremity vein and then threaded into the superior vena cava (nontunneled); used for long-term therapy.
Tunneled CVC	Catheter inserted into the central vascular structures and then pulled through subcutaneous tissue (tunneled) for a short distance before exiting the skin. The catheter also has a cuff where the catheter is tunneled.
Implanted Port	A tunneled catheter attached to a device with a hollow core, or port, implanted into the subcutaneous tissue. This port permits percutaneous access for intermittent or continuous infusions of fluids or medications.
Implanted Pump	A tunneled catheter attached to a pump implanted into a subcutaneous pocket. The pump permits continuous infusion of medications, with percutaneous access for refilling.

Catheters may be composed of polyurethane, silicone, and elastomeric hydrogel. **Polyurethane** is firm, allows for ease of insertion, softens after insertion, and is biocompatible so that tissues do not react to the material. It is less thrombogenic than earlier materials. A thrombus forms as a result of intima irritation and reaction; softer materials are less irritating to the vein wall. The strength of the polyurethane allows for a thinner catheter wall and larger internal diameter when compared with same-sized silicone catheters. **Silicone** is more flexible, thus requiring special insertion techniques, and has increased biocompatibility. **Elastomeric hydrogel** catheters combine hydrogel and polyurethane to obtain the lowest coefficient of surface friction of the catheter, thus allowing for less thrombogenicity and decreased mechanical tissue trauma. The hydrogel allows the catheter to soften, whereas the polyurethane provides strength and prevents absorption of the infusate into the catheter (Greene, 2000). Catheters had been composed of polyvinylchloride/Teflon, but this material was discontinued owing to its lack of flexibility and resultant vein wall damage. A summary of catheter materials is presented in Box 14–2.

BOX 14–2   Catheter Materials and Characteristics

Polyurethane	• Rigid during insertion but softens at body temperature • Less thrombogenic
Silicone Elastomer/Silastic	• Very flexible • Minimal thrombus formation • Biocompatible • Good for long-term use • Dramatic fibrin sheath formation when particulate matter is present; rinse gloves and catheter before insertion
Elastomeric Hydrogel	• Available in peripheral lines • Combines stretchable polymer with hydrophilic substance (water absorbing and similar to extended-wear contact lenses) • Rinse with normal saline solution; easier to insert

Catheter Properties

Advancements in technology related to catheter materials and properties are aimed at reducing complications of catheter-related infections and thrombosis. Catheter-related infections (CRI) occur when micro-organisms adhere to catheter materials and promote formation of a biofilm allowing cell proliferation, intercellular adhesion, and colonization (von Eiff, Jansen, Kohnen, & Becker, 2005). There are conflicting reports on whether catheter materials of polyurethane or silicone influence the risk of infection. One study compared silastic and polyurethane catheters and bacterial adherence and CRIs in rats. In the presence of a fibrin sheath, silastic catheters were associated with significantly more infection than polyurethane catheters (Mehall, Saltzman, Jackson, & Smith, 2001). A retrospective study examined risk factors for removal of implanted venous access devices in a sample of cystic fibrosis patients. Multivariate analysis indicated that removal of catheters, for whatever reason, was more often associated with polyurethane than silicone catheters (Munck, Malbezin, Bloch, et al., 2004).

Thrombosis associated with central venous catheters has many contributing factors. Any foreign material in the bloodstream becomes coated with a protein and fibrin deposit. This in turn activates internal coagulation, causing platelet activation and platelet adherence to the catheter. Damage to endothelial cells at the puncture site also promotes platelet activation. Patients requiring central venous catheters often have activated coagulation systems because of trauma or severe disease, both of which promote the development of thrombosis. Thrombosis may be limited to a fibrin sheath formation or may be severe enough to occlude the vein. It may have no clinical significance, or it may result in a fatal pulmonary embolism. Fibrin sheaths can lead to loss of function of the catheter and mediate bacterial adherence (Bagnall-Reed, 1998;

Krzywda, 1999; Mayo, 2001; McKnight, 2004; Mehall, Saltzman, Jackson, & Smith, 2002; Metheny, 2000).

Catheter properties aimed at reducing the complications of thrombosis and catheter-related blood stream infection (CRBSI) include bonding with heparin or cefazolin; impregnating with silver sulfadiazine and chlorhexidine or small silver particles; and coating with minocycline and rifampin, or silver. Multiple studies have demonstrated the effectiveness of these catheters at decreasing at least short-term CRIs. The short-term effect can be explained by the duration of release of the antimicrobial substance (von Eiff et al., 2005). Few studies have evaluated the use of heparin-coated catheters, but when examined, these catheters have demonstrated a decrease in CRBSIs (Marin, Lee, & Skurnick, 2000).

Most of the literature has focused on chlorhexidine and silver sulfadiazine (CHSS) or minocycline and rifampicin (MR). Studies have demonstrated decreased CRIs when compared with control catheters. Comparisons of MR and CHSS catheters have demonstrated a lower incidence of infection with MR catheters; however, those studies were based on first-generation CHSS catheters (Hanna, Benjamin, Chatzinikolaou, et al., 2004; Marin et al, 2000; Mermel, 2000; Veenstra, Saint, Saha, Lumley, & Sullivan, 1999). First-generation catheters were coated only externally, whereas the newer catheter is coated both internally and externally. A significant reduction in catheter colonization has been shown with the newer generation CHSS catheter (Gaonkar & Modak, 2003; Sampath, Saborio, Yaron, & Modak, 2001; vonEiff et al., 2005; Volkow, Vazquez, Tellez, et al., 2003). Studies evaluating various silver technologies have also been inconclusive (Bong, Kite, Wilco, & McMahon, 2003; Harter, Salwender, Bach, Egerer, Goldschmidt, & Ho, 2002; Ranucci, Isgro, Biomarelli, et al., 2003).

Evaluating the cost effectiveness of antimicrobial and antiseptic catheters has had mixed results. The higher cost of these catheters is weighed against the high cost of treating CRBSIs. Some studies have implied that the use of maximal sterile barrier precautions and appropriate subsequent management should precede the use of the more expensive catheters (Garland, Henrickson, & Maki, 2002; Hu, Lipsky, Veenstra, & Saint, 2004; Marciante, Veenstra, Lipsky, & Saint, 2003; Mermel, 2000; Saint, Veenstra, & Lipsky, 2000). The use of CHSS and MF catheters has also raised concerns over the possibility of microbial resistance against these agents and has been demonstrated in animal and in vitro studies (Crnich & Maki, 2002a; Garland et al., 2002; Mermel, 2001; Tambe, Sampath, & Modak, 2001; von Eiff et al., 2005).

The Centers for Disease Control and Prevention (CDC; 2002) recommends use of antimicrobial or antiseptic-impregnated central venous catheters when the expected duration is for >5 days; however, all other strategies to reduce CRBSIs should be in place. Strategies to achieve a low rate of CRBSI include maximal sterile barrier precautions during insertion, strict hand washing, patient skin preparation, and education and training of personnel in insertion and management of catheters (Braun, Kritchevsky, Wong, et al., 2003; Gnass, Barboza, Bilicich, et al., 2004). Last, almost all catheters are radiopaque, which means they can be visualized by radiologic means. This property is required to confirm catheter tip placement after insertion.

Catheter Designs

CATHETER WITH REMOVABLE INTRODUCER

Catheters with removable introducers are frequently made of polyurethane; a wide variety of products are available from today's manufacturers. These products have been developed with safety standards in mind in an effort to minimize the incidence of needlestick injury.

The unit consists of an introducer catheter or syringe and needle and a catheter with stylet. A catheter with a removable introducer is a single-lumen catheter with a fairly easy method of insertion. Because thrombus formation can be a problem with polyurethane, this may not be the catheter of choice for long-term therapy. However, minimal thrombus formation has been reported with hydromer-coated polyurethane and long-term use.

To insert the catheter, venipuncture is performed with the needle and syringe. The syringe is removed and the catheter threaded through the needle. The needle is withdrawn from the vein and removed from the catheter by splitting the needle into two parts.

CATHETER WITH INTRODUCER AND GUIDEWIRE

A safety catheter with an introducer and guidewire allows for the insertion of a multiple-lumen silicone catheter. The unit consists of a syringe and needle or an over-the-needle catheter (ONC), a long central catheter, and a guidewire.

To insert the catheter, venipuncture is performed with the syringe and needle or safety-type ONC. The syringe or stylet is removed. The guidewire is threaded through the short catheter or needle, and the short catheter or needle is withdrawn (usually into a self-contained locking cover to avoid needlestick injury). The puncture site may be enlarged with a no. 1 scalpel blade. The long catheter is threaded over the guidewire, which is then withdrawn, leaving the long catheter in the vein.

Cuffs and Valves

Tunneled catheters are available with one or two cuffs. Within weeks, the Dacron cuff becomes enmeshed in fibrous tissue securing the catheter in place. It lies within the subcutaneous tunnel 1 to 2 inches from the exit site. The cuff also inhibits migration of micro-organisms into the tunnel (CDC, 2002). These measures reduce the risk of infection. VitaCuff is an antimicrobial cuff that provides stability while reducing the risk of infection. The cuff contains a collagen matrix that exhibits antimicrobial activity attributed to silver ions that are active for 4 to 6 weeks until the matrix is absorbed (Camp-Sorrell, 2004).

Catheters are available with open-ended, closed-ended, and pressure-activated safety valves. Open-ended catheters have a blunt tip. They require clamping when not in use. Positive pressure devices, with or without positive fluid displacement, are recommended to prevent occlusion (Fig. 14–2).

Closed-ended catheters have a rounded closed tip. The Groshong has a rounded, closed tip and features a patented Groshong valve that opens inward for blood aspiration and outward for infusion, but remains closed when not in use (Fig. 14–3). Advantages of this type of catheter tip include

- Decreased risk of bleeding or air emboli
- Elimination of catheter clamping
- Elimination of the use of heparin in the catheter
- Reduction of flushing between use; weekly flushing is all that is required.

Catheters also are available with a pressure-activated safety valve (PASV; Catheter Innovations, Sandy, UT) that is located in the catheter hub. Other similar products are the CLC2000 Adapter Valve (ICU Medical, San Clemente, CA) and the PASV (Boston Scientific Corporation, Natick, MA). The patented valve (Catheter Innovations) opens with minimal positive pressure for infusion, yet requires four times as much negative pressure for aspiration. The PASV also reduces the reflux of blood into the end of the catheter during periods of increased central venous pressure and decreases difficulties with poor blood return. Weekly saline-only flushing is needed, and the product is consistent with needleless systems. The valve may also be used with peripherally inserted central catheters and midline catheters (Camp-Sorrell, 2004; Lamont, McCarthy, Stephens, et al., 2003). It is important to note that the nurse's technique must change when these valves are used. The catheter must not be clamped until after the syringe is removed or the valve will not function to prevent reflux. When the catheter is not in use, the catheter hub can be taped to the chest wall above heart level. This minimizes blood pressure at the catheter tip.

Central Venous Access Device Selection

Central venous access device selection requires a collaborative approach between the health care team members and the patient. Considerations in access device

FIGURE 14–2.   Pressure-activated safety valve (PASV; Catheter Innovations).

FIGURE 14–3.   Groshong valve (Davol, Inc., a subsidiary of CR Bard, Inc., Salt Lake City, UT).

selection include patient assessment, type of therapy, duration of therapy, patient's values and preferences, and catheter materials and properties, as reviewed above (Halderman, 2000).

Device selection is guided by the principles of the least invasive, fewest lumens, and smallest gauge catheter that are appropriate for the therapy and able to last for the duration of the therapy. The risk of adverse events decreases with less invasive insertion techniques, and decreased risk of infection may be associated with fewer CVC lumens (CDC, 2002; Dezfulian, Lavelle, Nallamothu, Kaufman, & Saint, 2003; Zurcher , Tramer, & Walder, 2004). A large external catheter diameter can cause damage to the intima, impede venous flow around the catheter, and interfere with appropriate dilution of medications. The internal diameter of the catheter can affect flow rate and ability to draw blood samples (Camp-Sorrell, 2004; CDC, 2002; Greene, 2000). The types of prescribed medication and nutrition therapy influence device selection. Multiple therapies that are incompatible require multiple lumens. Therapies that are irritants or of high osmolality, acidity, or alkalinity can cause endothelial damage and increase risk of phlebitis and thrombosis. An algorithm assists with matching the appropriate device to the specific criteria (Fig. 14–4).

Patient Assessment and Informed Consent

Patient values and preferences are as important in device selection as the other considerations. Patient assessment includes health history and physical assessment.

FIGURE 14–4. Algorithm for central venous catheter device selection.

Medical conditions of concern include allergies, coagulation status, diabetes, renal disease, and previous central venous catheters. Other conditions to note are previous arm, neck, or chest trauma; surgery; or radiation. Physical assessment is needed for circulatory status, lymphedema, and skin integrity. Patient activity level and lifestyle, mental status, and capacity to manage long-term care of the device must be assessed. Any limitations of patient activity the device may create should be thoroughly discussed. If the patient will be performing any self-care, this should be completely explained and agreed to by the patient before insertion. Commitment to therapy as well as the ability to financially manage the long-term costs of maintenance and drugs also need to be considered (Barton, Danek, Johns, & Coons, 1998; Galloway, 2002; Registered Nurses Association of Ontario [RNAO], 2004).

Any central venous catheterization procedure has inherent risks. The patient's informed consent, in writing, is essential before placement of any central venous catheter device.

 SAFE PRACTICE ALERT If peripheral veins are adequate and can be used for the desired treatment, a central venous catheter should not be inserted.

Preparation for CVC Insertion

Educating the Patient About the Procedure and the Device

Some of the information about central venous access devices and insertion technique would have been explained to the patient during device selection with the patient. However, once the type of device has been selected, specific education about this device and the insertion is necessary. Explaining the reasons for the central venous device and the procedure will allay fears and help the patient participate as he or she is able.

Patient education should include a description of the procedure, expected post-procedure discomfort, and the need for comfort measures. It may be necessary to use some form of premedication sedation for the procedure depending on type of device, insertion site, and individual patient needs (Box 14–3). If a tunneled catheter, implanted port, or pump device is being inserted, seeing and touching the device that will remain in the body helps to reassure most patients. Explain to the patient that she or he may be covered with a sterile drape, and the nurse and physician both wear gowns, masks, and gloves. Ensure that informed consent has been obtained.

Patient Positioning

If the catheter will be inserted by a subclavian approach, explain to the patient that he or she is positioned flat in bed with the head lowered and knees bent (Trendelenburg

---

**BOX 14–3   Teaching Guide for Patients Preparing for Central Venous
Access Catheter (CVC) or Device**

Features of an effective patient teaching plan include

- Appropriate level of information for the patient's age and language
- Identification of learning barriers and patient's preferred learning method
- Purpose and rationale for CVC or device placement and alternatives
- Delineated responsibilities of the patient or caregivers and health care providers
- Explanation of routine risks and complications of treatment
- Discussion of prognosis (procedure-specific)

Follow-up evaluation of teaching includes

- Documented assessment of patient or caregiver comprehension
- Documentation of consent for procedure and method of consent (verbal/ nonverbal/written)
- "Survival" information includes what to do if the external catheter is cut, breaks, or cracks; whom to call in an emergency; and when to return for maintenance of the device
- Support materials provided to patient (illustrated, audio, printed materials, as appropriate)

---

position). This position facilitates entry to the vein by distending the vein and increasing central venous pressure and the venous blood supply. A rolled towel is placed under the back along the spinal cord and between the shoulders to hyperextend the neck and elevate the clavicle. For the jugular approach, the head is turned to the opposite direction and extended. This stretches and stabilizes the vein and accentuates the muscular landmarks. During a cephalic or brachial insertion, abduction of the arm may be required to pass the catheter past the shoulder area. Explaining this to the patient before the procedure promotes patient cooperation when the uncomfortable position must be maintained.

Valsalva Maneuver

Practicing the **Valsalva maneuver** before the insertion also promotes cooperation when the patient is asked to hold her or his breath and bear down when the catheter is open to the air (INS, 2005).

Laboratory Studies

Before catheter insertion, several laboratory studies are needed. These include platelet count, prothrombin time, and partial thromboplastin time. Any abnormal findings may require correction with vitamin K, fresh frozen plasma, or platelet concentrates before catheter insertion is attempted. This should be explained to the patient.

Contraindications for a central venous access device include

- Abnormal coagulation studies
- Septicemia

BOX 14–4   Best Practices for Insertion of Central Venous Catheters

- The subclavian vein poses less risk than either internal jugular veins or the femoral veins in preventing CRBSI.
- Maximal barrier precaution requires strict aseptic technique and adherence to hand washing during vein selection and prior to donning sterile gloves. This also requires the use of protective equipment, ie, mask, sterile surgical gown, and gloves for all personnel, and complete sterile draping of the patient (IHI, 2005; Rubinson & Diette, 2004).
- The CDC (2002) recommends the use chlorhexidine gluconate (CHG) to cleanse the area of the insertion site prior to the procedure. Strict hand washing and adherence to institutional policy for site care and management also decreases the risk of subsequent complications.

- Anomalies of the central venous vascular structures
- Thrombosis of the subclavian or brachiocephalic veins or the superior vena cava.

Infection Control

Almost 90% of CRBSIs are related to CVCs (Mermel, 2000). For this reason, increased scrutiny is being focused on CVCs (Institute for Healthcare Improvement [IHI], 2005). Aseptic technique minimizes the risk of infection in the patient receiving a CVC. Hand hygiene is paramount to prevent infection; it should be practiced before and after insertion site palpation, before and after insertion, and before and after donning and removing gloves for the procedure.

The skin at the insertion site should be cleansed consistent with institutional policy (Krau, 2003), guidelines issued by the CDC (2002) and by the INS (2000). The recommended solution for site preparation is 2% chlorhexidine and 70% isopropyl alcohol (CDC, 2002). This solution is applied using a back-and-forth friction scrub for a minimum of 30 seconds; it must be allowed to air dry completely before inserting the catheter. Do not apply acetone or ether to the skin before CVC insertion (CDC, 2002).

Maximal barrier precautions are another critical component to prevent infection (Hu et al., 2004; IHI, 2005). These precautions require the patient to be covered from head to toe with a sterile drape (IHI, 2005). Best practices for CVC insertion are identified in Box 14–4.

Insertion of the Central Venous Catheter

CVC insertion is a medical act. Insertion of some types of catheters, such as PICCs, may be delegated to specially trained nurses according to each state's Nurse Practice Act. There are three basic approaches for central venous catheter insertions. The veins used for entry are the subclavian and the internal or external jugular veins for central insertion, and the cephalic, basilic, or median cubital vein for peripherally inserted central catheter insertion.

Subclavian Approach

The subclavian vein is the entry site of choice for centrally inserted and catheters and is recommended, if not contraindicated, to minimize risk of infection (IHI, 2005; Ruesch, Walder. & Traner, 2002). It requires the shortest catheter because it uses the most central vein, thus creating a high blood flow around a large portion of the catheter. This results in minimal irritation or obstruction by the catheter, which lowers the risk of complications and results in a longer catheter life.

Subclavian entry can foster major complications both during and after insertion (see Complications section of this chapter). The subclavian entry may be performed using the infraclavicular or supraclavicular approach. In both approaches, the catheter is inserted under the clavicle, aiming for the jugular notch. For the infraclavicular approach, the catheter is inserted at approximately the midpoint of the clavicle. For the supraclavicular approach, the catheter is frequently inserted at the base of the triangle formed by the sternal and clavicular heads of the sternocleidomastoid muscle. Contraindications to the subclavian approach may include

- Radiation burns at intended insertion site
- Fractured clavicle
- Hyperinflated lungs
- Malignant lesion at the base of the neck or apex of the lungs.

Internal Jugular Vein Approach

The internal jugular vein is preferred by many practitioners as the site of first choice for inserting a central venous catheter. The constant anatomic location of the internal jugular vein makes it easier to catheterize than the subclavian vein. The right internal jugular vein is usually chosen because it forms a straighter, shorter line to the superior vena cava. It also avoids the higher left pleura and thoracic duct. This insertion is frequently performed by first locating the vein with a small-gauge needle. After making a small skin incision to facilitate entry, a larger-gauge catheter is inserted, following the same direction as the locator needle, aiming for the ipsilateral nipple.

External Jugular Vein Approach

The external jugular vein is observable and easily entered. Insertion complications are rare. The external jugular vein varies in size, and its junction with the subclavian vein is acutely angulated. It contains two pairs of valves: the uppermost pair is 4 cm above the clavicle; the lower pair is located at the vein's entrance to the subclavian vein. Because of these factors, central catheterization can be difficult. Because a short catheter may be inserted easily, central catheterization may be achieved by using an introducer with a guidewire. Entry into the superficial vein is performed by directing the catheter toward the ipsilateral nipple.

The main objections to any jugular catheterization are the following:

- Catheter occlusion, resulting from the patient's head movement, is a persistent problem.

- Vein irritation also results from head movement, with a shorter catheter life as a consequence.
- Maintaining an intact dressing on the area is difficult.
- The idea of having a catheter in the neck may be aesthetically and psychologically disturbing to many patients and families.

CVC Insertion Complications and Tip Placement Verification

Prevention is the best intervention to deal with CVC insertion complications. Patient safety initiatives include using two identifiers to ensure having the right patient, doing a preprocedure verification, and having systems in place for high-alert medications.

However, there are several potential complications that result from CVC catheter insertion. Nursing surveillance during and after the procedure with prompt recognition of signs and symptoms of a complication and rapid response to the complication can keep patients safe. Table 14–1 outlines the major potential complications of CVC insertion with appropriate interventions.

SAFE PRACTICE ALERT The risk of air embolism is always present during catheter insertion because central venous pressure (CVP) can be negative. Placing the patient in the Trendelenburg position increases CVP. If possible, the patient should perform the Valsalva maneuver whenever the catheter is opened to the air. If the catheter stylet has been removed, the hub should be occluded either with a syringe or a gloved finger to prevent air entry.

Verifying the CVC tip placement also prevents potential complications from mechanical trauma of the catheter against the cardiac wall or infusion of fluids, medications, or nutrition into nonvasculature or inappropriate vasculature. The preferred tip placement for all CVCs is at the junction of the superior vena cava and the right atrium. If the tip lies in the right atrium, atrial arrhythmias may occur as a result of the catheter irritating the chamber. Proper placement also decreases the incidence of dislodgment, vessel wall erosion and stenosis, and device dysfunction.

A chest radiograph or fluoroscopy is used to confirm tip placement. Fluoroscopy can be used to verify tip placement if this method is being used to insert the catheter. The chest radiograph, if used, is always obtained immediately after catheter insertion to rule out pneumothorax and to document tip placement. The catheter should not be used until tip placement is confirmed. The site should be observed for any signs of excess bleeding or swelling, and the patient's breathing should be monitored for any signs of respiratory distress. Unexpected observations should be reported to the physician immediately, as should complications associated with central line placement.

Uses for Central Venous Catheters

CVCs are used for fluid, medication, and nutrition administration as well as for monitoring pressure or volume changes to detect potential problems or evaluate patient improvement.

TABLE 14–1   Complications of Central Venous Catheter or Device Insertion

Complication	Intervention
Air Embolism Symptoms: chest pain, dyspnea, hypoxia, apnea, tachycardia, hypotension, or a precordial murmur	• A potential danger whenever a central venous catheter is open to air: a result of intrathoracic pressure becoming less than atmospheric pressure. During insertion, placing the patient in the Trendelenburg position increases central venous pressure (CVP). Placing a sterile gloved finger over the catheter hub, between catheter stylet removal and IV system connection, can prevent air from entering the catheter. • Use of the PASV (pressure-activated safety valve) as an add-on device helps prevent air embolism. This device reduces the risk of air embolism or bleed-out resulting from an accidental disconnection of the tubing. • Immediately cap catheter or clamp the catheter proximal to the opening; place patient in supine position on the left side with the feet elevated (this position is used in an attempt to trap the air in the right atrium, where it can be aspirated with an intracardiac needle); administer oxygen.
Arterial Puncture Symptoms: rapid hematoma, bleeding at insertion site, pallor, weak pulse, tachycardia, hypotension	• The puncture of an artery requires the immediate application of digital pressure for at least 5 min. If the patient has a coagulation abnormality, digital pressure must be maintained until all bleeding stops. Catheter and introducer must be removed. • If the artery puncture is not recognized and treated early, a massive hematoma with tracheal compression or respiratory distress can occur.
Brachial Plexus Injury Symptoms: tingling of fingers, shooting pains down arm, paralysis	• Nerve damage, including the phrenic and laryngeal nerves • Occurs when advancing the catheter into the jugular vein • Symptoms usually resolve in minutes to hours after insertion; offer analgesics; catheter may have to be removed.
Catheter Embolism Symptoms: chest pain, cardiac arrhythmia	• A risk whenever a through-the-needle device is inserted or left in situ; results from catheter being withdrawn from introducer needle. Never withdraw the catheter back through the needle. • A severed catheter may require cardiac catheterization to retrieve the embolism. Breakaway needles minimize this hazard.
Pneumothorax, Hemothorax, and Hydrothorax Symptoms: difficult breathing, chest pain, cyanosis, tachypnea	• Occurs as a result of pleural puncture, after which the patient may experience symptoms. However, a pneumothorax that does not produce symptoms may be disclosed by radiography. A chest tube may be required. • Hemothorax may result if the subclavian or adjacent veins have been traumatized or transected during catheter insertion. • Hydrothorax results when IV fluid infiltrates into the chest. The symptoms and treatment of hemothorax and hydrothorax are identical to those of pneumothorax.

(Sources: Camp-Sorrell [2004].)

Medication and Nutrition Therapy

Central lines inserted in the subclavian vein were first used for administering total parenteral nutrition. Then, with the advent of catheter tunneling techniques, antithrombogenic catheter materials, new designs, and lowered infection rates, central venous catheters increased in popularity for patients with cancer. They may be used for administering antineoplastic agents over the long term, blood or blood components, and antibiotics, as well as for obtaining specimens of venous blood.

In a hospitalized patient who requires venous access and whose peripheral veins cannot be catheterized, a long-term central catheter may be used. The same is true for many home care patients, including those who have learned to self-administer continuous or intermittent medications through a centrally placed device.

Measuring and Interpreting Central Venous Pressure

Central venous pressure relates to an adequate circulatory blood supply. Pressure depends on blood volume, cardiac contractility (myocardial status), and vascular tone.

BLOOD VOLUME

Changes in blood volume alter the tone of the blood vessels and the ability of the heart to circulate the blood. Reduced blood volume results in less pressure at the right atrium, indicated by a drop in CVP; an increased blood volume produces more pressure at the atrium, with a rise in CVP (Metheny, 2000).

In managing inadequate circulation, the clinician must first establish a normal blood volume. If the inadequate circulation results from deficient blood volume, pressure may be manipulated by administering blood volume expanders. In instances of increased volume, phlebotomy may be used to reduce volume. If circulation is still insufficient, the clinician needs to evaluate the remaining two essential components: cardiac contractility (myocardial status) and vascular tone.

CARDIAC CONTRACTILITY

Cardiac contractility may be affected by disease, drugs, fluids, or anesthetics. Because the CVP is a measure of the capacity of the myocardium as well as the blood volume, it is invaluable in monitoring the effects of anesthesia and surgery on elderly patients with arteriosclerosis or patients with myocardial insufficiency. The CVP rises if the heart muscle is impaired. The pressure of the volume of blood at the heart increases because the heart muscle can no longer pump an adequate flow of blood out of the right atrium (Metheny, 2000). A high CVP may suggest cardiac failure, which is one of the most common causes of elevated CVP in shock. Drugs or chemicals are administered to improve myocardial response, thus increasing cardiac output and lowering the CVP.

VASCULAR TONE

The third essential component, vascular tone, depends on the arterial pressure and on external and internal pressures on the veins. The arterial pressure arises from the contractile force of the left ventricle and is transmitted through the capillaries to the veins.

The external pressures on the veins result from muscular and fascial pumping action in the extremities, the intra-abdominal pressure from straining and distention, and the intrathoracic pressure from contraction of the diaphragm and chest wall. CVP of patients on positive-pressure respirators is usually increased by 4 cm H_2O; patients on negative pressure show a decreased CVP (INS, 2000).

The blood volume, myocardial response, and sympathomimetic amines (epinephrine, norepinephrine) produce internal pressure on the veins. By stimulating contraction of the venous wall, vasopressors decrease the capacity of the venous system and improve vascular tone. Various methods are used to detect change in a patient's blood volume, including hematocrit, changes in patient weight, and blood volume computations. CVP is a parameter used to assess blood volume.

Central Venous Pressure Monitoring

Central venous pressure reflects the pressure of blood in the right atrium or vena cava. The CVP catheter is used to measure the filling pressures of the right side of the heart. During diastole, when the tricuspid valve is open and the blood is flowing from the right atrium to the right ventricle, the CVP accurately reflects fluid volume pressures in the right ventricle. (Urden, 2004). The CVP waveform reflects the contraction of the atria and the concurrent effect of the ventricles and surrounding major vessels. Normal parameters vary with the patient's clinical condition and the measurement methodology; as discussed previously, values are affected by circulating volume, cardiac contractility, and vascular tone.

Central venous pressure monitoring may be accomplished by using a water manometer, which records pressure in units of centimeters of water (between 4 and 12 cm H_2O), or by transducer and monitor, which records pressure in units of millimeters of mercury (between 0 and 8 mm Hg). CVP readings indicate changes in preload (filling pressure in the right ventricle). Abnormal readings may indicate inadequate or increased preload, decreased contractility, or increased afterload (pressure against which the left ventricle contracts). Abnormal pressures may appear in many patients.

USE OF WATER MANOMETER TO MEASURE CENTRAL VENOUS PRESSURE

Although CVP measurements are more commonly done in critical care units using a pressure transducer system, a method of obtaining a CVP measurement for patients who are on general hospital units is to place a water manometer with a three-way stopcock between the IV solution and the patient's IV catheter. Most facilities use CVP sets that are available with disposable water manometers and graduated unit measures. The nurse adjusts the zero mark of the water manometer so that it is level with the patient's right atrium. The pressure is measured at either the superior vena cava by introducing the catheter through the antecubital, jugular, or subclavian vein or at the inferior vena cava through the femoral vein.

The superior vena cava is the most commonly used insertion site because more complications have been associated with catheters placed in the inferior vena cava.

Use of the femoral vein and the length of time the catheter is in the vein increase the risk of thrombotic complications. A second disadvantage is the accompanying abdominal distention that interferes with accurate right atrial pressure readings. Once the central line is in place, the nurse needs to ensure that equipment is available to set up the manometer. The pressure reading can then proceed.

Pulmonary Artery Pressure Monitoring

Pulmonary artery catheters (or balloon flotation catheters) are used to assess several hemodynamic parameters including right ventricular function, pulmonary vascular status, and indirectly, left ventricular function (Gonce Morton, Fontaine, Hudak, & Gallo, 2005). These catheters advance through the right side of the heart into the pulmonary vessels. Inflation of the balloon at a specified point in the vessel secures (wedges) the catheter in a pulmonary artery. By this means, the pulmonary artery catheter is exposed to left atrial pressure and can reflect left ventricular function.

These vascular lines are used in caring for patients undergoing major surgery, trauma patients, and those with acute respiratory and cardiac impairment. The catheters are multiluminal and can measure CVP, pulmonary artery pressure, pulmonary artery wedge pressure, cardiac output, and mixed venous oxygen saturation; this kind of line may also be used for temporary heart pacing.

Assessing and Documenting Pressure

Central venous pressure is usually read at intervals directed by the patients' condition and/or therapy. When obtaining a CVP reading, the patient must be quiet, not coughing or straining, and in a supine position with the zero point on the manometer at the mid-atrial level. The procedure involves turning the stopcock off to the patient, so that the solution flows from the IV infusion into the manometer. The fluid is allowed to fill the manometer until reaching a level of 20 cm, at which point the nurse turns the stopcock off to the IV fluid infusion and turns the stopcock open to the patient, allowing the fluid in the manometer to flow to the patient. The fluid in the manometer should drop rapidly, reaching a level point in approximately 15 seconds. A slight fluctuation in the fluid column may occur, which corresponds with the patient's respiratory rate. CVP is measured at the high point of the fluctuation. Following measurement of the CVP, the nurse readjusts the stopcock to resume the infusion by turning the stopcock off to the manometer.

Note: The catheter is presumed to be in the thoracic cavity when the manometer fluid fluctuates 3 to 5 cm during breathing and when coughing and straining cause the column of water to rise. If the catheter is inserted too far and reaches the heart, higher pressure waves synchronous with the pulse are seen (Metheny, 2000).

Central Venous Access Device Descriptions, Insertions, and Considerations

An extensive description of nontunneled CVCs, PICCs, tunneled CVCs, and implanted ports and pumps is presented in Table 14–2. The table also includes

KEY INTERVENTIONS: Setting Up the Manometer and Measuring Central Venous Pressure

Equipment

- IV pole
- IV solution as ordered
- IV or transfusion tubing
- Central venous manometer set

- Tape
- Arm board with cover or commercial securement device
- Venous pressure level (optional)

Action	Rationale
1. Wash and dry hands thoroughly.	1. Ensures a clean field
2. Close the three-way stopcock.	2. Ensures a closed system
3. Hold and squeeze the drip chamber while inserting the tubing spike into the upright IV solution container. Be sure to use Luer-lock tubing.	3. Ensures stable connection
4. Relax the hold on the drip chamber and allow the chamber to fill from one fourth to one third.	4. Equalizes pressure and thereby eliminates air bubbles
5. Assemble the manometer. If the manometer requires permanent attachment to the IV pole, tape the centimeter strip onto pole and make sure that the zero point is at mid-atrial level. Also make sure that the patient is supine and the bed flat.	5. Promotes accuracy of pressure readings
6. Making sure the manometer setup is taut, tape the manometer to the IV pole with the zero point at the patient's mid-atrial level.	6. Promotes consistent measurements
7. Turn the stopcock off to the manometer and flush entire length of tubing (IV and manometer setup) with IV fluid.	7. Allows IV tubing to be cleared of air
8. Using air embolism precautions, connect manometer and IV tubing to catheter.	8. Prevents complications
9. Secure the catheter hub and tubing connection or use Luer-locking connections.	9. Prevents separation of device
10. Measure central venous pressure.	10. Provides base reading
11. Turn the stopcock off to the patient and fill the manometer halfway.	11. Allows solution to flow into manometer
12. Turn stopcock off to the IV fluid infusing (this is a 180-degree turn).	12. Allows fluid column in manometer to settle to a pressure equivalent to the vena cava pressure
13. Turn stopcock off to manometer.	13. Allows solution to be infused to patient
14. Secure the catheterized arm to an arm board or apply a commercial securement device.	14. Ensures consistent pressure readings and prevents kinking of the catheter

insertion technique descriptions and considerations for uses, replacement, and recommendations. Since many nurses insert PICCS, a more complete description is included below, as well as more information on implanted ports and pumps. Once a CVC or device is inserted, accurate documentation is critical to ensure communication of the infusion, patient tolerance of the procedure, and a record of the actual device specifications (Box 14–5).

Peripherally Inserted Central Catheter (PICC): Considerations and Insertion Information

The PICC has many advantages for patients and healthcare providers. These include the following:

- May be inserted at the bedside or in radiology under fluoroscopy by either RNs or physicians
- Decreased risk of insertion-related complications associated with other CVCs
- Lower infection rates than other CVCs
- Better suited for young children or the elderly because of the small gauge
- Cost-effective when compared with surgically placed CVCs and devices.

A PICC does require patient-related and therapy-related cautions. It is not suitable for rapid, high volume infusions, and blood sampling may be difficult. A PICC may

---

BOX 14–5 Documentation of CVC or Device Insertion and Procedure Outcomes

Documentation supports the continuity of care within and among caregivers and organizations or institutions and on discharge to continuing care or home care. Document the following information as appropriate for each type of device:

- Patient's informed consent (consent obtained prior to insertion)
- Date and time of catheter or device insertion, number and location of attempts, specific vein used, insertion methodology, use of ultrasonography, sedatives or local anesthetic
- Catheter or device information: type, lumens, composition, manufacturer, lot number, size/original length, actual length inserted, external length
- Function of catheter—ease of flush and quality of blood return
- Flush solution used and amount
- Appearance of catheter site, site care, and dressing applied
- Method of verifying catheter tip location
- Infusate, flow rate, and method of administration (if any)
- Patient's response to placement
- Patient/caregiver teaching and verification of their understanding with materials given
- A manufacturer's registration card or a hospital information card should be completed for the patient to carry at all times. This card should contain all information about the CVC or device, such as name of device, serial and model number, type of catheter material, gauge, tip position, frequency of maintenance procedures (eg, flushing, capping, or refills), and a number to call in case of questions.

TABLE 14–2   Central Venous Access Device Descriptions, Insertion Techniques, and Considerations

Central Venous Catheter (CVC) or Access Device	Insertion Techniques	Considerations

Nontunneled CVC
Large-bore catheter percutaneously inserted into the subclavian, jugular, or femoral vein using a guidewire or stylet
• Length ≥8 cm
• Size: 14–22 gauge
• Single to multiple lumens
• Silicone, polyurethane
• Distal tip openings are open or closed ended
• Options: radiopaque, antimicrobial, or heparin impregnated
	• Inserted by physician, trained nurse practitioner, or physician assistant
	• Anatomical landmarks of clavicle and sternocleidomastoid muscle used
	• 15° Trendelenburg position assists with vein distension and prevention of air emboli.
	• Needle inserted percutaneously until flashback of blood is observed
	  ○ Guidewire is advanced and needle is removed.
	  ○ Catheter is advanced over the guidewire and the guidewire is removed.
	• Peel-away sheath or introducer may also be used.
		• Recommended for short-term placement (≤6 wk) for
		  ○ Continuous or intermittent infusions
		  ○ Multiple infusions as well as incompatible infusions
		  ○ Central venous pressure monitoring
		  ○ Emergency or critical situations—this catheter can accept rapid and high-volume fluid or medication infusions
		• Subclavian site recommended to minimize infection risk
		• Routine replacement not performed
		• Accounts for most CRBSIs

Peripherally Inserted Central Catheter (PICC) Nontunneled CVC inserted through peripheral arm vein into superior vena cava • Length: 15–27 inches • Size: 16–28 gauge • Single and double lumen • Silicone, polyurethane, or elastomeric hydrogel • Distal openings may be open or closed ended • Options: radiopaque, peripheral port	• Inserted by specially trained nurses or physicians at the bedside or under fluoroscopy • Peripheral veins in antecubital fossa area used: basilic, cephalic, median cubital	• Recommended for therapy of >7 d • Can remain in place for at least 6 mo or indefinitely until complications • Appropriate for all infusion therapies other than rapid, high-volume infusions; especially appropriate for long-term antibiotic therapy in the home setting, frequent intermittent IV medications, or blood draws in a person with limited peripheral venous access • Gravity flow rates will vary based on the gauge size and the PICC material, with flow rates through a silicone catheter being slower than through one made of polyurethane. When a positive-pressure infusion pump is used for administration, flow rates are equal.

TABLE 14–2   Central Venous Access Device Descriptions, Insertion Techniques, and Considerations (*Continued*)

Central Venous Catheter (CVC) or Access Device	Insertion Techniques	Considerations
Tunneled CVC Flexible catheter inserted into the subclavian or internal jugular vein with tip in the superior vena cava; after tunnel, distal catheter tip exits skin. • Length: 35–100 cm • Size: 2.7–12.5 French • Single to triple lumen • Polyurethane, silicone, or combination • Dacron cuff +/− antimicrobial cuff • Distal tip openings are open or closed ended • 3-way safety valve (PASV) available	• Performed by physician in a minor operating room or interventional radiology suite using a local anesthetic and sedative. • Cutdown or percutaneous puncture is used to access the vasculature. • From central vasculature, the catheter is tunneled 3–5 cm through subcutaneous tissue to an exit site on the chest. A catheter cuff lies within the subcutaneous tunnel securing the catheter. Catheter is secured with absorbable sutures at the exit site • Typical exit sites are below the nipple or in the abdomen.	• Recommended for frequent or continuous therapy or long-term therapy (>6 mo) • Fibrous tissue forms around the Dacron cuff of the catheter. The cuff and the tunnel anchor the catheter, and the cuff inhibits migration of micro-organisms. • Lower rate of infection than nontunneled. • Open-ended catheters require clamping; closed-ended or valved catheters do not. • May have integral catheter clamp and a reinforced segment of catheter to reduce the risk of silicone fatigue after repeated clamping • The external end has a threaded Luer-lock adapter for capping. When a dual-lumen catheter is used, the lumens should be labeled to indicate the purpose and function of each.
Implanted Ports Tunneled CVC is attached to an implanted port with a self-sealing septum. The port is implanted into the subcutaneous tissue. • Length: 19.7–34.5 cm • Gauge: 4–12 French • Single or double lumen • Silicone or polyurethane • Catheter can be preattached or separate. • Port is made of plastic, titanium, polysulfone, stainless steel, or a combination. • The port houses a self-sealing silicone septum. • Diameter of the port body is 16.5–40 mm	• Insertion is similar to tunneled catheter insertion with the additional step of creating a pocket through blunt dissection to accommodate the port. CVC is kept sterile and buried subcutaneously with the implanted port. • The port is sutured in the pocket. Because the center of the port will be punctured repeatedly (septum area), when the pocket is closed the suture line is lateral, medial, superior, or inferior to the port septum.	• Septum can withstand 1,000–3,600 punctures, depending on the product. • Port is accessed with special noncoring needle (Huber). • Access with the smallest needle gauge and length. • Vascular access ports may be side entry or top entry. In a side-entry port, the needle is inserted almost parallel to the reservoir. In a top-entry port, the needle is inserted perpendicular to the reservoir. • Lowest risk for CRBSI • The port does not need site care when not in use. • Infrequent flushing maintenance (4 wk). • Port device can cause artifact on diagnostic imaging studies.

(*Continued*)

TABLE 14–2 Central Venous Access Device Descriptions, Insertion Techniques, and Considerations (*Continued*)

Central Venous Catheter (CVC) or Access Device	Insertion Techniques	Considerations

Implanted Pumps
Infusion device with a power source, refillable drug reservoir, and catheter that allows drug delivery to an artery, vein or anatomical space
• Length: 76–114 cm
• Size: 6.5 French
• Single lumen silicone catheter; may have separate port for direct access to the CVC. Port is attached to the pump housing.
• Titanium pump and reservoir.
• Pump powered via pressurized gas or lithium battery
• Reservoir volume: 10–60 mL
• Flow rate preset or programmable
• Flow rate: 0.3 mL/d to 21.6 mL/d
• Silicone septum to refill reservoir
• Dose titration: reprogrammable or remove drug and replace with new concentration
• Designed for continuous, low volume, long-term therapy
• Some uses: intra-arterial infusion to the liver, intrathecal morphine, intrathecal baclofen, intravenous insulin
Product examples:
IsoMed and SynchroMed
	• The pump is implanted surgically under anesthesia, usually in the abdomen, in a subcutaneous pocket just above or below the beltline. The catheter is connected to the pump and tunneled under the skin to the intended delivery site in the body.
	• Pump preparation in the surgical suite is dependent on the type of pump and planned infusate.
		• The patient is evaluated at regular intervals depending on his or her therapy protocol for pump refills and response to therapy.
		• Factors that influence flow rate:
		  ○ Viscosity of solution
		  ○ Arterial pressure on the catheter tip
		• Several factors influence gas-powered pumps.
		  ○ Body temperature
		  ○ Changes in altitude
		  ○ Pump reservoir volume
		• Magnetic resonance imaging should not be done with implanted pumps.
		• Patient education: Importance of returning for refill as scheduled, pump alarms, avoiding hot tubs >102°F; avoid traumatic physical activity around pump site, discuss high- and low-altitude conditions with physician, symptoms of pump malfunction (symptoms related to type of drug, such as withdrawal symptoms, excessive sedation, increase in underlying symptoms of the disorder, delivery of medication into the pump pocket, increased pain)
		• Use strict aseptic technique when accessing pump.
		• Use only access and refill kits designed for the pump with noncoring needles.
		• Refill procedures are specific to pump.
		• Know the pump model, reservoir size, and flow rate.

(From: Camp-Sorrell [2004]; CDC [2002]; Gorski & Czaplewski [2004]; Greene [2000].)

restrict arm movement as well as the patient's lifestyle and activities. Also, blood pressures and blood sampling should not be taken from the arm with a PICC insertion. The presence of any of the following conditions may be a contraindication for a PICC:

- Arm contractures, injury, or other musculoskeletal or vascular condition
- Axillary lymph node dissection, such as in breast cancer surgery, is considered a lifetime precaution for avoiding vascular access in that extremity.
- Vein preservation for possible future arteriovenous fistula for patients with chronic renal insufficiency should be considered.

Implanted Peripheral Port

An implanted peripheral port is an option when continuous infusions are not required, but frequent venous access is needed. The device consists of a small, flat port with a self-sealing septum, accessible by percutaneous needle puncture, and a catheter for the parenteral delivery of medications and fluids. These ports are accessed in the same manner as other implanted vascular access devices located on the chest wall.

Nurse-inserted PICCs: Training

Most state boards of nursing permit nurses with specialized training and demonstrated competency to insert PICCs with a physician's or authorized prescriber's order as a delegated medical act. Many training programs are available; these programs should include

- 4- to 8-hour class with didactic content
- Observation of insertion with three PICC insertion demonstrations by the learner
- Supervision as requested by the learner until ease of insertion and comfort are present.

Content should include anatomy and physiology of pertinent structures and vasculature, patient assessment, insertion technique, contraindications to the PICC, possible complications and appropriate interventions, and PICC product information. Last, a thorough understanding should be demonstrated of the state Nurse Practice Act. A skills checklist may be used to determine competencies of nurses who have completed the PICC training program. An annual supervised demonstration of competency ensures ongoing quality and safety for both patient and nurse. Providing patients with information on what to do when at home or in the community empowers patients to participate in their own care (Box 14–6).

PICC Insertion Techniques

VEIN SELECTION

The basilic and cephalic antecubital fossa veins are the preferred sites for PICC placement. The basilic vein is usually the first choice for the peripheral insertion of

---

BOX 14–6   Patient and Caregivers' Guide to Managing PICC Problems

Problem	Signs and Symptoms	Action
Air enters bloodstream	Shortness of breath, coughing, chest pain	Clamp catheter. Patient should lie on left side with head down. Call Emergency Medical Services (EMS) for assistance.
Catheter breaks or is accidentally cut	Noticeable damage or leakage	Clamp catheter. Notify nurse or physician.
Injection cap disconnects	Blood inside cap or leakage	Clamp catheter and notify nurse. Apply sterile cap. Flush catheter as directed.
Evidence of infection	Pain, redness, swelling, fever, drainage at site	Notify nurse or physician. Avoid infection by using sterile technique as instructed. Keep dressing dry and intact.
Occluded catheter	Resistance is met when infusing drugs	Stop infusion immediately; do not force it. Call nurse or physician.
Central vein thrombosis	Swelling around hand, arm, or neck	Call nurse or physician.
Phlebitis	Small area of redness 7 cm in diameter surrounding insertion site; evidence of tenderness or swelling	Call nurse or physician; early treatment is necessary (may include warm, moist compresses for 20 minutes four times daily). If no improvement within 24 hours, contact nurse or physician.

---

a central venous catheter. It ascends obliquely in the groove between the biceps brachii and pronator teres and perforates the deep fascia slightly distal to the middle of the upper arm. With the arm held at a 90-degree angle, it forms the straightest, most direct route into the central venous system.

The median cubital vein is the second choice. Ascending on the ulnar side of the forearm, the vein may be divided into two vessels, one joining the basilic vein and the other the cephalic vein. This vein varies substantially, and the proper branch must be ascertained before venipuncture for PICC placement. The median antecubital basilic is preferred.

The cephalic vein runs proximally along the lateral side of the antecubital fossa in the groove between the brachioradialis and the biceps brachii. It becomes a deep vein at the clavipectoral fascia, ending in the axillary vein immediately caudal to the clavicle. It is much more tortuous than the basilic vein and presents a greater potential for catheter tip malposition. It is not preferred because it may also be difficult to thread.

KEY STEPS FOR PICC INSERTIONS

There are several key steps for PICC insertions. Anatomical measurements are taken to determine the length of the catheter required to ensure catheter tip placement in the superior vena cava. Maximal sterile barrier precautions are used. The preferred site preparation is with a 2% chlorhexidine preparation, 3 mL, applied vigorously with friction for 30 seconds and then allowed to air dry completely before insertion.

BREAKAWAY NEEDLE TECHNIQUE

Use of a breakaway needle facilitates venipuncture with an introducer needle. The catheter, with or without a guidewire, is threaded through the introducer. The introducer is removed from the venipuncture site, broken in half, and peeled away. Catheterization technique involves using an introducer needle to place a plastic catheter (peel-away sheath) into the vein. The catheter is then threaded through this sheath. The sheath is removed from the insertion site and peeled away from the catheter.

MICROINTRODUCER ALTERNATIVE TECHNIQUE

As with the guidewire, a modified Seldinger technique is used for inserting a central catheter with the microintroducer. A hydrophilic coating facilitates vascular access device exchanges. Disadvantages include the need for specialized training and additional components compared with standard PICC placement. Potential complications associated with this technique include venous rupture or perforation, arterial puncture, hematoma, and embolization. The clinician should consult product literature and institutional guidelines before using any PICC product.

ULTRASONOGRAPHY

The use of portable ultrasound device for placing peripheral IV catheters has increased the success of PICCs inserted at the bedside. With ultrasonography, the nurse may identify arterial vessels by applying pressure with the probe against the patient's arm and noting the relative ease of vein compression compared with artery compression. The ultrasound device also facilitates visualization of solid material in the lumen of the vessel, such as catheters or thrombus formations. Thus, a comprehensive assessment of cannulated and uncannulated veins is ensured. Ultrasonography requires sterile lubricant and a sterile plastic cover over the ultrasound probe.

CATHETER SECUREMENT

The PICC must be secured to stabilize the catheter to prevent inadvertent dislodgment and catheter migration. Evidence does not support one method over another, but options include sutures, sterile tape strips, or manufactured securing devices (eg, Stat-Lock, Venetec International; K-Lock, Zefon International). Sutures are intended for short-term use. They can be a source of infection, cause inflammation and discomfort, and may cause catheter occlusion if they are too tight. Sterile tape secures the catheter

KEY INTERVENTIONS:	Steps Used in Placement of Percutaneously Inserted Central Catheters

Placement of a percutaneously inserted central, nontunneled catheter is a delegated medical act.

1. Wash hands with antiseptic soap.
2. Identify known patient allergies.
3. Explain the procedure and rationale to the patient.
4. Obtain consent.
5. Assess patient.
6. Assemble equipment and don personal protective equipment as appropriate.
7. Observe Standard Precautions throughout the procedure.
8. Position patient.
9. Remove excess hair from intended insertion site with scissors.
10. Cleanse intended insertion site with antimicrobial solution.
11. Stabilize access device after placement; suturing is the preferred method. Use of sterile surgical strips, sterile tape, or stabilizing device is also appropriate.
12. Dress access site with sterile gauze and cover with sterile, transparent, semipermeable dressing.
13. Secure connection junctions.
14. Before initiating therapy, radiographically confirm catheter placement in superior vena cava.
15. Initiate prescribed therapy.
16. Discard used equipment in appropriate receptacles.
17. Document procedure in the clinical record.

well, but can be difficult to remove. The adhesive can make the catheter sticky and may harbor micro-organisms that could contaminate if used on the catheter itself. Securement devices are specifically designed to stabilize catheters and are safe and effective.

VERIFICATION OF TIP PLACEMENT WHEN INSERTING PICCS

INS recommendations include that radiographic confirmation of the tip location should be obtained in the following clinical situations: difficulty with catheter advancement, pain or discomfort after catheter advancement, inability to obtain positive aspiration of blood, inability to flush the catheter easily, and difficulty in removing guidewire or guidewire bent on removal (INS, 2000).

Implanted Ports

Components and Features

An implanted port allows access to the central venous system without a catheter exiting the skin. It is the least visible and intrusive device for the patient. Maintenance is monthly, and minimal surveillance is necessary.

The port may have one or two portals with a separate self-sealing septum for each portal, accessed with a noncoring needle. The port can be connected to a catheter

FIGURE 14–5.   Single-lumen implanted port.

that accesses the superior vena cava as well as other structures, such as the peritoneum or pleural cavity. When the port is connected to a CVC, the same potential complications exist as for other CVCs.

The port comes with preattached or separate catheters. It is important that surgical staff know that special noncoring needles should be used to verify patency of the port (Figs. 14–5 and 14–6). Additionally, a needle guard covers the area where the

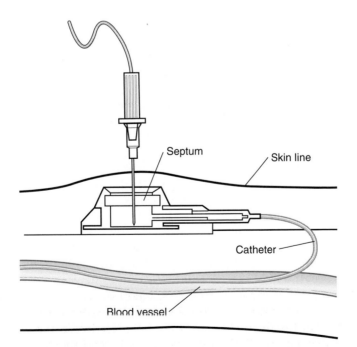

FIGURE 14–6.   Cross-section of implanted port with noncoring needle inserted.

catheter connects to the port, protecting the catheter from inadvertent puncture during access. Magnetic resonance imaging should not be done with most implanted ports; however, the MRI Port designed by Davol eliminates interference caused by metal ports during magnetic resonance imaging or computed tomography.

Noncoring Needles

Implanted ports or pumps should be accessed only by noncoring needles. A noncoring needle has an angled or deflected point that slices the septum on entry. When removed, the septum reseals itself. Noncoring needles are available in straight and 90-degree angle configurations, with or without extension sets. Some clinicians recommend the use of an ONC with needleless connector for continuous access to an implanted port.

Straight safety needles are used for heparin flush, bolus injection, or blood drawing. Needles bent to a 90-degree angle are used for continuous or frequent intermittent infusions. The bent needle may also be used for heparin flush, bolus injection, or blood drawing. Noncoring needles are also available with a permanently attached extension tubing and clamp.

Needles are available with metal or plastic hubs, in gauges 24 to 19, and in lengths from 0.5 to 2.5 inches. The required needle length depends on how superficially or deeply the septum lies. The needle gauge depends on the type and rate of infusate to be given. Packed red blood cells may require a 19-gauge needle, whereas a 24-gauge needle may be adequate for flushing. The needle must meet safety specifications; caution should be used to avoid injecting the drug into the subcutaneous tissue. An angular motion or twist of the needle must be avoided once the needle is seated in the septum to prevent cutting the septum and creating a path for drug leakage. If the heparin flush is performed without extension tubing, 3 mL heparin (100 U/mL) is used. If extension tubing is used, 5 mL heparin may be required. Again, the manufacturer's recommendations assist in developing institutional policy.

Access an implanted port or pump with the smallest needle gauge appropriate for therapy and length sufficient to touch the backstop of the port housing. Needles that are too short can become dislodged and lead to infiltration and extravasations.

Implanted Pumps

Components and Features

The pump contains a power source and refillable drug reservoir; many times there is a programmable mechanism as well. In a gas-powered implanted pump, there are two chambers separated by flexible metal bellows. One chamber is the drug–infusate compartment. The vapor pressure of the charging fluid exerts a constant pressure on the bellows, forcing the drug out of the reservoir through an outlet filter and flow restrictor into a silicone catheter. When the pump is refilled, the increasing pressure in the drug chamber exerts a pressure on the charging fluid, causing the fluid vapor to condense to its liquid state, and thereby storing energy for the next pumping cycle. Another pump is powered by a replaceable battery. The

FIGURE 14–7.   Exterior front and side view of Synchromed II implanted pump. (Courtesy of Medtronic.)

battery lasts for up to 2 years, depending on the volume of infusion, frequency of reprogramming, and other factors.

Various models are available. Most pumps have an infusion from the drug reservoir as well as a direct-access side port that bypasses the reservoir for administering bolus injections (Fig. 14–7). Another model has double catheters, which can be used to administer a drug to more than one site. The silicone catheter results in a low incidence of thrombus formation. Delivering solution by pump is an excellent method for continuous long-term administration of low-volume narcotics or antineoplastic agents to patients with cancer. Because there are no external parts, the pump requires no care between refills.

Several factors influence the pump flow rate. If the catheter site is arterial and arterial blood pressure increases significantly, the flow rate can decrease by as much as 15%. Hypotension can increase the rate by as much as 6%. When the patient moves from one altitude to another, the rate can increase by as much as 38%. Fever can increase the flow rate by as much as 13%. The amount of drug in the reservoir also affects the flow rate. The pump flow rate is established with the reservoir half full. At full volume, the rate is approximately 3% faster and at low volume 3% slower than the mean flow rate.

Never attempt to aspirate fluid from the pump. This causes blood to be drawn back into the catheter, resulting in occlusion. If no fluid is returned into the syringe barrel, either the septum has not been penetrated or the pump is completely empty of infusate. To test for septum penetration, remove the syringe barrel and connect a 5-mL syringe with normal saline solution. Inject the solution and release the plunger to allow the fluid to return to the syringe. If the fluid does not return, again attempt to locate and penetrate the septum, using 5 mL normal saline solution to test penetration. If this is not successful, the physician should be notified because pump failure may have occurred. Accurate fill and refill records are essential to ensure that the pump is refilled at the required intervals; these records also document appropriate pump functioning.

Contraindications

Contraindications to the implanted pump include body size that cannot support the size and weight of the pump; severe emotional, psychiatric, or neurologic disturbances;

and a lifestyle that involves extensive travel. Frequent altitude changes would affect only the gas-powered pump. In addition, an implanted pump can deliver only small volumes of drugs, so the device is unsuitable for patients needing greater volumes of medication.

Care and Maintenance of Central Venous Access Devices

Site Care and Dressings

Maintaining a clean, dry, and occlusive dressing is one of the most important mechanisms to prevent infection. CVCs are associated with a higher rate of CRBSIs than other catheters, and most of the organisms appear to originate from the patient's skin (Gillies, O'Riordan, Carr, Frost, Gunning, & O'Brien, 2005). Thus, antisepsis with the appropriate solution and adherence to the correct procedure is paramount. A 2% chlorhexidine-based preparation is recommended for site care (CDC, 2002; Chaiyakunapruk, Veenstra, Lipsky, & Saint, 2002).

SITE ASSESSMENT

The catheter–skin junction site should be inspected and palpated for tenderness daily through the intact dressing. Regular site inspection and standardized disinfection and dressing change should minimize the incidence of catheter-related sepsis. If there is tenderness at the site, fever without known source, or symptoms of local or systemic infection, the dressing should be removed and the site inspected directly. Signs of central venous access device (CVAD)-related complications include pain, redness, swelling, induration, tenderness, fever, chills, and inability to infuse or withdraw. Documentation should reflect routine assessment. Patient/caregiver education on assessment parameters can be provided as assessment is being performed.

DRESSINGS

A sterile dressing is applied and maintained to central line catheter sites (INS, 2000). Sterile gauze, with edges secured with occlusive material, or sterile transparent semipermeable membrane (TSM) dressings are appropriate dressings. Evidence is inconsistent to support a recommendation of one dressing over the other.

If gauze dressings are used, they should be changed every 48 hours. If transparent dressings are used, they should be changed weekly. The dressing should also be changed immediately if the integrity of the dressing is compromised (it becomes wet, soiled, or loose). The routine use of antimicrobial ointment at the insertion or catheter exit site is not recommended (CDC, 2002; INS, 2000).

Frequently there is bleeding at the insertion site (or exit site for a tunneled catheter) within the first 24 hours, so a gauze dressing is often put under the transparent dressing. When a gauze dressing is used under a transparent dressing, it is considered a gauze dressing and must be changed every 48 hours. However, with bleeding and oozing, it is critical to visually inspect the site and change the dressing if needed. After this first dressing change, it may not be necessary to put gauze under the transparent dressing. When transparent dressings are used alone, they may be changed every 7 days.

The dressing change procedure may be modified for the tunneled catheter. If the patient is immunosuppressed or if site healing is not complete, the same care given to the nontunneled catheter may be used for this catheter. If the patient is not immunosuppressed and site healing is complete, site care may be limited to daily inspection and cleansing with soap and water while bathing. Site preparation prior to accessing the port includes 2% chlorhexidine for a 30-second friction rub and aseptic technique. If the access needle is left in place, a sterile transparent semipermeable membrane dressing is used to cover the port/pump access site.

Biopatch is a quarter-sized disk placed around a central line exit site. It contains polyurethane, an absorptive foam, and chlorhexidine gluconate, a well-known antiseptic agent with antimicrobial and antifungal properties. Highly absorbent, this site cover stays in place and inhibits growth of bacteria for up to 7 days. When applied to a CVC site, the dressing helps reduce catheter tip colonization and bloodstream infection (Banton & Banning, 2002; Bhende & Spangler, 2004; Crawford, Fuhr, & Rao, 2004). Biopatch is covered with a transparent dressing to hold it in place. Follow manufacturer's directions for application and easy removal. Table 14–3 summarizes the most common care and maintenance procedures for central venous catheters and devices.

Changing Injection/Access Caps or Connectors

The injection/access connector or intermittent injection cap must be changed at routine intervals, but no more frequently than every 72 hours (CDC, 2002). These devices should also be changed when they are removed for an infusion or blood withdrawal, when residual blood remains within the connector or cap, or when integrity of the port is compromised (eg, leaking from the cap). The integrity of the cap septum should be confirmed before and immediately after each use. If compromised, it should be immediately replaced. Otherwise, the cap should be changed when the tubing is changed. It is generally recommended that injection/access caps on central access devices and catheters be changed at least as frequently as the administration set changes, usually every 96 hours (CDC, 2002). Using an injection cap that has a very small amount of dead space eliminates the need to preflush the cap, which minimizes the risk of touch contamination. Caps and connectors vary with manufacturer, so changes should be performed in accordance with the manufacturer's instructions.

If the catheter has more than one lumen, the nurse needs to change the caps/needleless connectors on all unused lumens. If the catheter is made of a material that cannot be clamped without catheter damage, the patient needs to lie flat in bed and perform the Valsalva maneuver whenever the catheter is open to the air.

CATHETER CLAMPS

Smooth-jaw clamps are used when tunneled silicone catheters are placed to prevent damage to the catheter material. Ideally, the clamp is applied to the distal two-thirds portion of the external catheter. If clamp damage should occur, catheter repair is

TABLE 14–3   Central Venous Catheter (CVC) or Device: Dressing Changes, Flushing, and Capping

Venous Access Device	Dressing Changes	Flushing: Solution/Frequency	Special Instructions and Blood Discard Amount for Blood Sampling
Nontunneled CVC *Use Biopatch*	Change transparent dressing every 7 d or gauze dressing every other day and PRN	2 mL, 0.9% NaCl every 24 h or after intermittent therapy (INS 2000; Newell-Stokes et al., 2001)	Do not routinely replace catheters unless evidence of local or systemic complications (CDC, 2002) 2 mL discard
Tunneled CVC Open tip	Use 3 mL 2% chlorhexidine solution, friction scrub for 30 s; sterile technique and sterile gloves Biopatch used *only* for nontunneled CVCs. Change every 7 d.	5 mL, 10 units/mL, heparin per lumen 3 times weekly or after intermittent therapy or blood draws (Buswell & Beyea, 1998)	May remain in place indefinitely if no complications. Can be removed only by a physician Use 10 mL or larger syringe for all IV injections.
Tunneled CVC Valve tip Groshong	Change catheter securement device every 7 d.	5 mL, 0.9% NaCl every wk or after intermittent therapy	5 mL discard
PICC Non-Groshong (open tip) *Use Biopatch*	For new catheters, if soiled, change after first 24 h. Home dressings may differ for tunneled catheters.	3 mL, 10 units/mL heparin q12h and after intermittent therapy or blood draws. Flush with 10 mL normal saline before and after IV medication.	May remain in place indefinitely if no complications (CDC 2002). Flush with 10 mL normal saline before and after blood administration. 2 mL discard Vacutainer may collapse catheter.
PICC Groshong *Use Biopatch*		5 mL, 0.9% NaCl every wk and after intermittent therapy	Use 10 mL or larger syringe for all IV injections.
Implanted Ports (including PAS-Port [arm implanted]) Non-Groshong (Open end)		5 mL, 10 units/mL heparin every 24 h while needle capped and after each intermittent IV therapy. Heparin 100 units/mL, 5 mL, prior to discontinuing Huber needle and every mo	Noncoring (Huber) needle to be changed every 7 d 20 mL normal saline flush after blood drawn Use 10 mL or larger syringe for all IV injections.
Groshong		Groshong: Flush vigorously with 0.9% NaCl 5 mL every wk and after intermittent therapy.	5 mL discard

(Sources: Buswell & Beyea [1998]; Centers for Disease Control & Prevention [2002]; Infusion Nurses Society [2005]; Newell-Stokes, Broughton, Guiliano, & Stetler [2001]; Oncology Nursing Society [2004]; and product information.)

KEY INTERVENTIONS:	Dressing Change and Site Care for Central Venous Catheters or Devices

 1. Obtain dressing materials or prepackaged kit and prepare a clean table for a work area.
 2. Position the patient comfortably on the bed.
 3. Put on the mask, wash hands thoroughly, and dry. Put on gloves.
 4. Carefully remove the old dressing. Gently lifting the tape from the outside edges inward toward the center prevents stress at the insertion site.
 5. Inspect the catheter insertion site for signs of discharge or leakage. Inspect the catheter to ensure that the sutures are intact, that the length of the external portion has not increased, that any needle protective cover is in place and locked, and that the catheter and hub are intact.
 6. Rewash the hands if they become contaminated during the dressing removal. If the procedure is performed with two pairs of gloves, the first pair is worn to remove the old dressing.
 7. Open kit. The overlay provides a sterile field.
 8. Put on the sterile gloves.
 9. Clean all debris from the insertion site and from the portion of the catheter close to the site with an alcohol swab, if necessary. Clean the site with 2% chlorhexidine in back-and-forth fashion with friction scrub for 30 seconds; allow to dry completely.
10. Apply an adhesive cover to maintain an occlusive dressing (transparent dressings may be used). Several types are available. Foam adhesive bandage or transparent tape is frequently used. Place the sterile tape directly over the site with the catheter exiting from the bottom of the tape. This position prevents stress at the catheter hub–tubing connection when the patient moves. Be sure this connection is outside the tape to facilitate tubing changes.
11. Inspect the catheter hub–tubing connection to ensure that it is locked and taped. Then loop the tubing and tape it to the chest wall to prevent stress at the connection or insertion site when the tubing is pulled or stretched.
12. Sign and date the dressing-change label and apply it to the dressing.

---

easily facilitated in this area. Clamp sites should be alternated to prevent weakening an area on the catheter itself. Second-generations silastic catheters use integral, soft-jaw clamps.

Tubing Changes

All tubing should be aseptically changed according to INS Standards of Practice (INS, 2005). The IV nurse must always keep in mind the possibility of negative pressure with a central catheter. Therefore, the risk of an air embolism is always present when the catheter is open to the air. If the patient cannot perform the Valsalva maneuver, extension tubing with a clamp that can be closed during the tubing change may be needed. Many practitioners use this system, especially for critically ill patients. Care must be taken to maintain the sterility of the extension tubing during each IV tubing change.

The extension tubing is changed at least weekly or more frequently as needed. Many times the extension set is attached during the sterile procedure of CVC insertion.

If this is the case, the extension set may not need to be changed since it is integral with the CVC. Between changes of components, the system should be maintained as a closed system. All entries into the system should be made through injection ports that have been disinfected immediately before use.

Looping the tubing and taping it to the chest wall prevents any related stress to the connection or insertion site when the tubing is pulled or inadvertently stretched. All connections should use junction securement devices or Luer-locking connections, consistent with INS Standards of Practice.

Intravenous Containers and Admixtures

All recommendations for peripheral containers or admixtures should be strictly adhered to for central catheter usage. To prevent risks of contamination, all manipulations for admixture and container changes must be performed with strict adherence to aseptic technique.

Catheter Patency

After using the catheter and at routine intervals, flushing with saline or heparin solution maintains catheter patency. For tunneled or nontunneled catheters, the frequency and heparin strength vary considerably depending on the agency or institution. The volume of the capping solution with heparin should be twice the internal volume of the CVC and any connector sets (INS, 2000). The strength of heparin may depend on the patient's condition; usually, it is 10 to 100 U/mL. Many practitioners find every-other-day flushing maintains catheter patency; see Table 14–3 for regular maintenance and flushing procedures.

Using a prefilled syringe reduces the risk of touch contamination during preparation and ensures administering the correct heparin dose. A saline flush solution may also be used. Whenever a flush solution—or any solution—is injected into ports or intermittent injection caps, using a needleless system, or at a minimum a short needle, prevents the risk of accidental puncture of the tubing or catheter. Ideally, the system used incorporates safety standards consistent with current technology.

Venous Sampling

Many central venous catheters are placed in patients who do not have peripheral veins available or who need minimal peripheral venipunctures. Therefore, drawing blood specimens through central catheters is common practice. Because each catheter is different, the nurse must follow the manufacturer's instructions for use and adhere to institutional policy that should be evidence based (Frey, 2003). The withdrawal of blood through a CVC can contribute to thrombotic catheter occlusion when the catheter is not flushed adequately.

To withdraw a blood sample, the syringe can be attached directly to a catheter to withdraw blood samples, or it can be attached to a needleless adapter and blood withdrawn through the injection port. The blood must be cleared from the injection cap after flushing and the cap changed if the blood sample is drawn through it. An evacuated tube (eg, Vacutainer) can be used to draw blood samples with most catheters. The specific catheter's specifications should be checked to confirm that it can withstand the pressure without collapsing.

The first aspirate of blood is discarded to reduce the risk of drug concentration or a diluted specimen. Reinfusion of this aspirate is not recommended owing to the risk of introducing clots into the system (Frey, 2003). The following key steps should be part of each agency's policy and procedure:

- If IV fluids are infusing, stop the infusion in *all* lumens while samples are drawn.
- Flush the catheter with normal saline prior to blood withdrawal.
- Withdraw an aspirate of 4 to 5 mL (or approximately three times catheter volume) of blood to discard before drawing laboratory sample.
- Withdraw laboratory sample.

Flush catheter vigorously with a sufficient amount (10 to 20 mL) of normal saline to adequately clear blood from the catheter. Use a push/pause technique to create turbulent flow to better clear catheter.

CVCs that have been flushed with heparin or that have heparin as a solution additive should be a secondary source for drawing blood samples for prothrombin time or partial thromboplastin time. Because heparin adheres to the catheter, falsely elevated test values may result. Coagulation studies should be drawn peripherally when possible. If the patient has no peripheral venous access, some institutions have procedures that allow for withdrawal of coagulation studies after a larger amount of blood has been withdrawn. The laboratory results should be evaluated for the possibility of false results.

Catheter Flushing and Capping

Adequate flushing is the most important factor in preventing blood, fibrin, and drug precipitates from building up and causing occlusions. The push/pause flushing technique, rather than even syringe pressure, is recommended to create a turbulent flow. Using a positive-end pressure technique while flushing, such as clamping catheter while continuing pressure on syringe, minimizes blood reflux into the lumen that may result in catheter clotting (INS, 2000). This technique involves injecting the flush solution and clamping the catheter before the syringe is completely empty. Then, the syringe and needle are removed while pressure is applied on the plunger. Of course, this technique changes when a positive-pressure access valve is in place.

Care must be taken when administering solutions and flushing through a central venous catheter because excessive pressure can be generated from a small syringe. The manufacturer of the specific device outlines the maximum recommended pressure in pounds per square inch (psi). The smaller the size of the syringe used to flush the catheter, the greater the pressure in pounds per square inch exerted on the catheter. Pressure in excess of 40 psi may cause catheter rupture with possible embolization. A wide-barrel syringe (diameter of 10 mL), which exerts <10 psi, is recommended for use with all central venous catheters to avoid excessive pressure when administering medication and flushing the catheter.

FLUSH SOLUTIONS

Flushing the catheter routinely and after each use maintains patency of the catheter. Flushing solutions and frequencies depend on the devices' characteristics, uses, and institutional policy. Heparin sodium is a protein that inhibits the conversion of prothrombin to thrombin and fibrinogen to fibrin, thus inhibiting coagulation. Controversy exists regarding the lowest dose of heparin that is effective. Newer evidence indicates that 10 units/mL may be as effective as 100 units/mL and avoids the cumulative total dose of heparin that could lead to heparin-induced thrombocytopenia or over-heparinization.

Sodium chloride (normal saline) has approximately the same osmotic pressure and composition as extracellular fluid and is thus an ideal solution for flushing blood and infusate from catheters. Sodium chloride is the only flush solution used for Groshong catheters that have the specialized closed-tip three-way valve.

Flush solution should be at least two times the internal volume of the catheter (INS, 2000). For almost all central catheters, 3 mL is an adequate amount to use as a flush solution. Using a prefilled syringe reduces the risk of touch contamination during preparation.

Implanted ports require heparin flushing after each use and monthly when not in use. This is almost universally done with 5 mL of 100 U/mL heparin (Table 14–3). A syringe or IV administration set is attached to a special noncoring needle, and the needle is primed with normal saline. The skin is prepared and punctured directly over the septum. The nurse then advances the needle through the septum until it makes contact with the bottom of the portal chamber. Without tilting or rocking the needle, the nurse flushes the device and administers the injection or infusate. The device is flushed again with 5 mL of heparinized saline solution to maintain patency. Positive pressure must be maintained when withdrawing the needle to avoid reflux of blood into the catheter.

A potential problem of over-heparinization exists when devices are capped frequently with heparin solution, ranging from one to six times per day. The nurse needs to recognize this increased risk. It is recommended to cap the device with normal saline when the device is accessed this number of times. Special note should be made on the care plan to revert to the usual capping order when the frequency matches the recommended capping regime.

Electronic Infusion Devices and Power Injection of Contrast Media

Electronic infusion pumps should be used to maintain flow accuracy and catheter patency. The diversity of electronic infusion devices today ensures availability for patients with central venous access devices. When a positive-pressure instrument is used, the pressure must not exceed that recommended for the type of catheter or electronic infusion device in use.

The question is often raised as to whether a tunneled catheter can be used for power injection of contrast media for computerized tomography (CT) examinations. The primary concern with power injection is catheter rupture. Manufacturers specify the psi that a catheter should be able to tolerate. Variables that affect or increase the psi are internal diameter, outer diameter, partial or complete occlusion, catheter material, and catheter length. Power injectors should not be used on VADs that are difficult to flush (Camp-Sorrell, 2004).

Polyurethane PICCs have been shown to tolerate higher flow rates than silicone catheters. A recent study found polyurethane PICCs tolerated power injection at the rate required for routine CT examinations of 2 mL/second (Coyle, Bloomgarden, Beres, Patel, Sane, & Hurst, 2004). Another study found that silicone PICCs were not able to withstand the higher flow rates required for CT arteriography, but many polyurethane catheters could safely be used for this purpose (Salis, Eclavea, Johnson, Patel, Wong & Tennery, 2004). Power injectors should be used cautiously with tunneled catheters and only by health care professionals who understand power injection and the properties of the specific catheter.

Complications of Indwelling Central Venous Catheters or Devices

Excellent care of patients with CVCs and devices requires skilled staff who are knowledgeable about the devices, their care, and the potential complications. Ongoing monitoring will assist in identifying problems or undesirable trends before an adverse event occurs. Risks and complications associated with central venous catheterization may be reduced when a team of qualified nursing specialists assumes responsibility for assisting with insertions, maintaining catheters and devices, and providing ongoing IV therapy care and education (INS, 2000). Astute nursing assessment and a comprehensive understanding of the vascular access device in place may avert complications such as dislodgment, migration, pinch-off syndrome, and occlusion. Potential complications and their definition, signs and symptoms, and treatment are outlined in Table 14–4. As needed, more specific information is provided below for some complications.

Catheter Occlusion

Catheter-related obstructions are categorized as nonthrombotic and thrombotic. Nonthrombotic catheter occlusions include clamped or kinked tubing, pinch-off syndrome, catheter fracture, catheter migration, and precipitation of drug. Thrombotic occlusions occur with the initiation of the coagulation process. Contributing factors include vessel wall trauma, venous stasis, and enhanced coagulation (see section on catheter properties). Risk factors for these conditions include dehydration, hypotension, atrial fibrillation, disease states (chronic renal failure, sepsis, malignancy), medications, traumatic insertion, large diameter catheters, and catheter malposition (Gorski, 2003a, 2003b; Mayo, 2001; McKnight, 2004).

It is estimated that thrombotic catheter occlusions account for about 60% of occlusions. Four categories of thrombotic catheter occlusions are commonly described in the literature:

- *Fibrin tail* is a layer of fibrin encasing the CVC at its tip. Flushing is easy, but withdrawal of blood is not possible as the "tail" acts as a one-way valve as it closes over the CVC tip.

TABLE 14–4   Potential Complications of Indwelling Central Venous Access Catheters and Devices

Complications	Signs/Symptoms	Treatment
Embolus of Catheter, Thrombus, or Air An embolus can be caused by catheter shearing, dislodgment of a thrombus, or air drawn into the central venous circulation during tubing disconnection.	Dyspnea, tachypnea, hypoxia, cyanosis, tachycardia, hypotension, precordial murmur, chest pain	Emergency Situation • For a catheter embolus, apply tourniquet to upper arm. • For thrombus, anticoagulants and thrombolytic agents are ordered. • For air embolus, position patient on left side in Trendelenburg position and give patient oxygen (may require air aspiration from right atrium). *Notify physician immediately.*
Catheter Occlusion • Catheter tip positioned against vein wall or valve • Mechanical: clamped or kinked catheter; tight sutures • Precipitate or lipid buildup • Thrombotic: fibrin tail, fibrin sheath, intraluminal occlusion, mural thrombus—may be due to inadequate flushing	Inability to infuse and/or aspirate; sluggish infusion or aspiration	• Have patient cough, raise arm, and change position, • Alleviate mechanical cause. • Flush catheter with normal saline using 10-mL syringe. • Consider flow study or other radiologic exam to determine source and site of occlusion. • Consider instillation of precipitate-clearing agent or instillation of thrombolytic agent for clot after discussion with physician and obtaining order.
Pinch-off Syndrome Mechanical compression of a CVC catheter by the clavicle and first rib at the costoclavicular space; results in catheter compression or possibly catheter fracture with resultant catheter embolism. Catheter fracture may occur as the catheter weakens owing to the scissoring action of the clavicle and first rib on the catheter (Gorski, 2003).	Difficulty infusing or withdrawing fluids until patient repositions shoulder or lies supine. Symptoms of catheter fracture and embolism may include chest pain, palpitations, swelling, or pain with flushing.	Chest radiography with patient upright and arms at side; confirmation is luminal narrowing. Catheter may be removed and reinserted carefully to stay within vein.
Thrombosis Related to CVC Compromising Blood Flow Through Superior Vena Cava (Also Known as Superior Vena Cava Syndrome [SVCS]) May be caused by malposition of catheter, intima damaged on insertion, irritating drugs, venous stasis, increased blood viscosity, or hypercoagulability.	Edema of the entire extremity, upper chest and neck; tenderness or pain in affected extremity; inability to aspirate blood and/or infuse through the catheter; discoloration of extremity	Venogram to establish diagnosis; thrombolytics, anticoagulants, and elevate extremity. CVC may have to be removed.
Catheter-Related Infections May result from contamination during insertion and/or	Local: erythema, induration, tenderness, purulent drainage from site	Blood culture from catheter and a peripheral site; remove catheter if indicated; warm moist compresses

TABLE 14–4   Potential Complications of Indwelling Central Venous Access Catheters and Devices (*Continued*)

Complications	Signs/Symptoms	Treatment
maintenance; seeding from another site; migration of micro-organisms along catheter	Systemic: fever, chills.	Appropriate antibiotic therapy may be ordered.
Damaged Catheter May occur owing to small syringe used with excessive force; use of pins or scissors near catheter; needle puncture; hemostat with teeth used on catheter	Fluid leak from catheter; ruptured catheter; popping sound heard while flushing; burning or pain with flush or infusion	Notify physician if internally ruptured. Remove catheter. If damage is external, clamp catheter proximal to tear and apply sterile dressing over tear. Repair if possible.
Catheter Tip Migration May happen because of coughing, vomiting, or excessive activity	Referred pain in jaw, ear, or teeth, distended veins on side of malposition; flushing or sense of fullness in head during rapid infusions	Radiograph or flow study to verify tip placement. Consult with physician to determine next steps.
Mechanical Phlebitis For PICCs, phlebitis at the insertion site is common during the first wk after insertion. Redness at the IV site usually appears within the first 48 h after insertion and may last the first wk. The incidence is 12.5%–23%.	Redness along the catheter line without induration, warmth, tenderness, or inflammation. The clinical signs will occur anywhere between the insertion site and the catheter tip location. Other complications (infection, infiltration, or loss of catheter integrity) should be ruled out.	• Warm moist compresses for 60 min three times daily to the affected area for 72 h • Rest and elevation of the extremity • Physician prescription for PO anti-inflammatory drugs, unless contraindicated For mechanical phlebitis, the catheter may continue to be used for IV therapy. *Observe for improvement within the first 24 h.* Continue heat application until complete resolution occurs, usually within 72 h. • Restrict movements to mild arm activity.
Extravasation From Implanted Port or Pump During Infusion or Cracked Catheter Occurs if noncoring needle not completely inserted into reservoir or it becomes loose or dislodged during infusion of vesicant or irritant drugs; CVC may have cracked owing to excessive flush pressure or scissors/pins used near catheter.	May have pain or burning in area, depending on the infusate May have redness, edema, or difficulty infusing solution	• Prevention is best intervention: use external catheter for vesicant solutions, infuse only if blood return present or correct needle placement is verified. • Stabilize needle during infusion; check infusion frequently. • Teach patient signs and symptoms of extravasation with instructions to call nurse if a problem. • If extravasation is suspected: Stop infusion. Aspirate residual drug. Give appropriate antidote. Apply heat or cold as indicated. Notify physician. Follow up with patient for observation of site, measure and photograph site for evaluation.

(Sources: Andris, Krzywda, Schulte, et al. [1997]; Arrants, Awillis, Stevens, et al. [1999]; Bagnall-Reed [1998]; Camp-Sorrell [2004]; CDC [2002]; Forauer & Alonzo [2000]; Gorski [2003a, b].)

- *Fibrin sheath* is a layer of fibrin that forms around the external surface of the catheter and can potentially extend to the entire exterior wall of the vessel. Any infusate administered may travel in a retrograde fashion along the fibrin sheath and could cause tissue irritation or necrosis depending on the nature of the infusate.
- *Intraluminal occlusion* occurs when the fibrin accumulates within the lumen of the CVC. Flow becomes sluggish and may progress to a complete occlusion. Causes include insufficient flushing, frequent blood withdrawal, or reflux of blood into the catheter.
- *Mural thrombus* is caused by catheter tip irritation against the inner lining of the vein. An accumulation of fibrin from the injury attaches to the fibrin buildup on the catheter surface causing the CVC to adhere to the vessel wall.

Symptoms of catheter occlusions include sluggish infusion, resistance to flushing, inability to aspirate blood, inability to infuse, or ability to infuse or aspirate dependent on patient positioning. Adherence to proper insertion and flushing technique according to institutional policy and guidelines decreases the incidence of catheter occlusion. Catheter occlusions can interfere with therapy and lead to CRBSI, pulmonary emboli, vein thrombosis, or superior vena cava syndrome (SVCS). Symptoms of serious complications include edema in the neck, chest, or upper extremities, jugular vein distension, or difficulty breathing. Descriptions of radiologic testing for possible catheter occlusions are given in Box 14–7.

CATHETER DECLOTTING

Clots develop when thrombin, an enzyme made from prothrombin, converts fibrinogen to fibrin, a collagen. The fibrin forms the clot. Activated plasminogen forms plasmin, an enzyme that dissolves the clot and keeps fibrinogen from reforming fibrin; this process is known as **fibrinolysis.** Within the lumen of a CVC, a clot or fibrin sheath occludes the line, and fibrinolytic agents are often used to restore patency. Thrombolytic agents dissolve clots by stimulating the conversion of plasminogen to plasmin, thereby triggering fibrinolysis. When alteplase (tPA), for example, is used

BOX 14–7   Radiologic Confirmation of Catheter Occlusions

Test	Evaluation	Indication for Test
Chest radiograph	Catheter placement	Suspected malposition—**pinch-off syndrome**, which may result from the patient's position whereby the pressure of the clavicle against the first rib pinches the catheter closed
Contrast study	Flow at distal tip of catheter	Suspected fibrin sheath formation
Venogram	Vessel patency	Suspected superior vena cava thrombosis

as directed for CVC clearance, therapeutic serum levels are not observed, because only minute amounts of the drug enter the bloodstream.

INTRALUMINAL PRECIPITATES OR LIPID BUILDUP

Precipitate may form from the mixing of incompatible drugs or solutions within the catheter or port and lead to occlusion of the catheter. Crystallization or drug-to-drug or drug-to-solution incompatibilities may exist, or an alteration in pH may cause precipitation. Precipitates may build up gradually or occur suddenly. It is uncommon when IV practice principles of adequate flushing technique and inspection for visible signs of precipitate or unusual appearance are followed. A registered pharmacist should be consulted on issues of compatibility.

In assessing occlusion, other more common causes such as mechanical obstruction and patient's position should be ruled out first. The infusate and other IV solutions are evaluated for compatibility and potential for precipitate. Intervention is initiated only after careful assessment of these factors (Krzywda, 1999). Depending on the nature of the precipitate, treatment may be possible with the use of a precipitate clearing agent specifically indicated for dissolving medication and/or solution precipitate.

Measures to restore patency from nonthrombotic occlusions are considered investigational. The instilled volume of the precipitate clearing agent solution is no greater than the internal volume of the catheter. It is allowed to dwell in the lumen of a catheter for a designated period of time, and the contents of the catheter are then aspirated. The nurse using a precipitate clearance agent should have knowledge of dosage, contraindications, side effects, and mechanism of instillation. Occlusions resulting from precipitates may result in catheter removal. Examples are included in Table 14–5. An algorithm assists the clinician to determine the best course of action; this is illustrated for catheter occlusions in Figure 14–8.

 SAFE PRACTICE ALERT For safe patient care, the clinician is urged to follow the manufacturer's recommendations for the individual thrombolytic product used.

TABLE 14–5   Solutions Causing Intraluminal Precipitates and Possible Clearing Agents

Drug/Solution	Precipitate	Clearing Agent
Total parenteral nutrition (TPN) formula with high amount calcium	Calcium/phosphorus	Hydrochloric acid (0.1% N HCl)
Low-pH drugs (eg, vancomycin)		
High-pH drugs (eg, phenytoin)		Sodium bicarbonate ($NaHCO_3$)
Lipids (eg, in 3-in-1 TPN)	Waxy buildup	70% ethanol solution

(Adapted from Gorski [2003a, b].)

KEY INTERVENTIONS: Declotting a Central Venous Catheter

Internal volume for specific catheters:

- 11-French Hickman = 0.8–0.9 mL
- 6-French = 0.5–0.7 mL
- Port-A-Cath = 1.3 mL

EQUIPMENT:

Gloves, alcohol wipe
Alteplase (r-tPa) 1 mg/mL drawn up into
    a 3-mL syringe
Sterile needle
Blue plastic catheter clamp (for use with
    silicone plastic type catheters)
10-mL syringe (empty; 2)
10-mL syringe containing 10 mL sterile
    normal saline
Luer-lock injection cap (2)

1. Disconnect IV tubing or cap from catheter. Swab catheter hub with alcohol.
2. Attach empty 10-mL syringe to hub of catheter.
3. Draw back gently on plunger to aspirate blood from catheter. If no blood is obtained, the catheter is occluded; proceed to step 5.
4. Reattach IV tubing to catheter or attach injection cap and flush central line.
5. Notify physician that catheter is occluded and obtain order for use of Alteplase to declot the catheter.
6. Obtain Alteplase from pharmacy (1 mg/mL). Only the specified amount of drug is to be used to surround and dissolve the clot. If required, follow the Alteplase with 0.9% sodium chloride to fill the remaining volume of the catheter.
7. Disconnect the IV tubing or cap at the catheter hub. *Remember:* any time the catheter hub is open to air, the line must be clamped. If clamping is not possible, instruct patient to exhale and then hold breath during the time that the catheter is open.
8. Attach the 3-mL syringe filled with 0.5 mL of Alteplase (r-tPa; 1 mg/mL). Inject the drug *slowly* and gently into the catheter. If required, follow the Alteplase with 0.9% sodium chloride to fill the remaining volume of the catheter. *Never* forcefully push on the syringe. Excessive pressure should be avoided when injecting a fibrinolytic drug into the catheter because such force could cause rupture of the catheter or expulsion of the clot into circulation. When the drug is injected slowly, the catheter can expand, allowing the drug to surround the clot.
9. Attach a Luer-lock injection cap to the catheter and wait 60 minutes.
10. Draw back *gently* on an empty 10-mL syringe to attempt to aspirate the drug and residual clot with the attached syringe.
11. If blood is not aspirated: Attempt to aspirate the first Alteplase (r-tPa) dose, discard it, and instill 1 mL of Alteplase 1 mg/mL. If required, follow Alteplase with 0.9% sodium chloride to fill the remaining volume of the catheter. Attach a Luer-lock injection cap to the catheter and wait an additional *60 minutes.*
12. Remove injection cap. Attach empty 10-mL syringe. Draw back gently on an empty 10-mL syringe to attempt to aspirate the drug and residual clot with the attached syringe.
13. Notify the physician if catheter remains occluded.
14. When the blood can be aspirated, aspirate clot into 10-mL syringe.
15. Disconnect 10-mL syringe. Attach an empty 10-mL syringe and withdraw 5–10 mL of blood. *Do not reinfuse this blood; it contains the thrombolytic.*
16. Remove blood-filled syringe and discard.

17. Connect syringe containing 10 mL normal saline. Flush catheter gently with 10 mL normal saline. Remove syringe from catheter. Reconnect IV tubing or replace injection cap and flush with appropriate solution.
18. Assess patient's tolerance to the procedure; document patient's response and outcome of intervention.

Infection

The use of central venous catheters is indispensable, especially in critical care. However, it puts patients at risk for local and systemic infections. These infectious complications include local site infections, catheter-related bloodstream infections, septic thrombophlebitis, endocarditis, and other infections such as osteomyelitis.

LOCAL INFECTION

The CDC's National Nosocomial Infection Surveillance System (NNIS) defines exit site infection as erythema or induration within 2 cm of the catheter exit site, in the absence of concomitant bloodstream infections (BSI), and without concomitant purulence (CDC, 2002; Emori, Culver, Horan, et al., 1991). There may also be tenderness at the site. Neutropenic patients may not produce a typical inflammatory response. These infections may be treated with local wound care and oral antibiotics. If signs of bacteremia are present, additional treatment may be necessary. In addition, catheter removal may be necessary.

SYSTEMIC OR CATHETER-RELATED BLOODSTREAM INFECTIONS (CRBSI)

The NNIS defines a catheter-related BSI as bacteremia-fungemia in a patient with an intravascular catheter who has at least one positive blood culture obtained from a peripheral vein, clinical manifestations of infection (ie, fever, chills, or hypotension), and no apparent source for the BSI except the catheter (CDC, 2002; Emori et al., 1991). The incidence of CRBSI varies by type of catheter, frequency of catheter access, and patient-related factors such as medical condition (Crnich & Maki, 2002b). Most serious catheter-related infections are associated with central venous catheters, especially those that are placed in critical care units. The most common type of organism that causes hospital-acquired BSIs is now coagulase-negative staphylococci, followed by enterococci. Common infectious organisms are listed in Box 14–8. These infections are costly in terms of patient morbidity and in financial resources (CDC, 2002).

Whenever a patient with a central venous catheter has an unexpected high fever, IV-related sepsis must be suspected. The insertion site should be inspected for signs of infection. A blood specimen may need to be drawn through the catheter and cultured. To rule out all sources of contamination, all tubings and containers should be changed immediately and sent promptly for bacteriologic culturing. A complete fever workup must be performed to rule out any other obvious source of infection.

Catheter Occlusion Treatment Algorithm

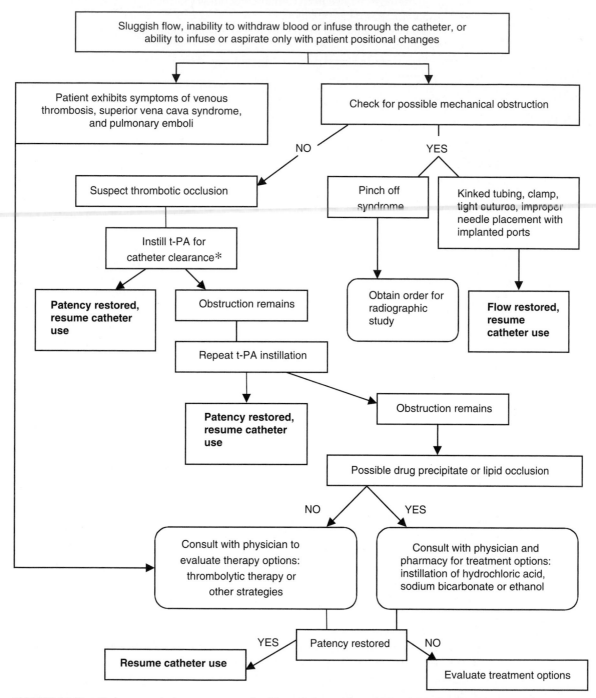

FIGURE 14–8. Catheter occlusion treatment algorithm. (Adapted from Haire & Herbst [2000]; McKnight [2004]).

BOX 14–8   Organisms Associated With Central Venous Catheter Infection

Escherichia coli
Klebsiella pneumoniae
Pseudomonas aeruginosa
Candida albicans
Staphylococcus epidermidis

If the fever remains and no other possible source can be established, catheter removal may be necessary.

Some practitioners perform a catheter exchange with a guidewire. If the blood culture is positive or the semiquantitative culture of the catheter tip yields 15 or more colonies, the new catheter is removed and the patient is considered to have catheter sepsis. If both culture results are negative, then the catheter can be used despite the fever. In cases of septic shock, shaking chills, recent positive blood cultures for *Staphylococcus* or *Candida,* or local infection of the catheter entry site, the catheter must be removed immediately. In some facilities, in situ treatment of catheter-related sepsis with a combination of systemic antibiotics and local thrombolytic agents has been reported.

Of primary importance in preventing IV-related infection is maintaining strict aseptic technique during insertion, admixture, and IV catheter manipulations. The nurse must also perform recommended site dressing and tubing changes using aseptic technique.

SINGLE LUMEN VERSUS MULTILUMEN CATHETERS

Single-lumen catheters are recommended when adequate for the required therapy (INS, 2000). A recent meta-analysis indicated that although many studies found multilumen CVCs to be associated with a slightly higher risk of infection when compared with single-lumen catheters, this relationship diminishes when only high-quality studies that control for patient differences are considered (Dezfulian et al., 2003). In many patient circumstances, especially in critical care, the advantages of using a multilumen catheter outweigh the slight increase in infectious risk.

Other strategies shown to be effective in preventing infection include

- Staff education
- Standardization of aseptic technique—good hand hygiene, maximal sterile barrier precautions (eg, cap, mask, sterile gown, sterile gloves, large sterile drape) during insertion of CVCs)
- Specialized IV teams
- Adequate staffing—infection risk increases with nursing staff reductions below a critical level.

Catheter Repair

Catheters can be damaged by excessive pressure with flushing, accidental cutting by scissors or clamps, or dislodgment of the catheter from an implanted portal body. Implanted ports need to be removed in the event of catheter damage. Nontunneled catheters can be replaced with guidewire exchange. "Survival" knowledge for the patient includes being able to identify a leak and knowing how to clamp or fold over the catheter until the patient can be seen. Some patients have been able to fold over the catheter and secure it with a rubber band.

Catheter repair kits are available for tunnelled catheters and PICC lines from individual manufacturers. Select a repair specific to the manufacturer and size of the catheter. Repair kits are sterile and include at least the replacement catheter, syringe, and Luer-lock plug. They are also available to repair double- and triple-lumen catheters. It is important to follow manufacturer instructions when repairing a catheter. Because catheter repairs are extremely rare, it is often helpful to have two people do the procedure: one to do the repair and one to assess the patient and read the directions. The following are general guidelines:

- Provide a sterile field: Assemble supplies including a sterile scissors.
- The catheter should already be clamped proximal to the rupture.
- Prep the site.
- Cut the damaged catheter to remove the damaged portion and provide a clean edge.
- Apply the repair sleeve, blunt connector, and adhesive as directed by the manufacturer.
- Secure the repaired area per manufacturer's directions.

A sterile repair kit, specific to the individual type of catheter, should be readily available. Repairing the external portion of a tunneled catheter is a sterile procedure requiring surgical gloves, gown, mask, and cap. (Note that some manufacturers provide catheter repair kits that may be used for most catheters.)

Once the catheter repair is achieved, taping a Luer-lock 0.2-µm air-eliminating filter directly to the catheter hub reduces the risk of connection separation and air infusion that could result in a fatal embolism. If a separation occurs distal to the filter, this device prevents air infusion and an inadvertent bleed. The 0.2-µm filter can also prevent any particulate matter, fungi, bacteria, and endotoxins from entering the system through the filter.

Removal of PICCs and Nontunneled CVCs

PICC REMOVAL

PICCs may be removed by a nurse with a physician's or authorized prescriber's order. The procedure involves removing the sutures, if present, and gently pulling the catheter out using precautions to prevent air embolism. Instruct the patient to take a deep breath and hold it as you gently pull the catheter out, 2 to 3 inches at a time. Pressure is held over the site with sterile gauze and a gloved finger until hemostasis is achieved; then antiseptic ointment and a sterile occlusive dressing should be applied to the access site. Application of ointment may occlude the skin tract and prevent air embolism (INS, 2005). The catheter tip should be inspected to ensure it is smooth and intact.

If resistance occurs during removal, *do not force removal*. Wait 30 minutes and try again. Apply heat to the upper arm, axilla, and hand; warming the extremity may decrease vasospasm and allow catheter removal. Try relaxation techniques or have the patient drink warm liquids. Flush the catheter gently with 10 mL 0.9% NaCl. If all of the above fail, notify the physician, who will consult an interventional radiologist.

After PICC removal, the dressing should be changed and the access site assessed every 24 hours until the site is epithelialized. Documentation of discontinuation of therapy includes catheter length and integrity, site appearance, dressing applied, and patient tolerance.

Nontunneled CVC Removal

A nurse may remove nontunneled CVCs with a physician or prescriber order. Explain to the patient what will happen and risks of removal; this will enable the patient to understand why it is important to lie still. Assist the patient to a supine position. Remove sutures if present. Instruct the patient to take in a deep breath and then hold it while withdrawing the catheter. If the patient is on a ventilator, withdraw the catheter during the expiratory cycle. Grasp the catheter with the dominant hand and steadily withdraw the catheter in one continuous motion while stabilizing the site with gauze in the other hand. Note that the distal end of a multilumen catheter should be removed quickly, since the exposed proximal and medial openings could permit air entry. Apply pressure with sterile gauze over the insertion point until bleeding has stopped. Apply pressure for a minimum of 1 minute or until bleeding stops. Cover site with an occlusive dressing. Instruct patient to notify the nurse if any bleeding is noted. Evaluate the catheter tip for signs of breakage; it should be smooth and intact. If you suspect that the catheter has been broken, have the patient lie still on the left side and notify the physician *immediately*. Document removal of catheter and any significant findings.

Nursing Practice: Skilled, Knowledgeable, and Safe

A focus on system safe practices and a nonpunitive environment for safe reporting is paramount for continually improving practice. Evidence-based practices, policies and procedures based on the best evidence, continuing education and annual skill demonstrations will provide practitioners with the tools to care for patients with these technologies. Competency checklists ensure thorough training and accurate return demonstrations. A documentation record that lists all the steps for accessing and maintaining long-term venous access assists family members and skilled technicians in consistently following safe practices and record their actions if follow-up is necessary.

BOX 14–9   Research Questions Still to Be Answered and Outcome Studies Needed

- What is the optimal dose for t-PA for central venous catheter occlusion?
- Does 2% chlorhexidine friction scrub using back and forth/up and down improve antisepsis versus back and forth only?
- What is the ideal capping solution and frequency for PICCs and nontunneled CVCs?
- CVC CRBSI rates for both ICU and medical/surgical units in adults and infants
- Occlusion rate for PICCs per 1,000 catheter days
- 100% of CVC dressings are dry, intact, applied correctly, and changed per policy.
- Complication rates for indwelling CVCs and devices per 1,000 catheter days are tracked and continually improved.

Nursing can impact patient-centered care by developing a multidisciplinary team to systematically select products and benchmark patient outcomes (Ault, Ng, & Artal, 2001; Galloway, 2002; Gorski, 2004; Hornsby, Matter, Beets, Casey, & Kokotis, 2005; McMahon, 2002; Moureau, Poole, Murdock, Gray, & Semba, 2002). Products should be reviewed annually and updated based on a body of sound research. Nurse-sensitive and health care team outcomes for CVCs and devices have been identified by the American Nurses Association, National Quality Forum and Institute for Healthcare Improvement (IHI, 2005). Outcomes for these indicators need to be measured, collected, and reported regularly to the Infections Control Committee, the IV Team, and to staff nurses on ICU and medical/surgical units. Data need to be reported so that improvements may be tracked and communicated. Questions for study to provide evidence for best practice and outcomes that need to be tracked are identified in Box 14–9, and legal and safety issues are highlighted in Box 14–10. Generating knowledge to improve nursing practices and using data to improve care and system processes advances quality care for all patients.

BOX 14–10   Legal and Safety Issues for Central Vascular Access Devices

- National and professional association guidelines, evidence-based practice, and health care–related agencies provide best practices that must be considered and adopted in agencies and institutions.
- Caregiver skill demonstration, policies, technology, and outcomes need to be reviewed regularly and on an appropriate basis that addresses the rapid changes in evidence and technology and helps maintain competent practitioners.
- Safety initiatives, including patient identifiers, infection prevention, and high-alert medications, need to become standard in agencies and institutions.
- Patients need to be involved in their own care, knowledgeable about care-related decisions and expected outcomes (Institute of Medicine, 2004).

References and Selected Readings

Asterisks indicate references cited in text.

*Andris, D.A., Krzywda, E.A., & Schulte, W., et al. (1997). Catheter pinch-off syndrome: Recognition and management. *Journal of Intravenous Nursing, 20*(12), 233–237.

*Arrants, J., Willis, M., Stevens, B., et al. (1999). Reliability of an intravenous intermittent port (saline lock) for obtaining blood sample for coagulation studies. *American Journal of Critical Care, 8,* 344–348.

*Ault, M., Ng, P., & Artal, R. (2001). The changing use of peripherally inserted central catheters: A review of 5000 insertions at a single hospital. *Journal of Clinical Outcomes Management, 8*(9), 17–23.

*Bagnall-Reed, H. (1998). Diagnosis of central venous access device occlusion: Implications for nursing practice. *Journal of Intravenous Nursing, 21*(Suppl. 5), S115–S117.

Banton, J., & Banning, V. (2002). Impact on catheter-related bloodstream infections with the use of the Biopatch dressing. *Journal of the Association for Vascular Access, 7*(3), 27–32.

*Barton, A., Danek, G., Johns, P, & Coons, M. (1998). Improving patient outcomes through CQI: Vascular access planning. *Journal of Nursing Care Quality, 13,* 77–85.

Bhende, S. (2004). In vitro assessment of chlorhexidine gluconate-impregnated polyurethane foam antimicrobial dressing using zone of inhibition assays. *Infection Control and Hospital Epidemiology, 25,* 664–667.

*Bong, J.J., Kite, P., Wilco, M.H., & McMahon, M.J. (2003). Prevention of catheter related bloodstream infection by silver iontophoretic central venous catheters: A randomized controlled trial. *Journal of Clinical Pathology, 56,* 731–735.

*Braun, B.I., Kritchevsky, S.B., Wong, E.S., et al., & Evaluation of Processes and Indicators in Infection Control (EPIC) Study Group. (2003). Preventing central venous catheter-associated primary bloodstream infections: Characteristics of practices among hospitals participating in the evaluation of processes and indicators in infection control (EPIC) study. *Infection Control and Hospital Epidemiology, 24*(12), 926–935.

*Buswell, L., & Beyea, S. (1998). Flushing protocols for tunneled central venous catheters: An integrative review of the literature. *Online Journal of Knowledge Synthesis for Nursing, 5*(Doc. No. 3).

*Camp-Sorrell, C. (Ed.). (2004). Access device guidelines: Recommendations for nursing practice and education (2nd ed.). Pittsburgh, PA: Oncology Nursing Society.

*Centers for Disease Control and Prevention. (2002). Guidelines for the prevention of intravascular catheter-related infections. *Morbidity and Mortality Weekly Report 51* (No. RR-10), 1–29. Erratum and correction for Appendix B in: *MMWR, 51*(32), 711.

*Chaiyakunapruk, N., Veenstra, D., Lipsky, B., & Saint, S. (2002). Chlorhexidine compared with povidone-iodine solution for vascular catheter-site care: A meta-analysis. *Annals of Internal Medicine, 136,* 792–801.

*Coyle, D., Bloomgarden, D., Beres, R., Patel, S., Sane, S., & Hurst, E. (2004). Power injection of contrast media via peripherally inserted central catheters for CT. *Journal of Vascular Interventional Radiology, 15,* 809–814.

*Crawford, A., Fuhr, J., & Rao, B. (2004). Cost-benefit analysis of chlorhexidine gluconate dressing in the prevention of catheter related-bloodstream infections. *Infection Control and Hospital Epidemiology, 25,* 668–674.

*Crnich, C.J., & Maki, D.G. (2002a). New technology for reducing infection and resistance in the ICU. *The Journal of Critical Illness, 17*(2), 48–50.

*Crnich, C., & Maki, D. (2002b). The promise of novel technology for the prevention of intravascular device-related bloodstream infection. *Clinical Infectious Diseases, 34,* 1232–1242.

Darouiche, R.O., Raad I.I., Heard, S.O., et al. (1999). A comparison of two antimicrobial-impregnated central venous catheters. *New England Journal of Medicine, 240,* 1–8.

*Dezfulian, C., Lavelle, J., Nallamothu, B,. Kaufman, S., & Saint, S. (2003). Rates of infection for single-lumen versus multi-lumen central venous catheters: A meta-analysis. *Critical Care Medicine, 31,* 2385–2390.

*Emori, T., Culver, G., Horan, T., Jarvis, W., et al. (1991). National nosocomial infections surveillance system (NNIS): Description of surveillance methods. *American Journal of Infection Control, 19,* 19–35.

*Forauer, A., & Alonzo, M. (2000). Change in peripherally inserted central catheter tip position with abduction and adduction of the upper extremity. *Journal of Vascular Interventional Radiology, 11*(10), 1315–1318.

*Frey, A. (2003). Drawing blood samples from vascular access devices: Evidence-based practice. *Journal of Infusion Nurses, 26*(5), 285–293.

*Galloway, M. (2002). Using benchmarking data to determine vascular access device selection. *Journal of Intravenous Nursing, 25*(5), 320–325.

*Gaonkar, T.A., & Modak, S.M. (2003). Comparison of microbial adherence to antiseptic and antibiotic central venous catheters using a novel agar subcutaneous infection model. *Journal of Antimicrobial Chemotherapy, 52,* 389–396.

*Garland, J.S., Henrickson, K., & Maki, D.G. (2002). The 2002 hospital infection control practices advisory committee centers for disease control and prevention guideline for prevention of intravascular device-related infection. *Pediatrics, 110*(5), 1009–1013.

Geerts, W., Jeit, J., Clagett, G., et al. (2001). Prevention of venous thromboembolism. *Chest, 119*(suppl 1), 132S–175S.

*Gillies, D., O'Riordan, L., Carr, D., Frost, J., Gunning, R., & O'Brien, I. (2005). Gauze and tape and transparent polyurethane dressings for central venous catheters. *Cochrane Database of Systematic Reviews, 1.*

*Gnass, S.A., Barboza, L., Bilicich, D., et al. (2004). Prevention of central venous catheter-related bloodstream infections using non-technologic strategies. *Infection Control and Hospital Epidemiology, 25*(8), 675–677.

*Gonce Morton, P., Fontaine, D., Hudak, C., & Gallo, B. (2005). *Critical care nursing: A holistic approach.* Philadelphia: Lippincott Williams & Wilkins.

Goode, C., Kleiber, C., Titler, M., et al. (1993). Improving practice through research: The case of heparin vs. saline for peripheral intermittent infusion devices. *MEDSURG Nursing, 2,* 23–27.

*Gorski, L.A. (2003a). Central venous access device occlusions, pt. 1: Thrombotic causes and treatment. *Home Healthcare Nurse, 21*(2), 115–121.

*Gorski, L.A. (2003b). Central venous access device occlusions, pt. 2: Non-thrombotic causes and treatment. *Home Healthcare Nurse, 21*(3), 168–171.

*Gorski, L.A. (2004). Central venous access device outcomes in a homecare agency: A 7-year study. *Journal of Infusion Nursing, 27*(2), 104–111.

*Gorski, L.A., & Czaplewski, L.M. (2004). Peripherally inserted central catheters and midline catheters for the homecare nurse. *Journal of Infusion Nursing, 27*(6), 399–409.

*Greene, D. (2000). Venous access devices. In V. Fieler & P.A. Hanson (Eds.). *Oncology nursing in the home*, pp. 13–32. Pittsburgh, PA: Oncology Nursing Society.

Griffiths, V., & Philpot, P. (2002). Peripherally inserted central catheters (PICCs): Do they have a role in the care of the critically ill patient? *Intensive Critical Care Nursing, 18*, 37–40.

*Halderman, F. (2000). VAD: selecting a vascular access device. *Nursing, 30*(11), 59–61.

*Hanna, H., Benjamin, R., Chatzinikolaou, I., et al. (2004). Long-term silicone central venous catheters impregnated with minocycline and rifampin decrease rates of catheter-related bloodstream infection in cancer patients: a prospective randomized clinical trial. *Journal of Clinical Oncology, 22*(15), 3163–3171.

*Harter, C., Salwender, H.J., Bach, A., Egerer, G., Goldschmidt, H., & Ho, A.D. (2002). Catheter-related infection and thrombosis of the internal jugular vein in hematologic-oncologic patients undergoing chemotherapy: A prospective comparison of silver-coated and uncoated catheters. *Cancer, 94*(1), 245–251.

Holmes, K.R. (1998). Comparison of push-pull versus discard method from central venous catheters for blood testing. *Journal of Intravenous Nursing, 21*(5), 282–285.

Horattas, M., Trupian, J., Hopkins, S., et al. (2001). Changing concepts in long-term venous access: Catheter selection and cost savings. *American Journal of Infection Control, 28*, 32–40.

*Hornsby, S., Matter, K., Beets, B., Casey, S., & Kokotis, K. (2005). Cost losses associated with the 'PICC, stick, and run team' concept. *Journal of Infusion Nursing, 28*(1), 45–53.

*Hu, K.K., Lipsky, B.A., Veenstra, D.L., & Saint, S. (2004). Using maximal sterile barriers to prevent central venous catheter-related infection: A systematic evidence-based review. *American Journal of Infection Control, 32*(3), 142–146.

*Institute for Healthcare Improvement (IHI). (2005). 100k Lives Campaign at http://www.ihi.org/IHI/Programs/Campaign/Campaign.htm. (Accessed 8/17/2005.)

*Institute of Medicine. (2004). *Keeping patients safe: Transforming the work environment of nurses.* Washington, DC: National Academies Press.

*Infusion Nurses Society. (2000). Revised standards of practice. *Journal of Infusion Nursing, 23*(Suppl. 1).

*Infusion Nurses Society. (2005). Revised standards of practice. *Journal of Infusion Nursing, 28*(Suppl. 1).

Intravenous Nurses Society. (2004). *Core curriculum for infusion nursing* (3rd ed.). Philadelphia: Lippincott Williams & Wilkins.

Jackson, D. (2001). Infection control principles and practices in the care and management of vascular access devices in the alternate care setting. *Journal of Intravenous Nursing, 24*(Suppl. 3), S28–S34.

*Krau, S. (2003). Review: chlorhexidine gluconate is more effective than povidone-iodine for preventing vascular catheter related bloodstream infections. *Evidence Based Nursing, 6*(1), 18.

*Krzywda, E.A. (1999). Predisposing factors, prevention, and management of central venous catheter occlusions. *Journal of Intravenous Nursing, 22*(Suppl. 6), 11–14.

*Lamont, J.P., McCarty, T.M., Stephens, J.S., et al. (2003). A randomized trial of valved vs nonvalved implantable ports for vascular access. *Baylor University Medical Center Proceedings, 16*(4), 384–387.

LaRue, G.D. (1999). Efficacy of ultrasonography in peripheral venous cannulation. *Journal of Intravenous Nursing, 23*(1), 29–32.

Lenhart, C. (2001). Preventing central venous access device occlusions with saline only flush by use of an adapter. *Journal of Vascular Access Devices, 6*(4), 29–31.

Lin, B.S., Kong, C.W., & Tarng, D.C. (1998). Anatomical variation of the internal jugular vein and its impact on temporary haemodialysis vascular access: An ultrasonographic survey in uraemic patients. *Nephrology Dialysis Transplant, 143*, 134–138.

*Marciante, K.D., Veenstra, D.L., Lipsky, B.A., & Saint, S. (2003). Which antimicrobial impregnated central venous catheter should we use? Modeling the costs and outcomes of antimicrobial catheter use. *American Journal of Infection Control, 31*(1), 1–8.

*Marin, M.G., Lee, J.C., & Skurnick, J.H. (2000). Prevention of nosocomial bloodstream infections: Effectiveness of antimicrobial-impregnated and heparin-bonded central catheters. *Critical Care Medicine, 28*(9), 3332–3338.

Masoorli, S., & Angeles, T. (2002). Getting a line of central venous access devices. *Nursing, 32*(4), 36–43.

Mayo Clinic Proceedings. (2000). Complications and cost associated with parenteral nutrition delivered to hospitalized patients through either subclavian or peripherally inserted central catheters. *Clinical Nutrition, 19*, 237–243.

*Mayo, D.J. (2001). Catheter-related thrombosis. *Journal of Intravenous Nursing, 24*(3), S13–S22.

Mayo, D., Dimond, E., Kramer, W., & Horne, M. (1996). Discard volumes necessary for clinically useful coagulation studies from heparinized Hickman catheters. *Oncology Nursing Forum, 23*(4), 671–675.

*McKnight, S. (2004). Nurse's guide to understanding and treating thrombotic occlusion of central venous access devices. *Medsurg Nursing, 13*(6), 377–382.

*McMahon, D. (2002). Evaluating new technology to improve patient outcomes. *Journal of Infusion Nursing, 25*, 250–255.

*Mehall, J.R., Saltzman, D.A., Jackson, R.J., & Smith, S.D. (2001). Catheter materials affect the incidence of late blood-borne catheter infection. *Surgical Infection, 2*(3), 225–229.

*Mehall, J.R., Saltzman, D.A., Jackson, R.J., & Smith, S.D. (2002). Fibrin sheath enhances central venous catheter infection. *Critical Care Medicine, 30*(4), 908–912.

*Mermel, L.A. (2000). Prevention of intravascular catheter-related infections. *Annals of Internal Medicine, 132*(5), 391–402. Erratum, *133*(5), 5.

*Mermel, L.A. (2001). New technologies to prevent intravascular catheter-related bloodstream infections. *Emerging Infectious Diseases, 7*(2), 197–199.

*Metheny, N.M. (2000). *Fluid and electrolyte balance* (4th ed.). Philadelphia: Lippincott Williams & Wilkins.

*Moureau, N., Poole, S., Murdock, M., Gray, S., & Semba, C. (2002). Central venous catheters in home infusion care: Outcomes analysis in 50,470 patients. *Journal of Vascular Interventional Radiology, 13,* 1009–1016.

*Munck, A., Malbezin, S., Bloch, J., et al. (2004). Follow-up of 452 totally implantable vascular devices in cystic fibrosis patients. *European Respiratory Journal, 23*(3), 430–434.

National Kidney Foundation. (2000). NKF-K/DOQI clinical practice guidelines for vascular access: Update 2000. *American Journal of Kidney Disease, 37*(1 Suppl), S137–181.

National Kidney Foundation. (2002). *K/DOQI clinical practice guidelines for chronic kidney disease: Executive summary.* New York: Author.

*Newell-Stokes, V., Broughton, S., Guiliano, K., & Stetler, C. (2001). Developing an evidence-based procedure: Maintenance of central venous catheters. *Clinical Nurse Specialist, 15,* 199–204.

Penne, K. (2002). Using evidence in central catheter care. *Seminars in Oncology Nursing, 18*(1), 66–70.

Penney-Timmons, E., & Sevedge, S. (2004). Outcome data for peripherally inserted central catheters used in an acute care setting. *Journal of Infusion Nursing, 27*(6), 431–436.

Perry, A., & Potter, P. (2004). Clinical Nursing Skills and Techniques (5th ed.). St. Louis, MO: Mosby.

Pinto, K. (1994). Accuracy of coagulation values obtained from a heparinized central venous catheter. *Oncology Nursing Forum, 21*(3), 573–575.

Powers, J. (1999). Obtaining blood samples for coagulation studies from a normal saline lock. *American Journal of Critical Care, 8,* 250–253.

Raad, I., Darouiche, R., Dupuis, J., et al. (1997). Central venous catheters coated with minocycline and rifampin for the prevention of catheter-related colonization and blood stream infections. *Annals of Internal Medicine, 128,* 267–274.

*Ranucci, M., Isgro, G., Biomarelli, P.P., et al., & the Catheter Related Infection Trial (CRIT) Group. (2003). Impact of oligon central venous catheters on catheter colonization and catheter-related bloodstream infection. *Critical Care Medicine, 31*(1), 52–59.

*Registered Nurses Association of Ontario. (2004). *Assessment and device selection for vascular access.* Toronto: Author.

*Rubinson, L, & Diette, G.B. (2004). Best practices for insertion of central venous catheters in intensive-care units to prevent catheter-related bloodstream infections. *Journal of Laboratory & Clinical Medicine, 143,* 5–13.

*Ruesch, S., Walder, B., & Tramer, M. (2002). Complications of central venous catheters: Internal jugular versus subclavian access—a systematic review. *Critical Care Medicine, 30*(2), 454–460.

Saad, T.F., & Vesely, T.M. (2003). Venous access for patients with chronic renal failure or end-stage renal disease: What is the role for peripherally inserted central catheters? *The Journal of the Association for Vascular Access, 8*(4), 27–32.

*Saint, S., Veenstra, D.L., & Lipsky, B.A. (2000). The clinical and economic consequences of nosocomial central venous catheter-related infection: Are antimicrobial catheters useful? *Infection Control and Hospital Epidemiology, 21*(6), 375–380.

*Salis, A., Eclavea, A., Johnson, M., Patel, N., Wong, D., & Tennery, G. (2004). Maximal flow rates possible during power injection through currently available PICCs: An in vitro study. *Journal of Vascular Interventional Radiology, 15,* 275–281.

*Sampath, L.A., Saborio, D.V., Yaron, I., & Modak, S. (2001). Safety and efficacy of an improved antiseptic catheter impregnated intraluminally with chlorhexidine. *Journal of Infusion Nursing, 24*(6), 395–403.

Sampath, L.A., Tambe, S.M., & Modak, S.M. (2001). In vitro and in vivo efficacy of catheters impregnated with antiseptics or antibiotics: Evaluation of the risk of bacterial resistance to the antimicrobials in the catheters. *Infection Control and Hospital Epidemiology, 22*(10), 640–646.

Schutz, J., Patel, A., Clark, T., et al. (2004). Relationship between chest port catheter tip position and port malfunction after interventional radiologic placement. *Journal of Interventional Radiology, 15,* 581–587.

*Tambe, S.M., Sampath, L., & Modak, S. M. (2001). In vitro evaluation of the risk of developing bacterial resistance to antiseptics and antibiotics used in medical devices. *Journal of Antimicrobial Chemotherapy, 47,* 589–598.

*Urden, L., Stacy, K., & Lough, M. (2004). Priorities in critical care nursing. St. Louis, MO: Mosby.

*Veenstra, D.L., Saint, S., Saha, S., Lumley, T., & Sullivan, S. (1999). Efficacy of antiseptic-impregnated central venous catheters in preventing catheter-related bloodstream infection: A meta-analysis. *Journal of the American Medical Association, 281*(3), 261–267.

Veenstra, D.L., Saint, S., & Sullivan, S. (1999). Cost-effectiveness of antiseptic-impregnated central venous catheters for the prevention of catheter-related bloodstream infection. *Journal of the American Medical Association, 282*(2), 554–560.

Vesely, T. (2003). Central venous catheter tip position: A continuing controversy. *Journal of Vascular and Interventional Radiology, 14*(5), 527–534.

*Volkow, P., Vazquez, C., Tellez, O., et al. (2003). Polyurethane II catheter as long-indwelling intravenous catheter in patients with cancer. *American Journal of Infection Control, 31*(7), 392–396.

*Von Eiff, C., Jansen, B., Kohnen, W., & Becker, K. (2005). Infections associated with medical devices: Pathogenesis, management, and prophylaxis. *Drugs, 65*(2), 179–214.

Walshe, L., Malak, S., Eagan, J., & Sepkowitz, K. (2002). Complication rates among cancer patients with peripherally inserted central catheters. *Journal of Clinical Oncology, 20*(15), 3276–3281.

Woodrow, P. (2002). Central venous catheters and central venous pressure. *Nursing Standard, 16*(2), 45–52, 54.

*Zurcher, M., Tramer, M., & Walder, B. (2004). Colonization and bloodstream infection with single- versus multi-lumen central venous catheters: A quantitative systematic review. *Anesthesia & Analgesia, 99,* 177–182.

Review Questions

Note: Questions below may have more than one right answer.

1. Which of the following statements is true of hydrothorax?
   A. Results when IV fluid infiltrates into the intravascular space
   B. Results when IV fluid infiltrates into the chest
   C. Has signs and symptoms identical to pneumothorax
   D. Has life-threatening implications

2. To accurately measure central venous pressure, the zero point on the manometer should be adjusted to what level?
   A. Right atrium
   B. Patient's heart
   C. Left lung
   D. Substernal notch

3. Air embolism may be avoided by using which of the following procedures?
   A. PICC insertion
   B. Valsalva maneuver
   C. Pneumocentesis
   D. Fluoroscopy

4. Radiologic testing for catheter occlusion includes all of the following tests *except:*
   A. Chest radiograph
   B. Air-contrast study
   C. Venogram
   D. Duplex scan

5. Which of the following statements concerning central venous catheter patency is correct?
   A. Patency includes ability to infuse through and aspirate blood from the catheter.
   B. Risk for occlusion increases with dehydration and atrial fibrillation.
   C. Occlusions can lead to CRBSI or SVCS.
   D. All of the above

6. The most common cause of catheter occlusion is:
   A. Clumping of particulate matter in the infusate
   B. Catheter defects
   C. Infection
   D. Thrombosis

7. Pain with infusion is a sign of which of the following?
   A. Catheter malposition
   B. Pinch-off syndrome
   C. Fibrin sheath occlusion
   D. External compression

8. The central vein used for CVCs with the least risk for CRBSI is:
   A. Brachiocephalic
   B. Femoral
   C. Internal jugular
   D. Subclavian

9. The chest radiograph is a test for:
   A. Fibrin sheath formation
   B. Pinch-off syndrome
   C. Superior vena cava syndrome
   D. Tip placement verification

10. Which of the following statements are true of air embolism?
    A. PASV reduces risk
    B. Trendelenberg position is indicated if air embolism is suspected.
    C. Digital pressure on the artery for 5 minutes is one treatment.
    D. Pneumothorax occurs at the same time.

CHAPTER 15

Alternate Access

KEY TERMS

Arterial Blood Gas (ABG)
  Analysis
Arterial Pressure Monitoring
Base Bicarbonate
Bicarbonate Excess

Hemoglobin Desaturation
Intraosseous Infusion
Oxyhemoglobin Dissociation
Total Pressure of Atmosphere
Ventricular Reservoir

Role of Arterial Blood Gas Analysis

Arterial blood with all its nourishing elements supplies all body tissues; thus, arterial blood is used routinely for diagnosing abnormalities and assessing patients' conditions. Intra-arterial therapy may involve one-time or daily blood sampling to analyze the concentration of gases, such as oxygen, and other components, or it may involve inserting an indwelling catheter to obtain serial or daily samples for **arterial blood gas (ABG) analysis** and continuous **arterial pressure monitoring**.

Although venous, arterial, and capillary blood all contain comparable levels of carbon dioxide and **base bicarbonate**, the levels of oxygen in venous and capillary blood vary significantly from the level of oxygen in arterial blood.

Oxygen in Plasma

Oxygen moves through the circulatory system in plasma and hemoglobin; because the small amount of oxygen dissolved in plasma cannot be measured directly, its presence is expressed as the tension or partial pressure it exerts on plasma (PaO_2—the letter P symbolizes the pressure value; the letter a signifies that the partial pressure of oxygen measured is that in arterial blood).

Oxygen in Hemoglobin

The major portion of blood oxygen is bound to hemoglobin and measured as a percentage of the hemoglobin saturated with oxygen (SaO_2). Tissue is adequately oxygenated when the partial pressure of oxygen in arterial blood (PaO_2) ranges between 80 and 100 mm Hg and when hemoglobin saturation (SaO_2) ranges from 93% to 100% (Horne & Derrico, 1999).

Under normal circumstances, when the PaO_2 value decreases slightly, there is an incremental drop in the SaO_2 value. However, when PaO_2 falls below 60 mm Hg, the association is disturbed, and minute decreases in partial pressure cause significant drops in SaO_2, known as **hemoglobin desaturation**. The **oxyhemoglobin dissociation** curve is illustrated in Figure 15–1.

FIGURE 15–1. Normally, PaO_2 and SaO_2 values are closely related. When PaO_2 decreases slightly, so does SaO_2. However, when PaO_2 drops below 60 mm Hg, the close association is disrupted. The disruption is represented graphically as the oxyhemoglobin dissociation curve, which illustrates the relationship between PaO_2 and SaO_2 values known as the 30–60–90 rule. When PaO_2 measures 30 mm Hg, SaO_2 is usually 60%, and when PaO_2 is 60 mm Hg, SaO_2 is usually 90%. (Adapted from Horne, C., & Derrico, D. [1999]. Mastering ABGs: The art of arterial blood gas measurement. *American Journal of Nursing, 99*[8], 26–33.)

TABLE 15–1 Choosing the Site of an Arterial Blood Sample

Site	Advantages	Disadvantages
Radial artery	Close to the surface Easily palpable Easy to check site	Pulsation is difficult to palpate on obese patients with short arms
Brachial artery	Largest artery in lower arm Close to surface Extension of arm stretches the artery Easily accessed Easily observed after puncture	May lie deep in muscular or obese patients Traumatic puncture may damage adjacent nerve and ligaments
Ulnar artery	Fairly close to surface and therefore accessible Good alternative to radial artery	Palpation difficult if artery is small or deep Difficulty in extending wrist if patient is uncooperative
Femoral artery	Relatively large artery Easily palpated Allows direct, perpendicular approach Incidence of arterial spasms is rare	Risk of contamination at site (groin) Possible to puncture femoral vein accidentally during procedure

Access Sites for Arterial Blood Analysis

The blood vessel of choice for obtaining an arterial blood sample is the radial artery, primarily because it is superficial and easily entered and located at the wrist, which makes it easy to stabilize for a quick entry. (See Table 15–1 for more information on choice of sites.) In addition, if thrombosis should occur, the ulnar artery will, by collateral circulation, supply blood to the entire hand, and it is easy to apply a pressure dressing after arterial puncture at this site.

Second and third site choices vary according to institution and personal preference. The brachial artery at the antecubital fossa lies deep, close to nerves and tendons, and is difficult to stabilize. If thrombosis should occur in the brachial artery, the blood supply to the forearm and hand may be compromised (Fig. 15–2). The ulnar artery is usually much deeper and more difficult to stabilize than the radial artery, so, although it may be larger, it is usually not the first choice as an entry site. (Most nurses agree that if the radial artery has been entered, the ulnar artery of the same arm should not be used.)

The femoral artery, located midway between the anterior superior spine of the ilium and the symphysis pubis (see Fig. 15–2), is the largest accessible artery and is easily palpated, stabilized, and entered. However, digital pressure is required for postpuncture pressure. If postpuncture thrombosis should occur in the femoral artery, a limb- or life-threatening condition may result.

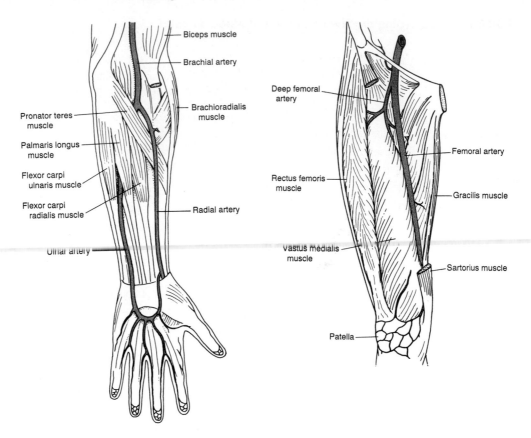

FIGURE 15–2.   Location of radial, ulnar, and brachial arteries (*left*) and location of the femoral artery in the leg (*right*).

One-Time Arterial Blood Sampling

To draw an arterial blood sample, the nurse needs first to assess and prepare the patient and the equipment.

Patient Preparation

To start, the nurse reviews the physician's order, which should specify the fraction of inspired oxygen (FIO_2) if the patient is receiving oxygen therapy or the fraction of oxygen in room air (21% O_2). The patient should be at this steady state continuously for 15 to 20 minutes before the blood sample is drawn. Unless a postexercise blood sample is ordered, the patient also should be at rest for this period.

Next, the nurse considers the patient's position, which can affect the ABG measurement. A patient in a supine position may have more difficulty breathing than would a patient in sitting position. The position most comfortable for the patient should be used for all blood sampling procedures.

⚠ **SAFE PRACTICE ALERT** While positioning the patient, the nurse fully explains the procedure to alleviate anxiety and fear, which can cause hyperventilation and hence an alteration of the blood analysis findings. Of course, the person performing the arterial puncture should be competent for the same reason. Undue trauma causes pain, often leading to hyperventilation by the patient and resulting in alteration of the blood values.

Equipment

The laboratory requisition form should have all identifying patient information plus the oxygenation status of the patient, time of day (important when drawing serial samples), and, if the patient is on a ventilator, all pertinent settings. In some institutions, the patient's temperature and hemoglobin count are also required. In any institution, the nurse follows recommended institutional policy.

Arterial blood samples can be drawn with existing equipment, such as a syringe and needle, or a prepackaged kit may be used. An ABG kit is inexpensive, and the kit contains, except for ice and tape, all equipment needed to perform a one-time arterial puncture. If the kit contains a heparinized prefilled syringe, the nurse removes the syringe cap, places and secures the appropriate-size needle, wets the inner walls of the syringe with heparin (to prevent blood clotting), and expels excess heparin with the same method used for a syringe that is not prefilled. Most ABG kits contain a plastic bag for the iced blood sample.

To heparinize the syringe, the nurse attaches a needle other than the one to be used for puncture to the syringe, cleanses the top of the heparin vial or neck of the ampule with an alcohol swab, and opens the vial or ampule. One milliliter (1 mL) of heparin is withdrawn into the syringe. The nurse then moves the plunger back and forth several times to coat the plunger with heparin and rotates the plunger to eliminate dry spots. To eliminate air bubbles, the nurse holds the syringe with the needle upright and gently taps the sides of the syringe or turns the syringe with the needle pointed downward and slowly inverts the syringe upright. The needle used for heparin is discarded.

The nurse replaces the needle used for heparinization with a sterile, tightly secured needle selected for arterial puncture. Then with the syringe in inverted position, the plunger is pushed up and all excess heparin expelled. The only heparin remaining should be in the dead space of the needle and on the walls of the syringe. Excess heparin or air bubbles alter the results of the ABG analysis.

Puncture Sites and Procedure

Before performing the procedure, arterial assessment should be completed and the blood withdrawal site selected (see Table 15–1).

RADIAL PUNCTURE

As with any invasive procedure, the nurse begins by putting on gloves. The site is palpated for a pulse and the condition of skin and surrounding tissues is inspected, particularly for previous arterial puncture marks. Allen's test is performed to ensure the adequacy of collateral circulation (Fig. 15–3).

FIGURE 15–3.   Performing Allen's test to determine circulatory adequacy. **A.** Patient clenches fist while nurse applies pressure. **B.** Patient opens hand and nurse releases pressure while watching to see how long it takes for hand to color (signifying circulation and patency of vessels). **C.** Evaluating pulse and blood return.

A rolled towel may be placed under the wrist, causing hyperextension of the hand to stretch and stabilize the artery. The skin is prepared with iodophor by wiping the area in concentric circles and allowing at least a 30-second contact time with the intended puncture site. Again, gloves are required and Occupational Safety and Health Administration standards should be met.

A local anesthetic is not always necessary for an arterial puncture with a needle. With it, the chances for a quick, successful entry are less, and the anesthetic does not ameliorate the discomfort of arterial entry. However, if a difficult entry is anticipated or multiple attempts are necessary, a local anesthetic injected at the intended entry site may eliminate skin discomfort.

To perform a radial puncture, the nurse uses one hand to palpate the artery and aligns two or three fingertips along the direction the artery follows. Holding the syringe at an angle no higher than 30 degrees with the needle pointed directly toward the artery, the nurse uses the other hand to enter the skin and artery smoothly in one quick motion. Arterial pressure usually causes the blood to pulsate spontaneously back into the syringe. If blood pressure is low or the syringe not free flowing, however, the nurse may need to pull back gently on the plunger. The plunger should be withdrawn 1 to 2 mL before the stick, for two reasons: if the sample is indeed arterial and not venous, the patient's pressure causes a brisk and often pulsatile reflux of blood into the syringe (unless the patient is severely hypotensive), and it prevents complications such as arterial spasm and blood hemolysis.

The blood return stops when the blood reaches the automatic shutoff level. If the equipment does not have a shutoff feature, a volume of 1 to 2 mL blood is a sufficient quantity for the blood gas analyzer.

Immediately after quickly withdrawing the needle and blood-filled syringe, the nurse applies digital pressure to the puncture site with a 2 × 2-inch sterile sponge folded to form a pressure point. Then, taking precautions not to encircle the entire wrist, a pressure dressing is firmly secured with tape.

If the syringe will be capped, the nurse removes the needle from the syringe and attaches the cap quickly and securely. If a rubber stopper is used, the nurse sticks the needle tip into the center of the stopper. The nurse next rolls the syringe back and forth between the hands for 5 to 10 seconds to ensure that the blood mixes with the heparin lining the syringe. The unit is then placed in an iced container and taken to the laboratory immediately for analysis. A small amount of cold water added to the ice provides for even cold distribution and facilitates placement of the sample so that all the blood in the barrel is chilled by iced water.

SAFE PRACTICE ALERT An ABG sample that is not placed immediately on ice can produce faulty results on analysis because red blood cells continue to metabolize oxygen and give off carbon dioxide. Ice retards the process.

FEMORAL PUNCTURE

The femoral artery is usually easily palpated with the patient in the supine position. If the patient is obese, assistance may be needed to hold the abdomen away, or the patient's buttocks may be placed on an inverted bedpan. A pendulous abdomen may be taped up and away to provide easier access and maintain sterility. Procedures for wearing gloves and preparing the skin are the same as for a radial artery puncture.

The following two techniques may be used for a femoral arterial puncture:

- The artery is located and kept between two fingers, allowing pulsation to be felt on both fingers, but at the same time allowing enough room between them for the needle entry. The syringe and needle are held almost straight down. When the puncture is made in this manner, care must be taken not to pierce through the other wall of the artery.
- The entry may be performed with the same techniques used for a radial artery puncture. Two or three fingertips are placed along the direction of the femoral artery, and the syringe and needle are held at an angle no higher than 30 degrees. This method must be used for femoral artery catheter placement; if used for a one-time needle and syringe sample, there is less chance of artery perforation.

Regardless of the method used, when pulsation is strong, it is relayed up through the needle and syringe as the needle touches and penetrates the artery. The walls of the femoral artery are usually thick and resistant to puncture, so feeling pulsations can be a good guide to needle tip placement. When the artery is entered, the blood usually pulsates back into and fills the syringe without any traction being applied on the plunger.

Postprocedural Patient Interventions

When the needle and syringe are removed, digital pressure is needed because a pressure dressing with tape is difficult to maintain in the femoral artery area. The pressure should be maintained for at least 10 minutes and for 20 minutes or longer in a patient who has received anticoagulant therapy. It is helpful to remember to release pressure slowly. A sudden release may cause undue pressure against the arterial wall, and the patient will begin bleeding. The care of the blood sample is the same as

---

BOX 15-1   Postprocedural Patient Interventions

- Determine if the oxygen status of the patient has been altered only for the blood sampling.
- If so, resume presampling status as soon as the blood sample is drawn.
- Maintain pressure dressing long enough—usually between 10 and 20 minutes depending on the access site—to prevent excessive seepage of blood into the tissue. Be sure that the pressure dressing is not so tight that blanching occurs or that venous blood flow in the hand is severely restricted.
- If the patient is receiving anticoagulation therapy, apply digital pressure. Digital pressure is also preferable to the use of a C-clamp at the femoral site because significant occult bleeding into the retroperitoneal space can occur rapidly and may result in unnecessary blood loss and discomfort for the patient.
- Remove pressure dressing after bleeding stops.

---

that outlined for a radial artery puncture. Postprocedural patient care and nursing responsibilities are described in Box 15–1.

Use of an Indwelling Arterial Catheter

In many situations, serial or daily blood samples are needed for ABG analysis. To avoid multiple punctures, an indwelling catheter may be inserted to obtain the blood samples. The radial artery is usually the site of first choice because it is the easiest to enter, is the easiest to maintain with intact sterile dressings, and allows the patient the greatest freedom of movement. It is imperative that Allen's test be performed before placing any indwelling catheter in the radial artery because the long-term placement with decreased blood flow increases the risk of thrombosis.

SAFE PRACTICE ALERT   If at all possible, use of the brachial artery for indwelling catheter placement should be avoided because the catheter easily fractures or bends in this site, which significantly increases the chance of embolization.

The femoral artery may be a favorable site because it can accommodate a catheter of substantial diameter to achieve consistent blood sampling and monitoring. Care must be taken at all times not to leave the patient in bed at a 30-degree angle or less. Frequent pedal pulse checks for strength of pulsatile flow and color of limb should be maintained and documented. The patient's skin should be appropriately prepared and shaved before the procedure so that a sterile occlusive dressing may then be maintained intact. If the catheter is to be maintained for a substantial period, it may be prudent to suture it in place. This is also true with arterial lines to be maintained in the radial artery.

When inserting any indwelling arterial catheter, extra precautions must be taken to wash hands thoroughly. Skin preparation in this instance may include an acetone defatting as well as a complete iodophor preparation. In some institutions, sterile gloves are mandatory for this procedure and should always be used when probing is anticipated.

A local anesthetic may be injected at the insertion site, especially if an 18-gauge or larger catheter is being used. It is preferable that only experienced personnel perform this procedure; a successful entry on the first attempt is highly desired because the availability of suitable arteries is limited.

Catheter Insertion and Blood Sampling

When using a catheter with an obturator, the procedure outlined in the accompanying Key Intervention display should be followed.

KEY INTERVENTIONS:	Inserting a Catheter With an Obturator and Obtaining a Blood Sample

Catheter Insertion

1. Put on gloves. Insert catheter at a 30-degree angle, using the same techniques as those used to perform venipuncture of a superficial vein without a tourniquet.
2. As the catheter tip touches and enters the artery, pulsation can be felt through the catheter. Keep in mind that the arterial wall is thicker and more resistant to entry than a venous wall, making this procedure painful if not performed quickly and expertly.
3. When the artery is fully entered, blood pulsates back into the stylet. The catheter then can be fully advanced.
4. To maintain a sterile field while removing the stylet and placing the obturator, place an iodophor swab or sterile 2 × 2-inch sponge under the catheter hub.
5. To facilitate the stylet–obturator change, temporarily shut off the arterial blood flow either by digital pressure at the catheter tip or by adequate placement of a tourniquet proximal to the insertion site.
6. After the obturator is removed from its protective shield, the stylet is removed from the catheter and the obturator inserted and locked by twisting in place. Pressure on the artery may now be released.
7. Dress and label the arterial entry site. Include the date and time of insertion and the initials of the person performing the procedure on the dressing.
8. Document the procedure, stating the date, time, type, and gauge catheter used, insertion site, any patient reactions, name of person performing procedure, and pertinent data regarding distal extremity, including color, pulse, warmth.

Obtaining Arterial Blood Sample for Arterial Blood Gas Analysis

1. Wearing gloves, prepare a heparinized syringe without a needle.
2. Apply digital or tourniquet pressure over the artery.
3. Place iodophor swab or sterile 2 × 2-inch sponge under the catheter hub.
4. Remove obturator.
5. Connect heparinized syringe to catheter hub.
6. Release arterial pressure.
7. Allow syringe to fill with required amount of blood.
8. Reapply arterial pressure.
9. Remove syringe from catheter.
10. Insert and lock new sterile obturator.
11. Release arterial pressure.
12. Cap syringe and treat blood sample the same way as for a one-time puncture for arterial blood gas sample.

The procedure for inserting an intermittent catheter with an injection cap, or port, is similar to inserting a catheter with an obturator, with some exceptions. For example, pressure to stop arterial blood flow is not needed because there is no stylet–obturator change. The catheter is, however, flushed with a dilute heparin solution. Dressing, label documentation at the site, and documentation in the medical record are the same as for a catheter with an obturator.

To obtain a blood sample for ABG analysis from a catheter with a heparin lock device, the nurse puts on gloves and prepares three syringes:

- A heparinized syringe with a 1-inch, 22-gauge needle
- A plain syringe with a 1-inch, 22-gauge needle for withdrawal of dilute heparin from the injection port
- A syringe and needle with dilute heparin solution for flushing the catheter after drawing the blood sample.

Next, the nurse cleanses the injection site of the catheter with antiseptic, securely anchors the catheter hub with the free hand to prevent excessive pressure at the insertion site, and inserts the needle of the plain syringe. Approximately 0.5 mL blood with dilute heparin is withdrawn from the catheter and discarded.

The injection port is recleansed, the needle in the heparinized syringe inserted, the syringe allowed to fill with enough blood for the analysis, and the syringe removed with the needle. Finally, the injection port is recleansed, and the nurse, still securely anchoring the catheter hub, inserts the needle of the syringe containing dilute heparin, flushes the catheter, and removes the syringe and needle. The blood sample is treated in the same manner as the sample obtained for a one-time analysis.

SAFE PRACTICE ALERT When entering any intermittent catheter with a needle, extreme care must be taken to use a needle that is short—too short to pass beyond the catheter hub into the catheter itself. If the needle tip does enter the catheter, the catheter can be pierced and broken off by the needle tip. The result is a catheter embolus. In addition, the needle gauge must be small enough to allow postpuncture closure of the entry site. Otherwise, blood leakage and risk of contamination increase.

Close site monitoring is required after placement of any type of indwelling arterial catheter.

KEY INTERVENTIONS: Postarterial Catheter Insertion Care

1. Observe the catheter site for signs of arterial thrombosis, hematoma formation, arterial perforation, and catheter kinking or dislodgment.
2. Check the patient's hand for adequate blood supply by noting color and temperature.
3. Maintain secure, clean, and intact dressings.
4. Avoid placing undue stress at the insertion site by using the unaffected arm for blood pressure monitoring and venipunctures.

Continuous Arterial Pressure Monitoring

Continuous arterial pressure monitoring requires inserting an indwelling arterial catheter, which permits the IV nurse and other health care personnel to obtain continuous systolic, diastolic, and mean arterial pressure readings; to assess the cardiovascular effects of vasopressor or vasodilator drugs during the treatment of shock and, at the same time, to draw arterial blood for ABG measurements.

EQUIPMENT

A cardiac monitor with a module for measuring arterial pressure is required. The monitor is connected by cable and a transducer to a special IV setup (Fig. 15–4). The IV system consists of a 500-mL bag of normal saline solution that has been heparinized (usually 500 to 2,000 U/500 mL) to inhibit catheter clotting and thrombus

FIGURE 15–4. System for continuous arterial pressure monitoring.

formation at the catheter tip. *Klebsiella, Enterobacter,* and *Serratia* species and *Pseudomonas cepacia* show rapid growth within 24 hours with dextrose 5% in water. The bag is connected to IV tubing and placed inside a pressure infuser bag with a gauge and inflation bulb, the same one used to pump blood transfusions. Some institutions prefer microdrip tubings, but air bubbles are more persistent with this size drip. Other hospitals prefer macrodrip tubings; this size allows a larger volume of fluid to be infused.

The IV tubing is connected by a high-pressure extension tubing, a continuous-flush attachment, and three-way stopcocks to a transducer dome. Most of these systems deliver 3 to 5 mL of solution. The entire system is flushed. All connections must be secured and all air bubbles eliminated. The transducer is covered with the dome and secured on a plate attached to an IV pole at the level of the patient's right atrium. Each manufacturer provides detailed instructions for this setup. The instructions should be carefully followed.

GENERAL PROCEDURE

Any indwelling catheter may be used for this procedure, and the insertion procedure is the same as for serial or daily blood sample drawings. The catheter is connected to the primed IV tubing by placing an iodophor swab or sterile 2 × 2-inch sponge under the catheter hub, applying digital or tourniquet pressure over the artery distal to the site, removing the stylet, connecting and securing the tubing adapter, and releasing pressure on the artery. The pressure infuser bag is inflated to 300 mm Hg to deliver automatically a designated volume of fluid (depending on the drip size) hourly.

A sterile dressing is applied to the insertion site and taped securely. The site is labeled clearly to denote arterial access, date, time, type and gauge of catheter, and initials of person performing the insertion. A short hand board may be required to limit wrist motion. If restraints are necessary, they should be applied around the hand board, not the patient's wrist, because this could interfere with arterial pressure and thereby increase the risk of catheter kinking or dislodgment.

AFTERCARE

Aftercare of the insertion site is the same as that for an indwelling catheter used for drawing blood samples for serial or daily ABG analysis.

OBTAINING BLOOD FOR ABG ANALYSIS

When an ABG sample is needed, a sampling port provides an easy arterial access. Another method is to attach a three-way stopcock connection as close as possible to the site. The sampling site should be capped with a heparin lock (intermittent infusion cap). The nurse removes the cap when sampling and attaches an appropriate syringe. The stopcock is turned off to pressure or to the sampling site, and the nurse gently withdraws the sample and handles it consistent with institutional policy. The port is then flushed and the stopcock turned back to its original position.

TABLE 15–2   Malfunctions Occurring in Arterial Pressure Monitoring

Malfunction	Intervention
• Air bubbles may distort wave patterns.	• Eliminate air from system in setup; avoid entry of air in manipulation.
• Near-exsanguination has been reported.	• Secure all connections.
• Damped pressure tracing (almost flat) may occur if tip lies against artery wall.	• Secure catheter hub; ensure use of intact dressings.
• Catheter clotting can occur if pressure is <300 mm Hg.	• Check pressure bag to ensure that it is maintained.
• Abnormally high or low reading may occur if height of transducer is at zero reference point or is the type placed with a plate on an IV pole.	• Identify type of system used on the control switch of patient's bed.

MALFUNCTIONS AND COMPLICATIONS

Common malfunctions occurring in arterial pressure lines are listed in Table 15–2. Common complications related to arterial pressure lines include thromboses, hematomas, pseudoaneurysms, and prolonged arterial spasms. These problems may be reduced by clinical expertise during catheter insertion and by careful monitoring of insertion sites.

Infection is a serious complication as well. Arterial pressure monitoring is associated with up to 13% of reported cases of nosocomial bacteremia. Incidences of contaminated transducers, transducer domes, and flush solutions are well documented. Sterilizing the transducer after each use, using disposable domes, and changing the entire monitoring system except for the catheter every 2 days helps reduce infection rates. As with any invasive procedure, thorough hand washing before catheter insertion and maintenance of aseptic technique during setup of the system, during insertion, and during all manipulations of the line are mandatory.

Use of Swan-Ganz Catheters

Although a Swan-Ganz catheter is inserted into a vein, it is important to intra-arterial therapy because it enters the pulmonary artery and measures arterial pressures. Whereas central venous pressure lines assess only right heart pressure, Swan-Ganz catheters allow the health care team to assess both right and left heart pressures. This makes a Swan-Ganz catheter suitable for diagnosing and managing heart failure resulting from myocardial infarction and cardiogenic shock. In cardiogenic shock treatment, the Swan-Ganz catheter serves many purposes. It guides the administration of IV therapy and provides the site. At the same time, it facilitates the evaluation of any therapeutic drugs given and provides information regarding the cause of shock.

Basic Swan-Ganz catheters have double or triple lumens. Catheters are approximately 110 cm long and come in sizes 5-, 6-, 7-, and 7.5-French. Each has a balloon tip that is inflated with 0.8 to 1.5 mL air, depending on the size and manufacturer.

A double-lumen catheter contains a larger port that is connected to an IV system and monitor to measure pulmonary artery wedge pressure and a smaller port with a two-way stopcock for inflation and deflation of the balloon. Triple-lumen catheters contain a third proximal port, which is connected to another IV system and may be used to monitor right atrial pressure.

The IV system contains a heparinized bag, pressure infuser bag, pressure tubings with stopcocks, and transducer with cable connected to a monitor. This equipment is the same as that used for arterial monitoring except that for Swan-Ganz catheters, the lines may be color-coded blue to differentiate them from arterial lines, which may be color-coded red.

INSERTION

The Swan-Ganz catheter may be inserted either percutaneously or by a cutdown procedure in any accessible vein large enough to allow passage of the catheter. As the catheter is threaded and the tip passes the superior vena cava, the balloon is inflated. Normal blood flow then assists catheter advancement. The tip enters the right atrium and passes through the tricuspid valve, entering the right ventricle. It then passes through the pulmonic valve into the pulmonary artery. Use of a cardiac monitor is essential during insertion because the waveform pattern defines changes with each advancement, thereby providing a guide for tip location, and simultaneously monitoring the patient's condition throughout the procedure. The catheter tip placement must be confirmed by radiography.

Pulmonary capillary wedge pressure, which reflects left heart pressure, is measured intermittently by inflating the balloon to its recommended level (Fig. 15–5). Care should be taken not to overinflate the balloon and not to inflate it too frequently. Typically, the balloon is inflated every 4 hours, with the inflation pressure maintained no longer than 1 to 2 minutes.

Complications

Possible complications include the following:

- Cardiac arrhythmias, which may occur during insertion—lidocaine hydrochloride and defibrillation equipment must be readily available. Serious dysrhythmias during insertion are rare.
- Catheter knotting, which may occur with the 5-French catheter when it is advanced too far for the chamber whose pressure is being registered.
- Balloon rupture, which is possible in a patient without intracardiac shunting of blood.
- Pulmonary damage, which may result from obstructed pulmonary artery blood flow caused by peripheral migration of the catheter to a wedged position. This is avoidable with constant monitoring and by following recommendations regarding balloon inflation.
- Infection, which is always a threat. The use of disposable equipment has minimized the occurrence of infection. Strict adherence to aseptic technique is mandatory.

FIGURE 15–5. Pulmonary capillary wedge pressure.

Intra-Arterial Parameters and Interpretation

Arterial blood gas measurements are used to detect and cope with respiratory imbalances. Specific uses include diagnosing and regulating oxygen therapy and evaluating all other therapy and metabolic imbalances. In particular, ABG levels assess the effectiveness of the therapy. To interpret ABG values, the nurse must understand the physiologic, chemical, and physical processes that influence each parameter.

pH

The pH value refers to the degree of acidity or alkalinity of the blood. It is not an absolute measurement, but gives an approximation of hydrogen ion concentration. The pH scale is as follows (numbers are inversely related to the degree of acidity): the range compatible with life is roughly 6.8 to 7.8, and the normal range lies between 7.35 and 7.45. A pH increase represents a decrease in acidity and a pH decrease represents an increase in acidity. A pH decrease of 0.3 shows a doubling of hydrogen concentration. Blood pH 7.10 has twice the hydrogen concentration of blood pH 7.40.

Blood pH is directly proportional to the ratio of carbonic acid to bicarbonate (HCO_3^-). When there is 1 part carbonic acid to 20 parts bicarbonate, the resultant pH is 7.35 to 7.45. If only carbonic acid increases or only bicarbonate decreases, the ratio becomes closer (1:5 to 16) and acidosis results. Conversely, when only carbonic acid decreases or only bicarbonate increases, the ratio widens (1:25 to 50) and alkalosis results.

Carbonic acid or bicarbonate changes themselves produce no toxic effects. It is the ratio alteration and resultant pH change that interfere severely with enzyme activity.

Hydrogen

Cell metabolism produces hydrogen, which combines with bicarbonate to form carbonic acid. This breaks down into water, which is excreted by the kidneys, and carbon dioxide, which is excreted by the lungs.

Because waste products of metabolism are mainly acidic, humans are by nature acid-producing animals. The body generates and processes 15,000 to 20,000 mEq of hydrogen daily. Most (99.8%) is nonfixed or volatile acid, which means it can change into a gaseous form. The remainder (0.2%) is fixed or nonvolatile.

Body processing of hydrogen is accomplished with no appreciable change in blood concentration by elimination of volatile acid as carbon dioxide by the lungs, by excretion and reabsorption of fixed acid and bicarbonate by the kidneys, and by chemical buffering.

Buffers

A *buffer* is a solute that resists pH change when acids or bases are added. The buffer base consists of bicarbonate and all nonbicarbonate buffers. The bicarbonate buffer system cannot buffer volatile acids, but does buffer approximately 75% of all the fixed acid generated by the body. The nonbicarbonate buffer system consists primarily of proteins, hemoglobin, and phosphate. It buffers volatile nonfixed acids.

BICARBONATE

The primary metabolic parameter, bicarbonate, may be reported as carbon dioxide content, carbon dioxide combining power, carbon dioxide, or standard bicarbonate, any of which refers to the same factor. Bicarbonate is measured by concentration and reported as milliequivalent per liter (mEq/L). It is universally related to the quantity of fixed acid excess and therefore is more a controlled than a controlling factor.

Sources of fixed acids include organic and inorganic dietary acids, lactic acid as a by-product of cell metabolism without oxygen, and ketoacids as by-products of cell metabolism without glucose or insulin.

The normal excretion rate of fixed acid by the kidneys is 50 mEq/day. However, the excretion and reabsorption of both hydrogen and bicarbonate can be greatly increased or decreased by body demands.

The normal bicarbonate range is 24 ± 3 mEq/L. The minimum level compatible with life is 1 mEq/L; the maximum level is 48 mEq/L.

BASE EXCESS

The base excess (BE) parameter is the sum total in concentration of all the buffer anions (bicarbonate and nonbicarbonate) in a sample of whole blood, equilibrated with a normal PCO_2 (40 mm Hg). Because BE is equilibrated with a normal PCO_2, it is not affected by primary respiratory imbalances.

Normal BE is 48 ± 3 mm/L but is reported as plus or minus zero. In metabolic acidosis, BE is minus; in metabolic alkalosis, BE is plus.

Physics of Gas

The parameters discussed so far are measured by concentration. The two respiratory parameters measured by pressure (intensity) warrant a brief review of the physics of gas.

Gas has volume, which refers to the space the gas occupies, and is measured in milliliters (mL). Gas has pressure, which is measured mathematically as force per unit area by noting the height to which the force can support a column of mercury. This measurement is expressed in millimeters of mercury (mm Hg). Gas has temperature, which is generated by gas molecules in constant motion and is measured in degrees Celsius (°C) or Fahrenheit (°F). Dalton's law regarding the behavior of gas in a mixture, as applied to oxygen in the atmosphere (room air), indicates the following:

- The total pressure of the gas mixture equals the sum of the partial pressures of each gas, or **total pressure of atmosphere** (P_{atm}) = partial pressure oxygen (PO_2) + partial pressure nitrogen (PN_2) + partial pressure carbon dioxide (PCO_2).
- Each gas acts independently, as if it alone occupied the total space.
- Each gas contribution to the total pressure depends solely on the percentage of the total gas it occupies. The contribution of oxygen to the total atmospheric pressure is 21%. (Other variables not discussed here can exist.)
- The partial pressure of each gas depends on the number of molecules existing in the fixed space. At high elevations, the number of oxygen molecules is decreased; therefore, PO_2 is decreased.
- Each gas is unaffected by any changes in other gas molecules. The PO_2 does not increase or decrease because PCO_2 is increased or decreased.

PARTIAL PRESSURE OF CARBON DIOXIDE

The PCO_2 value reflects the adequacy of alveolar ventilation. It is the primary respiratory parameter. Carbon dioxide is eliminated by the lungs at the same rate it is formed by the tissues and at the same time maintains constant blood levels.

Arterial PCO_2 is inversely related to the level of ventilation. With hypoventilation, carbon dioxide is retained and the PCO_2 elevates; with hyperventilation, carbon dioxide is blown off and the PCO_2 decreases.

The normal range for PCO_2 is 40 ± 4 mm Hg. The minimum value compatible with life is 9 mm Hg; the maximum value is 158 mm Hg.

PARTIAL PRESSURE OF OXYGEN

The PO_2 value is also an intensity factor, measured in millimeters of mercury. It tells how fast and for how long oxygen passes from blood into tissue. The PO_2 is usually not a direct influence in acid–base balance.

Normal PO_2 values are oxygen and age dependent. When the FIO_2 is 21% (room air) and the patient is 60 years of age or younger, the PO_2 should be at least 80 mm Hg. With each 10-year advance in age, the normal PO_2 decreases by 10 mm Hg. If the PO_2 is 50 mm Hg or lower in a patient younger than 60 years of age, respiratory failure is present. A PO_2 between 50 and 75 mm Hg reflects moderate hypoxemia.

HYPOXEMIA

Hypoxemia is insufficient oxygenation of the blood and can be measured directly by the PO_2. Hypoxia—insufficient oxygenation of the tissues—cannot be directly measured, but is presumed if the partial pressure of oxygen in venous blood ($P\overline{v}O_2$) is 30 mm Hg or lower. To avoid hypoxia when hypoxemia is present, the cardiovascular system must increase the rate of tissue perfusion or the hemoglobin content must be elevated (Ryabov, 1995).

Shunting is a common cause of hypoxemia. *Shunting* is any impediment in the blood transport system that results in blood not coming in contact with oxygen. This can be seen in vascular lung tumors, a right-to-left intracardiac shunt, or capillary shunting in which pulmonary capillary blood comes in contact with totally unventilated alveoli (dead space).

OXYGEN SATURATION

Oxygen saturation (SaO_2) is the parameter that tells the amount of oxygen taken up by hemoglobin when fully saturated. It is a quantity factor and is measured in percentage. It may also be called PO_2%. The normal adult values are 96% to 97% before 65 years of age and 95% to 96% in older patients. Oxygen saturation

- Depends on PO_2. When the pressure exceeds a certain value, the amount of oxygen taken in no longer increases.
- Is altered by pH. If PO_2 remains constant, oxygen saturation decreases when the pH decreases and increases when the pH increases.
- Is altered by temperature. If the PO_2 is constant, oxygen saturation decreases when the temperature increases and increases when the temperature decreases.

This indicates that hyperthermia causes metabolic acidosis and hypothermia causes metabolic alkalosis. In hypothermia, the oxygen need is decreased, but the oxygen is bound so tightly to the hemoglobin that the ability to deliver it is greatly decreased. Inhalation of carbon dioxide may be used to cause acidosis and release the bound oxygen.

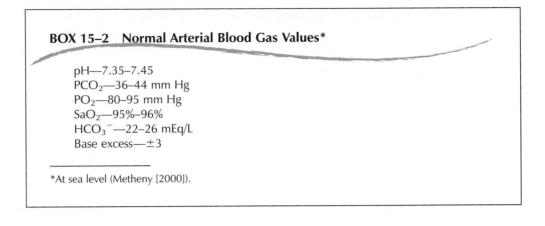

BOX 15–2   Normal Arterial Blood Gas Values*

pH—7.35–7.45
PCO_2—36–44 mm Hg
PO_2—80–95 mm Hg
SaO_2—95%–96%
HCO_3^-—22–26 mEq/L
Base excess—±3

*At sea level (Metheny [2000]).

Chemoreceptors and Primary Acid–Base Imbalances

Chemoreceptors located peripherally in aortic and carotid vessels and centrally in the brain play a role in body responses to abnormal PCO_2 and PO_2 values. Chemoreceptors signal the brain to stimulate or depress ventilation, according to body needs. The response to an elevated PCO_2 is greater than to a decreased PO_2 because PCO_2 elevation is a danger signal of respiratory failure. At high altitudes where oxygen supply is decreased, oxygen need is greater than PCO_2 constancy; the chemoreceptors stimulate hyperventilation to obtain more oxygen, but this hyperventilation results in a decreased PCO_2. Box 15–2 summarizes normal ABG values.

METABOLIC ACIDOSIS

Metabolic acidosis results from an excess of fixed acids or a primary bicarbonate deficit. The primary causes are

- Increased production of fixed acids, including ketoacids, which are evident in diabetic acidosis or starvation when glucose and insulin are unavailable for cell metabolism, and lactic acid, which is evident in cardiopulmonary failure when oxygen is unavailable for cell metabolism
- Failure of kidneys to excrete fixed acid
- Primary bicarbonate deficit—severe diarrhea or bowel or biliary fistula

This is a metabolic imbalance because bicarbonate is the parameter primarily affected. Acidosis is present because the carbon dioxide level has not changed, but the decrease in bicarbonate has caused the ratio to go closer than 1 part acid to 20 parts base. It can be between 1:16 and 1:5, depending on the degree of bicarbonate deficit. Because pH depends on the acid–base ratio, and this ratio has now narrowed, acidosis is present. BE is minus because there is not enough bicarbonate to buffer the fixed acid.

Arterial blood gas values in metabolic acidosis:

pH: <7.35
HCO_3^-: <22 mEq/L
PCO_2: normal (40 ± 4 mm Hg)
BE: <−3

If the metabolic acidosis is of renal origin, the kidneys cannot respond. If it is of nonrenal origin, the kidneys increase the excretion of hydrogen and the reabsorption of bicarbonate. This response is slow, but once started, can be maintained for weeks or months.

The chemoreceptors are sensitive to the increase in hydrogen and stimulate compensatory hyperventilation to blow off carbon dioxide, decreasing the PCO_2 less than 40 mm Hg to obtain an acid–base ratio closer to normal (1:20) needed for a normal pH. This compensatory respiratory response is prompt and predictable; it occurs within minutes, but becomes less effective with time. The limit of compensatory hyperventilation occurs when the PCO_2 reaches 12 mm Hg.

After the kidneys and lungs respond, bicarbonate increases to a level closer to normal. PCO_2 decreases, and the acid–base ratio comes closer to 1:20 with a resultant pH closer to normal. Compensation thus occurs.

With bicarbonate administration, the bicarbonate level reverts to normal and the lungs stop hyperventilation. Therefore, PCO_2 reverts to normal, resulting in a 1:20 acid–base ratio and allowing a normal pH (7.35 to 7.45). Correction thereby is achieved.

METABOLIC ALKALOSIS

Metabolic alkalosis results from a decrease in body content of fixed acids or a primary **bicarbonate excess**. The primary causes are

- Excessive loss of fixed acids resulting, for example, from prolonged vomiting, gastric suctioning, potassium deficit
- Primary bicarbonate excess resulting, for example, from excessive administration of sodium bicarbonate, sodium citrate, or chloride deficit, whereby bicarbonate increases to maintain cation–anion balance or sodium deficit, with bicarbonate excretion dependent on sodium.

This is a metabolic imbalance because the primary parameter affected is bicarbonate. Alkalosis occurs because the acid–base ratio has widened to 1 part acid to 25 to 50 parts base. This ratio results in a pH elevation. Because there is an excess of bicarbonate, the BE is plus.

Arterial blood gas values in metabolic alkalosis:

pH: >7.45
HCO_3^-: >26 mEq/L
PCO_2: normal (40 ± 4 mm Hg)
BE: > ± 3

Whether the kidneys respond to metabolic alkalosis depends on several factors. An increase in bicarbonate causes bicarbonate excretion to increase, provided there is no deficit of chloride or potassium. If a chloride depletion is present, bicarbonate is reabsorbed as the accompanying anion for sodium. Because a bicarbonate increase is usually accompanied by an increase in sodium, a decrease in chloride, and a potassium deficit, bicarbonate is not excreted but reabsorbed.

Compensatory respiratory response to metabolic alkalosis is variable. The degree of hypoventilation that occurs depends on the causative factors. Regardless of the cause, hypoventilation as a compensatory response is rarely sufficient to bring the $PCO_2 > 55$ mm Hg because an elevated PCO_2 causes the chemoreceptors to stimulate breathing to prevent respiratory failure.

When the lungs and kidneys do respond, some compensation occurs: bicarbonate falls, PCO_2 rises, and the acid–base ratio comes closer to 1:20. The pH thus decreases to a level closer to normal.

Correction occurs with the administration of solutions containing chloride and potassium. In assessing and treating respiratory imbalances, ABG measurements are an absolute clinical necessity because ventilation is reflected in PCO_2 and oxygenation in PO_2. Furthermore, acute respiratory failure may occur with slight changes in pulse, blood pressure, or alertness until cardiopulmonary collapse occurs.

RESPIRATORY ACIDOSIS

Respiratory acidosis is always caused by carbon dioxide retention from hypoventilation. This is rarely seen without hypoxemia ($PO_2 < 60$ mm Hg). The causes of hypoventilation include

- Anesthesia, narcotics
- Central nervous system disease such as polio, spinal cord lesions
- Severe hypokalemia
- Intrathoracic collection of blood, fluid, or air
- Pulmonary diseases, both restrictive (congestive heart failure, tumors, atelectasis) and obstructive (bronchitis, emphysema, asthma, or foreign body)

The acidosis process is respiratory because the PCO_2 is the primary parameter involved. Nonfixed, volatile acid (PCO_2) is in excess but the base (bicarbonate) is normal. The acid–base ratio is closer than 1:20; it is between 1:5 and 1:20, resulting in acidosis.

Arterial blood gas values in respiratory acidosis:

pH: <7.35
PCO_2: >44 mm Hg
HCO_3^-: normal (24 ± 2 mEq/L)

Because the lungs are always the primary cause of respiratory acidosis, they cannot play a role in compensation. Renal compensation is always slow in onset but effective once started: generation and reabsorption of bicarbonate increase, excretion of hydrogen increases, and the excretion of chloride increases, resulting in a chloride deficit.

With renal response, bicarbonate rises above normal and PCO$_2$ remains unchanged. The acid ratio comes closer to 1:20, allowing for somke compensation, with a pH closer to normal.

Correction of respiratory acidosis is possible only by correction of the pulmonary cause. Chloride solutions are usually given to treat the chloride deficit.

RESPIRATORY ALKALOSIS

Respiratory alkalosis is always caused by a carbon dioxide deficit owing to hyperventilation. Factors causing hyperventilation include the following:

- Chemoreceptor response to hypoxemia. The chemoreceptors sense the decrease in oxygen and send a message to the brain to stimulate ventilation. This hyperventilation results in carbon dioxide being blown off, thus decreasing PCO$_2$. This is normal at high altitudes.
- Respiratory response to metabolic acidosis. This response can persist for several hours or days after the metabolic acidosis is corrected because of higher levels of hydrogen excess in cerebrospinal fluid and the fact that chemoreceptors are more responsive to cerebrospinal fluid than to blood.
- Central nervous system malfunctions (trauma, infection, brain lesions)
- Anxiety, pain, fever, shock
- Anemia, carbon monoxide poisoning
- Epinephrine, salicylates, and progesterone
- Improper mechanical ventilation. Any patient with chronic obstructive pulmonary disease who is overcorrected by mechanical ventilation so that the PCO$_2$ decreases faster than 10 mm Hg/hour will have respiratory alkalosis.

This hyperventilation process is respiratory because PCO$_2$ is the primary parameter affected. Alkalosis is present because carbon dioxide is decreased and the bicarbonate value is normal, resulting in an acid–base ratio between 1:25 and 1:50. This ratio results in a pH above 7.45.

Arterial blood gas values in respiratory alkalosis:

pH: >7.45
PCO$_2$: <36 mm Hg
HCO$_3$$^-$: normal (24 ± 2 mEq/L)

Because the lungs are the primary cause of respiratory alkalosis, they cannot respond for compensation. Renal response occurs after several hours or days. The kidneys decrease excretion of hydrogen and increase excretion of bicarbonate. The urine cannot become more alkaline than pH 7.0. This renal response creates some compensation. The bicarbonate value drops <24 mEq/L. The acid–base ratio comes closer to 1:20, allowing the pH to come closer to normal.

Respiratory alkalosis can be corrected by administering chloride solutions to replace the bicarbonate ion load. However, the buffering capacity of the plasma has been compromised as a result of the alkalosis and any additional insult to the balance is poorly tolerated.

Mixed Acid–Base Imbalances

In the hospital setting, two or more primary imbalances may coexist in the same patient. The following combinations sometimes occur:

- Metabolic acidosis and metabolic alkalosis in a patient who has diabetic acidosis and who is vomiting
- Metabolic acidosis and respiratory acidosis in a patient with severe pulmonary edema, followed by cardiogenic shock
- Metabolic acidosis and respiratory alkalosis in a patient with both kidney and liver failure
- Respiratory acidosis and metabolic alkalosis in a patient who has chronic respiratory insufficiency and who is on a salt-poor diet and taking diuretics
- Respiratory alkalosis and metabolic alkalosis are usually seen as a result of mechanical overventilation.

Respiratory acidosis and respiratory alkalosis cannot coexist because a person cannot hypoventilate and hyperventilate at the same time.

Intraosseous Access Devices

Intraosseous infusion may be considered when instances of venous collapse in shock, anatomic scarcity of veins, and thrombosis of venous sites preclude the ability to establish peripheral venous access. First proposed in 1922 by Drinker, intraosseous infusion of IV fluids was initiated in 1934, particularly for shock, pediatric emergencies, adults with mutilated skin, and transport of uncooperative patients. The technique has endured, despite dwindling interest after the advent of disposable needles and catheters. Commonly administered fluids were colloids, crystalline solutions, plasma, blood products, antibiotics, epinephrine, morphine, and glucose. A renewed acceptance and interest in the technique as a viable alternative to peripheral or central venous access has grown since the 1970s.

Current indications for intraosseous infusion are anaphylaxis, burns, cardiac arrest, coma, dehydration, drowning, respiratory arrest, septic shock, hypovolemia, diabetic acidosis, status epilepticus, status asthmaticus, trauma, and sudden infant death syndrome. Standard protocol calls for establishing an intraosseous line in children if percutaneous peripheral venous access cannot be established within 60 to 120 seconds. It may be the route of choice in event of cardiac arrest or hypotension.

Bones are vascular structures with dynamic circulation capable of accepting large volumes of fluid and rapidly transporting fluids or drugs to the central circulation (Fuentes-Afflick, 1990; Metheny, 2000). Long bones consist of a shaft called the *diaphysis* with a very dense cortex, the *epiphysis* (or the rounded ends of the bone), and the *metaphysis* (the transitional zone). The epiphysis and the metaphysis have a much thinner cortex and contain cancellous, or spongy, bone. The iliac crest is made of a thin cortex and is filled with cancellous bone. The hollow core of the shaft of long bones and the spaces within the cancellous bone are referred to as the *medullary space,* which contains the marrow.

FIGURE 15–6. Possible insertion sites of percutaneous intraosseous infusion device in the lower extremity.

The marrow cavity has been appropriately called the *noncollapsible vein* (Fuentes-Afflick, 1990). Comprising a highly interconnected network of venous sinusoids, analogous to a sponge, the intramedullary space is an integral part of the vascular system. Nutrient arteries that penetrate the cortex of the bone supply the marrow. Many bone sites have been used for intraosseous infusions, including the sternum, the tibia (Fig. 15–6), the femur, and the iliac crest. In children younger than 5 years of age, the site of choice is the flat anterior medial surface of the proximal tibia just below the tibial tubercle or the distal tibia, followed by the distal femur (Fuentes-Afflick, 1990). In adults, the iliac crest or sternum is the bone of choice. Strict asepsis is essential and the skin preparation should be consistent with INS Standards of Practice (INS, 1998, 2000a). Local anesthetics may be used for conscious patients.

INTRAOSSEOUS NEEDLES: OSTEOPORT

Components and Features

Appropriate access needles include standard steel hypodermic, spinal, trephine, sternal, and standard bone marrow needles. The needle must be able to stand without support once the stylet is removed and it must facilitate aspiration of blood and marrow. The standards throughout the industry for intraosseous needles have been the Kormed/Jamshidi bone marrow biopsy needle, the Osgood needle, and the Cook intraosseous infusion needle. These products come in several sizes and with various tips. A needle with a short shaft prevents dislodgment.

The osteoport was developed by Von Hoff and colleagues, who patented the device as an intramedullary catheter (Fig. 15–7). Threads were added to the needle so that it could be placed precisely within the marrow and at the same time decrease complications of insertion. The device is made of medical implant–grade titanium, with thread size and shape identical to those of commonly accepted orthopedic devices. The membrane is a medically implantable grade of Silastic (the same material commonly used in IV catheters and other implanted ports).

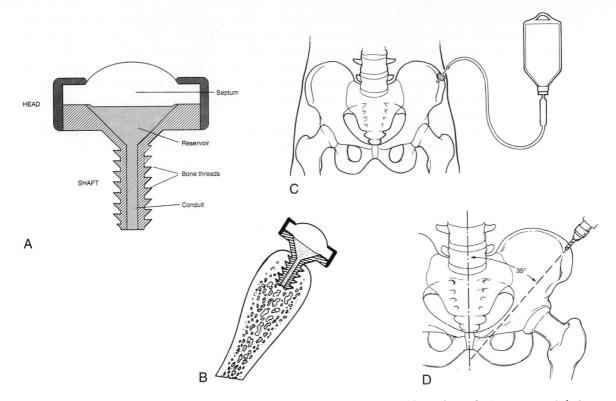

HEAD

SHAFT

A

Septum

Reservoir

Bone threads

Conduit

B

C

D

35°

FIGURE 15–7.   (**A, B**) Osteoport and osteoport in place in a bone. (**C, D**) Additional sites for intraosseous infusion.

To decrease leakage, a cone was added to provide a tight seal between the bone and the osteoport. To decrease the rate of osteomyelitis and cellulitis, the osteoport was made implantable, thereby eliminating any direct conduit from outside the body into the bone marrow. To increase patient comfort, the osteoport has a low profile and does not require a stiff needle protruding through the skin. Rather, the port is a hollow, 1-inch titanium or stainless steel needle with a self-sealing cap. It resembles a partially threaded bolt (see Fig. 15–7). Repeated bone punctures are not required for repeated use (Fuentes-Afflick, 1990).

To initiate the flow of fluids, a needle attached to the IV tubing is inserted through the skin into the cap of the osteoport. The physician locates the device by feeling it under the skin. Because it is implanted in bone, the device promotes rapid absorption by the blood from the marrow cavity, eliminates clotting and lung puncture problems, and reduces the risk of infection. It is indicated for patients who require access to the vascular system but who have exhausted all other reasonable IV sites. The recommended duration of implant is <30 days (Fuentes-Afflick, 1990).

Insertion Technique

After the patient receives a local or general anesthetic, the intraosseous needle is quickly advanced through the skin to the bony cortex. With firm pressure and a rotary motion, the needle is further advanced into the marrow cavity. Insertion resistance decreases as the needle penetrates the cortex (known as the "trap-door effect"). The stylet is removed and the correct position is verified by observing the needle standing without support and the ability to aspirate blood and marrow contents. In adults, the device is usually implanted in a large bone of the hip or leg. Once the incision is closed, the device is ready for use and a continuous infusion can begin (Metheny, 2000).

If the attempt at implantation is unsuccessful, further attempts must be undertaken in other bones. If an infusion was established in the same bone, the infused fluid would leak from the original abandoned hole in the cortex.

Ventricular Reservoirs

The implanted **ventricular reservoir** provides direct access to the cerebrospinal fluid (CSF) without performing a spinal tap. The reservoir is also used to measure CSF pressure, obtain CSF specimens, and instill medication. Implanted surgically, it is positioned in the right frontal region's lateral ventricle, sutured to the pericranium, and covered with a skin flap (see Chap. 20).

Major complications associated with ventricular reservoirs include infection, malfunction, and displacement. Infection is characterized by tenderness, redness, drainage, fever, neck stiffness, and headache with or without vomiting.

Malfunction typically results when the catheter is obstructed by the distal subarachnoid blockage of CSF. This is characterized by the inability to aspirate or inject the port and slow refilling of the reservoir after manual expression of fluid.

Catheter displacement or migration is also characterized by slow or absent refilling of the reservoir after manual expression of fluid. The complication is confirmed by computed tomography and change in neurologic status.

References and Selected Readings

Asterisks indicate references cited in text.

American Association of Blood Banks. (1999). *Technical manual* (13th ed.). Bethesda, MD: Author.

Bennett, J.V., & Brachman, P.S. (1998). *Hospital infections* (4th ed.). Philadelphia: Lippincott Williams & Wilkins.

*Fuentes-Afflick, E. (1990, March 12). *Use and management of intraosseous infusions.* Presented at the Bay Area Vascular Access Nurses (BAVAN) Fourth Annual Conference, San Francisco, CA.

*Horne, C., & Derrico, D. (1999). Mastering ABGs: The art of arterial blood gas measurement. *American Journal of Nursing, 99*(8), 26–33.

*Metheny, N.M. (2000). *Fluid and electrolyte balance* (4th ed.). Philadelphia: Lippincott Williams & Wilkins.

*Ryabov, G. (1995, November). *Hypoxia: Incidence, identification, and interventions.* Lecture presented at the Mount Sinai Hospital Medical Center/Finch University of Health Sciences, New York, NY.

Spivey, W.H. (1987). Intraosseous infusions. *Journal of Pediatrics, 3,* 639–643.

West, V.L. (1998). Alternate routes of administration. *Journal of Intravenous Nursing, 21*(4), 221–231.

Review Questions

Note: Questions below may have more than one right answer.

1. Which of the following tests should be performed before insertion of an indwelling catheter in the radial artery?
   A. Allen's
   B. Swan-Ganz
   C. Serial
   D. Dalton's

2. Oxygen dissolved in plasma is expressed as:
   A. PaO_2
   B. PO_2
   C. PCO_2
   D. pH

3. ABG values may be altered by:
   A. Bicarbonate
   B. Air bubbles
   C. Excess heparin
   D. Dry spots

4. Which of the following is true of the ulnar artery?
   A. It is deep.
   B. It is difficult to stabilize.
   C. It lies close to nerves.
   D. A and B only

5. Mixed acid–base imbalances may coexist in the same patient. Which of the following are examples?
   A. Metabolic acidosis and metabolic alkalosis in a patient who has diabetic acidosis and who is vomiting
   B. Metabolic acidosis and respiratory acidosis in a patient with severe pulmonary edema
   C. A only
   D. A and B

6. Constant arterial monitoring is used for:
   A. Systolic, diastolic, and mean arterial pressure readings
   B. Assessment of cardiovascular effects of vasopressor or vasodilator drugs during shock
   C. Simultaneous ABG sampling
   D. All of the above

7. Blood pH is directly proportional to the ratio of:
   A. Carbonic acid to bicarbonate
   B. Bicarbonate to carbonic acid
   C. Base excess
   D. Alkalinity of the blood

8. In metabolic acidosis, base excess is:
   A. Plus
   B. Minus
   C. Zero
   D. Minimal

9. Which of the following is *not* an advantage of intraosseous infusion?
   A. Fluids are rapidly absorbed.
   B. Clotting and lung puncture problems are eliminated.
   C. Fluids are absorbed slowly.
   D. The risk of infection is reduced.

10. A ventricular reservoir may be used for which of the following?
    A. Access to CSF
    B. Measurement of CSF pressure
    C. Instillation of medication
    D. All of the above

UNIT 4

Patient-Specific Therapies

Parenteral Nutrition

KEY TERMS

Drug–Nutrient Interaction
Enteral Nutrition
Hyperalimentation
Kwashiorkor
Malnutrition
Marasmus

Nutrients
Nutritional Screening
Nutritional Support
Parenteral Nutrition
Protein Malnutrition
Total Nutrient Admixture

History of Parenteral Nutrition

Development of **parenteral nutrition** (PN), formerly known as *hyperalimentation*, began in the early 1960s in the Harrison Department of Surgical Research at the University of Pennsylvania. Dr. Stanley Dudrick devised a system of feeding by central venous routes that resulted in the normal weight gain and growth of beagle puppies that were fed only by vein (Dudrick & Wilmore, 1968). His animal experiments quickly led to human applications; he successfully used hyperalimentation to feed a severely ill infant who was unable to sustain herself with any type of gastrointestinal (GI) feeding because of small bowel atresia (Wilmore & Dudrick, 1968).

Further applications followed in the adult population. The term **parenteral hyperalimentation** was coined by Dr. Jonathan E. Rhoads and Dr. Dudrick and defined as "the intravenous administration of nitrogen, calories, and other nutrients sufficient to achieve tissue synthesis and anabolism in patients with normal or excessive nutritional needs" (Dudrick & Wilmore, 1968). These accomplishments led to further research and application as other clinicians and researchers realized their potential. Hyperalimentation soon became a recognized specialty resulting in nutritional support teams being formed. **Nutritional support** provides specially formulated or delivered parenteral or enteral nutrients to maintain or restore optimal nutrition status.

JoAnne Grant became the first nurse hired exclusively for work with this new form of nutritional support at the University of Pennsylvania, in 1967. In 1976, a multidisciplinary group of professionals (physicians, nurses, dietitians, and pharmacists) was organized, and the American Society for Parenteral and Enteral Nutrition (ASPEN) held its first clinical congress in Chicago.

Hyperalimentation evolved as a science in the 1980s and became more commonly known as total PN or simply PN, the term used throughout this chapter. Disease-specific formulas were developed to address the particular needs of patients with renal, cardiac, or hepatic disease and became commercially available. Multiple organizations, such as the Oley Foundation and hospital-based support groups, have grown for the rehabilitation of patients surviving catastrophic illnesses by maintenance on home PN (HPN). A January 2005 Web search yielded almost 800 sites of information links or support groups for parenteral nutrition. Parenteral nutrition has evolved into a sophisticated field of therapeutic intervention that has its own multidisciplinary specialists and a large body of established knowledge.

With the changing health care environment and emergence of care management in the 2000s, additional changes and challenges came to the field of nutritional support. Among the challenges were a growing focus on home care, home nutritional support, and nutritional support in long-term care facilities, together with increasingly stringent restrictions on reimbursement for home nutritional support. In light of this, nutritional support teams are also moving into the outpatient setting or being eliminated. Additionally, evaluation is always focused on the need for PN versus other avenues of nutritional support.

RESEARCH ISSUES: Current Investigations

- Reduced morbidity and mortality with enteral versus parenteral nutrition in critical care units
- Use of practice guidelines for nutritional support in different care settings
- Use of PN and outcomes in different patient populations, such as low-birth-weight infants; patients with HIV, pancreatitis, short bowel syndrome, and other conditions
- Usage of glutamine (an amino acid)
- Trials of designer lipid emulsions, for example, soybean oil, medium chain triglycerides, olive oil, and fish oil
- Infusion-related support for PN: administration set changes, dressing guidelines, prevention of infection and extravasation, rate of infusion, and thrombosis prevention

Indications for Parenteral Nutrition

Parenteral nutrition (PN) is an invasive therapy with inherent risks. It is intended to provide nutrition for individuals without adequate gastrointestinal (GI) function (ASPEN, 2002). Inappropriate use and monitoring of PN has been attributed to additional risks for infection and increased health care costs (Kirby, 2001; Trujillo, Young, Chertow, et al., 1999). Additionally, Medicare has changed its payment schedule for PN, and more evaluation studies are being done (Centers for Medicare & Medicaid Services, 2001). An early study revealed an annual excess of more than $500,000 in patient charges when PN was ordered and not indicated or its use was preventable (Trujillo, Young, Chertow, et al.). Central parenteral nutrition (CPN), also known as total parenteral nutrition (TPN), can provide the entire nutrient needs of a patient. It is indicated when the GI tract is not functional or cannot be accessed and in patients who cannot be adequately nourished by an oral diet or enteral nutrition over a 7- to 10-day period (ASPEN, 2002). Peripheral parenteral nutrition (PPN) is reserved for patients with a nonfunctioning GI tract and a need for short-term nutrition of <2 weeks. Patients must have adequate peripheral access and be able to tolerate 2 to 3 liters of fluid per day (Aihara, Schoepfel, Curtis, et al., 2002).

The standard rule is still appropriate: "When the gut works, use it!" The enteral route is preferred whenever possible because it is more physiologic—that is, it maintains the integrity and function of the GI tract. The enteral route is also less expensive, less invasive, and easier to manage, generally with fewer complications. PN is contraindicated for patients without severe malnutrition when treatment is anticipated to be <5 days (Aihara et al., 2002). General guidelines for the appropriate use of PN are outlined in Box 16–1.

Nutritional Assessment

Nutritional assessment is necessary because inadequate nutrition increases the complications of disease, especially infection; decreases the ability to heal wounds; prolongs length of hospital stay; and contributes to anorexia and weakness. **Malnutrition** is determined through a nutritional assessment reviewing body weight, body composition, somatic and visceral protein stores, and laboratory values. Early nutritional intervention is recommended to avoid additional complications of malnutrition including impaired respiratory muscle function, renal failure, and nonhealing wounds.

Two common types of protein-energy malnutrition include marasmus and kwashiorkor. **Marasmus** is characterized by catabolism of fat and muscle tissue, lethargy, generalized weakness, and weight loss. Visceral proteins are relatively preserved with serum albumin >3 g/dL. Patients are generally <80% of standard weight for height (Hammond, 2004). **Kwashiorkor** is characterized by edema, catabolism of muscle tissue, weakness, neurologic changes, secondary infections, stunted growth in children, and changes in hair. Visceral proteins are depressed with serum albumin <3 g/dL. Patients are generally >90% of standard weight for height (Hammond, 2004).

Another type of protein-energy malnutrition is characterized by a combination of marasmus and kwashiorkor symptoms. Patients are generally <60% of standard weight for height and have depressed visceral proteins with serum albumin <3 g/dL. This type of malnutrition usually occurs when a patient with marasmus is exposed to stress.

Nutritional Screening and Assessment Standards

Starting in 1995, the Joint Commission on the Accreditation of Healthcare Organizations (JCAHO) standards for both hospital and home care mandated screening and

---

BOX 16–1   Guidelines for the Use of Parenteral Nutrition (PN)

1. Patients who are candidates for PN support cannot, should not, or will not eat adequately to maintain their nutrient stores. These patients are already malnourished or have the potential of becoming malnourished.
2. Peripheral parenteral nutrition (PPN) may be used to provide partial or total nutrition support for up to 2 weeks in select patients who cannot ingest or absorb oral or enteral tube-delivered nutrients, or when central vein parenteral nutrition is not feasible.
3. PN support is necessary when parenteral feeding is indicated for longer than 2 weeks, peripheral venous access is limited, nutrient needs are large, or fluid restriction is required, and the benefits of PN support outweigh the risks.

Use PN when:

1. Patient has failed EN trial with appropriate tube placement (postpyloric).
2. EN is contraindicated or the intestinal tract has severely diminished function owing to underlying disease or treatment. Specific applicable conditions are as follows:
   - Paralytic ileus
   - Mesenteric ischemia
   - Small bowel obstruction
   - GI fistula except when enteral access may be placed distal to the fistula or volume of output (<200 mL/day supports a trial of EN).
3. In postoperative nutrition support, the exact duration of starvation that can be tolerated without increased morbidity is unknown. Expert opinion suggests that wound healing is impaired if PN is not started within 5 to 10 days postoperatively for patients unable to eat or tolerate enteral feeding.
4. The patient's clinical condition is considered in the decision to withhold or withdraw therapy. Conditions in which nutrition support is poorly tolerated and should be withheld until the condition improves are severe hyperglycemia, azotemia, encephalopathy, hyperosmolality, and severe fluid and electrolyte disturbances.

(From ASPEN [2002]).

---

nutritional assessment as part of the specific nutritional care standards. The standards emphasize an interdisciplinary approach. In many settings, the nutritional screen is completed by a health professional other than the dietitian. The goal of **nutritional screening** is to identify individuals who are at nutrition risk, as well as to identify those who need further assessment (Hammond, 2004).

Many hospitals have established formal nutritional screening programs for all hospital admissions to identify those patients most at risk or already malnourished. An algorithm for nutritional screening is presented in Figure 16–1. A nutritional screening tool for use by registered nurses to classify the nutritional status of hospitalized patients appears in Figure 16–2. Once a nutritional screen is completed, patients who are at nutritional risk are usually referred to a dietitian.

A nutritional assessment should be included in the overall assessment of patients, particularly on admission to the hospital and periodically throughout the

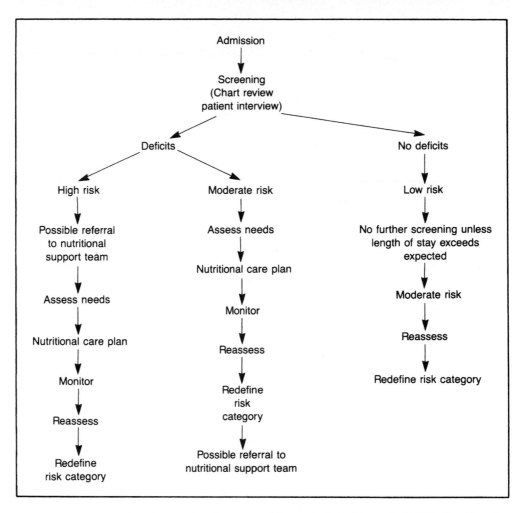

FIGURE 16–1. Nutritional screening (Courtesy of Grant, A., & DeHoog, S. [1999]. *Nutritional assessment, support and management* (2nd ed.). Seattle, WA: Authors).

hospital stay. It should also be a component of nursing assessment in all health care settings, with reassessment at appropriate intervals, depending on the patient's status. Studies indicate that when admitted to acute care facilities, between 33% to 65% of all patients have some degree of malnutrition and nutritional status deteriorates when patients are hospitalized >2 weeks (Hammond, 2004). Primary care, outpatient management, and the new standards have moved the role of nutritional assessment into the physician's office and home care setting as well. Mechanisms for documenting nutritional screening and assessment should be established and monitored. Suggested goals of nutritional assessment include the following:

- To identify individuals who require aggressive nutritional support
- To restore or maintain an individual's nutritional status

A. Diagnosis
   If the patient has at least ONE of the following diagnoses, circle and proceed to section E to consider the patient
      AT NUTRITIONAL RISK and stop here.
   Anorexia nervosa/bulimia nervosa
   Malabsorption (celiac sprue, ulcerative colitis, Crohn's disease, short bowel syndrome)
   Multiple trauma (closed-head injury, penetrating trauma, multiple fractures)
   Decubitus ulcers
   Major gastrointestinal surgery within the past year
   Cachexia (temporal wasting, muscle wasting, cancer, cardiac)
   Coma
   Diabetes
   End-stage liver disease
   End-stage renal disease
   Nonhealing wounds
B. Nutrition intake history
   If the patient has at least ONE of the following symptoms, circle and proceed to section E to consider the patient
      AT NUTRITIONAL RISK and stop here.
   Diarrhea (>500 mL × 2 days)
   Vomiting (>5 days)
   Reduced intake (<1/2 normal intake for >5 days)
C. Ideal body weight standards
   Compare the patient's current weight for height to the ideal body weight chart on the back of this form. If at
      <80% of ideal body weight, proceed to section E to consider the patient AT NUTRITIONAL RISK and stop
      here.
D. Weight history
   Any recent unplanned weight loss? No_____ Yes _____ Amount (lbs or kg)_____
   If yes, within the past _____ weeks or _____ months
   Current weight (lbs or kg) _____
   Usual weight (lbs or kg)_____
   Height (ft, in or cm)_____
   Find percentage of weight lost: usual wt − current wt × 100 = _____ % wt loss
                                     usual wt
   Compare the % wt loss with the chart values and circle appropriate value

Length of time	Significant (%)	Severe (%)
1 week	1–2	>2
2–3 weeks	2–3	>3
1 month	4–5	>5
3 months	7–8	>8
5+ months	10	>10

   If the patient has experienced a significant or severe weight loss, proceed to section E and consider the patient
      AT NUTRITIONAL RISK
E. Nurse assessment
   Using the above criteria, what is this patient's nutritional risk? (circle one)
   _____ LOW NUTRITIONAL RISK
   _____ AT NUTRITIONAL RISK

FIGURE 16–2.   Admission nutritional assessment tool. (Reproduced with permission from Kovacevich, D.S., Boney, A.R., Braunschweig, C.L., et al. [1997]. Nutritional risk classification: A reproducible and valid tool for nurses. *Nutrition Support in Clinical Practice, 12*[1], 20–25.)

- To identify appropriate medical nutrition therapies
- To monitor the efficacy of these interventions (Hammond, 2004)

A nutritional assessment traditionally begins with a complete history, which includes a diet history, anthropometric measurements, physical assessment, and complete medical history, including **drug–nutrient interactions,** and biochemical evaluation.

HEALTH AND DIET HISTORY

The patient's usual and current dietary intake is helpful in identifying the adequacy of **nutrients** (ie, protein, carbohydrate, lipid, vitamins, minerals, trace elements, and water) and possible nutritional deficiencies. Nutrients in the medical history should include any acute or chronic diseases that may have an impact on nutrient intake or utilization and conditions that increase metabolic needs or fluid and electrolyte losses. Surgical history, certain medications, and social factors also have an impact on nutritional status and should be evaluated. Multiple computerized programs for dietary assessment are available, each providing different endpoints of data (Probst & Tapsell, 2005). Benefits of a computerized assessment include standardized questioning, immediate micronutrient information, and possible recommendations; additionally, these programs may be used for practice or research. Box 16–2 lists some of the specific factors that may alter nutritional status.

PHYSICAL ASSESSMENT

A thorough physical assessment by an experienced clinician can detect signs and symptoms suggesting nutritional deficiencies. These include but are not limited to changes in hair, eyes, skin, nails, and all organ systems (Table 16–1).

ANTHROPOMETRICS

Anthropometric measurements consist of simple, noninvasive, inexpensive techniques for obtaining body measurements useful in evaluating for overnutrition or undernutrition. The patient's actual height and weight should be obtained and used to help determine nutritional status.

Body weight can by assessed by several methods including (a) body mass index, (b) comparison with usual body weight, and (c) comparison with ideal body weight. Body mass index (BMI) is a tool for judging body weight in relation to height and risks for weight-related health problems such as heart disease, diabetes, and certain types of cancer (Duyff, 2002). See Box 16–3 for an interpretation of BMI. BMI calculators are available on the following websites:

www.consumer.gov/weightloss/bmi.htm (accessed 8/22/2005)
www.nhlbisupport.com/bmi/bmicalc.htm (accessed 8/22/2005)

Usual body weight (UBW) is obtained from past medical records or subjectively from the patient or family member. Actual weight as a percentage of UBW is usually

BOX 16–2   Factors Influencing Food Intake

Diet
Food allergies, aversions, and intolerance
Fad diets
Diet modifications (low sodium, low fat)
Ethnic and cultural factors
Poor dentition or ill-fitting dentures
Oral sores or lesions
Alteration in taste or smell
Breathing difficulty
Inability to prepare food or feed self
Frequent fasting (NPO) status, clear liquid diet

Health Factors
Chewing or swallowing difficulty
Neurologic impairment
Malabsorption
Inflammatory bowel disease
Chronic illness (ie, chronic obstructive pulmonary disease, human immunodeficiency virus infection,
     liver disease, end-stage renal disease, cancer)
Increased losses from draining wounds, ostomies, fistulas, effusions, diarrhea

Surgical History
Small or large bowel obstruction
Surgical reconstruction (ie, gastrectomy, gastrojejunostomy, esophagogastrectomy, small intestine resection)
Head and neck surgery
Surgical procedure for morbid obesity

Medications (may alter dietary intake or nutrient utilization):
Analgesics
Antacids
Antibiotics
Anticonvulsants
Antineoplastic agents
Diuretics
Laxatives
Oral contraceptives

Psychosocial Factors
Alcohol or substance abuse
Income
Institutionalization
Psychologic or physical disabilities
Recent loss of spouse/partner
Religion

TABLE 16–1 Physical Assessment Findings in Nutritional Deficiencies

Physical Changes	Deficiency
Hair	
Lackluster, thin, sparse; pigmentation changes	Protein, calorie, zinc, linoleic acid
Mouth	
Angular stomatitis: cracks, redness at one or both corners of mouth	Vitamin B
Cheilosis—vertical cracks in lips	Riboflavin and niacin
Varicose veins under tongue	Vitamin C
Tongue	
May become purplish, red, or beefy red or may appear smooth and pale; one or more fissures, atrophy of taste buds	Vitamin B
Skin	
Dryness, flakiness	Vitamin A, essential fatty acids
Petechiae or easy bruising; hemorrhagic spots on skin at pressure points; may occur in presence of liver disease or during anticoagulation	Vitamins C and K
Musculoskeletal	
Muscle wasting (especially quadriceps, deltoids, and temporalis)	Protein, calorie
Kyphosis, osteoporosis	Calcium and vitamin D
Neurologic	
Confusion, listlessness	Protein malnutrition
Sensory-motor, vibratory	Thiamine and vitamin B_{12}

BOX 16–3 Interpreting Body Mass Index

Formula
  Metric formula: BMI = Weight (kg)/Height (m)^2

Recommended Classification
Underweight	<18.5
Normal	18.5–24.9
Obesity, grade I	25–29.9
Obesity, grade II	30–40
Obesity, grade III	>40

TABLE 16–2   Evaluation of Weight Change

Loss	Significant Weight Loss	Severe Weight Loss
1 wk	1%–2%	>2%
1 mo	5%	>5%
3 mo	7.5%	>7.5%
6 mo	10%	>10%

Values charted are for percent weight change:

$$\text{Percent weight change} = \frac{\text{Usual weight} - \text{actual weight}}{\text{Usual weight}} \times 100$$

(Reproduced with permission from Blackburn, G.J., Bistrian, B.R., Maini, B.S., Schlamm, B.A., & Smith, M.F. [1997]. Nutritional and metabolic assessment of the hospitalized patient. *Journal of Parenteral and Enteral Nutrition, 1*[1], 17.)

the most accurate determinant of weight loss. Minimum weight for survival is 48% to 55% of usual body weight (Hammond, 2004). Usual body weight can be calculated as follows:

$$\text{Usual weight} = \frac{\text{Actual weight}}{\text{Usual weight}} \times 100$$

Percentage of ideal body weight (IBW) may also be used, and can be determined with the preceding formula by substituting IBW for usual weight. This method is not as effective when assessing the nutrition risk of a critically ill patient. A normally thin person, with stable weight, may be incorrectly identified as malnourished if weight is less than IBW; the obese patient with significant recent weight loss may be overlooked if weight is still above IBW (Grant, 1992). See Table 16–2.

IBW can be determined from standard reference tables such as the Metropolitan Life Insurance tables, which are based on sex, height, and body frame. Body frame can be determined by measuring the wrist circumference just distal to the styloid process (Table 16–3). Ideal body weight can also be estimated using the Hamwi method, as follows:

Females: 100 pounds for the first 5 feet of height and 5 pounds for every inch over 5 feet
Males: 106 pounds for the first 5 feet of height and 6 pounds for every inch over 5 feet

An adjustment factor is made of $+/-10\%$ depending on frame size.

Other anthropometric measurements include triceps skinfold thickness, which estimates subcutaneous fat stores, and midarm muscle circumference, which estimates somatic protein stores (skeletal muscle mass). These measurements can be helpful in assessing individuals over time, but not in the critical and acute care settings because changes in body fluid and composition may influence the results (Hammond, 2004).

TABLE 16–3 Determination of Body Frame

Frame	Male	Female
Large	r*= >10.4 cm	r = >10.9 cm
Medium	r = 9.6–10.4 cm	r = 9.9–10.9 cm
Small	r = <9.6 cm	r = <9.9 cm

$$*r = \frac{\text{Height (cm)}}{\text{Wrist circumference (cm)}}$$

(Curtis, S. [1996]. Nutrition assessment of adults. In K.A. Hennesy & M.E. Orr (Eds.). *Nutrition support nursing core curriculum* (3rd ed., pp. 1-1–12). Silver Spring, MD: American Society for Parenteral and Enteral Nutrition.)

Reproducibility of accurate measurements requires strict adherence to protocol and may vary widely in the same individual with different examiners.

BIOCHEMICAL ASSESSMENT

A variety of biochemical tests are used to assess nutritional status, with a broad range of cost and sensitivity. The most commonly used, and most readily available, are visceral proteins and tests to evaluate immune function.

Visceral Proteins

Depletion of visceral proteins is characteristic of **protein malnutrition,** which occurs acutely in the hospitalized patient (hypoalbuminemia). An estimate of visceral protein status can be obtained from measurements of specific serum transport proteins that are synthesized in the liver. These include albumin, transferrin, prealbumin, and retinol-binding protein (Table 16–4). Serum albumin is useful for helping to determine nutritional status, but has limited value in assessing acute changes in nutritional status related to its long half-life (Carney & Meguid, 2002). It is recommended that serum albumin measurements be included in the initial chemical profile when screening for malnutrition. An albumin concentration of <3.5 g/dL is associated with increased morbidity in hospitalized patients (Carney & Meguid).

Transferrin has a shorter half-life than albumin, but does not respond rapidly enough to protein energy status to be useful in acute care settings (Carlson, 2004). Retinol-binding protein also has a shorter half-life, but does not accurately reflect protein energy status in acutely stressed patients. It is also not useful for patients with vitamin A deficiency or renal failure (Carlson). Prealbumin, with a shorter half-life, seems to be a more sensitive and specific indicator for monitoring the effectiveness of nutritional support. It is more expensive and may be limited in smaller hospitals. Consideration should also be given to assessing non-nutritional factors, such as inflammation, that may affect these visceral proteins. Even though these tests are useful, new nutritional markers are needed that better identify malnourished patients and precisely monitor the effectiveness of nutritional intervention on nutritional status. Other proteins are being investigated to determine their efficacy in nutritional assessment.

TABLE 16–4 Visceral Proteins

Visceral Protein	Half-Life	Normal Range	Causes of Decrease	Causes of Increase
Albumin Maintains plasma oncotic pressure Carrier protein (zinc, calcium, magnesium, fatty acids)	18–21 d	Normal: >3.5 g/dL Mild depletion: 2.8–3.5 g/dL Mod. depletion: 2.1–2.7 g/dL Severe depletion: <2.1 g/dL Reflects *chronic*, not acute change	Metabolic stress Infection, inflammation Liver disease ↑ Losses (wounds, burns, fistulas) Inadequate protein intake Fluid imbalance (ascites, edema, overhydration)	Dehydration may falsely ↑ levels Salt-poor albumin infusion
Transferrin Carrier protein for iron	8–10 d	Normal: >200 mg/dL Mild depletion: 150–200 mg/dL Mod. depletion: 100–150 mg/dL Severe depletion: <100 mg/dL	Malabsorptive states Chronic infection Inflammatory state Acute catabolic states ↑ Iron stores Liver damage Overhydration	Pregnancy Hepatitis Iron deficiency anemia Dehydration Chronic blood loss
Thyroxine-binding prealbumin (transthyretin) Carrier protein for retinol-binding protein Transport protein for thyroxine	2–3 d	Normal: >20 mg/dL Mild depletion: 10–15 mg/dL Mod. depletion: 5–10 mg/dL Severe depletion: <5 mg/dL Sensitive to acute changes in protein status Limited use in situation in which there is a sudden demand for protein synthesis	Infection Acute catabolic state Postsurgery (5–10 mg/dL drop first week) Liver disease Altered energy and protein balance Hyperthyroid	Chronic renal failure Corticosteroids
Retinol-binding protein Transport retinol (alcohol of vitamin A)	10–18 h	Normal: 3–5 mEq/dL Reflects acute change	Vitamin A deficiency Acute catabolic states Postsurgery Liver disease Hyperthyroid	Renal disease

Immune Function Tests

Alterations in the immune system may be influenced by stress, specific disease states, and malnutrition. The total lymphocyte count (TLC) is indicative of a patient's ability to fight infection and is known to decrease with malnutrition, especially inadequate calories and protein. TLC (total lymphocyte count) may be calculated using the complete blood count with differential: TLC = white blood cell count (WBC) × lymphocytes. Normal levels range from 1,500 to 1,800 mm^3. However, TLC is affected by many medical disease states and varies widely; thus it is of limited value.

Cell-mediated immunity is most frequently evaluated with delayed cutaneous hypersensitivity skin tests. Intradermal injections of specific recall antigens, such as *Candida*, mumps, or tuberculin, are used. Patients who are immunocompetent will exhibit a positive response within 24 to 48 hours; this response consists of a small, reddened area (5 mm) around the test site. Patients who are malnourished and possibly immunosuppressed may exhibit a delayed response, a response to only one of the antigens, or no reaction. These results are classified as normal or reactive if there is a response to two or more antigens, relatively anergic if only one response occurs, and anergic if there is no response to any of the antigens. These results must be weighed with other findings in the nutritional assessment because non-nutritional factors, such as infection, sepsis, cancer, liver disease, renal failure, immunosuppressive diseases, and immunosuppressive drugs, may also affect immunocompetence (Dudek, 2001).

DECISION FOR NUTRITIONAL SUPPORT

Many nutritional assessments are available for different health care providers (Brogden, 2004; Rodriguez, 2004), as well as emerging technologies that provide information on the individual's metabolic analyses (German, Roberts, & Watkins, 2003). There is no single indicator of nutritional status. A global assessment of many indices, and the patient's clinical status, is necessary to determine the incidence and degree of nutritional deficiency. Reassessment is individualized whenever the clinical status changes and periodically throughout the course of nutritional therapy. Once the nutritional assessment data have been collected and evaluated, the optimal method for nutritional support must be selected. This decision process is depicted in Figure 16–3.

Nutritional Requirements

The practical outcome of the nutritional assessment is to determine the caloric and protein needs of the patient. These requirements change in acute, catabolic illness, and in some chronic conditions.

Energy Requirements

Nutrient energy requirements are usually expressed in kilocalories (kcal). Numerous methods for determining a person's nutritional requirements are available, with

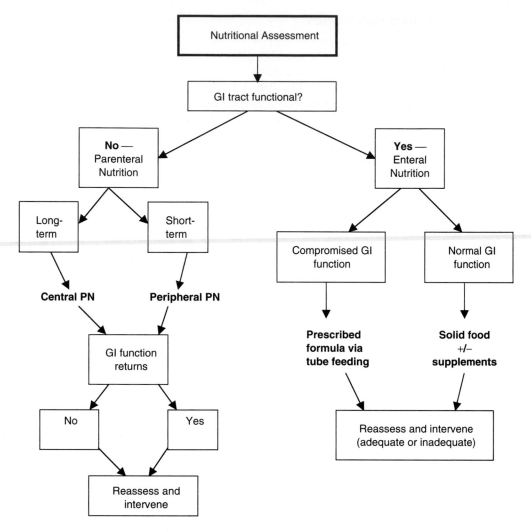

FIGURE 16–3. Decision-making process for nutritional support. (Adapted from Grant, J., & DeHoog, S. [1999]. *Nutritional assessment, support, and management* [2nd ed.]. Seattle, WA: Authors; and Livingston, A., Seamons, C., & Dalton, T. [2000]. If the gut works, use it. *Nursing Management, 31*[5], 39–42.)

varying degrees of sophistication. Indirect calorimetry is one of the most accurate ways of determining a patient's energy needs. In the clinical setting, metabolic carts are often used to determine the oxygen consumption and carbon dioxide production of the body over a period of time. This helps to determine actual energy expenditure. Indirect calorimetry requires expensive equipment and therefore is not available at all institutions (Hammond, 2004).

One of the most widely used equations to estimate energy expenditure is the Harris-Benedict equation, which was derived from healthy individuals. It estimates

TABLE 16–5   Correction Factors for Estimating Nonprotein Energy Requirements of Hospitalized Patients

Activity Description	Activity Factor
Chair or bed bound	1.2
Out of bed	1.3
Little movement and little or no leisure activity	1.4–1.5
Seated work with requirement to move but little strenuous leisure activity	1.6–1.7
Clinical Status	**Stress Factor**
Elective surgery	1–1.1
Peritonitis	1.05–1.25
Multiple/long bone fractures	1.1–1.3
Cancer	1.1–1.45
Severe infection	1.2–1.6
Closed head injury	1.
Infection with trauma	1.3–1.55
Multiple trauma	1.4
Burns	1.5–2.1

Actual energy requirements = basal energy expenditure (BEE) × activity factor (AF) × injury factor (IF).
(Information adapted from Rychlec, G., et al. [2000]. Nutrition assessment of adults. In: B. Hornick [Ed.]. *Manual of clinical dietetics* [6th ed., pp. 3–33]. Chicago: American Dietetic Association.)

basal energy expenditure (BEE) in kilocalories, using weight, height, age, and sex (Harris & Benedict, 1919) with the following equations:

$$\text{BEE (male)} = (66 + 13.8W + 5H) - 6.8A$$
$$\text{BEE (female)} = (655 + 9.6W + 1.8H) - 4.7A$$

where W is weight in kilograms, H is height in centimeters, and A is age in years.

UBW is most commonly used, although an adjusted body weight is often recommended if the patient is obese (BMI >30). Stress and activity factors are often added to predict energy expenditures of critically ill or injured patients, which can range from an addition of 30% to 50% above resting energy expenditure (Ireton-Jones, 2002). Actual energy requirements are then estimated by multiplying BEE × AF × IF. Correction factors (for activity [IF] and stress/injury [IF]) to estimate nonprotein energy requirements of hospitalized patients are listed in Table 16–5.

Another common way to estimate energy needs is by calculating energy per kilogram. It has been estimated that 25 to 35 kcal per kg body weight is needed for total energy expenditure in the nonobese population, whereas only 21 kcal per kg body weight is needed in the obese critically ill population (Rychlec et al., 2000).

Regardless of the method chosen, it is important to avoid overfeeding. The early adage of nutritional support "the more, the better," is no longer advocated. Overfeeding, which causes hyperglycemia and has deleterious effects on respiratory and hepatic function, should be avoided, especially in the acutely ill patient (Cerra, Benitez, & Blackburn, 1997; McMahon, 1997; Souba, 1997). Additional calories for desired weight gain should be held until the patient recovers.

Protein Requirements

Protein requirements for healthy people are based on the amount needed to maintain nitrogen equilibrium, assuming energy is being met by nonprotein kilocalories. The recommended daily allowance for healthy adults is 0.8 g/kg/day. Protein requirements are increased during illness to meet stress needs for wound healing, promote immune competence, and replace losses. Critically ill patients require an increased protein intake of 1.5 to 2.0 g/kg/day (Cresci, 2002).

CALORIE–NITROGEN RATIO

A nonstressed patient can achieve nitrogen balance with adequate calorie intake and protein accounting for 8% of calories. When a patient becomes stressed, both calorie and protein requirements increase. Protein should contribute 15% to 20% of energy in a stressed patient. The optimal calorie:nitrogen ratio for critically ill patients is 150:1 (Matarese & Gottschlich, 1998).

NITROGEN BALANCE

Nitrogen balance is an objective method of evaluating the efficacy of the patient's nutritional regimen. For a patient to be in a positive nitrogen balance or anabolic state, the amount of nitrogen taken in by the patient (IV and orally) needs to be more than that excreted. A 24-hour urine collection is needed to measure the amount of urinary urea excreted. A factor of 4 g is added (2 g for fecal losses and 2 g for integumentary losses) to measure total nitrogen excretion. A nitrogen balance of 2 to 4 grams of nitrogen per day indicates the patient is in an anabolic state. It is nearly impossible to achieve positive nitrogen balance immediately after a metabolic insult. Nitrogen balance studies are not accurate for patients with impaired creatinine clearance, severe hepatic failure, massive diuresis, or abnormal nitrogen losses through diarrhea or large draining wounds (Cresci, 2002). The nitrogen balance formula and measures that reflect the severity of the catabolic state can be found in Box 16–4.

Fluid Requirements

Individual fluid requirements vary greatly and can fluctuate on a daily basis. Fluid needs should be carefully assessed when designing the PN formula. The minimum daily requirement for healthy adults is 1 mL/kcal. Factors that may increase fluid needs include fever and increased losses from diuresis, diarrhea, vomiting, and drainage from wounds and fistulas. Environmental factors such as specialized high–air-loss beds, ultraviolet light therapy, and radiant warmers also increase fluid requirements. Humidified air reduces insensible fluid loss and results in lower fluid requirements. Pre-existing excess or deficiency states and cardiac and renal function must also be evaluated.

BOX 16–4 Nitrogen Balance

Formula

Nitrogen balance is calculated by subtracting the amount of nitrogen lost from the amount of nitrogen given or taken by the patient, as follows:

$$\text{Nitrogen balance} = \frac{\text{Protein intake}}{6.25} - (\text{urine urea nitrogen} + 4)$$

Interpretation

Normally at equilibrium, the following measures reflect the severity of the catabolic state:

Equilibrium   0 g/d
Mild   −5 to −10 g/d
Moderate   −10 to −15 g/d
Severe   >−15 g/d

Usual goal during nutritional support = +2/−4 g nitrogen/24 h

---

Fluids may be required in addition to the fluids provided by parenteral nutrition (PN). Because fluid requirements shift rapidly with changes in clinical status in hospitalized patients, this is best done by giving additional crystalloid IV fluids, such as dextrose 5% in water (D_5W) or dextrose 5% in 0.45% sodium chloride solution by a separate lumen or route. These can be frequently adjusted as necessary without affecting nutrient delivery. They can also be used as additional vehicles for electrolyte corrections, avoiding possible wastage of the PN solution. The PN solution can be formulated using concentrated nutrients (70% dextrose, 15% amino acids, 15% lipids) to provide adequate nutrients when fluid restriction is needed.

Parenteral Nutrition Solutions

The complex solutions used in PN can provide all the necessary nutrients to meet requirements for growth, weight gain, anabolism, and wound healing.

Components

Total nutrient admixtures (TNA) are formulations consisting of carbohydrates, amino acids, lipids, vitamins, minerals, trace elements, water, and other additives in a single container. The proportion of each component is individualized based on the patient's clinical status, chronic diseases, fluid and electrolyte balance, and specific goals of PN.

CARBOHYDRATES

Glucose is the primary energy source in most PN solutions. Concentrations from 10% to 70% glucose may be used with a final solution concentration of no more than 10%

to 12% for peripheral infusion and no greater than 35% for central venous infusion. A carbohydrate, parenteral glucose is hydrolyzed and provides 3.4 kcal/g. At least 150 to 200 g of glucose is needed to meet the obligate needs for glucose by the brain, central nervous system, red blood cells, white blood cells, active fibroblasts, and certain phagocytes, which normally require glucose as the sole or major energy source (Galica, 1997). No more than 5 to 7 mg/kg/minute (equals a maximum of 5 to 7 g/kg/day, which is easier to calculate) should be given, which is the maximum rate of glucose oxidation. Less is given to the diabetic, hyperglycemic, or critically ill patient—usually no more than 4 g/kg/day (Burke, Wolfe, Mullany, et al., 1979; Galica, 1997; Rosmarin, Wardlow, & Mirtallo, 1996). In excess of this amount, the incidence of hyperglycemia seems to increase. Overfeeding carbohydrates may result in conversion of excess glucose to fat, which requires energy (increased oxygen consumption and carbon dioxide production), and leads to fatty liver changes with prolonged use. From 50% to 70% of the daily nonprotein kilocalories usually are given as glucose.

LIPIDS

Lipids (fats) provide the second source of nonprotein calories for PN solutions. Lipids serve as integral structural components of cell membranes and are vital to support the synthesis of hormones and prostaglandins (Galica, 1997). IV lipid emulsions are given to prevent essential fatty acid deficiency (EFAD) and as a concentrated source of energy (each gram of fat provides 9 kcal). The only recommendation regarding specific fatty acids is that 1% to 2% of daily energy requirements should be derived from linoleic acid and about 0.5% of energy from α-linoleic acid to prevent essential fatty acid deficiency (Kris-Etherton, Taylor, Yu-Poth, et al., 2000). EFAD has been detected as early as 3 to 7 days after initiation of fat-free PN, although clinical signs of dietary inadequacy may take 3 to 4 weeks to become evident (Carpentier, VanGossum, Dubin, & Decklebaum, 1993). Clinical signs include dry or scaly skin, thinning hair, thrombocytopenia, and liver function abnormalities. Prevention of this deficiency state is desirable because EFAD is associated with decreased ability to heal wounds, adverse effects on red blood cell membranes, and a defect in prostaglandin synthesis.

> **LEGAL ISSUES:**   Lipid Administration
> - Prevention of essential fatty acid deficiency
> - Do not use in patients with severe egg allergies.
> - Prevention of adverse reactions related to inadequate or excess amounts and too-rapid infusion rates
> - Available formulations contain fatty acids that may be immunosuppressive.

Use of IV lipids with glucose in a daily PN solution decreases the glucose calories and minimizes insulin requirements. Lipids should provide 30% to 50% of the nonprotein calories in PN solutions, but should not exceed 60% or 2.5 g/kg, or an infusion rate of 1.7 mg/kg/minute (Galica, 1997). Some data support the use of a maximum of lipid 1 mg/kg/day intravenously, especially in critically ill patients (Battistella, Widergren, Anderson, Siepler, Weber, & MacColl, 1997). IV lipids are available in 10% (1.1 kcal/mL), 20% (2 kcal/mL), and 30% (3 kcal/mL) formulations. They provide fatty acids solely as long-chain triglycerides and contain egg phospholipid as an emulsifier. They should not be used in patients with severe egg allergies. In general, 20% and 30% solutions are used because less volume is needed. Adverse reactions may occur, although the incidence is <1%. Symptoms include dyspnea, cyanosis, nausea, vomiting, headache, dizziness, increased temperature, sweating, chest or back pain, pressure over eyes, and hyperlipidemia. Administration of IV fat emulsions is contraindicated in patients with disturbances in normal fat metabolism such as pathologic hyperlipidemia, lipoid nephrosis, or acute pancreatitis if accompanied by hyperlipidemia.

Because lipids are isotonic (300 mOsmol/L), up to 50% of nonprotein calories may be supplied as lipids in peripheral parenteral nutrition to decrease the incidence of phlebitis. Lipids are better tolerated and utilized if they are infused slowly, not to exceed 1.7 mg/kg/minute. Fast infusion rates have been associated with deleterious effects on pulmonary function and impairment of the reticuloendothelial system function, potentiating the inflammatory response by altering the ability of this defense system to respond to bacterial invasion.

PROTEIN

Protein is used in PN solutions to replete muscle mass and support immune functions. Unlike the other substrates, proteins are not stored. They are in a constant dynamic state of synthesis and breakdown that requires energy and adenosine triphosphate. In the absence of an adequate energy source, protein is used for energy. The protein or nitrogen source is provided by synthetic crystalline amino acid solutions. Whereas earlier amino acids were formulated as protein hydrolysates and were associated with toxicities, this is not a concern with the current crystalline amino acids (McMahon, 1997). These solutions contain a mixture of essential and nonessential amino acids. Special amino acid formulations for renal failure, hepatic failure, and neonates are available. There is some evidence that high–branched-chain amino acid formulas may be beneficial during sepsis and severe metabolic stress, but this remains controversial. Use of the special formulas is restricted because of the high cost and conflicting reports of efficacy (Galica, 1997). Protein requirements are determined by metabolic demands and underlying organ function. For the unstressed patient with adequate organ function, 0.8 gm/kg per day may be adequate, but requirements may rise with metabolic demands to 2 gm/kg per day (or, rarely, even higher; ASPEN, 2002, p. 23SA).

ELECTROLYTES

Electrolytes are essential to maintain normal metabolic function. They include sodium, potassium, chloride, calcium, magnesium, phosphorus, and acetate. A variety of standard electrolyte solutions are available, as well as individual electrolytes. The requirements of individual patients may vary depending on their nutritional status and underlying disease process. Table 16–6 provides standard ranges for electrolyte additions to PN solutions. The activity of electrolytes in the body is usually characterized by interrelated patterns; no one electrolyte can function, be deficient, or be overabundant in the body without affecting other electrolytes.

TABLE 16–6   Daily Electrolyte Additions to Adult Parenteral Nutrition Solutions*

Electrolyte	Parenteral Equivalent of Recommended Dietary Allowance	Standard Intake
Calcium	10 mEq	10–15 mEq
Magnesium	10 mEq	8–20 mEq
Phosphate	30 mmol	20–40 mmol
Sodium	N/A	1–2 mEq/kg + replacement
Potassium	N/A	1–2 mEq/kg
Acetate	N/A	As needed to maintain acid–base balance
Chloride	N/A	As needed to maintain acid–base balance

N/A, not applicable.
*Assumes normal organ function.
(Reproduced with permission of National Advisory Group on Standards and Practice Guidelines for Parenteral Nutrition. [1998]. Safe practices for parenteral nutrition formulations. *Journal of Parenteral and Enteral Nutrition, 22*[2], 49–66.)

VITAMINS

Vitamins are organic compounds essential for maintenance and growth that are not synthesized by the body (Andris, 1996). There are two main groups: fat soluble (A, D, E, K) and water soluble (B complex, C). Vitamins are sensitive to or become inactive with temperature changes and exposure to light. Therefore, they are added before administration and protected from direct light.

Parenteral multivitamins are available to meet the daily requirements set by the American Medical Association Nutrition Advisory Group. Usually, 10 mL of the multivitamins are added to the daily PN solution. Vitamin K, a fat-soluble vitamin necessary for clotting, is included in new formulations of parenteral multivitamins.

TRACE ELEMENTS

Trace elements are required in small amounts and are referred to as *micronutrients*. They are essential components of metabolic pathways. Those commonly added to PN solutions include zinc, copper, chromium, manganese, and selenium. They are available individually or as multitrace solutions. Requirements for individual trace elements may be increased in certain situations (Andris, 1996; Galica, 1997).

DRUGS AND MEDICATIONS

A variety of drugs and medications have been found to be compatible with PN solutions, although compatibility studies are lacking for many. Compatibility studies that have been done used specific PN and TNA solutions and specific concentrations of drugs tested. Compatibility results may be different if a different solution or medication dose or concentration is used. Compatibilities also differ depending on whether the medication is being added to a traditional dextrose and amino acid solution or to a TNA.

The most commonly added medications are heparin, regular insulin, and histamine-2 blockers. It is preferable not to add multiple drugs to the solution. For current information about drug compatibility with PN solutions, readers are referred to Trissel's *Handbook on Injectable Drugs,* which is updated and published yearly and available in hospital pharmacies. Caution is needed to avoid drug–nutrient interactions. The responsible pharmacist should verify that the coinfusion of drugs with PN either admixed in the solution or coinfused through the same IV tubing is safe, stable, and free from incompatibilities (Rollins, 1997). If no information exists in the literature, stability and compatibility should be discussed with the manufacturer.

> **⚠ SAFE PRACTICE ALERT** The feasibility of mixing drugs with PN solutions depends on various factors, including the physical compatibility of the admixed components, the chemical stability of the drug, the retention of drug concentration over time, and the bioactivity of the components after admixture. For safety, the nurse should check with the pharmacy when the compatibility of drugs and PN solutions is a concern.

Because a designated IV catheter port is recommended solely for PN, piggybacking medications to PN solutions usually is not recommended. A study of compatibility of medications during Y-site administration with TNA solutions found that 23 of 106 common medications were incompatible (Trissel, Gilbert, Martinez, et al., 1999).

Preparation of Total Nutrient Admixtures Solution

Safe preparation of solutions requires that trained personnel admix the solution under a laminar-flow hood using strict aseptic technique. Specific protocols covering all aspects of preparation, storage, and quality assurance should be established. Guidelines may vary from institution to institution but should meet established standards. The Board of Directors of ASPEN has recommended that the practice guidelines in the *Safe Practices for Parenteral Nutrition Formulations* document be the "standard of practice for the provision of parenteral nutrition" (National Advisory Group on Standards and Practices Guidelines for Parenteral Nutrition [National Advisory Group], 1998). Practice guidelines for labeling, formulation and nutrient ranges, nutrient prescription, compounding, quality assurance, stability and compatibility, and in-line filtration are included. These guidelines may have broad ramifications in changing clinical practice in many health care settings. Adoption of these standards should prevent future patient harm and also serve as a catalyst for future research.

Solutions may be prepared as traditional dextrose–amino acid solutions or as TNAs. If dextrose–amino acid solutions are used, the IV lipid emulsions are usually piggybacked to the PN or administered by a separate route. TNAs, also known as trimix or 3-in-1, consist of all components, including lipids, mixed together in one large bag. These solutions are used almost exclusively by home care companies and increasingly in many hospitals.

All additives should be added to the PN solution in the pharmacy under sterile conditions. Additives should not be added on the nursing unit or after the PN container has been spiked and hung. If additional additives are needed after the container is hanging, alternate methods or routes should be considered.

TABLE 16–7   Visible Phenomena in Total Nutrient Admixture Solutions

Phenomena	Characteristics	Considerations
Physical phenomena		
Aggregation (stratification)	Rare white streaks (early stages of creaming)	Readily reverses with *gentle* agitation Not harmful
Creaming	Dense white color at top of solution ("cream" layer) Aggregates migrate to top of the solution	Reverses with *gentle* agitation If creaming reappears in 1–2 h or decreases after agitation, it may indicate an unstable emulsion If left undistributed, may begin to coalesce (see below)
Chemical phenomena		
Coalescence/cracking (breaking/oiling out)	Oil globules on the surface of creamed emulsion coalesce or fuse to form larger oil droplets May appear as an oil layer on top of the solution, as large oil globules, or streaks of oil throughout the solution	Irreversible Cannot be dispersed Do not hang the container If coalescence appears during infusion, take container down and return it to pharmacy immediately

Total nutrient admixture solutions offer a significant advantage in the ability to provide cost effective, patient-specific nutrition support. Having only one solution container to hang each day saves nursing time. Pharmacy admixing is simplified by the use of computerized automixing systems, which also allow for more patient-specific formulations. Potential bacterial contamination of either the solution or line is decreased because of decreased accessing of the line. The increased use of TNA reflects the trend toward the daily use of lipid emulsions as a daily calorie source.

The stability of TNA is affected by many factors, including admixture contents, storage time and conditions, addition of non-nutrient drugs, pH of the solution, and variability in temperature (Rollins, 1997). A recent U.S. Food and Drug Administration (FDA) alert strongly advises pharmacists to use care in the compounding order of nutrients, and advocates, along with the safe practices guidelines, the use of a 1.2-μm filter during infusion to avoid problems with calcium and phosphate precipitation (National Advisory Group, 1998). A TNA solution is normally milky white and opaque, although a faint yellow hue may be evident with the addition of vitamins. The nurse should examine the solution for any signs of instability before hanging and periodically thereafter. Particulate matter is hard to detect because of the opacity of the solution. Other physical or chemical phenomena may occur and are outlined in Table 16–7. Nurses should be aware of these phenomena and be able to recognize a stable lipid emulsion or TNA solution (Rollins, 1997). A TNA solution is usually stable for 24 hours after admixing with the addition of vitamins, and for up to 7 days if vitamins are not added until the solution is ready to use.

Administration of Parenteral Nutrition

Administration of hypertonic PN solutions requires an easily placed, well-tolerated central venous access device (CVAD) that can be used for extended periods. Infusion into a large vein with high blood flow to dilute the solution rapidly is desirable to reduce phlebitis, venous thrombosis, pain, and hemolysis (Andris & Krzywda, 1997).

Vascular Access

A variety of CVADs are used for short-term and long-term access. Short-term access is usually obtained using percutaneously placed central catheters and peripherally inserted central catheters (PICCs). It is recommended that these devices have a minimum number of lumens and one lumen that is dedicated solely to the infusion of TPN (Krzywda, 2004; Penney-Timmons & Sevedge, 2004) to decrease the risk of contamination. Opinions about the use of PICCs for TPN infusion vary. Some studies suggest that PICCs may not be the best choice for TPN infusion because of reported problems with malposition, mechanical phlebitis, and breakage (Duerksen, Papineau, Siemens, & Yaffe, 1999; Mayo Clinic Proceedings, 2000). Penney-Timmons & Sevedge reported that PICCs could be used successfully for infusion of TPN based on their study findings that 83% of participants were able to complete TPN therapy with a PICC. This finding was based on 1,057 catheters used for TPN and 15,732 total catheter dwell days.

Tunneled catheters and implanted vascular access ports are suitable for long-term access. Tunneled catheters are most commonly used for long-term TPN administration and are available with single or multiple lumens. Swan-Ganz catheters usually are not recommended for infusion of PN. However, if no other access is available, the right atrium or proximal port can be used. The side arm of the introducer should not be used because it is short and located in the subclavian vein; additionally, the subclavian vein is not recommended for PN infusions because of the risk of thrombosis and inadequate dilution.

Nurses play a major role during the insertion and use of CVADs. They are responsible for the daily care and are held accountable for preventing or minimizing the many device-related complications, including those that are life threatening. Protocols for the insertion, care, and maintenance of CVADs should be established and followed according to current standards. For example, a CVAD should not be used until the location of the catheter tip has been determined to be in the distal superior vena cava and any complications of insertion have been ruled out. Parenteral nutrition should never be initiated until catheter tip placement has been confirmed. It is unacceptable for the tip to be located in the heart, inferior vena cava, or any extrathoracic vessel. Atrial rupture, valvular damage, myocardial irritability with arrhythmias, and cardiac tamponade are some of the reported complications when the catheter tip is located in the heart. An increased incidence of catheter-induced thrombosis and occlusion is associated with tip placement in the subclavian, jugular, inferior vena cava, or narrower extrathoracic vessels.

Complications are infrequent, but the patient should be closely monitored after catheter insertion, particularly for signs of respiratory distress, pain, slowly increasing hematoma, or any unexplainable symptom.

Protocols and Precautions

All institutions should have specific protocols for the administration, monitoring, and discontinuation of PN, which should be reviewed annually. ASPEN has published standards for nutritional support of hospitalized patients, hospitalized pediatric patients, home patients, residents of long-term care facilities, and nutritional support nurses (ASPEN Board of Directors, 1988, 1996a, 1996b, 1997, 1999; ASPEN Board of Directors and The Clinical Guidelines Task Force, 2002). It also has similar standards for nutritional support physicians and nutritional support dietitians. In addition, the Intravenous Nurses Society has published standards for IV therapy, which include PN (Intravenous Nurses Society, 2000). Safe administration of PN depends on strict adherence to these protocols and the safe practices guidelines (National Advisory Group, 1998).

Normally, PN solutions are refrigerated immediately after preparation or refrigerated at 4°C until used. The acceptable length of time for refrigeration is based on the stability of the admixture. Lipid emulsions can be refrigerated or stored at room temperature (Krzywda, 2004). The recommended maximum hang time for PN solutions is 24 hours. PN solutions should be inspected for signs of precipitate or instability before hanging. The label also should be matched with the PN orders to ensure accuracy. The volume and infusion rate are usually noted on the label by the pharmacy. Published guidelines for labeling are available (National Advisory Group, 1998).

TPN should be administered at a constant rate. Any changes in rate should be gradual. Current rate recommendations advise a gradual rate introduction of approximately 60 to 80 mL/hour for the first 24 hours with a 20 mL/hour incremental increase every 24 to 48 hours. Changes in the rate of administration should be gradual because fluctuations in glucose levels can occur if the infusion is interrupted or irregular in rate. An electronic infusion device should be used to maintain consistency and accuracy of the infusion.

Glucose tolerance may be compromised by sepsis, stress, shock, hepatic and renal failure, starvation, diabetes, pancreatic disease, and administration of some medications, particularly steroids and some diuretics. Age is another variable; the elderly and the very young are particularly susceptible to glucose intolerance and hyperglycemia. For these patients, administration of exogenous insulin is often necessary. It is preferable to add insulin to the PN solution because it provides a more constant serum insulin level than does periodic subcutaneous administration (McMahon, 1997). In addition, a sliding-scale subcutaneous insulin coverage schedule should be implemented. Box 16–5 outlines steps in managing and preventing hyperglycemia in patients receiving PN. The blood glucose level should continue to be monitored closely because insulin needs may decrease as the stress or sepsis subsides or as steroids are decreased and discontinued. Blood glucose should be maintained at <200 mg/dL during PN administration. One study also found that dextrose infusion rates >4 to 5 mg/kg/minute increase the risk of hyperglycemia (Rosmarin et al., 1996). Avoidance of the extremes of hyperglycemia and hypoglycemia is important.

Extra caution should be used when infusing PN in patients undergoing peritoneal dialysis or propofol infusions. Peritoneal dialysis can provide significant amounts of dextrose calories. The dextrose calories in dialysate solution should be

---

BOX 16–5 Managing Hyperglycemia in Patients Receiving Parenteral Nutrition

Goals

- Maintain serum glucose levels between 100 and 200 mg/dL, with an optimal range of 100–150 mg/dL.
- Avoid overfeeding.

Initiating Parenteral Nutrition

- Limit to no more than 200 g dextrose in the first few days until glycemic control is achieved.
- If baseline fasting blood glucose level is >180–200 mg/dL, or if the patient is a diabetic patient previously treated with insulin or oral agent, add 0.1 U regular insulin per gram of dextrose (ie, 15 U/L 15% dextrose [150 g/L]; 20 U/L 20% dextrose [200 g/L]).
- In general, do not increase dextrose concentration in PN until serum glucose level is consistently <200 mg/dL for 24 h.

Ongoing

- Adjust insulin accordingly whenever the concentration of dextrose increases or decreases.
- Check serum glucose level by reflectance meter every 4 to 6 h initially, then every 8 h once patient's levels are stable.
- Increase regular insulin in PN by 0.05 U/g dextrose daily if serum glucose was consistently >200 mg/dL in previous 24 h.
- Use subcutaneous (SQ) regular insulin to supplement PN insulin according to the following algorithm:

Glucose (mg/dL)	SQ Regular insulin dose (units)
200–250	2–3
251–300	4–6
301–350	6–9
>350	8–12

- If serum glucose is consistently >200 mg/dL with PN insulin and adherence to the SQ insulin algorithm, a separate IV infusion may be helpful in achieving glycemic control.
- Once the patient's glucose level is stable, frequency of glucose monitoring can be decreased.
- Monitor and assess daily to anticipate effects of PN on glucose level (ie, patient's clinical status, fluid status, medication/IV profile, peritoneal dialysis, and dextrose volume).

---

calculated and a comparable amount subtracted from the dextrose ordered in the PN solution to avoid overfeeding and hyperglycemia from excess dextrose. Propofol is a lipid-based sedative that provides 1.1 kcal/mL. It is widely used in critical care units. Infusion of propofol or any other lipid-based drug must be monitored closely when given with PN to avoid the pitfalls of overfeeding and hypertriglyceridemia (Lowrey, Dunlap, Brown, et al., 1996). PN solutions need to be manipulated when excessive calories are provided in these drugs. Daily calculation of dextrose or lipid calories provided by dialysate or lipid-based drugs with appropriate adjustments in the dextrose or lipids provided in PN should be mandatory.

Consideration should also be given to dextrose administered in crystalloid IV solutions. Many patients on PN need supplemental infusions of crystalloids to correct hypernatremia or because of medication compatibility. When possible, non–dextrose-containing crystalloids should be used. If significant amounts of dextrose-containing crystalloids are needed, insulin may be added to decrease the risk of hyperglycemia.

If PN solutions are interrupted or unavailable, standing orders should be available to infuse 5% dextrose solutions at the same rate, either through the central line or peripherally if the central line is removed or lost. This prevents the sudden hypoglycemia caused by the high endogenous insulin secretion that is associated with hypertonic PN solutions. Although some institutions and physicians still prefer to use a 10% dextrose solution in these situations, it has been deemed unnecessary.

Many institutions have established standard start times for PN (eg, 2 PM) to simplify management of infusions and promote clear communication among departments. This also allows the pharmacy to establish standard times for admixing the solutions and delivery to the nursing unit. Orders for PN are usually required in the pharmacy several hours before the established start time. A nurse should demonstrate core competencies in administering PN (Box 16–6).

INTRAVENOUS TUBING AND FILTERS

Primary IV tubing set changes should be established in organizational policy and procedures, based on appropriate guidelines (Centers for Disease Control and Prevention [CDC], 2002; INS, 2000). Tubing used to administer lipid emulsions and TNA solutions should be changed every 24 hours (CDC). If these solutions are administered in a cyclic regimen, the administration set should be discarded after each unit. If the solution contains only dextrose and amino acids, the administration set does not need to be replaced more frequently than every 72 hours (CDC). It is most efficient to standardize the time of tubing and filter changes to coincide with the daily start time for the day's solution. This eliminates additional breaks in the line. Luer-lock connections are optimal to avoid accidental disconnection. If not available, the tubing connection should be taped. The use of needleless systems is recommended.

The need for in-line filtration of PN solutions is apparent given the recommendations of the FDA and the safe practices guidelines of the National Advisory Group (1998). A 0.22-μm filter is recommended for traditional dextrose–amino acid solutions, with the lipids piggybacked below the filter. These filters effectively retain bacteria, fungi, and particulate matter. TNA solutions require use of a 1.2- or 5.0-μm filter that effectively eliminates microprecipitates, *Candida,* and some bacteria. Bacterial contamination of PN solutions is rare. The justification for use of in-line filters centers on the removal of microprecipitates rather than micro-organisms. Microprecipitates are commonly not visible on inspection, particularly in TNAs. A filter should not be used with only-lipid emulsion infusions (INS, 2000).

A risk of contamination always exists when IV tubing and filters are changed. Therefore, precautions need to be taken and aseptic technique strictly followed. All connections should be swabbed thoroughly with 2% chlorhexidine solution, povidone–iodine, or alcohol before the tubing is changed. It is also a good idea to swab the end of the catheter hub to remove any dried blood or sticky residue. The nurse must clamp the catheter before changing the tubing to avoid the risk of air

---

BOX 16–6 Core Competencies for Nurses Administering and Monitoring Parenteral Nutrition

- Demonstrates appropriate use of Standard Precautions and aseptic technique
- Verbalizes knowledge of nursing policies and procedures related to administering PN
- States awareness of the impact of other dextrose sources (IV infusions, IV medications), lipid-based medications (eg, propofol), and dialysate on the development and exacerbation of hyperglycemia
- Demonstrates correct procedure of PN administration
- Indicates knowledge of complications associated with PN administration and their management
- Verbalizes knowledge of pharmacy, nursing, and hospital policies related to PN ordering (who can order, when orders need to be received in pharmacy, what to do if changes are needed, start time)
- Verbalizes understanding that no medications or additives can be added to PN on the nursing unit (only in the pharmacy)
- Verbalizes knowledge of instances when the physician should be notified
- Demonstrates appropriate documentation of PN administration and patient response

Cycling Parenteral Nutrition

- Demonstrates appropriate use of Standard Precautions and aseptic technique
- Verbalizes understanding of nursing policies and procedure related to cycling PN
- Demonstrates appropriate use of glucose monitoring device
- States knowledge of acceptable glucose monitoring parameters and management of hypoglycemia and hyperglycemia
- Verbalizes knowledge of parameters to be monitored and the frequency (ie, intake and output, vital signs, weight, blood analyses, central venous access device site, infusion pump)
- Verbalizes knowledge of potential complications related to cycling and their management
- Expresses knowledge of instances when the physician should be notified
- Demonstrates appropriate documentation of cycling and patient response

Discontinuing Parenteral Nutrition

- Demonstrates appropriate use of Standard Precaution and aseptic technique
- Verbalizes knowledge of nursing policies and procedures related to discontinuing PN
- States understanding of monitoring patient for signs of rebound hypoglycemia during and after discontinuation of PN
- Displays knowledge of need to hang dextrose 5% in water solution at same rate as PN solution if PN must stop abruptly (ie, because of no orders, signs of complications, central venous access device malfunction)
- Verbalizes knowledge of instances when physician should be notified
- Demonstrates appropriate documentation of discontinuing PN and patient response

---

embolism. If a clamp is not available, the patient should be positioned flat in bed and advised to perform the Valsalva maneuver during the tubing change. PN should be infused through a dedicated line. PN lines should not be violated by pressure monitoring devices or transducers, stopcocks, blood drawing, or administration of blood or medications. This practice also reduces the risk of contamination and infection.

KEY INTERVENTION: Administration of Total Nutrient Admixture

Equipment

Total nutrient admixture (TNA) solution
IV administration set
1.2-μg filter

Povidone–iodine wipes
3-mL syringe filled with normal saline
Electronic infusion pump

Action	Rationale
Identify daily administration time with nursing and pharmacy: eg, 1400 (2 PM).	
Assemble equipment.	Gathering equipment in advance saves time.
Explain the procedure to the patient.	Explanations allay anxiety.
Maintain Standard Precautions and always use aseptic technique.	Deters spread of micro-organisms.
Check TNA container label against physician's orders—orders may change from previous day. • Check patient name, date, and rate of infusion. Also check expiration date on formula and time. • Notify pharmacy of any discrepancies or contact pharmacist with questions.	Ensures accuracy and patient safety.
Examine TNA solution for signs of instability (creaming, coalescence, cracking, particulate matter) and notify pharmacist if any signs of instability are observed.	Avoids adverse reactions.
Don clean gloves.	Prevents contamination from bodily fluids and prevents infection.
Attach 1.2 μg filter to end of standard IV tubing; attach to TNA solution, then prime and clamp.	Removes air from IV tubing and filter.
• Cleanse central venous access device (CVAD) lumen/IV tubing or lock connection with 2% chlorhexidine solution, povidone–iodine swab or alcohol swab for 30 seconds; allow to dry.	Cleans any solution residue and micro-organisms from catheter hub connection to prevent contamination.
Clamp catheter lumen; disconnect IV tubing or lock and discard.	
Flush CVAD lumen with 3–10 mL normal saline solution.	Prevents TNA mixing with other drugs or fluids in catheter tubing; prevents incompatible fluids or drugs forming a precipitate.
Attach new primed TNA tubing to dedicated lumen of CVAD. If multilumen CVAD, designate a lumen for TNA and label that lumen. If single lumen, label lumen as TNA.	Ensures safety in that the same lumen is always used for TNA and not used alternately for medications or other fluids; additionally, blood sampling for some lab work is not recommended from lumens used for PN.

Attach primed tubing to infusion pump and set desired rate. Start pump just before opening clamp on CVAD lumen.

Accuracy in administering TNA helps to prevent fluctuations in rate and also backflow of blood into catheter hub.

If TNA is interrupted or stopped or unavailable, infuse dextrose 5% in water solution at the same rate as the ordered TNA.

Prevents rebound hypoglycemia from abrupt cessation of TNA.

Discard any solution left at the end of 24 hours and hang next TNA bag (1400 daily).

Maintains daily start time of 1400 or other designated start time.

Monitor patient frequently for any signs of adverse reactions or problems.

Avoids or identifies potential complications in a timely matter so that appropriate action can be taken.

Document the procedure: Include interventions, patient response and outcomes, pertinent laboratory findings, vital signs, intake and output and any problems or complications.

Accurate documentation is necessary to record nursing care given and ensure continuity of care.

Special notes:
- Medications cannot be added to TNA solutions on the nursing unit; they must be added in the pharmacy.
- TNA tubing and filter must be changed every 24 hours.
- TNA must be ordered daily.

Cycling Parenteral Nutrition

Long-term continuous PN can be associated with fatty liver, hepatic indices, and hepatomegaly caused by hyperinsulinism (Hammond, Szeszycki, & Pfister, 2001). Therefore, cyclic PN is widely used for those patients who require long-term PN support. This also allows for increased mobility during the day, giving the patient some time to participate in normal daytime activities and offering an improved sense of well-being and quality of life. Cycling may also benefit certain patients by allowing maximum freedom for ambulation and physical therapy. Cyclic administration is often indicated for patients who have been in stable condition on continuous TPN, patients who are on home TPN, and patients who require TPN for only a portion of their nutritional needs.

Once tolerance to 24-hour continuous TPN has been established, a transition to cyclic infusions can be initiated. Cycling from 24 hours of nutritional therapy to 12 to 16 hours is usually done over several days with a gradual reduction in the hours of infusion. The infusion time is decreased approximately 4 hours at a time as the infusion rate is increased to maintain nutrition goals for calories and protein. Cyclic TPN is usually not infused at a rate greater than 200 mL/hour. The patient's ability to tolerate the glucose and fluid volume determines the hourly rate. Close monitoring for fluid status and blood glucose alterations is essential. Most patients tolerate this well without development of rebound hypoglycemia.

Blood glucose levels during the accelerated infusion rates for cyclic PN may be up to 250 mg/dL. Normoglycemia is usually present during the hours when the patient is receiving PN.

Discontinuing Parenteral Nutrition

Parenteral nutrition should not be stopped without alternate plans for therapy so that nutritional status can be maintained or continue to improve. Nor should reductions in PN begin until an alternate source of nutritional intake, such as **enteral nutrition** (nutrition by the GI route), is initiated. Tapering of PN can begin when enteral nutrition is able to meet 33% to 50% of nutrient requirements. PN can be discontinued once enteral nutrition is tolerated and able to meet >75% of nutrient requirements (Charney, 2001). Accurate calorie counts are essential to the successful transition from PN to enteral or oral intake.

KEY INTERVENTION:	Discontinuing Parenteral Nutrition

Equipment
Syringe with appropriate amount of normal saline solution
Povidone–iodine wipes
Syringe with appropriate amount of heparin flush solution
Lock device (Luer lock, male adapter)

Action	*Rationale*
Explain procedure to patient.	Explanation allays anxiety.
Maintain Standard Precautions and aseptic technique.	Deters spread of micro-organisms.
Follow these principles when discontinuing PN:	Avoids abrupt cessation of nutrients in absence of any other source of glucose (oral, IV, or enteral) and avoids rebound hypoglycemia.
• Reduce PN infusion rate in conjunction with an increase in caloric intake by oral or enteral route.	Ensures adequacy of nutrient intake.
• Be sure the patient can take half of the estimated nutrient requirements either enterally or orally before PN discontinues.	Same as above.
• Fluid intake may also decrease as the PN is decreased, so provide adequate fluids by other routes.	Prevents dehydration.
• Decrease PN by 50% for 2 hours prior to discontinuation for unstable patients and patients with glucose intolerance or a high dextrose concentration.	Prevents rebound hypoglycemia.

Discontinue PN before surgery: Decrease rate to 40 mL/h the night before surgery, and discontinue infusion at least 4 hours before surgery. Any 5% dextrose solution can be infused. Keep in mind that potassium shifts may occur with hyperglycemia. Also ensure adequate preoperative hydration.	Stress of surgery may increase blood glucose levels, and signs and symptoms of hyperglycemia are not easily monitored or detected in the anesthetized patient.
Verify physician's order to stop infusion.	Ensures that PN is to be discontinued.
Hang dextrose 5% in water at same rate as PN if PN must stop abruptly (eg, no orders, suspected infection, central venous access device [CVAD] malfunction).	Prevents rebound hypoglycemia.
Cleanse CVAD lumen–PN tubing connection with povidone–iodine wipe for 30 seconds. Allow to dry.	Antibacterial and antifungal cleansing of hub deters spread of micro-organisms.
Disconnect PN tubing and discard. Then flush lumen per established protocol and attach lock device to end of CVAD.	Maintains patency and prevents occlusion.
Document procedure in appropriate records.	Accurate and comprehensive documentation reflects nursing care given.

Nursing Management in Parenteral Nutrition

Clinical assessment and monitoring are imperative for the safe administration of PN, which should be considered in the same manner as medication administration. The nurse should be familiar with the solution composition, the expected metabolic response, and the potential complications of therapy. A good knowledge base should enable the nurse to identify patients who are at risk for metabolic complications in order to monitor the patient's response. Catheter site care, dressing changes, and monitoring PN administration are also in the domain of nursing management. The importance of clear and thorough documentation of care cannot be overemphasized. Many hospitals and nutritional support teams have developed clinical pathways for PN, allowing patient outcomes to be tracked and adequacy of therapy to be monitored. ASPEN has also developed clinical pathways for PN. Institutions should tailor PN clinical pathways to reflect research or evidenced based practice. Patient outcomes should be reviewed quarterly with improvement strategies developed for the pathways that result in optimal patient care.

Catheter and Site Care

Skin care and catheter site care are some of the most important measures for preventing catheter-related infections, especially for PN, since these infusions are the nutritional source for patients. Strict adherence to hand washing and aseptic technique is critical. Clean skin should be disinfected at the time of insertion as well as during dressing changes. A 2% chlorhexidine-based solution is recommended (CDC, 2002), although povidone–iodine or 70% alcohol may be used. Ensure that site care materials and solutions are compatible with catheter material. The antiseptic should be allowed to dry prior to dressing. The insertion site should be palpated daily for tenderness and induration; it should be observed through the transparent dressing for erythema, swelling, or exudate. The catheter site should be directly inspected without the dressing if the patient has a fever without obvious source or symptoms of bloodstream infection. If symptoms are present, physician notification and further evaluation are warranted.

ANTIMICROBIAL OINTMENTS AND DRESSINGS

Routine use of prophylactic topical antibiotic ointments or creams on the insertion or exit site is not recommended because of their potential to promote fungal infections and antimicrobial resistance (CDC, 2002). (Hemodialysis catheters have different recommendations from CDC.)

A newer product has been shown to reduce nontunneled CVAD infections, a chlorhexidine-impregnated sponge. Biopatch is recommended for application at the insertion or exit site of arterial catheters and nontunneled CVADs. Several studies have demonstrated the efficacy of Biopatch with no adverse reactions and a reduction in colonization; Chapter 14 has a complete description of this product with current references. However, in 2002, the CDC made no recommendation for the use of a chlorhexidine sponge dressing to reduce the incidence of infection.

CATHETER DRESSING REGIMENS

Before a dressing is applied, determine if a sutureless catheter securement device is warranted. CDC has not made a recommendation for the use of such devices (2002). However, the complications and adverse effects of an inadvertent withdrawal of a CVAD far outweigh the cost of these devices. See information in earlier chapters regarding this type of equipment.

Transparent or gauze dressings are the two preferred materials for CVAD dressings. Transparent dressings allow the insertion site to be observed without disturbing the dressing. They are more comfortable for the patient and require dressing changes no more than every 7 days (CDC, 2002). Gauze and tape dressings preclude site inspection, are usually more uncomfortable for the patient, and require changing every 48 hours (CDC).

It is recommended that either gauze or transparent dressing be used to cover the catheter insertion site. Either type of dressing should be changed when the device is removed or replaced, when the dressing becomes damp, loose, or soiled, or any time the integrity of the dressing is compromised. CDC guidelines recommend gauze dressing when the patient is diaphoretic or when the site is oozing or bleeding. No recommendation has been made for a dressing on a well-healed exit site of a tunneled catheter (CDC, 2002), although a recent study demonstrated no difference in CRBSI rates when the exit site of a well-healed tunneled catheter had a dressing or no dressing (Olson, Rennie, Hanson, et al., 2004).

Site care and dressings are completed using sterile technique. Prepackaged sterile dressing change kits, which include all necessary equipment, are typically used. Some kits may include instructions as well. A careful review of the literature should be done when establishing dressing change protocols.

INJECTION PORT CARE

Injection port care is just as important as catheter site care. The injection port should be cleansed with 2% chlorhexidine solution, 10% povidone–iodine, or 70% alcohol before accessing the system (CDC, 2002). Minimizing manipulation of the hub and tubing connection can also decrease the risk of infection. All stopcocks must be capped.

MAINTAINING CATHETER PATENCY

Anticoagulant capping solutions may be used to maintain catheter patency. Some controversy still exists regarding the concentration of heparin, appropriate volume, and frequency of flush. However, the lowest effective concentration of heparin in a volume two times the internal volume of the catheter should be used (INS, 2000). A concentration of 10 U/mL, 3 mL, has been shown to maintain catheter patency (Buswell & Beyea, 1998). It is imperative to know specific information about the catheter being used, including catheter material, flushing volume, and pressure and syringe size limitations. Studies have found that normal saline is as effective as heparin in maintaining patency of peripheral catheters. There are no studies evaluating the use of saline in short- or long-term CVADs.

Surveillance

Nurses play a vital role in monitoring patients on PN. Patient monitoring is as important as proper administration in preventing serious metabolic complications. Accurate measurements of the patient's daily body weight, measured at the same time of day, using the same scale, and with the patient wearing the same amount of clothing, are important. A baseline weight should be obtained, then weigh daily thereafter. Intake and output records should also be scrupulously maintained and recorded. These measures are necessary to assess fluid balance and adequacy of the prescribed nutrients.

Vital signs should be obtained and recorded at least every shift and more often if the patient is unstable or the temperature is >100°F (37.7°C) orally or 101°F (38.3°C) rectally. Certain drugs and disease states suppress the normal febrile response, and affected patients must be assessed individually.

- Blood glucose levels should be monitored according to physician order, the patient's level of glycemic control, or minimally every 6 hours. This practice

TABLE 16–8   Laboratory Monitoring of Parenteral Nutrition

Frequency	Daily until stable, then Monday, Wednesday, Friday			
Test	Blood sugar	BUN	Creatinine	Electrolytes
Frequency	Baseline, then weekly (eg, every Monday)			
Test	CBC	PT	Albumin	ALT
	AST	Alkaline phosphatase		Calcium
	Cholesterol	LDH	Magnesium	Phosphorus
	Transferrin	Total bilirubin	Total protein	Triglycerides

ALT, alanine transaminase; AST, aspartate transaminase; BUN, blood urea nitrogen; CBC, complete blood count; LDH, lactic dehydrogenase; PT, prothrombin time

has become easier with the use of glucose monitors on nursing units. Biochemical monitoring is also important to assess the adequacy of the PN regimen and the presence of any metabolic complications. Nutritional profiles or standing laboratory tests are recommended for routine PN monitoring. Routine laboratory tests and their frequency are outlined in Table 16–8. Ideally, a full chemical profile, including glucose, electrolytes, urea nitrogen, creatinine, albumin, transferrin, calcium, magnesium, phosphorus, liver function, prothrombin time, and complete blood count, should be obtained before initiating PN. Critically ill and unstable patients may require more frequent monitoring. Other studies may be warranted depending on the clinical status of the patient.

 LEGAL ISSUES: Legal and Safety Considerations

Nurses need to demonstrate core competencies when monitoring patients receiving PN; some competencies need initial successful demonstration whereas others need regular skill or knowledge demonstration.

- Demonstrate appropriate use of Standard Precautions and aseptic technique.
- Demonstrate appropriate use of blood glucose monitoring device.
- Verbalize knowledge and understanding of acceptable blood glucose parameters and management of hypoglycemia/hyperglycemia.
- Verbalize knowledge of parameters to be monitored and frequency, (ie, intake/output, vital signs, weight, blood analyses, central venous access device care, infusion pump).
- Verbalize knowledge of abnormal assessments and when the physician should be notified.
- Demonstrate appropriate documentation.

Complications of Parenteral Nutrition

Complications associated with PN are divided into three categories: catheter related, metabolic, and infectious. These complications can be minimized or even avoided with the establishment of and adherence to strict protocols as well as knowledgeable surveillance.

KEY INTERVENTION:	Monitoring Parenteral Nutrition

Action	*Rationale*
Explain procedures to patient.	Patient understanding will allay anxiety.
Check vital signs every shift. If temperature >100.5°F, take vital signs q4h and monitor blood glucose (BG) level q4–6h. BG level should be maintained at <200 mg/dL.	Discloses signs of complications or infection during PN infusion; notify physician if critical value.
After 1 week, stable patients (BG <200 mg/dL) can be monitored less frequently if ordered by physician.	Determines need to increase or decrease insulin if added to PN and patient not receiving other types of insulin.
Monitor blood work as ordered. Notify physician of any critically abnormal values.	Assesses need to adjust PN regimen and detects complications early.
Strictly measure intake and output:	Monitors fluid balance and avoids complications; notify physician of significant changes.
• Intake includes PN, other IV solutions, IV medication volume, and any oral intake. • Output includes urine and any other output (nasogastric tube, ostomy, fistula, drainage); unplanned diuresis.	
Obtain baseline weight, then weigh daily. (Stable patients on prolonged PN can be weighed weekly.)	Points to adequacy of therapy (weight maintenance or weight gain).
Observe central venous access device (CVAD) site for and notify physician if:	Discloses complications early and establishes patency of sutures, if present.
• Erythema, edema, exudate • Intact dressing or sutures • Pain at insertion site • Securely taped catheter and PN tubing that relieves tension on CVAD	
Monitor infusion rate and pump for signs of possible malfunction.	Ensures ordered infusion and prevents complications.
Monitor for and notify physician:	Identifying and treating complications early avoids more serious effects.
• If patient's temperature >101°F • If BG >200 mg/dL, or for critical laboratory values • Presence or increase in edema • Weight gain ≥2 lb/wk • Edema over insertion site, neck, face, chest, either arm	

(Continued)

KEY INTERVENTION:	Monitoring Parenteral Nutrition *(Continued)*
• Any significant changes in clinical status: vital signs, intake or output, mental status, convulsions, or coma	
Adhere to all polices related to PN administration and CVAD management.	Maintains established standards of care.
Culture catheter tip if signs/symptoms of infection are present.	Identifies catheter as source of infection for suspected catheter sepsis.
Accurately document all monitoring activities in appropriate patient medical records. Also document any abnormal laboratory results and adverse reactions. Include actions taken and patient's response to treatment.	Documentation should be accurate and comprehensive to reflect nursing care given, actions taken, and patient's response to treatment.

Catheter-Related Complications

Catheter-related complications are related to the insertion or maintenance of CVADs and may be immediate or delayed. Insertion complications are infrequent when a physician is knowledgeable about anatomy and skilled in the technique. Insertion complications and complications of indwelling CVADs are addressed in Chapter 14.

CATHETER TIP PLACEMENT

Because of the nature of PN infusions, having this infusate flowing into areas other than the central vasculature is a serious complication. Considerations include verification of catheter tip placement before use and any time there is a question of tip position. Displacement may occur during insertion from coiling or misdirection, overinsertion or underinsertion, aberrant route on catheter advancement, venous thrombosis or stenosis, and venous or atrial perforation. The catheter tip may become displaced spontaneously at any time, from days to months later because of a change in intrathoracic pressure as with coughing or vomiting, a rapid infusion, or random body movement.

AIR EMBOLISM

Air embolism is fortunately rare because its occurrence is the most lethal complication of catheter insertion or maintenance. Air embolism is a potential danger whenever the central venous system is open to the air, such as during insertion, IV tubing or cap changes, accidental disconnection, or through a tract left after catheter removal. This is most likely to occur on deep inspiration when the patient is in an upright position, dehydrated, or hypovolemic. Symptoms occur with an air entry rate of 20 mL/second. Death can occur with an air entry rate of 75 to 150 mL/second; a 70- to 300-mL air volume may be lethal (Drewett, 2000). Signs and symptoms vary depending on the severity; they may include dyspnea, apnea, hypoxia, disorientation, tachycardia, hypotension, pulmonary wheeze, or a precordial murmur. Severe neurologic deficits, including hemiplegia, aphasia, seizures, and coma, are associated with air embolism. This is attributed to direct access of air into the cerebral circulation in most situations.

Immediate treatment aims to prevent obstruction of the right ventricular outflow tract by air. The patient should immediately be placed on the left side in deep Trendelenburg position (right side up). This keeps the air in the right atrium and out of the pulmonary circulation. Needle aspiration of air through the catheter or by direct intracardiac approach may be necessary. Oxygen therapy should be initiated.

Precautions should be taken during catheter insertion, tubing and cap changes, and catheter removal to prevent air embolism. Tubing junctions should be properly secured. Catheter removal should be immediately followed by placement of occlusive gauze dressing with an ointment over the site. The ointment occludes the tract and assists with healing. This dressing is usually needed for 24 to 48 hours or until the tract is totally closed.

CATHETER OCCLUSION

Partial or complete catheter occlusion may result from fibrin sheath formation or thrombus at the tip of the catheter, blood clots, lipid deposits, precipitates, kinking or malposition, pinch-off syndrome, and rupture or breakage of the device. Increased difficulty in infusing fluids may be the first indication of fibrin sheath formation. The fibrin sheath may cause a partial occlusion of the catheter by acting as a "flap valve" to prevent withdrawal of blood but allow infusions. It may eventually encase the entire catheter, causing complete occlusion of all lumens. The sheath may also become seeded with micro-organisms, serving as a focus for infection.

Occlusion of the CVAD may also occur from drug precipitates or lipid deposition. Precipitate occlusion may occur from inadequate flushing between medications, simultaneous administration of incompatible medications or solutions, and medications admixed in concentrations exceeding that required for stability. Calcium and phosphorus precipitates are a common cause of occlusion with PN solutions. Occlusions from drug precipitates or lipid deposition typically result in sudden occlusion of the catheter either during or immediately after an infusion. Occlusion with lipid depositions is also a liability, especially with the use of TNAs. Chapter 14 outlines interventions for catheter occlusions.

VENOUS THROMBOSIS

The development of venous thrombosis may occur with any type of CVAD secondary to injury to the vein wall during insertion, or by movement of the catheter against the vein wall after insertion. Catheter thrombogenicity may depend on the type of catheter material and the surface characteristics (Drewett, 2000). Predisposing risk factors for venous thrombosis include hypovolemia, venous stasis, and hypercoagulable states (eg, pregnancy, cancer, hypovolemia, bone marrow transplantation). Chemically induced thrombosis can result from infusion of hypertonic solutions, including PN, and small-volume antibiotics or chemotherapy admixtures and vesicants administered through CVADs whose tips are in the upper arm, subclavian, or innominate veins. Intermittent or long-term infusion of these solutions should be delivered through catheters whose tips terminate in the superior vena cava. A lower incidence of thrombosis has been noted in catheters whose tips lie in the distal superior vena cava (Drewett).

Patients with venous thrombosis may be asymptomatic, making careful observation for early signs imperative. Signs may include increased anterior chest venous pattern, arm or neck swelling, external jugular distention, or fluid leaking from the insertion site during infusion (caused by backflow). Diagnosis may be made by arm venography, contrast studies through the catheter, Doppler duplex imaging, magnetic resonance imaging, and radionucleotide studies (Drewett, 2000). Treatment of catheter-induced venous thrombosis remains controversial and depends on the extent of thrombus formation, the severity of the symptoms, the current clinical conditions, and the future access needs of the patient (Hamilton, 2004). Conservative treatment without device removal consists of IV anticoagulant therapy followed by warfarin therapy for 3 or more months. Catheter removal followed by anticoagulant therapy may be necessary for more severe symptoms. Some practitioners advocate using prophylactic low-dose warfarin to reduce the risk of thrombosis for patients who are at increased risk (Drewett).

The major complication of catheter-associated venous thrombosis is pulmonary embolism. This complication should be treated with catheter removal plus standard therapy for that disorder, including anticoagulation or thrombolysis at the discretion of the treating physician.

Metabolic Complications

Metabolic complications are the most frequently observed adverse effects with PN and can be avoided when PN orders are written by knowledgeable physicians and laboratory studies are meticulously monitored. Frequent metabolic monitoring can ensure that potential metabolic complications are prevented or documented and treated. The nurse is in a key position to monitor for these changes and report them to the appropriate physician. Table 16–9 cites the most frequently observed metabolic complications. Only the most life threatening are discussed more fully in the following sections.

COMPLICATIONS RELATED TO GLUCOSE LEVEL

Glucose intolerance has already been discussed. The sudden development of hyperglycemia in a patient who was previously glucose tolerant may indicate impending infection or sepsis. Hyperglycemia and glycosuria may precede clinical signs of sepsis by 12 to 24 hours. Patients with pre-existing diabetes or significant physiologic stress may develop hyperglycemia on initiation of PN. Because hyperglycemia has been shown to be associated with decreased immune function and increased risk of infectious complications, efforts to monitor and control blood glucose during specialized nutritional support are prudent (McMahon & Rizza, 1996). Blood sugars should be maintained between 100 and 150 mg/dL. Studies have demonstrated that tighter control (80 to 120 mg/dL)may decrease mortality in ICU patients (Van De Berghe, Wouters, Weekers, et al., 2001).

TABLE 16–9 Potential Metabolic Complications of Parenteral Nutrition

Cause(s)	Prevention	Treatment
Hyperglycemia		
Carbohydrate intolerance	Accuchecks q6h	Decrease PN rate or dextrose concentration/amount
Too rapid infusion of PN	Be aware of meds that may cause glucose intolerance (ie, steroids)	Increase proportion of calories as lipids
Too much carbohydrate load	Start PN infusion slowly	Add insulin to the solution or use sliding-scale insulin coverage
Insulin resistance—stress, sepsis, diabetes, steroids		Maintain blood glucose 100–150 mg/dL
Hypoglycemia		
Abrupt decrease or cessation of PN	Wean or slow down PN infusion when stopping	Hang $D_{10}W$ at same rate of PN if unable to hang PN
Excessive insulin administration	Hang $D_{10}W$ at same rate of PN if unable to hang PN	Give IV glucose STAT; 50% dextrose may be needed; maintain proper flow rate
Weaning steroids	Maintain infusion rate; use an infusion pump	
	Monitor serum glucose levels	
Hyperglycemic hyperosmolar nonketotic coma		
Untreated glucose intolerance causes hyperosmolar diuresis, electrolyte imbalances, coma, death (40%–50% mortality rate)	Appropriate glucose monitoring	Monitor closely
	Frequent chemistry profiles to assess electrolytes, osmolarity	Discontinue PN
		Rehydrate with normal saline or other isotonic solution
Increased risk in elderly, diabetes malnourishment, steroid therapy, and with stress or sepsis		Correct electrolyte imbalances, especially potassium and bicarbonate
		Monitor ABGs
		Insulin as needed
Hyperkalemia		
Excessive potassium replacement	Monitor serum potassium and renal function	Stop or decrease potassium in solution
Renal disease—potassium cannot be excreted	Accurate I/O to evaluate fluid balance	Assess for other sources of potassium
Leakage of potassium from cells after severe trauma		Monitor for arrhythmias
		Administer infusion of $D_{50}W$
Hypokalemia		
Excessive potassium losses (increased GI losses with diarrhea, fistulas)	Monitor serum potassium	Add potassium to PN solution
	Anticipate potential potassium depletion with large GI losses	May need additional IVPB potassium run over 4–6 h to correct severe deficiency
Diuretic therapy	Monitor I/O	Monitor pulse for tachycardia/arrhythmia

(Continued)

TABLE 16–9   Potential Metabolic Complications of Parenteral Nutrition   (Continued)

Cause(s)	Prevention	Treatment
Large doses of insulin Increased requirement with anabolism Refeeding severely malnourished patients	Be aware of drugs that cause excessive potassium loss Be aware that patients severely malnourished are susceptible (refeeding syndrome)	Monitor for metabolic alkalosis (potassium loss may cause sodium retention)
Hypernatremia		
Dehydration Diarrhea Diabetes insipidus Excessive replacement	Maintain I/O Monitor serum sodium Be aware of drugs that cause sodium retention (ie, steroids)	Decrease sodium or provide salt-free solution until corrected Provide enough free water to meet needs Treat or correct cause
Hyponatremia		
Diuretics GI losses (vomiting, fistula) Congestive heart failure, renal failure, cirrhosis Water intoxication	Accurate I/O Urine specific gravity Accurate weights (assess fluid shifts)	Fluid restriction Add sodium to PN Minimize GI loss if possible Close metabolic monitoring
Hyperphosphatemia		
Renal failure Excessive replacement	Accurate I/O Monitor serum levels and renal status	Low or no phosphate added May need dialysis
Hypophosphatemia		

Inadequate in PN
 	
Insulin therapy
 	
Disease states:
  Alcoholism
  Respiratory alkalosis
  Renal problems
  Severe diarrhea
  Malabsorption associated with low calcium and magnesium levels
  Increased requirements
  Refeeding severely malnourished patients
	Be aware of potential disease states that cause low phosphate levels
	
	Frequent laboratory monitoring, especially if low levels/depleted
	
	Be aware of medications that may lower phosphates (carafate, magnesium and aluminum hydroxide, steroids)
		Replace phosphate in PN
		
		May need additional IVPB of phosphate over 4–6 hours
		
		Replace calcium as needed (repletion of phosphate may cause calcium to drop)
		
		Discontinue PN if patient symptomatic

Hypocalcemia		
Vitamin D deficiency Insufficient replacement Pancreatitis Hypomagnesemia	Monitor serum levels Be aware of disease states, medications, malnutrition that can cause hypocalcemia	Replace by adding calcium to PN May require IVPB of calcium to correct severe deficiency Correct hypomagnesemia

TABLE 16–9 Potential Metabolic Complications of Parenteral Nutrition *(Continued)*

Cause(s)	Prevention	Treatment
Hyperphosphatemia		Monitor ionized calcium
Hypoalbuminemia		
Hypomagnesemia		
Insufficient magnesium in PN	Monitor serum levels closely	Increase magnesium in PN
	Be aware of disease states or drugs that can cause hypomagnesemia	If very low, IVPB replacement
Excess GI or renal losses (diarrhea, fistula, diuretics)		Discontinue PN if patient symptomatic
Certain drugs (aminoglycosides, diuretics, cisplatin)		Monitor for cardiac arrhythmia
Disease states (chronic alcoholism, pancreatitis, diabetic acidosis, sepsis/infection, burns)		
Hypermagnesemia		
Excess magnesium in PN	Monitor serum levels	Decrease or delete from PN
Renal failure	Monitor renal function	Calcium salts
Metabolic acidosis		
Renal insufficiency; acute/chronic renal failure	Monitor ABGs, electrolytes	Give bicarbonate or replace some or all of chloride with acetate in PN
Diabetic ketoacidosis	Monitor renal function	Monitor vital signs
Diarrhea	Be aware of disease states that may cause metabolic acidosis	
Lactic acidosis (shock)		
Potassium-sparing diuretics		
Massive rhabdomyolysis		
Metabolic alkalosis		
Gastric losses	Replace GI losses	Increase chloride content
Thiazide and loop diuretics	Monitor ABGs	Decrease acetate content
Mineralocorticoids	Be aware of acetate content of amino acids	
Amino acid solutions		

ABGs, arterial blood gases; D$_5$W, dextrose 5% in water; GI, gastrointestinal; I/O, intake and output; IVPB, intravenous piggyback.

Progressive hyperglycemia, if not detected or if inadequately treated, can lead to the life-threatening complication of hyperglycemic hyperosmolar nonketotic coma. If untreated, marked hyperglycemia and glycosuria may lead to an osmotic diuresis accompanied by dehydration, electrolyte imbalance, and a decreasing level of consciousness that can result in seizures and coma and death. Reversal of this state requires immediate discontinuation of the PN solution, aggressive fluid and electrolyte replacement, correction of hyperglycemia by insulin administration, and correction of acidosis with bicarbonates. During treatment, frequent monitoring of blood glucose, electrolyte, and arterial blood gas levels and vital signs is essential (Goff, 1997).

Hypoglycemia is chemically defined as a serum glucose level of <50 mg/dL. Many patients may be asymptomatic at this level. Symptoms include weakness, headache, chills, tingling in the extremities or mouth, cold and clammy skin, thirst, hunger, apprehension, diaphoresis, decreased levels of consciousness, and changes in vital signs. Hypoglycemia during PN may occur with excess insulin administration. Insulin needs decrease when steroids are tapered and discontinued, and as sepsis resolves, and should be adjusted in the PN solution accordingly. Abrupt cessation of PN may also result in rebound hypoglycemia. Unstable patients and those with glucose intolerance may benefit from a 1- to 2-hour taper to avoid rebound hypoglycemia. If a PN solution must be discontinued abruptly, D_{10} should be infused for 1 to 2 hours to avoid possible rebound hypoglycemia (Bloch & Mueller, 2004).

COMPLICATIONS RELATED TO ELECTROLYTES

The infusion of hypertonic dextrose results in the intracellular shift of potassium, magnesium, phosphorus, and calcium. Requirements for these electrolytes, particularly potassium and phosphorus, may be increased. Increased losses or requirements related to the patient's clinical status or treatment may also increase electrolyte requirements. Conversely, renal failure may require restriction of potassium, magnesium, and phosphate. Careful monitoring of electrolyte levels and adjustments to the PN solution are essential to maintain electrolyte balance.

The refeeding syndrome describes metabolic complications seen when severely malnourished patients receive aggressive administration of nutritional support. Rapid infusion of carbohydrate calories can result in hypophosphatemia, hypokalemia, and hypomagnesemia. A rapid expansion of extracellular volume can result in heart failure. Alternatively, significant hyperglycemia may cause osmotic diuresis and dehydration. Hypophosphatemia is considered a hallmark of the refeeding syndrome. Careful initiation and close monitoring of serum phosphate, magnesium, potassium, and glucose is imperative when providing specialized nutritional support to chronically malnourished patients (Marik & Bedigian, 1996).

COMPLICATIONS RELATED TO LIPIDS

Essential fatty acid deficiency and potentiation of inflammatory response by rapid infusion were discussed previously. Elevated liver enzyme levels may be commonly observed in patients receiving PN. Causes are multifactorial and include drugs, sepsis, shock, surgery, and anesthetics. Mild elevations may appear on days 9 to 14 of PN infusion, usually returning to normal once PN is discontinued (Goff, 1997). Overfeeding of calories is often responsible and should be avoided. Slow, continuous infusion of lipids over 16 to 24 hours has also been associated with better tolerance and clearance of lipids.

Hypertriglyceridemia usually is owing to an alteration in lipid clearance and occurs most frequently in critically ill patients and those with sepsis. It has been identified as a possible etiologic factor in the development of pancreatitis, immunosuppression, and altered pulmonary hemodynamics in patients receiving PN. Acceptable serum triglyceride levels are <400 mg/dL for continuous lipid infusion. For levels >400 mg/dL, lipid and dextrose amounts should be reduced and/or eliminated from the PN solution. If serum triglyceride levels remains >400 mg/dL for >2 weeks, provide approximately 1 g/kg of lipid emulsion twice each week to prevent essential fatty acid deficiency (Seidner & Fuhrman, 2001).

COMPLICATIONS RELATED TO PROTEIN

Adjustments in protein concentrations should be made according to the patient's tolerance, clinical response, and laboratory results. Pre–renal azotemia can occur if excess protein is administered, causing a rise in blood urea nitrogen because of excess urea production. The amount of amino acid in PN should be reduced for patients who develop amino acid intolerance such as pre–renal azotemia, hepatic encephalopathy, or hyperammonemia. Special solutions are available for patients with liver disease and renal disease.

Infectious and Septic Complications

Catheter-related sepsis associated with PN is a serious and potentially lethal complication, particularly in high-acuity patient populations. An estimated 250,000 to 500,000 intravascular device-related bloodstream infections (BSIs) occur in the United States each year, associated with mortality rates of 12% to 25% (Crnich & Maki, 2002; Maki, 2003). Central venous catheters (CVCs) pose the greatest risk of BSI. It has been reported that up to 75% of catheter-related BSIs originate from CVCs of various types. Catheter-related BSIs increased continuously in the 1980s but declined 30% to 40% in the 1990s through increased adherence to Center for Disease Control Guidelines for the Prevention of Intravascular Device-Related Infections. The current version of the Guidelines were published in 2002.

Most catheter-related BSIs are associated with short-term, noncuffed, single-lumen or multilumen catheters inserted into the subclavian or internal jugular vein (Crnich & Maki, 2002; Darouiche, Raad, Heard, et al, 1999). Migration of skin organisms at the insertion site is the most common route of infection for short-term percutaneously inserted catheters. Hub contamination is the most likely source of infection in long-term catheters. Other causes of catheter-related infections include multiple line violation and manipulation, improper technique during catheter insertion and hematogenous seeding of the catheter by bloodborne organisms from infection at a distant site.

Meticulous admixing protocols make the incidence of solution contamination rare. PN solutions are poor growth media for bacteria owing to the low pH and hypertonicity of amino acid and dextrose solutions. PN may also contain large quantities of acetate, which is bacteriostatic. When albumin is added to a solution, bacteria and fungi growth increase (Krzywda, 2004). *Candida albicans* is a common fungus in standard solutions. Resistance of *Candida* spp. to commonly used antifungal agents is increasing (CDC, 2002). Data from the Surveillance and Control of Pathogens of Epidemiologic Importance (SCOPE) Program documented that 10% of *C. albicans* bloodstream isolates from hospitalized patients were resistant to fluconazole (Pfaller, Jones,

Messer, Edmond, & Wenzel, 1998). Another 48% of *Candida* BSIs were caused by non-albicans species that are more likely to demonstrate resistance to fluconazole and itraconazole. Three-in-one solutions have significantly higher micro-organism growth than standard solutions. Lipid emulsions support growth of gram-positive, gram-negative, and fungal species at room temperature (Krzywda, 2004).

Descriptions and treatment options for catheter-related infections are presented in Table 16–10. Catheter-related BSI is indicated by bacteremia/fungemia in a patient with an intravascular catheter with at least one positive blood culture obtained from a peripheral vein, clinical manifestations of infections, and no apparent source for the bloodstream infection except the catheter. One of the following should be present: a positive semiquantitative or quantitative culture whereby the same organism is isolated from the catheter segment and peripheral blood; simultaneous quantitative blood cultures with a 5:1 ratio CVC versus peripheral; differential period of CVC culture versus peripheral blood culture positivity of >2 hours (Krzywda, 2004).

The most common organisms causing catheter-related infection from 1992 to 1999 include coagulase-negative staphylococci (37%), *S. aureus* (12.6%), enterococci (13.5%), *Candida* spp. (8%), and gram-negative bacilli (14%; CDC, 2002). Catheter site infections should not be confused with catheter-related sepsis. Erythema or exudate at the site may indicate a localized infection and not necessarily a catheter infection. Conversely, patients may have sepsis without signs at the catheter site.

TABLE 16–10 Catheter-Related Infections

Infection Type	Description	Treatment
Insertion site infection	Erythema, induration, tenderness, and purulence localized to an area within 2 cm of the catheter insertion site	Daily site care Warm, moist compresses Possibly oral antibiotics
Pocket site infection	Erythema, tenderness, and induration over the port reservoir site; possibly necrosis; purulent exudate from the subcutaneous pocket	Warm, moist compresses Oral or IV antibiotics Port removal
Tunnel infection	Erythema, tenderness, induration or purulence extending more than 2 cm from the site along the course of the subcutaneous tunnel	Catheter removal Infection may respond poorly to other treatment attempts
Catheter-related bloodstream infection	Isolation of the same organism (identical species, antibiogram) from semiquantitative or quantitative cultures of the catheter tip and peripheral blood of a patient with clear signs of bloodstream infection and no other identifiable sources of infection (selected symptoms include temperature ≥101.5°F, chills, rigors, malaise, and temperature defervesence with catheter removal)	Catheter removal Systemic antibiotics by catheter Antibiotic lock

Catheter-related sepsis may present in the patient as fever, chills, hypotension, change in mental status, and leukocytosis. Metabolic acidosis and hyperglycemia may be early signs of sepsis in critically ill patients receiving PN. A complete fever workup is necessary. All potential sources of infection need to be cultured.

Options for managing catheter-related sepsis include exchange of the catheter over guidewire, catheter salvage, and catheter removal. The decision is determined by the patient's clinical status, culture results, and the nature of the offending organism. Catheter removal remains the treatment of choice for short-term catheters. Guidewire exchange is indicated only if the catheter is malfunctioning and there is no sign of catheter site infection (Whitman, 1996). If infection is suspected and if there is no evidence of catheter site infection and the patient is not floridly septic, the catheter may also be exchanged over a guidewire and the catheter tip sent to the laboratory for culture. If the culture results are positive for colonization or infection, the catheter should be removed and a new catheter inserted in a different location. If the patient is floridly septic, the catheter should be removed immediately (Jones, 1998; Whitman, 1996). In either situation, empiric antibiotics are often started once all appropriate specimens for culture are obtained.

Tunneled catheters and implanted ports pose additional problems because they cannot be changed over a guidewire or readily replaced, and they often serve as life-lines for patients with limited sites for central venous access. Catheter salvage is a desired option in these instances. Many of these infections can be successfully treated with antibiotics without removing the catheter (Andris & Krzywda, 1997). The use of an antibiotic lock technique has been successful in several instances (Andris & Krzywda). Various drugs in a wide range of concentrations for varying durations have been used. Prophylactic vancomycin is not recommended, and in many institutions, *Candida* infection is automatic grounds for catheter removal, regardless of type.

A recent strategy to decrease catheter-related BSI, the chlorhexidine-impregnated sponge (Biopatch), placed over the insertion site of short-term CVCs, is supported in the literature (Banton & Banning, 2002; Maki, 2003; Maki, Mermel, Kluger, Narans, Knasinski et al., 2000). A striking decline in the incidence of catheter-related BSI has been documented coincident with the adoption of this simple and cost-effective dressing.

Vigilant observation of protocols for insertion, use, and maintenance of CVADs is necessary to minimize the incidence of infection and catheter-related sepsis. A recent study supported the use of a dedicated team for PN and care of those catheters used solely for PN; colonization was lower for those short-term CVADs used for PN and cared for by a team (Dimick, Swoboda, Talamini, Pelz, Hendrix, & Lipsett, 2003). Nurses are legally accountable for providing safe and appropriate care to patients. This includes knowledge of and adherence to established guidelines, standards of care, and institutional policies and procedures. Literature should be evaluated and policies and procedures reviewed annually with staff nurse participation.

Home Parenteral Nutrition

Advanced technology, care management, and consumer demand have contributed to making home parenteral nutrition (HPN) a successful alternative for many patients who require prolonged or lifelong PN. The emergence and growth of "high-tech" home care infusion companies facilitated the safe administration of PN in the home environment. The results are shorter hospital stays, reduced costs, and improved patient well-being, both psychologically and physically. Referrals for HPN are increasingly being made from the community (ie, physician's offices, home care screening, medical clinics) as patterns of health care change. Care provided in long-term care facilities has also become increasingly complex and includes PN.

Regardless of the health care setting, all patients should be evaluated to determine their eligibility for and the appropriateness of home PN. Standards for home nutrition support (ASPEN, 1999) have been established and should be used. HPN is expensive, and strict policies have been established for reimbursement. The Health Care Financing Administration has published specific eligibility criteria for HPN. Permanent impairment, defined as a condition of long and indefinite duration (minimum of 3 months), is one requirement, and additional care must be taken in determining eligibility for HPN (Winkler, Watkins, & Albina, 1998).

Home PN may be provided as a continuous or a cyclic infusion. Cyclic infusion over 12 to 14 hours, as previously discussed, is preferred, especially for ambulatory patients. Most home infusion companies prefer to provide TNAs for HPN. Regardless of the method chosen for a particular patient, the teaching program should be individualized for a patient's learning needs, capabilities, and home care environment. Patients should be encouraged to assume as much responsibility for self-care as possible. Doing so enhances their sense of control.

Nurses have a primary role in preparing the patient for HPN (Evans-Stoner, 1997; Forloinses-Lynn & Viall, 1996; Winkler et al., 1998). The prospect of HPN may seem overwhelming to the patient and family or caregiver, and thorough preparation and teaching is essential because of the complexity of the procedures to be learned. Careful assessment of the patient's and caregiver's willingness and ability to perform the procedures and assume responsibility for managing this therapy should be a priority. One nurse should be selected as the primary teacher because a lack of consistency can confuse the learner and extend the learning period. Survival skills should be taught in the hospital and full education for PN initiated in the home.

Education should include verbal instructions and demonstration of all procedures. Return demonstration by the patient or primary caregiver is essential so that the instructor can assess competency. A manual of written instructions should be provided to all patients. The verbal and written instructions should include the following (Evans-Stoner, 1997; Forloinses-Lynn & Viall, 1996; Winkler et al., 1998):

- All appropriate procedures related to the administration of PN and care and maintenance of the CVAD
- Use, maintenance, and troubleshooting of the infusion pump
- Storage, management, and disposal of solutions and supplies
- Self-monitoring form for home PN (Fig. 16–4)
- Problem-solving techniques
- Emergency interventions
- Expectations of home care and follow-up plans.

A social worker, discharge planner, or case manager may be helpful to patients and families who have questions and concerns about financial considerations and

HOME PARENTERAL NUTRITION LOG

Instructions   Name:_____

Keep a daily log to record your results. Fill in the boxes. Put an "X" in the box when you do not
need the information. Your home care nurse will review this log with you on each visit.

	Sun	Mon	Tues	Wed	Thurs	Fri	Sat
Date							
Weight							
Temperature AM							
PM							
Blood sugar							
Urine sugar / acetone AM							
PM							
Rate / amount of PN infused							
Lipids (if separate)							
Oral / IV fluids taken							
Urine output							
Other output							
Stool							
Antibiotics							
Site (or dressing appearance): C = clean /dry D = drainage S = swelling R = red P = pain							
Comments							

FIGURE 16–4.   Self-monitoring form for home parenteral nutrition.

BOX 16–7   Principles for Self-Administration of Parenteral Nutrition

1. Patient/caregiver understands the disorder and rationale for therapy:
   - Agrees to home therapy and the associated benefits and risks
   - Understands alternatives, consequences if therapy not accepted, advantages and disadvantages
   - Understands short- and long-term goals and the expected duration of treatment
2. Patient/caregiver has the visual acuity, manual dexterity, cognitive ability, and mobility to perform procedures related to PN therapy:
   - A backup caregiver is identified and trained in case patient needs assistance.
   - Adaptive/assistive devices are available if needed.
3. Patient's physical environment is safe and appropriate for home therapy:
   - Adequate work area with water supply, refrigeration, storage area for supplies
   - Grounded outlets or adapters available
4. Patient/caregiver verbalizes and demonstrates knowledge and understanding of PN administration:
   - Aseptic technique
   - Solution storage and handling
   - Solution inspection, preparation, and addition of vitamins or other medications as ordered; attachment of administration set
   - Infusion pump operation, maintenance, and troubleshooting
   - Connection and disconnection from CVAD, including appropriate flushing and locking
   - Administration schedule and importance of compliance with established schedule and protocols (including written instructions provided)
   - Self-monitoring guidelines and record keeping
   - Recognition and treatment of potential complications
   - Emergency interventions
   - When/whom to call for questions or assistance
   - Identify emergency 24-hour on-call number.
   - CVAD care and monitoring
5. Patient/caregiver understands and agrees to follow-up care as scheduled by the physician/nutrition support team:
   - Home nursing visits
   - Follow-up in physician's office or clinic

---

community resources. Psychosocial support is also essential. Principles for self-administration of TNAs are given in Box 16–7.

Arrangements for a home infusion provider should be determined as early as possible (Snell & Randolph, 2004). Ideally, the home infusion nurse visits the patient and family in the hospital to establish rapport and discuss learning needs, feelings and concerns, health status, and the regimen prescribed by the physician. In many cases, the home infusion nurse provides all the teaching in the home.

Documentation should include patient eligibility data and the indication for therapy. It should also incorporate the patient's nutritional therapy objectives into the care plan. Short- and long-term goals should be included and updated as applicable. Patient progress and monitoring parameters, as well as any problems, should be carefully recorded. Evaluation of the nutritional prescription, readiness for transitional feeding, and periodic nutritional assessments also should be included in the documentation (Winkler et al., 1998).

An ongoing quality assessment and improvement program is important to identify variables and incorporate corrective actions to improve care and outcomes as identified in this transplant program's evaluation of sepsis, readmission, and days of therapy (Beerman, O''Bryan, Olesen, Grafe, & Warchall, 2000). The benefits of HPN clearly outweigh the risks, and patients today enjoy new freedoms and near-normal lifestyles as a result of this added dimension to nutritional support therapy.

References and Selected Readings

Asterisks indicate references cited in text.

*Aihara, R., Schoepfel, S.L., Curtis, A.R., et al. (2002). Guidelines for improving nutritional delivery in the intensive care unit. *Journal for Healthcare Quality, 24*(2), 22–29.

*American Society for Parenteral and Enteral Nutrition (ASPEN) Board of Directors. (1988). Standards of nutrition support: Hospitalized patients. *Nutrition in Clinical Practice, 3*(1), 28–31.

*American Society for Parenteral and Enteral Nutrition Board of Directors. (1996a). Standards of practice: Nutrition support nurse. *Nutrition in Clinical Practice, 11,* 127–134.

*American Society for Parenteral and Enteral Nutrition Board of Directors. (1996b). Standards for nutrition support: Hospitalized pediatric patients. *Nutrition in Clinical Practice, 11,* 217–228.

*American Society for Parenteral and Enteral Nutrition Board of Directors. (1997). Standards for nutrition support for residents of long-term care facilities. *Nutrition in Clinical Practice, 12,* 284–293.

*American Society for Parenteral and Enteral Nutrition Board of Directors. (1999). Standards for home nutrition support. *Nutrition in Clinical Practice, 14,* 151–162.

*American Society for Parenteral and Enteral Nutrition Board of Directors and the Clinical Guidelines Task Force. (2002). Guidelines for the use of parenteral and enteral nutrition in adult and pediatric patients (erratum appears in 2002, 26[2], 144). *JPEN: Journal of Parenteral & Enteral Nutrition, 26*(1 Suppl), 1SA–138SA.

*Andris, D.A. (1996). Substrate metabolism—micronutrients. In: K.A. Hennessy & M.E. Orr (Eds.). *Nutrition support nursing core curriculum* (3rd ed.). Silver Spring, MD: American Society for Parenteral and Enteral Nutrition.

*Andris, D.A., & Krzywda, E.A. (1997). Central venous access: Clinical practice issues. *Nursing Clinics of North America, 32,* 719–740.

*Banton, J., & Banning, V. (2002). Impact on catheter-related bloodstream infections with the use of the Biopatch dressing. *Journal of the Association for Vascular Access, 7*(3), 27–32.

*Battistella, F.D., Widergren, J.T., Anderson, J., Siepler, J., Weber, J., & MacColl, K. (1997). A prospective, randomized trial of intravenous fat emulsion administration in trauma victims requiring total parenteral nutrition. *Journal of Trauma-Injury Infection & Critical Care, 43*(1), 52–58; discussion 58–60.

*Beerman, L., O'Bryan, C., Olesen, M., Grafe, J., & Warchall, S. (2000). Clinical outcomes of intestinal transplant patients receiving home infusion services. *Tranplantation Proceedings, 32,* 1216–1217.

*Blackburn, G.J., Bistrian, B.R., Maini, B.S., Schlamm, B.A., & Smith, M.F. (1997). Nutritional and metabolic assessment of the hospitalized patient. *Journal of Parenteral and Enteral Nutrition, 1*(1), 17.

*Bloch, A.S., & Mueller, C. (2004). Enteral and parenteral nutrition support. In: K.L. Mahan & S. Escott-Stump (Eds.). *Krause's Food, Nutrition, & Diet Therapy* (11th ed., pp. 533–553). Philadelphia: W.B. Saunders.

*Brogden, B.J. (2004). Clinical skills: Importance of nutrition for acutely ill hospital patients. *British Journal of Nursing, 13*(15), 914–920.

*Burke, J., Wolfe, R., Mullany, C., et al. (1979). Parameters of optimal glucose infusion and possible hepatic and respiratory abnormalities following excessive glucose infusion. *Annals of Surgery, 190,* 379–385.

*Buswell, L., & Beyea, S. (1998). Flushing protocols for tunneled central venous catheters: An integrative review of the literature. *Online Journal of Knowledge Synthesis for Nursing, 5*(Doc. 3).

*Carlson, T.H. (2004). Laboratory data in nutrition assessment. In: K.L. Mahan & S. Escott-Stump (Eds.). *Krause's food, nutrition, & diet therapy* (11th ed., pp. 436–453). Philadelphia: W.B. Saunders.

*Carney, D.E., & Meguid, M.M. (2002). Current concepts in nutritional assessment. *Archives of Surgery, 137,* 42–45.

*Carpentier, Y.A., VanGossum, A., Dubin, E.Y., & Deckelbaum, R.J. (1993). Lipid metabolism in parenteral nutrition. In: J.L. Rombeau & M.D. Caldwell (Eds.). *Clinical nutrition: Parenteral nutrition* (pp. 35–74). Philadelphia: W.B. Saunders.

*Centers for Disease Control and Prevention (CDC). (2002). Guidelines for the prevention of intravascular catheter-related infections. *Morbidity and Mortality Weekly Report (MMWR). 51*(RR-10), 1–26. Erratum and correction in Appendix B. *MMWR, 51*(32), 711.

*Centers for Medicare and Medicaid Services (CMS). (2001). Medicare program: Replacement of reasonable charge methodology by fee schedules for parenteral and enteral nutrients, equipment and supplies. Final Rule. *Federal Register, 66*(167), 45173–45177.

*Cerra, F.B., Benitez, M.R., Blackburn, G.L., et al. (1997). Applied nutrition in ICU patients. *Chest, 111,* 769–778.

*Charney, P. (2001). Enteral nutrition: Indications, options, and formulations. In: M.M. Gottschlich (Ed.).

The science and practice of nutrition support: A case-based core curriculum (pp. 701–726). Dubuque, IA: Kendall/ Hunt Publishing.

*Cresci, G.A. (2002). Nutrition assessment and monitoring. In: S.A. Shikora, R.G. Martindale, & S.D. Schwaitzberg (Eds.). *Nutritional considerations in the intensive care unit* (pp. 21–29). Dubuque, IA: Kendall/ Hunt.

*Crnich, C.J., & Maki, D.G. (2002). The promise of novel technology for the prevention of intravascular device-related bloodstream infection, I: Pathogenesis and short-term devices. *Healthcare Epidemiology, 34,* 1232–1242.

*Curtis, S. (1996). Nutrition assessment of adults. In: K.A. Hennessy & M.E. Orr (Eds.). *Nutrition support nursing core curriculum* (3rd ed., pp. 1-1–12. Silver Spring, MD: American Society for Parenteral and Enteral Nutrition.

*Darouiche, R.O., Raad, I., Heard, S., et al. (1999). A comparison of two antimicrobial-impregnated central venous catheters. *New England Journal of Medicine, 340* (1), 1–8.

*Dimick, J.B., Swoboda, S., Talamini, M.A., Pelz, R., Hendrix, C., & Lipsett, P. (2003). Risk of colonization of central venous catheters: Catheters for total parenteral nutrition vs other catheters. *American Journal of Critical Care, 12,* 328–335.

*Drewett, S. (2000) Complications of central venous catheters: Nursing care. *British Journal of Nursing, 9*(3), 465–477.

*Dudek, S. (2001). *Nutrition essentials for nursing practice* (4th ed.). Philadelphia, PA: Lippincott Williams & Wilkins.

*Dudrick, S.J., & Wilmore, D.W. (1968). Long-term parenteral feeding. *Hospital practice, 3*(10), 65–78.

*Duerksen, DR., Papineau, N., Siemens, J., Yaffe, C. (1999). Peripherally inserted central catheters for parenteral nutrition: A comparison with centrally inserted catheters. *Journal of Parenteral Enteral Nutrition, 23,* 85–89.

*Duyff, R.L. (2002). *American Dietetic Association complete food and nutrition guide.* (2nd ed., pp. 21–24). Hoboken, NJ: John Wiley & Sons.

Elia, M. (1997). Assessment of nutritional status and body composition. In: J.L. Rombeau & R.H. Rolandelli (Eds.). *Clinical nutrition: Enteral and tube feeding* (3rd ed., pp. 155–192). Philadelphia: W.B. Saunders.

*Evans-Stoner, N. (1997). Nutritional assessment: A practical approach (pt. 1) and Guidelines for the care of the patient on home nutrition support: An appendix (pt. 2). *Nursing Clinics of North America, 32,* 637–650.

*Forloinses-Lynn, S., & Viall, C. (1996). Home care. In: K.A. Hennessy & M.E. Orr (Eds.). *Nutrition support nursing core curriculum* (3rd ed., pp. 24-1–14. Silver Spring, MD: American Society for Parenteral and Enteral Nutrition.

*Galica, L.A. (1997). Parenteral nutrition. *Nursing Clinics of North America, 32,* 705–718.

*German, J., Roberts, M., & Watkins, S. (2003). Personal metabolomics as a next generation nutritional assessment. *Journal of Nutrition, 133*(12), 4260–4266.

*Goff, K. (1997). Metabolic monitoring in nutrition support. *Nursing Clinics of North America, 32,* 741–754.

*Grant, J.P. (1992). *Handbook of total parenteral nutrition* (pp. 15–47, 107–136, 171–201). Philadelphia: W.B. Saunders.

*Grant, J., & DeHoog, S. (1999). *Nutritional assessment, support, and management* (2nd ed.). Seattle, WA: Authors.

*Hamilton, H. (2004). Central venous catheter: Choosing the most appropriate route. *British Journal of Nursing, 13*(14), 862–870.

*Hammond, K.A. (2004). Dietary and clinical assessment. In: K.L. Mahan & S. Escott-Stump (Eds.). *Krause's food, nutrition, & diet therapy* (11th ed., pp. 407–431). Philadelphia: W.B. Saunders.

*Hammond, K.A., Szeszycki, E., & Pfister, D. (2001). Transitioning to home and other alternate sites. In: M.M. Gottschlich (Ed.). *The science and practice of nutrition support: A case-based core curriculum* (pp. 701–726). Dubuque, IA: Kendall/Hunt Publishing.

*Harris, J.A., & Benedict, F.G. (1919). *A biometric study of basal metabolism in man* (Pub. 279). Washington, DC: Carnegie Institute of Washington.

*Intravenous Nurses Society. (2000). Infusion nursing standards of practice. *Journal of Intravenous Nursing, 23* (6S Suppl), S1–S88.

*Ireton-Jones, C.S. (2002). Estimating energy requirements. In: S.A. Shikora, R.G. Martindale, & S.D. Schwaitzberg (Eds.), *Nutritional considerations in the intensive care unit* (pp. 31–36). Dubuque, IA: Kendall/ Hunt Publishing.

Joint Commission on Accreditation of Healthcare Organizations. (2004). *Comprehensive accreditation manual for hospitals.* Oakbrook Terrace, IL: Author.

*Jones, G.R. (1998). A practical guide to evaluation and treatment of infections in patients with central venous catheters. *Journal of Intravenous Nursing, 21* (Suppl. 5), S134–S142.

*Kirby, D.F. (2001). Decision for enteral access in the intensive care unit. *Nutrition, 17*(9), 776–779.

*Kovacevich, D.S., Boney, A.R., Braunschweig, C.L., et al. (1997). Nutritional risk classification: A reproducible and valid tool for nurses. *Nutrition in Clinical Practice, 12*(1) 20–25.

*Kris-Etherton, P.M., Taylor, D.S., Yu-Poth, S., et al. (2000). Polyunsaturated fatty acids in the food chain in the United States. *American Journal of Clinical Nutrition, 71* (1 Suppl.), 179S–188S.

*Krzywda, E. (2004). Parenteral nutrition. In: M. Alexander & A. Corrigan (Eds.). *Core curriculum for infusion nursing* (3rd ed., pp.355–412. Philadelphia: Lippincott Williams & Wilkins.

*Livingston, A., Seamons, C., & Dalton, T. (2000). If the gut works, use it. *Nursing Management, 31*(5), 39–42.

*Lowrey, T.S., Dunlap, A.W., Brown, R.O., et al. (1996). Pharmacologic influence on nutrition support therapy: Use of propofol in a patient receiving combined enteral and parenteral nutrition support. *Nutrition in Clinical Practice, 11*(4), 147–149.

*Maki, D.G. (2003). Preventing intravascular catheter-related infections: An evidence-based approach. *Physician's Weekly, XX*(17).

*Maki, D.G., Mermel, L.A., Kluger, D., et al. (2000). The efficacy of a chlorhexidine-impregnated sponge (Biopatch) for the prevention of intravascular catheter-related infection—A prospective, randomized, controlled, multicenter study. Paper presented at the 40th Interscience Conference on Antimicrobial Agents and Chemotherapy. Toronto, Ontario, Canada.

*Marik, P., & Bedigian, M.K. (1996). Refeeding hypophosphatemia in critically ill patients in the intensive care unit: A prospective study. *Archives of Surgery, 131,* 1043–1047.

*Matarese, L.E., & Gottschlich, M.M. (1998). Protein in nutrition support. In: *Contemporary Nutrition Support Practice.* Philadelphia: W.B. Saunders.

*Mayo Clinic Proceedings. (2000). Complications and cost associated with parenteral nutrition delivered to hospitalized patients through either subclavian or peripherally inserted central catheters. *Clinical Nutrition, 19,* 237–243.

*McMahon, M. (1997). Management of hyperglycemia in hospitalized patients receiving parenteral nutrition. *Nutrition in Clinical Practice, 12,* 35–41.

*McMahon, M.M., & Rizza, R.A. (1996). Nutrition support in hospitalized patient with diabetes mellitus. *Mayo Clinic Proceedings, 71,* 587–594.

*National Advisory Group on Standards and Practice Guidelines for Parenteral Nutrition. (1998). Safe practices for parenteral nutrition formulations. *Journal of Parenteral and Enteral Nutrition, 22*(2), 49–66.

Newell-Stokes, V., Broughton, S., Guiliano, K, & Stetler, C. (2001). Developing an evidence-based procedure: Maintenance of central venous catheters. *Clinical Nurse Specialist, 15,* 199–206.

*Olson, K., Rennie, R.P., Hanson, J., et al. (2004). Evaluation of a no-dressing intervention for tunneled central venous catheter exit sites. *Journal of Infusion Nursing, 27,* 37–44.

*Penney-Timmons, E., & Sevedge, S. (2004). Outcome data for peripherally inserted central catheters used in an acute care setting. *Journal of Infusion Nursing, 27*(6), 431–436.

*Pfaller, M.A., Jones, R.N., Messer, S.A., Edmond, M.B., & Wenzel, R.P. (1998). National surveillance of nosocomial blood stream infection due to species of *Candida* other than *Candida albicans*: Frequency of occurrence and antifungal susceptibility in the SCOPE Program. *Diagnostic Microbiology & Infectious Diseases, 30,* 121–129.

*Probst, Y., & Tapsell, L. (2005). Overview of computerized dietary assessment programs for research and practice in nutrition education. *Journal of Nutrition Education & Behavior, 37*(1), 20–26.

*Rodriguez, L. (2004). Nutritional status: Assessing and understanding its value in the critical care setting. *Critical Care Nursing Clinics of North America, 16*(4), 509–514.

Rolandelli, R.H., & Ulrich, J.R. (1994). Nutritional support in the frail elderly surgical patient. *Surgical Clinics of North America, 74,* 79–92.

*Rollins, C.J. (1997). Total nutrient admixtures: Stability issues and their impact on nursing practice. *Journal of Intravenous Nursing, 20,* 299–304.

*Rosmarin, D.K., Wardlow, G.M., & Mirtallo, J. (1996). Hyperglycemia associated with high continuous infusion rate of total parenteral nutrition dextrose. *Nutrition in Clinical Practice, 11*(4), 151–156.

*Rychlec, G., Edel, J., Murray, M., Schurer, W., & Tomko, M.M. (2000). Nutrition assessment of adults. In: B. Hornick (Ed.). *Manual of clinical dietetics* (6th ed., pp. 3–33). Chicago: American Dietetic Association.

*Seidner, D.L., & Fuhrman, P.M. (2001). Nutrition support in pancreatitis. In M.M. Gottschlich (Ed.) *The science and practice of nutrition support: A case-based core curriculum* (pp. 553–565). Dubuque, IA: Kendall/Hunt Publishing.

*Snell, L., & Randolph, S. (2004). Home care management of intestinal transplant recipients. *Progress in Transplantation, 14,* 299–310.

*Souba, W.W. (1997). Nutritional support. *New England Journal of Medicine, 336,* 41–48.

*Trissel, L.A., Gilbert, D.L., Martinez, J.F., et al. (1999). Compatibility of medications with 3-in-1 parenteral nutrition admixtures. *Journal of Parenteral and Enteral Nutrition, 23*(2), 67–74.

*Trujillo, E.B., Young, L.S., Chertow, G.M., et al. (1999). Metabolic and monetary costs of avoidable parenteral nutrition use. *Journal of Parenteral and Enteral Nutrition, 23*(2), 109–113.

*Van de Berghe, G., Wouters, P., Weekers, F., et al. (2001). Intensive insulin therapy in the surgical intensive care unit. *New England Journal of Medicine, 345,* 1359–1367.

*Whitman, E.D. (1996). Complications associated with the use of central venous access devices. *Current Problems in Surgery, 33*(4), 311–378.

*Wilmore, D.W., & Dudrick, S.J. (1968). Growth and development of an infant receiving all nutrients exclusively by vein. *Journal of the American Medical Association, 203,* 860–864.

Wilson, J., & Jordan, N. (2001). Parenteral nutrition. In: J. Hankins, R. Lonsway, H. Hedrick, M. Perdue (Eds.). *Parenteral nutrition in infusion therapy in clinical practice* (2nd ed.), pp. 209–247). Philadelphia: W.B. Saunders.

*Winkler, M.F., Watkins, C.K., & Albina, J.E. (1998). Transitioning the nutrition support patient from hospital to home. *Infusion, 4*(7), 39–44.

Review Questions

Note: Questions below may have more than one right answer.

1. Which of the following visceral proteins is most useful in monitoring the effectiveness of nutritional support because of its shorter half-life and sensitivity to acute changes in protein status?

   A. Albumin

   B. Transferrin

   C. Prealbumin

   D. Total protein

2. What is the minimum amount of glucose needed to meet the obligate needs for glucose by the brain, central nervous system, red blood cells, white blood cells, active fibroblasts, and certain phagocytes?

   A. 50–75 g

   B. 150–200 g

   C. 250–300 g

   D. 350–400 g

3. All of the following are adverse reactions to IV lipids *except:*

   A. Dyspnea

   B. Chest pain

   C. Headache

   D. Leg cramps

4. As a general rule, the higher the stress, the lower the calorie-to-nitrogen ratio. Which of the calorie-to-nitrogen ratio ranges below is most often considered appropriate for the highly stressed patient?

   A. Between 60:1 and 90:1

   B. Between 90:1 and 100:1

   C. Between 90:1 and 150:1

   D. Between 100:1 and 150:1

5. Which of the following complications is not associated with placement of the central venous catheter tip into the heart?

   A. Thrombosis

   B. Cardiac tamponade

   C. Valvular damage

   D. Cardiac dysrhythmias

6. During parenteral nutrition administration, the serum blood glucose level should be maintained at less than

   A. 50 mg/dL

   B. 80 mg/dL

   C. 100 mg/dL

   D. 200 mg/dL

7. If symptoms of an air embolism occur, the patient should be placed in which of the following positions?

   A. On the back in semi-Fowler's

   B. On the left side, in deep Trendelenburg

   C. On the right side, in deep Trendelenburg

   D. On the left in semi-Fowler's

8. Symptoms of hyperglycemic hyperosmolar nonketotic coma include all of the following *except:*

   A. Glycosuria

   B. Seizures

   C. Coma

   D. Anuria

9. During parenteral nutrition administration, the refeeding syndrome is associated with which of the following electrolyte abnormalities?

   A. Hypophosphatemia

   B. Hypermagnesemia

   C. Hypercalcemia

   D. Hyponatremia

10. Infectious complications are more frequently associated with which type of central venous access device?

    A. Cuffed tunneled central catheter

    B. Cuffed tunneled port

    C. Noncuffed peripherally inserted central catheter

    D. Noncuffed, short term, multilumen catheter

CHAPTER 17

Transfusion Therapy

KEY TERMS

Allogeneic

Autologous

Factor V Leiden

Heterozygous

Homozygous

Immunohematology

Transfusion Therapy—21st Century Considerations

Opportunities are endless to transform and improve transfusion therapy. With transfusions increasing at the rate of 6% per year, transfusion therapy will need to become safer and address innovative therapeutics while being cost effective and efficient. More blood donors are needed, because less than 5% of healthy Americans eligible to donate actually do so (American Association of Blood Banks [AABB], 2005). And, it is imperative that nurses work closely with patients. There are better outcomes when patients are involved with their own care and with the decisions affecting them (Institute of Medicine [IOM], 2004).

Since the 2000 IOM report, *To Err Is Human: Building a Safer Health System*, there has been a national agenda focused on patient safety. This includes the Joint Commission on Accreditation of Healthcare Organizations' National Patient Safety Goals (JCAHO; 2005) and the National Quality Forum's focus on indicators of safe care. Dzik (2003) outlined three danger points in the transfusion process and proposed solutions for each point. Incorrect blood being transfused was the major cause of patient complications; therefore, the administration process needs the most examination and improvement (Dzik). With continuous monitoring and process changes, sustained evidence of safe blood administration can be achieved (Saxena, Ramer, & Shulman, 2004).

One of the most important steps is identification of the patient for each procedure in the transfusion process. A current mandate is that patients must be identified using two identifiers, and the room number cannot be used in either case (JCAHO, 2005). By 2006, all blood and blood products administered to patients in hospitals will have to be verified by a machine-readable bar code that matches the patient's information on a bar coded identification bracelet (U.S. Department of Health and Human Services, 2004). Initial studies support the safety and efficiency of bar coding. One research group reported no errors in 41,000 blood-sampling procedures and 27,000 units of blood administration in >3 years when bar coding was used (Chan, Chu, Young, et al., 2004). It was also found that bar coding reduced the number of transfusion steps from 27 to 16 and eliminated the need for another nurse to do the conventional double check (Dohnalek, Cuonac, Westcott, Langeberg, & Sandler, 2004; Turner, Casbard, & Murphy, 2003). Continued exploration of technology and decision-support processes are needed to make transfusion therapy safer and efficient at the bedside.

Nurses will also need to maintain their knowledge and competence with each new transfusion therapy product introduction. Hematopoietic growth factors, blood substitutes, cord blood, gene therapy, and cellular engineering are among the innovations in transfusion science and alternatives (Goodnough, 2003; McCullough, 2003; Rudnicke, 2003). Nurses are the last checkpoint to ensure safe administration of transfusion therapy. Along with the patient, nurses are the first to identify possible transfusion reactions and can intervene appropriately. Nursing care is the 24-hour surveillance, assessment, problem identification, and intervention that keeps patients safe.

Nurses will see changes in the indications for transfusions, a decrease in transfusion requirements, and analyses of cost-effectiveness of transfusion therapy (Goodman, Chan, Collins, Haught, & Chen, 2003; Porte & Leebeek, 2002; Ward & Levy, 2004). Novel methods to identify trends in incident reports may help with complex system issues (Tsatsoulis & Amthauer, 2003). Additionally, researchers are continually trying to reduce pathogen transmission via the blood supply. Nurses need to be aware of these innovations to explain to patients how blood is made safe and also need to be alert to the potential for patient reactions to a blood processing methodology. Patients perceive the risk of blood transfusion differently than do physicians (Lee, Mehta, & James, 2003). Understanding this difference can assist nurses in evaluating patient education materials and involving patients in the decision-making process. Care must be customized for each patient for his or her safety and personal engagement.

Nurses are integral health care partners in transfusion therapy. Along with providers in their own facilities, nurses work with many regulatory agencies to improve care. Some of these agencies in the United States include the Center for Disease Control and Prevention, the Food and Drug Administration, the Occupational Safety and Health Administration, the American Association of Blood Banks, the Clinical Laboratory Improvement Act, and the Joint Commission on Accreditation of Healthcare Organizations. The AABB sets standards that represent accepted performance guidelines for the provision of safe blood banking, transfusion, transplantation, and work environments for personnel. Professional organizations also assist in the maintenance of standards, both for professionals and health care agencies, such as the American Nurses Association, the Infusion Nurses Society, the Oncology Nursing Society, and the American Association of Critical-Care Nurses. Adhering to the standards of these agencies can keep health care providers and patients confident that care is current and policies and procedures are followed. The future for transfusion therapy is filled with opportunities. Nurses can provide the safest therapy for patients and minimize the risks when working collaboratively with all health care colleagues toward this common goal. "Nursing actions . . . are directly related to better patient outcomes" (IOM, 2004).

Basic Immunohematology

Immunohematology is the science that deals with antigens of the blood and their antibodies. Antigens (also called agglutinogens because they can cause blood cell agglutination, or clumping) are substances capable of stimulating the production of antibodies in response to the antigen's presence on the blood cell. An antibody is a protein in the plasma that reacts with this specific antigen. People who have been exposed to the red blood cells or leukocytes of other people through transfusion, transplantation, or pregnancy (maternal-fetal hemorrhage) may produce antibodies to the antigens carried on those foreign cells.

Antibodies are named for the antigen that stimulated their formation and with which they react. For example, an antibody against the Rh, or "D" antigen, formed after the transfusion of an Rh (D)-positive unit to an Rh (D)-negative recipient is called *anti-D*. Antibodies formed in response to exposure to foreign antigens are called *immune antibodies*.

Numerous antigens have been discovered on human blood cells, some more commonly encountered, such as Kell, Duffy, and Kidd. There are, however, hundreds of antigens that are rarer. Most of these are weak and of minimal importance in transfusion. Leukocytes also carry antigens on their surfaces, the most important being human leukocyte antigens (HLA). The groups most likely to cause transfusion reactions are the ABO and Rh systems of antigens.

The ABO system, discovered by Karl Landsteiner in 1901, is the most important group of antigens for transfusion as well as transplantation. The synthesis of these antigens, which are located on the surface of red blood cells, is under the control of the A, B, and O *genes*. There are four ABO blood types: In the presence of the A gene, a person makes A antigen and is classified as group A, group B people have B antigens on their red blood cells, group AB people have both, and group O people have neither. These antigens, inherited genetically, determine the person's blood group.

Some blood group antibodies are formed without exposure to **allogeneic** (from another person) red blood cells. The most important of these so-called naturally occurring antibodies, or isoagglutinins, are anti-A and anti-B. During the first few months of life, infants make antibodies to whichever of the ABO antigens they lack. For example, a group A infant makes anti-B (Table 17–1). These isoagglutinins can

TABLE 17–1   ABO Classification of Human Blood

Group	Cell Antigens		Plasma Antibodies		% U.S. Population
	A	B	A	B	
O	−	−	+	+	45
A	+	−	−	+	40
B	−	+	+	−	11
AB	+	+	−	−	4

produce rapid hemolysis of red blood cells with the corresponding antigen, forming the basis of ABO incompatibility.

The Rh system, discovered in 1940 by Stetson and Levine, is the second most clinically important system for transfusion. The Rh system is so called because of the discovery of this substance in the red blood cells of the Rhesus monkey. The antigens of the human Rh system are of great clinical significance because they often are responsible for transfusion incompatibility and hemolytic disease of the newborn. Approximately 85% of the white population has the D antigen on their red blood cells and are classified as Rh positive, and 95% of African Americans are Rh positive (Webert, Chan, Smith, Heddle, & Kelton, 2004). In the remainder of the population, the D antigen is missing; these people are classified as Rh negative and can readily form anti-D after exposure to the antigen. Severe hemolytic reactions and hemolytic disease of the newborn result from this antigen–antibody reaction.

Mechanism of Immune Response

When a patient is transfused with allogeneic blood bearing foreign (ie, nonself) antigens, the immune system may respond by producing antibodies. Phagocytic cells called *macrophages* play an important role in this response by capturing and processing foreign antigens. The macrophages then present the processed antigens to other members of the immune system, called *T and B lymphocytes*, which begin to produce antibodies specific for the antigens presented. Stimulated by the foreign antigen, the B cell swells, changes its internal structure, and differentiates into plasma cells that produce the antibodies to bind and aggregate foreign cells and ensure their removal (Sommer, 2002). Each plasma cell then produces large quantities of antibodies specific to the particular antigen as genetically programmed into the cell. The cells secrete the antibodies into a variety of body fluids, including the blood plasma. The T lymphocytes act as helpers or suppressors to B-lymphocyte function. The intertwined relationship between B and T lymphocytes regulates the type and sensitivity of the immune response.

Mechanism of Red Blood Cell Destruction

Two mechanisms of red blood cell destruction are known: intravascular hemolysis and extravascular hemolysis. Intravascular hemolysis occurs within the vascular compartment. This mode of red blood cell destruction results from the sequential binding of an antibody to a foreign antigen on the surface of a red blood cell. This reaction then activates the complement system. When the complement system cascade is triggered, a resulting lytic complex forms on the red blood cell membrane, which leads to rupture of the red blood cell and the release of hemoglobin into the intravascular compartment. The most frequent cause of this type of red blood cell destruction is transfusion of ABO-incompatible blood. Mostly immune globulin (IgM) antibodies, anti-A and anti-B are capable of engaging the complement, coagulation, and kinin systems when they bind with their corresponding antigens. The consequences of this type of hemolysis are usually immediate, severe, and often fatal.

The other mechanism of red blood cell destruction, extravascular hemolysis, is more commonly seen as a result of incompatibilities in blood group systems other than the ABO. In contrast to anti-A and anti-B, antibodies to these other blood group antigens are usually immune globulin G (IgG) and bind to red blood cells with the corresponding antigen. Phagocytic cells of the reticuloendothelial system, particularly in the spleen, bind the IgG-coated red blood cells, ingest them, and destroy them extracellularly—hence the term, *extravascular hemolysis*. These IgG antibodies also may fix some amount of complement, but not enough to lyse the red blood cells. Instead, the phagocytic cells of the liver, the Kupffer cells, clear the complement-coated red blood cells from the circulation and destroy them intracellularly. The consequences of extravascular hemolysis are less severe than those of intravascular hemolysis, but are recognizable by a drop in the hematocrit, an increase in the bilirubin level, and perhaps the clinical signs of fever or malaise.

Blood Group Systems

As discussed, the ABO system is the only system in which antibodies (anti-A and anti-B) are consistently and predictably present in the sera of people whose red blood cells lack the corresponding antigen(s). The ABO system is the foundation of pretransfusion testing and compatibility.

Antibodies to the Rh (D) antigen are not present unless a person has been exposed to D-positive red blood cells, either through transfusion or pregnancy. Because of the ease with which antibody D is made, grouping is done on all donors and recipients to ensure that D-negative recipients receive D-negative blood, except for reasonable qualifying circumstances. D-positive recipients may receive either D-positive or D-negative blood. People who develop Rh antibodies have detectable levels for many years. If undetected, subsequent exposure may lead to a secondary immune response. Occasionally, weak variants of the Rh (D) antigen are found, which are identified by special serologic tests. These people are termed weak D or Du positive, but they are considered Rh positive both as donors and recipients.

Other blood group systems have been defined on the basis of cells' reactions to antigens. Antibodies to antigens in the Kell, Duffy, Kidd, and Lewis systems are encountered frequently enough to be clinically important. Antibodies to the blood group antigens in most other systems are found so infrequently that they do not cause everyday problems. When present, these antibodies may produce hemolytic reactions. Once demonstrated, precautions must be taken to ensure that the patient receives compatible blood lacking the corresponding antigen. When difficulty arises in crossmatching or when a transfusion reaction occurs, these systems acquire special significance. Today, systems to identify, validate, and ensure ABO and Rh groupings are set up on computer databases. Confirmatory testing must be in place according to AABB guidelines.

Pre-Transfusion Testing, Blood Donation, and Blood Preservation

The Donor

A donor may donate blood no more than every 8 weeks. A donation shall be no more than 10.5 mL/kg body weight. In addition to ABO and Rh group determination and a screen for unexpected antibodies, several other tests are performed on donor blood. These tests must be negative for the antibodies identified (Box 17–1) before any blood or component is released for patient use.

The Recipient

Tests performed on the intended transfusion recipient include ABO and Rh group determination and screening for unexpected antibodies. Before the administration of

---

BOX 17–1   Donor and Recipient Blood Testing Requirements for Transfusion Therapy

Allogeneic Donor

ABO group
Rh type
Antibodies to HbsAg (hepatitis B surface antigen)
Antibodies to HBc (hepatitis B core antigen)
Antibodies to HCV (hepatitis C virus)
Antibodies to HIV-1 and -2
STS (serologic test for syphilis)
Antibodies to HTLV I/II (human T-cell lymphotropic virus)
Antibodies to CMV (cytomegalovirus) [Performed on cellular blood component donated for immuno-compromised patient]

Recipient

ABO group
Rh type
Unexpected antibodies to red cell antigens
Crossmatch against donor red cells

Adapted from American Association of Blood Banks (2004). *Primer of blood administration*. Bethesda, MD: Author.

whole blood or red blood cell components, a major crossmatch (combining donor red blood cells and recipient serum or plasma) is performed to detect serologic incompatibility. The AABB requires that if a patient has been transfused in the preceding 3 months with blood or a blood component containing red blood cells, has been pregnant within the preceding 3 months, or the history is uncertain or unavailable, the sample must be obtained from the patient within 3 days of the scheduled transfusion (AABB, 2004). This requirement is made to rule out the possibility of missing a newly formed antibody.

In situations in which delaying the provision of blood may jeopardize life, blood may be issued before completion of routine tests according to AABB standards (AABB, 2004). Recipients whose ABO group is not known must receive group O red blood cells. Physicians must indicate in the record that the clinical condition is sufficiently urgent to release blood before the completion of compatibility testing. The tag or label must conspicuously indicate that compatibility testing is not completed, and standard compatibility tests should be completed as promptly as possible. Recipients whose ABO group has been determined by the transfusing facility without reliance on previous records may receive ABO group-specific whole blood or ABO group–compatible red blood cell components before other compatibility tests have been completed (Box 17–1).

Directed Donations

The risk of transfusion-transmitted diseases has generated programs whereby prospective patients may designate their own blood donors. Blood centers and hospitals have increased the availability of this program, known as *directed donation*, for the public. Each donor enters the same process as any other, but the blood is labeled for a specific recipient provided screening tests are appropriate and the unit is compatible. Units are specifically labeled for the intended recipient.

The primary benefit of this program may be to reduce the fear of disease transmission in recipients, who feel reassured knowing who their donors are. If the donor is a blood relative of the recipient, the cellular components must be irradiated to prevent graft-versus-host disease (GVHD; AABB, 2004). These programs must address cost-effectiveness, staffing, quality assessment measures, and legal considerations.

Autologous Donation

Autologous transfusion is the collection, filtration, and reinfusion of a person's own blood; thus, the donor and recipient are the same individual. There are several types of autologous donation, all of which eliminate risk of disease transmission as well as immunosuppression, although other mechanical and nonhemolytic reactions can occur. *Autologous transfusion* takes on several different meanings and methods and is accepted practice for appropriate candidates in a specific setting based on the patient's clinical condition.

Autologous transfusion is a conservative approach. In the 1980s and early 1990s, the AIDS epidemic and increased awareness of bloodborne disease transmission created interest and demand for autologous blood collection. This interest, however, decreased in the late 1990s and early 2000s (Galel, Malone, & Viele, 2004) as a result of improved donor screening and public perception of a safe blood supply. As the possibility of new transfusion-transmitted diseases (eg, variant Creutzfeldt-Jakob disease or mad cow disease) are identified, there may be a renewed interest in autologous donation (Brecher & Goodnough, 2002).

Although receiving one's own blood is the safest transfusion, careful administration of autologous blood is still required. To avoid any errors, those administering the blood must verify all aspects of the component, including proper identification. Verification procedures should be identical to those for giving homologous transfusions. All products of autologous donation must be labeled "For Autologous Use Only."

The AABB endorses all modalities of blood conservation, including the goals of autologous transfusions. Autologous transfusion can be accomplished by preoperative donation, acute normovolemic hemodilution, intraoperative salvage, and postoperative blood salvage.

PREOPERATIVE AUTOLOGOUS DONATION

This technique is best used when a patient is planning an elective surgical procedure that normally would cause the loss of a significant number of units of blood. The patient may plan periodic visits to a donor center for phlebotomies to store his or her own blood for later use.

ACUTE NORMOVOLEMIC HEMODILUTION

In this procedure, the patient's blood is collected, stored at room temperature for up to 8 hours in the operating room, and returned to the patient at the time of blood loss. Deterioration of platelets and coagulation factors is minimal in this time frame. To maintain plasma volume, the patient receives infusions of a crystalloid or colloid solution. The benefit of this technique is that it reduces the patient's hematocrit by dilution before surgical blood loss so that the patient loses a smaller number of red cells. Frequently used in cardiac surgery, hemodilution may be limited by the patient's blood volume or other hemodynamic considerations. Because the hematocrit is reduced, patients with lung disease or hypo-oxygenation require close monitoring.

INTRAOPERATIVE BLOOD COLLECTION

This frequently used method of autologous transfusion involves recovering blood during surgical procedures associated with significant blood loss from clean wounds. Blood is aspirated from the operative site, washed by using cell-washing machines, and reinfused back to the patient. The process may be performed completely in the operating room. It is most frequently used in cardiovascular, thoracic, orthopedic, neurologic, and hepatic surgery, including transplantations. The technique makes large volumes of blood immediately available when bleeding occurs in a clean operative procedure. The procedure is contraindicated in patients with malignancy or infection because reinfusion of contaminated cells may disseminate the tumor cells or infectious organism.

Sterile technique is mandated to prevent infectious agents from entering the system. Initial equipment and personnel costs can be high, but improved medical care outweighs the disadvantages. The program's success requires (a) availability of responsible staff 24 hours a day, (b) preferably dedicated operators for each machine, (c) a quality improvement program, and (d) physician support and public awareness programs. Some hospitals have developed programs that have established a break-even point for using this method of autologous transfusion. Others may hire outside agencies to do traveling intraoperative autologous transfusions.

POSTOPERATIVE BLOOD COLLECTION

This technique involves collecting shed blood from surgical drains after cardiac, trauma, orthopedic, and plastic surgery. Other clinical conditions also may be appropriate. The advantage of this technique is that it can be done for planned surgery or emergency operations and trauma. Postoperative shed blood is collected through special equipment for reinfusion. If the blood in the sterile canister is not reinfused within 6 hours, it must be discarded. This technique is safe, simple, and cost effective. Combined with other methods of autologous transfusions described, the goal of avoiding homologous blood transfusions is closer.

Blood Preservation

Blood is routinely collected in sterile plastic bags that contain different anticoagulant–preservative solutions. Whole blood may be collected in anticoagulant citrate phosphate dextrose solution (CPD), citrate phosphate double dextrose solution (CP2D), or anticoagulant citrate phosphate dextrose adenine solution (CPDA-1). Since patients may suffer an adverse reaction to an anticoagulant–preservative, it is important to be knowledgeable of chemicals used in the solutions. Citrate is an anticoagulant that binds with free calcium in the donor's plasma. Since blood requires calcium to clot, the presence of citrate inhibits the coagulation cascade. Phosphate buffers the pH, preventing a decrease in 2,3-DPG, thus facilitating the oxygen-carrying capacity of the blood. Dextrose (glucose) prolongs the life of the red blood cells by providing a nutrient source. Blood cells may be stored in CPD for 21 days at 1°C to 6°C. CPDA-1 contains adenine, which helps the RBCs synthesize adenosine triphosphate (ATP) during storage and lengthens the shelf life of the blood to 35 days. The red blood cell depends on ATP to maintain cell surface ion pumps (AABB, 2004).

The duration for storage is based on the standard that a minimum of 75% of the transfused red blood cells (stored for 35 days) must be present in the bloodstream of the recipient 24 hours after the transfusion. Providing a nutrient biochemical balance to red blood cells during storage is important to maintain viability and function of the components in the blood and to prevent physical changes. To minimize bacterial proliferation, specific temperatures must be maintained.

A second group of anticoagulant–preservative systems is similar to CPDA-1. They differ, however, in that once the platelet-rich plasma is removed from the unit within 8 hours, an additive solution of 100 mL containing saline, dextrose, and adenine is added to the packed red blood cells. These additive systems permit storage for up to 42 days. FDA-approved solutions include AS-1 (Adsol), AS-3 (Nutricel), and AS-5 (Optisol).

Whole Blood

Whole blood contains red blood cells, white blood cells, platelets, plasma (blood proteins, antibodies, water, and waste), and electrolytes. The usual volume is 450 to 500 mL/unit. Transfusions of whole blood are rare and indicated only in acute, massive blood loss for the purpose of expanding blood volume and increasing oxygen-carrying capacity. If possible, blood loss should be managed with other blood components, crystalloids, or colloidal solutions.

Administration of whole blood subjects the patient to the possibility of complications such as fluid volume excess, especially in patients with a compromised cardiac status. In addition, after 24 hours of storage, cell breakdown can result in elevated potassium levels, the formation of microaggregates, nonviable platelets and granulocytes, and decreased levels of the clotting factors, factor V and factor VIII. In patients with a severely damaged liver, massive whole blood transfusions can result in a calcium deficit owing to the presence of citrate anticoagulant. Monitoring of the patient's potassium level before and after the transfusion is important. Hemoglobin and hematocrit levels may be inaccurate owing to fluid shifts during active bleeding. Whole blood transfusion must be ABO *identical* with that of the recipient because of the presence of antibodies. One unit of whole blood increases hemoglobin by about 1 gm/dL and hematocrit by about 3 to 4 percentage points (AABB, 2002a).

Whole blood is stored at a temperature of 1°C (34°F) to 6°C (43°F). Expiration depends on the anticoagulant–preservative. The rate of administration for whole blood should be as rapid as necessary to correct and maintain hemodynamic status. In massive hemorrhage, one or more large-gauge catheters, such as 14 or 16 gauge, allows a free-flow infusion of blood, although whole blood can be administered through either an 18- or 20-gauge catheter. Electronic infusion devices do not deliver high enough rates to meet the needs of a clinical crisis. In this instance, pressure cuffs applied to the bag of blood may be required for rapid infusion. Further information is in the section on Blood Administration.

Whole Blood, Irradiated

Irradiated whole blood and blood components have been exposed to a measured amount of radiation in order to prevent lymphocytes from replication. Irradiated blood components are used to prevent graft-versus-host-disease (GVHD) in patients with Hodgkin's or non-Hodgkin's lymphoma, acute leukemia, congenital immunodeficiency disorders, patients with malignant tumors who are being treated with immunosuppressive therapy such as chemotherapy or radiation, low-birth-weight neonates, and intrauterine infusions (AABB, 2004). Irradiated units pose no risk to a transfusionist or the recipient. Because irradiation may damage and reduce the viability of red blood cells, the original expiration date of the component prevails.

Red Blood Cells

Packed Red Blood Cells

Packed red blood cells are prepared by removing approximately 225 to 250 mL (70% to 80%) of platelet-rich plasma from a unit of whole blood, either by centrifugation, sedimentation, or apheresis. These processes pack the red blood cells and separate most of the platelet-rich plasma (Fig. 17–1). The red blood cell concentrate contains the same red blood cell mass as whole blood, 20% to 30% of the original plasma, and some leukocytes and platelets. Depending on the anticoagulant-preservative used, red blood cells (RBCs) usually have a hematocrit of between 60% and 80%; thus, the viscosity of the unit is increased. Each unit of RBCs contains about 60 g of hemoglobin or 180 mL of pure red cells. A unit designated as a low-volume collection will contain at least 50 g of hemoglobin. One unit of packed red blood cells provides the same amount of oxygen-carrying red blood cells as a unit of whole blood, but at a reduced volume. Each unit of packed red blood cells is expected to raise the hematocrit by 3 percentage points and the hemoglobin level 1 gm/dL in the average 70-kg person.

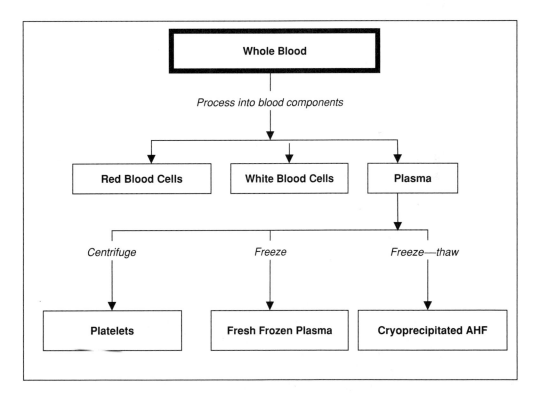

FIGURE 17–1. Identification of blood components from whole blood. Adapted from American Association of Blood Banks (2004). *Primer of blood administration*. Bethesda, MD: Author.

The major indication for packed red blood cells is to restore or maintain oxygen-carrying capacity as in cases of acute or chronic blood loss, symptomatic anemia, trauma, and chemotherapy when nutrition, drug therapy, and treatment of the underlying disease cannot achieve an improved RBC count (AABB, 2004). Criteria for transfusion are based on patient's symptoms, time frame, amount of blood loss, and levels of hemoglobin and hematocrit. Patients with chronic anemia usually adjust to a lower hemoglobin level and are transfused only when symptomatic. RBCs should not be given to treat anemia that responds to iron or recombinant erythropoietin.

Because of the reduced volume of a unit of RBCs, the danger of circulatory overload is decreased with advantages for the patient with renal failure or heart failure and for the elderly or debilitated patients (AABB, 2004). Because approximately two thirds of the plasma is removed, less citrate is infused and there are fewer byproducts of cell breakdown such as potassium and ammonia.

The expiration time of packed red blood cells is 35 to 42 days, depending on the anticoagulant–preservative used. RBCs may be frozen for extended storage (AABB, 2004). Typing and crossmatching is still required. Group O may be given to other blood groups. In emergencies, when time does not permit ABO determination, group O red blood cells may be given (Table 17–2).

TABLE 17–2   ABO Compatibilities for Red Blood Cell Components, Fresh Frozen Plasma, and Whole Blood

	Donor: Red Blood Cell Components Universal donor is O− and Universal recipient is AB+		
Recipient	First Choice	Second Choice	Third Choice
O+	O+	O−	—
A+	A+	O+, A−	O−
B+	B+	O+, B−	O−
AB+	AB+	AB−, A+, B+	O+, A−, B−, O−
O−	O−	—	—
A−	A−	O−	—
B−	B−	O−	—
AB−	AB−	A−, B−, O−	—
Recipient	**Donor: Fresh Frozen Plasma**		
O	O, A, B, or AB	—	—
A	A or AB	—	—
B	B or AB	—	—
AB	AB	—	—
Recipient	**Donor: Whole Blood** (must be ABO identical)		
O	O	—	—
A	A	—	—
B	B	—	—
AB	AB	—	—

Adapted from American Association of Blood Banks (2004). *Primer of blood administration.* Bethesda, MD: Author.

Red Blood Cells, Leukocytes Reduced

Red blood cells, leukocytes reduced, are used in patients with symptomatic anemia who have previously experienced febrile reactions from leukocyte antibodies and cytokines released during storage (AABB, 2004). This component prevents recurrent febrile, nonhemolytic transfusion reactions and also reduces the incidence of HLA alloimmunization and the risk of transfusion-transmissible cytomegalovirus (CMV; AABB, 2002a). Leukocyte-reduced RBCs are not to be used to prevent graft-versus-host disease.

A unit of leukocyte-reduced RBCs contains fewer than 5×10^6 white blood cells as compared with a unit of whole blood, which contains ≥ 1 to 10×10^9 cells. Leukocyte reduction may be accomplished either at the bedside by filtering blood with a special filter that can remove as much as 99% of the white blood cells, or during processing. Washing the red blood cells will also remove the leukocytes, but may also reduce the number of red blood cells by 20% and is an expensive and time-consuming process. Washed RBCs must be used within 24 hours. The ABO compatibility is the same as for packed red blood cells.

Red Blood Cells, Rejuvenated, and the Use of Anticoagulants

Red blood cells prepared from whole blood and collected with appropriate anticoagulants can be rejuvenated at any time during storage for up to 3 days after expiration. The FDA-approved rejuvenating solution consists of inosine, phosphate, and adenine, which restore 2,3-diphosphoglycerate and ATP to normal levels. They must be washed before infusion to remove the inosine, which may be toxic. If not administered within 24 hours, these red blood cells must be glycerolized and frozen (AABB, 2002a). The ABO compatibility is the same as for packed red blood cells.

Red Blood Cells, Deglycerolized

Deglycerolized red blood cells are prepared for freezing by removing plasma and adding glycerol, which enters the cell and protects it from cell dehydration and ice formation in its frozen state. The purpose of this process is to preserve rare units of blood or autologous donor units. They may be frozen for up to 10 years. At the time the unit is needed, it is thawed and the glycerol is removed by washing the cells with successively lower concentrations of sodium chloride until the final suspension is 0.9% sodium chloride injection (USP). Deglycerolized red blood cells carry the risk of hemolysis if the deglycerolization process is inadequate (AABB, 2002a). After thawing, the component should be administered within 24 hours of the washing process. The finished product has virtually all the leukocytes, plasma, and platelets removed. It contains less than 5% of the original donor platelets and leukocytes and has a hematocrit of approximately 80%.

This component is not used as a routine red cell replacement, but is useful to preserve blood from donors with rare blood groups. It is also useful to patients who are sensitized to IgA or other plasma proteins because the cellular components have been removed. The major disadvantage is the substantial additional cost related to the process of preparing and storing the component. The ABO compatibility is the same as for packed red blood cells.

Platelets

Platelets are indicated for the control or prevention of bleeding in the presence of thrombocytopenia or abnormal platelet function. There are two preparations for platelets: random donor concentrates made from pooled units of platelets from several donors, and concentrates obtained by platelet apheresis of a single donor. Units may be combined into a single bag before release from the blood bank. Platelets should not be infused through the same tubing as RBCs since some platelets are not ABO specific and may cause coagulation in the tubing. Platelets contain factor III, a phospholipid that enhances the conversion of prothrombin to thrombin, which forms one of the most important steps in the coagulation process.

Platelets, Pooled

Clinical conditions that adversely affect platelet function include sepsis, diseases of the liver and kidney, drugs, cardiopulmonary bypass, some bone marrow disorders, and congenital and acquired platelet disorders (AABB, 2004). Platelet transfusions are indicated for thrombocytopenia caused by hemorrhage with platelet counts of $<50,000/\mu L$, patients undergoing surgery with a platelet count of $<100,000/\mu L$, chemotherapy patients with platelet counts of $\leq10,000/\mu L$, and patients without bleeding whose counts are $<15,000$ to $20,000/\mu L$ and are rapidly decreasing. Major invasive procedures require platelet counts of at least 40,000 to $50,000/mm^3$.

The decision to transfuse platelets must be based on the clinical condition of the patient, the cause of the thrombocytopenia, and the ability of the patient to produce platelets. Platelet transfusions should not be given on the basis of the number of red blood cells infused, but by the platelet count and signs and symptoms of hemorrhage. Stable patients with thrombocytopenia may tolerate platelet counts of $<5,000/\mu L$ with minor (but not serious) bleeding. Platelets are not routinely indicated for patients with conditions in which rapid platelet destruction occurs such as in idiopathic thrombocytopenic purpura (ITP) or untreated disseminated intravascular coagulation, except in the presence of life-threatening bleeding (AABB, 2004). For patients with thrombotic thrombocytopenic purpura (TTP) and heparin-induced thrombocytopenia with thrombosis (HITT), transfusion with platelets should be avoided owing to the risk of fatal thrombosis, except in the setting of life-threatening hemorrhage.

Platelet concentrate prepared from whole blood contains a minimum of 5.5×10^{10} platelets in 40 to 70 mL of plasma (AABB, 2002a). Each unit is expected to increase the platelet count of a 70-kg adult by $5,000/\mu L$ to $10,000/\mu L$. The usual dose in an adult is 4 to 8 units and may be repeated in 1 to 3 days owing to the short lifespan of 1 to 3 days. Routinely, random donor platelets (usually 6 units) are pooled and transfused. Patients are subjected to multiple allogeneic donors (AABB, 2002a).

Since ABO antigen is present on the platelet membrane, it is ideal to give ABO identical platelets. However, if a matching unit is not available and prompt transfusion is required, patients may receive any ABO group (AABB, 2004). Platelet concentrates do not require crossmatching before infusion; however, documentation of the patient's ABO and Rh status is necessary to make appropriate selection decisions. D-negative patients should receive compatible platelets, however, if available. Platelets may be infused as fast as the patient tolerates, but must be infused within 4 hours after release from the blood bank (AABB, 2004). Platelets may be stored at room temperature for 5 days with gentle agitation. Platelets are never put into a refrigerator or cooler.

Platelets, Single Donor

Because of immune or nonimmune mechanisms, as many as 70% of patients who receive repeated platelet transfusions will become refractory to platelet transfusions and will not have an adequate sustained rise in their platelet counts after transfusion. This is owing to the destruction of platelets by HLA antibodies soon after the transfusion is completed (AABB, 2004). Causes of refractoriness to platelets also include disseminated intravascular coagulation (DIC), drug therapies, ITP, and sepsis (AABB, 2004). These patients are more likely to benefit from single-donor platelets.

Obtained by the process of platelet pheresis, these platelets are collected from a single donor who is HLA compatible with the recipient. Family is often a more suitable match; however, a non-related donor may be found. Pheresis platelets contain approximately 4.5×10^{11} per bag in about 250 mL of plasma. The platelet infusion volume may be between 100 and 500 mL supplied in a large plastic pack or in two connected packs to improve platelet viability by providing more surface area for gas exchange. The exact number of platelets in the unit can be obtained from the blood bank. Reactions to platelets may include disease transmission, graft-versus-host disease, alloimmunization, febrile or allergic effects, and circulatory overload.

Platelets, Leukocytes Reduced

Leukocyte-reduced platelets are used to prevent recurrent febrile, nonhemolytic transfusion reactions that are caused when donor white cell antigens and/or cytokines released during storage react to recipient white cell antibodies (AABB, 2004). Leukocyte removal may be accomplished by filtration resulting in the removal of 99% of the leukocytes at the bedside. The manufacturer's guidelines for priming the filter must be adhered to for effective administration. Leukocyte-reduction RBC filters and leukocyte-reduction platelet filters are not interchangeable (AABB, 2004). Leukocyte-reduced platelets are also used to decrease the incidence of HLA alloimmunization in patients who may require long-term platelet replacement or transplantation in the future.

Granulocytes

Granulocytes, administered infrequently, are obtained from a single donor by the process of apheresis or the centrifugation of whole blood (AABB, 2004). Previously prescribed for gram-negative sepsis, the emergence of new antibiotic regimens, new recombinant growth factors, and improved management of infections have greatly decreased the use of this component. Granulocytes are used in neutropenic patients with counts >500/μL (AABB, 2002a). Granulocytes migrate toward, phagocytize, and kill fungi and bacteria. Patients receive granulocytes when they have infections not responsive to antibiotics and have a reasonable chance of recovery of bone marrow function (AABB, 2004). Cultures to identify the offending organism should be done. Granulocyte transfusion is not effective in localized infections or infections caused by agents other than bacteria. These transfusions only temporarily improve the patient's condition. Granulocyte infusion only rarely is associated with an increase in the patient granulocyte count, possibly owing to consumption or sequestration of the granulocyte in the infectious process (AABB, 2002a).

Granulocytes are stored at 20°C to 24°C (68°F to 75°F) for no more than 24 hours, and preferably <6 hours without agitation (AABB, 2004). Granulocytes should be administered as soon after collection as possible because of the deterioration of granulocyte function during short-term storage. Granulocytes are never put into a refrigerator or cooler.

Patients undergoing granulocyte transfusions are acutely ill, and adverse effects are common. Fever, chills, allergic reactions, and pulmonary reactions may occur and can be managed with diphenhydramine, non-aspirin antipyretics, steroids, meperidine, and slow administration of the unit. The transfusion should not be stopped unless severe respiratory symptoms occur. If the recipient is seronegative and severely immunosuppressed, donor CMV-seropositive granulocytes should not be given. Granulocytes are generally irradiated to prevent graft-versus-host disease (AABB, 2002a).

A unit of granulocytes contains variable amounts of lymphocytes, platelets, and RBCs suspended in 200 to 300 mL of anticoagulant and plasma. The granulocyte donor must be ABO and Rh compatible because a unit of granulocytes is heavily contaminated with donor red blood cells (AABB, 2004).

Hydroxyethyl starch (HES) may be used as a red cell sedimenting agent and will be present in the final component (AABB, 2002a). Granulocytes are administered through a standard blood filter over a 4-hour period for both adult and pediatric patients. Depth-type microaggregate filters and leukocyte-reduction filters should not be used.

Plasma

Plasma is the liquid content remaining after the red blood cells have been removed from a unit of whole blood. It contains water, electrolytes, proteins (principally albumin), globulin, and coagulation factors. Plasma plays an important role in the treatment of burns by supplying plasma proteins that are lost from the wound.

Liquid Plasma

Liquid plasma is indicated for patients who have a deficit of stable coagulation factors such as factor IX and fibrinogen. However, this component has reduced amounts of factors V and VIII, which limits its use in some patients (AABB, 2004). Single-donor liquid plasma is stored at 1°C to 6°C for no more than 26 days in CPD or 40 days in CPDA-1, or 5 days after the expiration of whole blood (AABB, 2004). Some of the clotting factor activity may be lost during storage.

Under ordinary circumstances, single-donor plasma should be compatible with the recipient's red blood cells. Because it lacks anti-A and anti-B agglutinins, AB plasma may be used for all ABO groups and in emergencies when the patient's blood group is unknown.

Fresh Frozen Plasma

Fresh frozen plasma (FFP) is used to replace coagulation factors in patients with coagulation disorders or deficiencies secondary to DIC, liver disease, or dilutional coagulopathy resulting from volume replacement or volume overload. It is also used to reverse warfarin sodium overdose in patients who are to undergo an invasive procedure when there is not adequate time to administer vitamin K or to stop the drug. Patients with antithrombin III deficiency, TTP, C-1-esterase deficiency, protein S deficiency, and those with deficiencies for which there are no concentrates available may also receive FFP. It is beneficial to patients with demonstrated multiple coagulation deficiencies, inherited or acquired bleeding disorders, and, on occasion, to treat active bleeding owing to vitamin K deficiency.

Fresh frozen plasma contains albumin, globulins, antibodies, and clotting factors in addition to 200 to 400 mg fibrinogen. It has a shelf life of 1 year when stored at a temperature of −18°C, or 7 years at −65°C when frozen within 8 hours of collection and stored in CPD, CP2D, or CPDA-1. Plasma stored in ACD or 2% to 3% sodium citrate must be frozen within 6 hours at −18°C or colder (AABB, 2004). The volume is dependent on the anticoagulant solution used, but is usually 200 to 250 mL. Kept frozen until the time of transfusion, FFP is then thawed in a water bath at 30°C to 37°C (98.6°F) and gently agitated or kneaded up to 30 minutes. FFP should be administered within 6 hours, but no more than 24 hours after thawing to minimize the loss of the most labile clotting factors, factor V and factor VIII. To provide factors V and VIII, the component should be used within the first year of storage for treatment of coagulation disorders.

Because FFP is an isotonic volume expander, patients receiving multiple units should be monitored closely to prevent fluid overload. FFP should never be used for volume expansion or as a nutrient supplement; these is more safely treated with crystalloid or colloid solutions that lack the risk of transmitting disease and are less expensive than FFP. Other safer volume expanders are albumin and plasma substitutes, which do not carry the risk of viral disease transmission.

FFP may be administered over 30 to 60 minutes through a standard blood filter (AABB, 2004). The unit must be ABO compatible, but Rh matching is not required. If the recipient's blood type is unknown, group AB can be safely given (Table 17–2). Although a crossmatch is not required, the component should be compatible with the recipient's red blood cells. Generally, 5 to 20 mL/kg are needed to bring coagulation factor levels up to sufficient concentrations to achieve hemostasis and to bring fibrinogen levels and activated partial thromboplastin time levels within the normal hemostatic range (generally ≤1.5 time the midrange of the normal value).

Solvent–Detergent-Treated Plasma

Somewhat controversial, a newly licensed plasma component is available. Referred to as PLAS + SD (pooled plasma, solvent–detergent treated) or SDP, this plasma component is prepared from ABO blood group–specific donor-pooled plasma. The solvent–detergent process inactivates the viruses by stripping away their lipid coating (AABB, 2002b). It is the only human blood plasma product treated to inactivate HIV, HCV, and hepatitis B virus (HBV). It is thought that the process used to treat the plasma adds another layer of protection for the public from disease transmission.

Clinical indications include treatment for patients with clotting factor deficiencies when factor concentrates are not available. The two disadvantages of SDP are cost and a potential greater risk of non-enveloped virus transmission such as hepatitis A virus (HAV) and parvovirus because of pooling of plasmas.

An alternative to SDP is non-pooled FFP, donor-retested. This method requires the donor to be retested after a minimum of 90 days after collection. Used extensively in Europe, advantages and disadvantages are still being weighed in the United States because, to date, the risk/benefit and cost/benefit ratios are not favorable compared with a single unit of FFP. Table 17–3 contains a summary of the blood and blood components described.

Plasma Derivatives and Plasma Substitutes

NORMAL SERUM ALBUMIN AND PLASMA PROTEIN FRACTION

Albumin and plasma proteins are referred to as *protein colloids* and are the most abundant solutes in plasma; albumin is the most abundant, making up 54% of the plasma proteins (Gaspard, 2005). These protein colloids are collected from blood, serum, and human placentas and are heated at 60°C (140°) for 10 hours to inactivate viruses including HIV, HBV, and HCV. Albumin is available in two concentrations, 5% in 250 mL saline and 25% in 50 mL saline. It may replace plasma in many clinical conditions.

Albumin 5% is isotonic. Available in 250 mL, it is osmotically equivalent to an approximately equal volume of citrated plasma and may be used to provide volume and colloid in the treatment of shock and burns. Initially after a burn, large volumes of crystalloid solution are needed to correct extracellular fluid losses because of fluid leakage into the intracellular compartment. Smaller amounts of colloid are required at this time. After 24 hours, increased amounts of albumin may be used to maintain intravascular volume and avoid hypoproteinemia while smaller amounts of crystalloid are then infused.

Albumin 25% is hypertonic and depends on additional fluids, either drawn from the tissues or administered separately, for its maximal osmotic effect; 50 mL of 25% albumin is osmotically equivalent to 250 mL citrated plasma. Albumin 25% is also available in 100 mL. In either case, it must be administered with caution because a rapid infusion may cause an increase in intravascular oncotic pressure. This may result in circulatory overload and pulmonary edema, or in the development of interstitial dehydration unless adequate amounts of supplemental fluids are

TABLE 17–3 **Blood Components and Whole Blood: Action and Use, Volume and Infusion Guide, and Special Considerations and Risks**

Blood Component	Action and Use	Volume and Infusion Guide	Special Considerations and Risks
Red blood cells	• Increases oxygen-carrying capacity • For symptomatic anemia, aplastic anemia, or bone marrow failure caused by malignancy or antineoplastic therapy • Expected to increase the hematocrit 3% and the hemoglobin level 1 g/dL in the average 70-kg person	250–300 mL As tolerated but no longer than 4 h from the time of release from blood bank	Hemolytic, allergic, and febrile reactions GVHD Infectious disease transmission
Red blood cells, leukocyte reduced	• To prevent recurrent febrile, nonhemolytic transfusion reactions • Reduces the incidence of HLA alloimmunization and the risk of transfusion-transmissible CMV	250–300 mL	Infectious disease transmission
Red blood cells, deglycerolized	• To preserve rare units of blood or autologous donor units • Used in patients sensitized to IgA/plasma proteins causing anaphylaxis • Expected to increase the hematocrit 3% and the hemoglobin level 1 g/dL in the average 70-kg person	200–250 mL	Hemolytic, allergic, and febrile reactions GVHD Infectious disease transmission Substantial cost related to preparation
Platelets, pooled	• Thrombocytopenia or platelet function abnormality • Improves hemostasis • Increases platelet count by 5,000/mL per each unit (30,000 to 60,000/mL for 6-unit pool)	50–70 mL/unit Usual dose 6–8 units As fast as tolerated: 1 unit/10 min or less	Infectious disease transmission GVHD Allergic/febrile reactions May need to be repeated every 1–3 days
Platelets, single donor	• To prevent platelet destruction • Platelets are from single donor who is HLA compatible • Increase as above	100–500 mL As fast as tolerated: 1 unit/10 min or less	GVHD Febrile/allergic reactions

(Continued)

TABLE 17–3   Blood Components and Whole Blood: Action and Use, Volume and Infusion Guide, and Special Considerations and Risks   *(Continued)*

Blood Component	Action and Use	Volume and Infusion Guide	Special Considerations and Risks
Platelets, leukocyte reduced	• To prevent recurrent febrile, nonhemolytic transfusion reactions • Reduces the incidence of HLA alloimmunization and the risk of transfusion-transmissible CMV • Increase as above	30–50 mL/U Usual dose 6–8 units As fast as tolerated: 1 unit/10 min or less	Infectious disease
Granulocytes or irradiated granulocytes	• Rarely used • Infection unresponsive to antibiotic	200–300 mL Administer slowly over 2–4 h	Allergic/febrile reactions common; requires premedication to control reactions GVHD
Fresh frozen plasma	• Replace coagulation factors in patients with DIC, liver disease, factor V or XI deficiencies, reversal of warfarin	200–250 mL May be infused rapidly or as fast as tolerated: 30–60 min or within 2 h	Infectious disease Allergic reactions Does not provide platelets
Cryoprecipitated AHF (antihemophilic factor)	• Von Willebrand's disease • Hemophilia A • Factor XIII deficiency • Fibrinogen deficiency	Pooled units contain several units of about 15 mL Administer as rapidly as tolerated	Infectious disease Allergic reactions
Whole blood	• Rarely used • Indicated for volume expansion in massive acute blood loss • Increases oxygen carrying capacity • Increases Hgb 1 gm/dL and Hct 3 to 4%	450–500 mL As fast as tolerated through large-gauge catheter	Volume overload Hyperkalemia Decreased clotting factors Hemolytic, allergic, and febrile reactions GVHD Infectious disease
Whole blood, irradiated	• As above and also used to prevent GVHD in patients with Hodgkin's, non-Hodgkin's lymphoma, and acute leukemia and in patients receiving immuno-suppressive therapy		All risks as above except no risk for GVHD

Adapted from American Association of Blood Banks (2004). *Primer of blood administration.* Bethesda, MD: Author.

administered. Controversy exists over its use for protein replacement in severe hypoalbuminemia. Other uses for specific patient conditions include therapeutic apheresis, large-volume paracentesis, diuresis, and subarachnoid hemorrhage. Albumin 25% is not appropriate for hypovolemia unless there is an associated condition such as hypoalbuminemia, malnutrition, chronic nephrosis or hepatic failure, or peripheral edema. The rate of administration for albumin varies depending on the indication of administration, the patient's blood volume, and the patient response.

Administration of 5% and 25% albumin requires strict aseptic handling. Once the container is entered, it must be used immediately or discarded because albumin has no preservatives. Drugs should not be added to albumin, nor should albumin be added to IV solutions. Albumin is a good culture medium, and bacterial contamination is rare. If a reaction is suspected, the product should be held, the lot number recorded, and the manufacturer and the FDA notified. More frequently, adverse reactions are caused by improper administration. Both products have been heat treated to eliminate transfusion-transmitted diseases.

| **KEY INTERVENTIONS:** | Administration of Albumin |

1. Assemble equipment: albumin 5% or 25%; vented administration set; blunt cannula, if connecting to primary IV; alcohol prep pad; equipment for performing IV access if patient does not have an IV line.
2. Verify written order for correct product (concentration) and prescribed rate of administration.
3. Verify signed transfusion consent form. Check your institution's policies; some health care facilities do not require a consent for albumin.
4. Make positive patient identification per institution policy.
5. Close clamp on albumin set.
6. Remove closure disk from the albumin bottle and prepare entry port with an alcohol pad.
7. Squeeze the drip chamber of the albumin set and insert spike of the set into the center of the stopper of the albumin bottle.
8. Suspend the albumin bottle from the IV pole, release the drip chamber, and flush all air from line. Close clamp.
9. Attach appropriate blunt cannula to the albumin set.
10. Do not administer through any IV containing any medications.
11. Scrub the injection site of the primary IV with alcohol pad and insert the blunt cannula into the injection site. Secure catheter tightly.
12. Regulate albumin to prescribed administration rate
13. Document vital signs before the start of and after the transfusion. Record date, time, and signature of transfusion on blood requisition that accompanies the blood component. Place in appropriate part of patient's record. Document the patient's response and record the volume of infusion.

NOTE: Procedure can be converted for institutions using multilead blood administration sets. This procedure also may be modified for the administration of plasma and single-donor platelets.

Plasma protein fraction (human) 5% is an isotonic solution of protein consisting of 83% albumin and 17% alpha- and beta-globulins. Similar to albumin, it is used for emergency treatment of shock or other conditions in which there is a circulatory volume deficit. Plasma protein fraction is given IV without dilution and is available as a 5% solution; each 100 mL contains 5 g of selected plasma proteins. Again, dose and rate of administration are dependent on the patient's condition, but should not exceed 10 mL/minute because too rapid administration may cause hypotension. For treatment of shock, the minimum effective dose is usually 250 to 500 mL, depending on the patient's condition and response.

Neither albumin nor plasma protein fraction has any clotting factors, nor should they be considered plasma substitutes. There is no ABO or Rh matching for albumin or plasma protein fraction.

PLASMA SUBSTITUTES

Several types of infusions are available to expand vascular volume, including crystalloids such as isotonic saline or plasma expanders such as dextran and colloidal solutions. Dextran 40, dextran 70, and hetastarch (hydroxyethyl starch) are nonprotein colloids that do not require blood typing and remain in circulation longer than the crystalloids.

CRYOPRECIPITATED ANTIHEMOPHILIC FACTOR

Cryoprecipitated antihemophilic factor (AHF) is a plasma precipitate containing fibrinogen, factor VIII:C, factor VIII:vWF (von Willebrand factor), factor XIII, and fibronectin (AABB, 2004). Cryoprecipitated AHF is indicated for treatment of fibrinogen and factor XIII deficiency. It is used for the treatment of von Willebrand's disease and hemophilia A (factor VIII:C deficiency) only if virus-inactivated factor VIII concentrates are not available.

Cryoprecipitated AHF is prepared by thawing FFP between 1°C and 6°C, gathering the precipitate, and refreezing within 1 hour (AABB, 2002a). Pooled units contain several units of cryoprecipitated AHF. This component should be kept at room temperature and transfused as soon as possible within 6 hours or 4 hours if units have been pooled. Each unit of cryoprecipitate should contain at least 80 IU of factor VIII:C and 150 mg of fibrinogen in about 15 mL of plasma (AABB, 2002a). ABO compatibility is preferred. For treatment of hemophilia A, a rapid loading dose may be required to produce the desired level of factor VIII:C followed by a maintenance dose every 8 to 12 hours. For fibrinogen deficiency, infusions every 3 days may be required (AABB, 2002a).

The patient must be closely monitored during and after the transfusion to assess and identify signs and symptoms of potential reactions. Most immediate adverse effects are preventable and caused by improper administration, failure to comply with standards, or lack of knowledge of the procedure or impact of the therapy. Thoroughly following written procedures and complying with policy are crucial for safe transfusion therapy.

ANTIHEMOPHILIC FACTOR (HUMAN)

Antihemophilic factor (AHF) is a sterile, purified, dried concentrate prepared from the cold-insoluble fraction of pooled FFP by a variety of methods, including fractionation by physiochemical techniques to provide factor VIII concentrates, and extraction and purification from plasma using monoclonal antibodies to factor VIII. These newer techniques offer a higher activity of AHF and are less likely to transmit disease. The levels of AHF vary depending on the technique used to make the component. Various processes used to inactivate viruses have yielded a safer product and greatly decreased the incidence of viral infection after transfusion. The discovery of the molecular structure of factor VIII has led to the creation of genetically engineered products that are produced using recombinant DNA technology. There are several concentrates of recombinant factor VIII available in the United States.

The clinical use of AHF concentrate is the treatment of hemophilia A, a hereditary bleeding disorder characterized by deficient coagulant activity. Infusions offer a temporary replacement of the deficient clotting factor to prevent bleeding episodes or provide coagulant activity when emergency or elective surgery is performed on hemophiliac patients. The stability of the component allows patients to treat themselves at home and maintain a more normal lifestyle than in the past.

Several commercial products using the cryoprecipitate of pooled donors are available and do not have the disadvantages of plasma or plasma cryoprecipitate. These are supplied as a lyophilized powder, and preparations are labeled in international units per bottle. The concentrate is provided with a sterile diluent, and users should adhere to guidelines supplied by the manufacturer. No ABO or Rh matching is required. The dosage to be administered is calculated based on knowing that one unit of factor VIII per kilogram of patient weight will raise the level of factor VIII in the blood by about 0.02 units/mL. Site and severity of hemorrhage are also considered in dosing (Roberts & Hoffman, 2001).

FACTOR IX CONCENTRATE

The clinical indication for factor IX concentrate is the prevention and control of bleeding in patients with hemophilia B, also known as Christmas disease. This disorder resembles hemophilia A. The cause of the deficiency of factor IX is an abnormal gene that leads to defective synthesis of factor IX, or an acquired factor IX deficiency. To achieve therapeutic levels of factor IX, large volumes of FFP would be required. Factor IX concentrates are the only treatment available for patients with this deficiency. The product, in conjunction with activated factor VIII, results in the conversion of prothrombin to thrombin. Thrombin then converts fibrinogen to fibrin, with clot formation as the end result.

Several preparations of factor IX concentrate are available. One product is available in the United States; it is produced by recombinant DNA technology and is free from the risk of transmission of human bloodborne pathogens such as HIV, hepatitis viruses, and parvovirus. The product is not derived from human blood and contains no preservatives or animal or human components. Other preparations are made from pooled human plasma and are processed by a solvent–detergent, ultrafiltration, or chemical treatment to reduce risks of transmission of viral infection (Roberts & Hoffman, 2001).

Preparation cautions vary from one product to another. It is important for users to adhere to preparation and administration guidelines supplied by the manufacturer. The number of units of factor IX is printed on each vial. The rate of administration is determined by the patient's condition, and the concentrate may best be infused by a push method not exceeding 10 mL/minute.

INTRAVENOUS IMMUNE GLOBULIN

Intravenous immune globulin (IVIG) is a highly purified solution of human IgG for IV use. Currently the most widely used plasma component in the world, plasma for the production of IVIG comes mostly (80%) from plasma donors with the remaining 20% in recovered plasma from whole blood donors (Knezevic Maramica & Kruskall, 2003). It is prepared from large pools of plasma (at least 1,000 donors) by a manufacturing process that eliminates contaminants such as bacteria and viruses.

Many different preparations are available from different manufacturers and are ordered for specific patient populations. One brand should not be substituted for another. The properties and side effects of IVIG can vary from patient to patient as well as between manufacturers (Schleis, 2000).

The primary use of IVIG is to supply sufficient amounts of IgG antibodies passively to patients who are unable to produce their own antibodies. The Food and Drug Administration (FDA) has control over IVIG as a drug and has approved its use for the following conditions: idiopathic thrombocytopenic purpura (ITP), primary immunodeficiencies, secondary immunodeficiency owing to chronic lymphocytic leukemia, pediatric human immunodeficiency virus (HIV), prevention of infection and rejection in adult bone marrow transplant, and in Kawasaki syndrome. Additionally, there are off-label uses for IVIG that have emerged through research, many of which are controversial. These uses require further large-scale controlled investigation (Knezevic-Maramica & Kruskall, 2003).

Some IVIG products are liquid, and some are powders that need to be reconstituted before administration. Some products need to be refrigerated. Follow the manufacturer's guidelines, and if provided, use the infusion kit supplied with the product. IVIG contains no preservatives and should be administered promptly after the vial is reconstituted. IVIG should not be mixed with other medications or IV solutions, and filtration is not required.

Dosage varies depending on the patient's response and may be repeated every 3 to 4 weeks. IVIG is not an irritant or a vesicant and may be administered by peripheral or central venous access by an electronic infusion device. The infusion of IVIG generally starts out slowly and is increased at specific intervals based on the patient's tolerance (Schleis, 2000). Most reactions are rate related, so caution is necessary. Other reactions are mild and self-limiting.

INTRAVENOUS CYTOMEGALOVIRUS (CMV) IMMUNE GLOBULIN (HUMAN)

Intravenous CMV immune globulin (CMV-IVIG) is a purified pooled plasma product containing a standardized amount of antibody to CMV. It is derived from plasma

---

KEY INTERVENTIONS: Administration of Intravenous Immune Globulin (IVIG)

1. Assemble equipment: IV immune globulin; vented IV administration set; infusion pump, if needed; alcohol prep pad; blunt cannula.
2. Allow product to warm to room temperature.
3. Verify written order for transfusion and rate of administration. (Note: Most adverse reactions are rate related.)
4. Make positive patient identification.
5. Calculate dosage based on weight of patient.
6. If product is not pooled, spike with IV tubing.

Techniques to administer:

7A. If infusion by gravity:
   a. Hang container on IV pole and half-fill drip chamber. Open clamp, flush air from the line. Close clamp.
   b. Scrub the injection site with alcohol and attach the blunt cannula into the injection site. Secure cannula tightly.

7B. If infusion with IV pump:
   a. Insert spike of IV pump set into bottle. Prime as directed.
   b. Secure catheter to injection site closest to IV site.

8. Initiate infusion at specified rate and monitor patient. Increase rate as indicated.
9. Record date, time, and signature on requisition, which accompanies the blood component. Place in appropriate part of patient's record. Document patient's response. Record volume of infusion.

---

selected for high titers of the antibody and is primarily indicated as an adjunct to antiviral therapy in organ transplantation or CMV pneumonia (Nichols & Boeckh, 2000). Solid organ transplant recipients who are seronegative for CMV and receiving an organ from a CMV-seropositive donor are at risk of CMV disease. The risk of actual virus transmission via this pooled product is considered low because of a solvent–detergent viral inactivation process used in its manufacture.

Because the product contains no preservatives, infusion should begin within 6 hours after preparing the dose and be completed within 12 hours after entering the vial. The recommended initial rate of infusion is 15 mg/kg/hour, increasing to a maximum of 60 mg/kg/hour at specified intervals if the patient experiences no adverse reactions. No infusion should exceed 75 mL/hour (Massachusetts Public Health Biological Laboratories, 2004). Use of an electronic infusion pump is usually necessary to maintain a constant infusion.

Most reactions are rare and are usually rate related. When flushing, chills, muscle cramps, nausea, back pain, fever, or hypotension are observed, the infusion should be slowed or temporarily stopped. Vital signs should be monitored on a scheduled basis.

RH IMMUNE GLOBULIN

Rh immune globulin (RIG) is a concentrate of anti-D immune globulin that is derived from plasma. It is used to prevent an Rh-negative individual from becoming sensitized (isoimmunized) to the Rh (D) antigen when exposed to the antigen by transfusion or, more commonly, pregnancy.

Rh antibody is produced by the Rh-negative mother in response to the D antigen in an Rh-positive infant and is the cause of Rh hemolytic disease of the newborn (HDN). Prophylaxis against this sensitization was developed in the sixties and seventies. Since antepartum administration of RIG became a standard of practice in 1983, the incidence of pregnancy-associated isoimmunization and HDN has decreased. Today the incidence of HDN is less than five cases per 10,000 births (Harrod, Hanson, VandeVusse, & Heywood, 2003). RIG is given at 28 weeks gestation and again at 72 hours postpartum. This reduces the risk of isoimmunization to 0.1% (AABB, 2002b). Mothers are not candidates for RIG if the fetus is Rh negative or there is evidence that the mother is already sensitized. A standard 300-μg dose of RIG will prevent maternal sensitization in most cases, but in some situations, the volume of fetomaternal hemorrhage may be higher and require more than one dose of RIG to prevent immunization (Harrod et al., 2003). In addition to antepartum and postpartum use, RIG is used for other outcomes of pregnancy (abortion, miscarriage) or amniocentesis when a fetomaternal hemorrhage could occur.

Use of RIG may be appropriate when an Rh-negative recipient receives Rh-positive red blood cells or components, such as platelets or granulocytes, which may contain sufficient cells to cause immunization. Individual situations dictate prophylaxis for red blood cell transfusions because the dose required is extremely large and causes discomfort.

Several commercial preparations of RIG are available. RIG is primarily administered by intramuscular injection; however, an IV preparation has been approved by the FDA and is suitable for patients who are at high risk for hematoma from intramuscular injections (AABB, 2002b). Although use of RIG is not associated with viral transmission, no drug is risk free, and informed consent may be required as this is a product that is derived from human plasma (Harrod et al., 2003). RIG is usually given intramuscularly in the deltoid, but manufacturer's recommendations for administration and patient observation should be followed closely.

Transfusion Reactions

Significant improvements in the collection, testing, and storage of blood and blood components, together with growing knowledge in the field of immunohematology, have increased the safety of transfusion therapy. An inherent risk still exists, however, with every unit of transfused blood. The transfusionist, the primary nurse, and the patient should be aware of the risks and remain alert for symptoms of untoward events. Since the patient is often the first person to recognize a change in how he or she feels, it is important to involve the patient in all aspects of the transfusion, if possible. ABO and Rh compatibility testing cannot eliminate all reactions to administered blood.

A transfusion reaction is defined as "any unfavorable event occurring in a patient during or following transfusion of blood or blood components that can be related to that transfusion" (AABB 2004, Chapter 5, p. 18). Any unfavorable sign or symptom experienced by the patient during or following a transfusion should be

---

BOX 17–2   Hemolytic Transfusion Reaction Signs and Symptoms

Objective Signs	Subjective Symptoms
Fever: temperature increase of 1°C or 2°F	Restlessness
Chills, rigor	Anxiety, feeling of impending doom
Hypotension, shock	Vague, uneasy feeling
Tachycardia	Pain in abdomen, chest, or back
Respiratory distress/extreme dyspnea	Headache
Hemoglobinuria, oliguria, anuria	Nausea, vomiting
Bleeding, generalized oozing	Pain at IV site or along vein
Rash, hives	

Adapted from Bryan, S. (2002). Hemolytic transfusion reaction: Safeguards for practice. *Journal of Perianesthesia Nursing, 17,* 399–403.

---

considered serious, the transfusion should be stopped, and the patient should be evaluated. Box 17–2 outlines the objective signs and subjective symptoms that may be observed, need assessment, and require intervention. Urticarial reactions need treatment, but may not require blood testing; they should be reported to the blood bank or transfusion service per institutional procedure. Institutional policy will outline the specific course of action that must be followed when a transfusion reaction is suspected (AABB, 2004). However, if a transfusion reaction is suspected, essential interventions are universal:

- Stop the transfusion.
- Keep the IV access open with normal saline.
- Notify the physician.
- Notify the blood bank or transfusion service.

KEY INTERVENTIONS: Suspected Transfusion Reaction

1. At initial sign or symptom of suspected transfusion reaction, *stop* the transfusion.
2. Immediately set up a 250-mL infusion of 0.9% sodium chloride. Flush the administration set with the 0.9% sodium chloride.
3. Disconnect the blood or component and blood administration set from the hub of the catheter and replace with the set primed with sodium chloride. Put a sterile cap on the tubing and save for possible restart of infusion. If using Y-tubing blood set, *do not open* lumen infusing sodium chloride because this causes more blood to be infused.
4. Begin infusion of sodium chloride solution.
5. Notify the physician and the blood bank or transfusion service of the patient's symptoms and vital signs.

(Continued)

KEY INTERVENTIONS: Suspected Transfusion Reaction   *(Continued)*

6. If the physician determines the need for a transfusion reaction evaluation, initiate the following steps: Gather remaining equipment to draw blood and package the blood administration bag and set.
7. Draw blood samples as directed by institutional protocol and send to the blood bank. Blood samples are tested to determine the cause of the reaction.
8. Confirm that blood component set is tightly clamped and distal end is covered to prevent leakage of blood. Place blood component bag with any residual fluid, attached administration set with intravenous solution, filter, and all related tags and labels in a plastic bag. Secure bag and send to blood bank or transfusion service with suspected transfusion reaction report and other related forms. Report must be on the outside of plastic bag.
9. Send a urine sample for hemoglobinuria if ordered by the patient's physician or institutional protocol.
10. Continue to monitor patient closely for any further signs and symptoms of reaction.
11. Document any signs and symptoms observed and the time of recognition. Note type of component, amount infused, amount remaining, and nursing interventions performed. Record that remaining component and suspected transfusion reaction report were sent to blood bank or transfusion service.

Transfusion reactions may be divided into two main classes: acute and delayed. These may each be further divided into immunologic and nonimmunologic (Box 17–3). Some reactions are common, and actions can be taken to reduce the patient's discomfort—for example, a mild allergic reaction—whereas other adverse effects need to be prevented, such as circulatory overload.

BOX 17–3   Acute and Delayed Immunologic and Nonimmunologic Transfusion Reactions

Acute Reactions

Immunologic

Acute hemolytic reaction
Febrile non-hemolytic reaction
Transfusion-related acute lung injury
Urticaria (mild allergic reaction)
Anaphylaxis

Nonimmunologic

Transfusion-associated circulatory overload
Air embolism
Citrate toxicity
Hypothermia
Electrolyte disturbances
Bacterial contamination

Delayed Reactions

Immunologic

Delayed hemolytic reaction
Transfusion-associated graft-versus-host disease

Nonimmunologic

Infectious organism transmission
Iron overload

Acute Reactions

Acute adverse effects of transfusion therapy usually occur during the transfusion or within hours (<24 hours) after the completion of an infusion. Therefore, the patient must be closely monitored during and after the transfusion to assess and identify signs and symptoms of impending reactions. Most immediate adverse effects are preventable and caused by improper administration, failure to comply with standards, or lack of knowledge of the procedure or impact of the therapy. Thoroughly following written procedures and complying with policy are crucial for safe transfusion therapy and to protect patients from harm.

ACUTE IMMUNOLOGIC REACTION

Antigen–antibody reactions from red blood cells, leukocytes, or plasma proteins are responsible for adverse effects in the recipient. They are usually produced by the body's response to foreign proteins.

Acute Hemolytic Reaction

Acute hemolytic transfusion reactions occur when an antigen–antibody reaction occurs in the recipient as the result of an incompatibility between the recipient's antibodies and the donor's red blood cells (intravascular). Incompatibilities in the ABO blood group system are responsible for most deaths from acute hemolytic transfusion reactions and may occur with the administration of as little as 10 to 15 mL of incompatible blood.

The interaction of the isoagglutinins and ABO-incompatible red blood cells activates the complement, kinin, and coagulation systems. The entire complement system is activated in the ABO mismatch, causing intravascular hemolysis. If the amount of free hemoglobin released from the destruction of red blood cells exceeds the quantity that can combine with haptoglobin in the plasma, the excess hemoglobin filters through the glomerular membrane into the kidney tubules and hemoglobinuria occurs. The kinin system is activated by the antigen–antibody complex and produces bradykinin, which increases capillary permeability, dilates arterioles, and decreases systemic blood pressure. The coagulation system activates the intrinsic clotting cascade, causing small clots in the circulation, and may trigger disseminated intravascular coagulation (DIC), which results in formation of thrombi in the microvasculature.

Intravascular hemolytic reactions are often fatal. Investigation of fatal hemolytic transfusion reactions shows that the most common causes are clerical or other errors in the identification of (a) the recipient sample sent to the blood bank, (b) the blood unit, or (c) the recipient. Hemolytic transfusion reactions may be accompanied by chills, fever, facial flushing, a burning sensation along the vein in which the blood is being infused, lumbar or flank pain, chest pain, frequent oozing of blood at the injection site and surgical areas, or shock. When reactions occur, the transfusion must be stopped at once and the vein kept open with 0.9% sodium chloride. When Y tubing is used, a new setup (container of fluid and a new administration set) should be connected directly to the patient's intravascular device (ie, peripheral IV or central venous catheter). The flow to the normal saline hanging with the Y tubing should not be opened; to do so could result in the patient receiving additional incompatible blood cells contained in the Y tubing.

Vigorous treatment of hypotension and promotion of adequate renal blood flow are imperative. Therapy may consist of administration of volume, diuretics, and volume expanders to promote diuresis and to minimize renal damage. Urinary flow rates in adults should be maintained above 100 mL/hour for at least 18 to 24 hours (AABB, 2002b). Vasopressors, such as dopamine in low doses (<5 μg/kg/minute), dilate the renal vasculature while increasing cardiac output (AABB, 2002b). Their use requires careful monitoring of the patient's urinary flow, cardiac output, and blood pressure. A diuretic agent such as furosemide is recommended to be given concurrently with adequate IV fluid replacement. The drug improves renal blood flow, thus minimizing the possibility of renal tubular ischemia and renal failure. Mannitol is infrequently used because, if ineffective, it may cause hypervolemia and pulmonary edema. The use of heparin therapy for the resulting DIC remains controversial and is addressed after evaluation of all consequences of the acute hemolytic reaction. Prevention is the hallmark of therapy for this severe reaction.

Extravascular hemolysis occurs when an antigen–antibody reaction occurs as an incompatibility between the recipient's red blood cells and the donor's plasma. Signs and symptoms of extravascular hemolysis are chills, fever (typically several hours after the transfusion is completed), and a positive direct antiglobulin test. Relief of symptoms is the goal of treatment.

Febrile Nonhemolytic Reaction

Febrile nonhemolytic reactions (FNHR) are usually the result of transfusion of cellular components in the absence of hemolysis, whereby anti-leukocyte antibodies in the recipient are directed against the donor's white blood cells. Even though some leukocytes break down rapidly during storage, the membrane fragments are still capable of sensitizing patients in the same manner as intact leukocytes. Patients who have been sensitized by numerous transfusions or multiple pregnancies are more likely to have a febrile nonhemolytic reaction.

A FNHR is defined as a rise in temperature of 1°C or 2°F or more without any other clinical reason and may occur immediately or within several hours of completion of the transfusion (Miller, 2004). Febrile reactions, which occur in 0.5% to 6% of transfusions (AABB, 2002b), may be accompanied by chills, rigors, and malaise. As the name implies, no red blood cell hemolysis occurs. Antipyretics are used for treatment. When this reaction is anticipated, give acetaminophen 30 minutes before the blood or component is started or as ordered by the physician. Antihistamines are not indicated because most febrile nonhemolytic reactions are not caused by release of histamine (AABB, 2004). Documentation of the reaction is important for prevention of future adverse effects. This reaction can be prevented through the use of leukocyte-reduced components, which usually are produced by filtration techniques. Deglycerolized red blood cells and washed red blood cells are also relatively depleted of leukocytes. All febrile responses should be clinically monitored because other reactions may occur.

Anaphylactic Reactions

Fortunately, anaphylactic reactions are rare, estimated to occur in 1 per 20,000 to 50,000 units (AABB, 2002b). The cause is unknown, but may be owing to sensitization to a foreign protein. They may occur in patients who are IgA deficient and who have developed anti-IgA antibodies. The two classic signs that an anaphylactic reaction is imminent are symptoms after only a few milliliters of blood or plasma have been infused, in the absence of fever. Bronchospasm, respiratory distress, abdominal cramps, vascular instability, shock, and perhaps loss of consciousness characterize the reaction. This medical emergency requires immediate resuscitation of the patient along with administration of epinephrine and steroids. Close observation during the first 15 minutes of the transfusion and continuing surveillance throughout the transfusion are important to monitor for signs of this reaction. Patient education will alert the patient to signs and symptoms that may occur once the patient is home and must be reported to the physician.

Prevention includes the use of autologous transfusions or obtaining units from donors who lack IgA. Reducing the plasma content of red blood cell and platelet transfusions may also be effective in reducing the severity of this reaction.

Allergic Reactions

These reactions are relatively common and are based on a hypersensitivity response to foreign plasma proteins in donor plasma. Allergic reactions can range from mild to severe. Reactions are characterized by local erythema, hives, itching, asthmatic wheezing, and laryngeal edema in varying degrees of intensity. Occasionally, fever may be present. Treatments for these reactions are based on the severity of the patient's symptoms. In mild allergic reactions, the transfusion may be stopped temporarily and then continued after the patient has responded to antihistamine therapy. In severe allergic reactions, the transfusion is stopped until a diagnosis is made. The goal of treatment is to alleviate the patient's symptoms. Washed or frozen, thawed, and deglycerolized red blood cells may be indicated for any future therapy (AABB, 2004).

Transfusion-Related Acute Lung Injury

Transfusion-related acute lung injury (TRALI) is a clinical syndrome associated with the transfusion of whole blood, packed red blood cells, fresh frozen plasma platelet concentrate, cryoprecipitate, and rarely, IGIV. It is often undiagnosed and under-reported. It is important to recognize the signs and symptoms of TRALI and treat it promptly and aggressively (Kopko, Marshall, Malcom, Holland, & Popovskey, 2002).

The usual cause of TRALI is a reaction between donor high-titer anti-leukocyte antibodies and recipient leukocytes. The reaction can result in leukoagglutination. The leukoagglutinins may become trapped in the pulmonary microvasculature and cause massive leakage of fluids and proteins into the alveolar spaces and interstitium (AABB, 2002a). This reaction causes severe respiratory distress unassociated with circulatory overload and without evidence of cardiac failure. The severity of the respiratory distress is usually disproportional to the volume of blood infused and is related to the degree of hypoxemia. Chest radiography reveals bilateral pulmonary infiltrates consistent with pulmonary edema but without other evidence of left heart failure. Clinical signs and symptoms other than respiratory distress include chills, fever, cyanosis, hypotension, and normal pulmonary capillary wedge pressure. These symptoms can occur during or within 1 to 2 hours after the transfusion, but are usually present by 4 to 6 hours post-transfusion. Treatment begins by discontinuing the transfusion and providing aggressive respiratory and blood pressure support measures. Once a donor has been implicated in such a reaction, that person's plasma should not be used for any plasma-containing components.

ACUTE NONIMMUNOLOGIC

Acute nonimmunologic adverse effects are caused by external factors in the administration of blood: bacterial infection of the patient, contamination of the donor blood, improper handling of blood, and administration of a hypertonic fluid with the transfusion. An antigen–antibody reaction is absent.

Circulatory Overload

Transfusion-associated circulatory overload (TACO) may occur when blood or its components are infused at a rate exceeding the recipient's cardiac output. The consequence is volume overload. Patients susceptible to this adverse effect are the young and elderly and those with cardiac or renal disease. Symptoms include a pounding headache, dyspnea, constriction of the chest, coughing, hypertension, engorged neck veins, pulmonary edema, and heart failure. The transfusion must be stopped and the patient placed in a sitting position. Rapid-acting diuretics and oxygen usually relieve the symptoms.

Prevention consists of lung auscultation at the initiation of the transfusion and frequent monitoring during the transfusion for those patients susceptible to heart failure, the administration of diuretics before and/or between units, and the administration of concentrated components slowly. Additionally, the blood bank can be requested to divide the unit into two aliquots for slower administration; each aliquot can be administered over 2 to 4 hours, thus decreasing the risk of fluid overload. This adverse effect is preventable.

Air Embolism

The use of plastic bags has dramatically reduced this complication of transfusion therapy, which may result from faulty technique in changing equipment or plastic bags, careless use of Y-type administration sets, air infused from one of the containers when fluid and blood are pumped together, or when infusing blood under pressure before the container is empty (AABB, 2004). If air does enter the patient, acute cardiopulmonary insufficiency occurs. Symptoms are the same as those for circulatory collapse: cyanosis, dyspnea, shock, and occasionally cardiac arrest. The infusion should be stopped immediately and the patient turned on the left side, with the head down. This position traps air in the right atrium, preventing it from entering the pulmonary artery; the pulmonic valve is kept clear until the air can escape gradually. It may be necessary for the physician to aspirate the air with a transthoracic needle. This adverse effect is emergent and preventable.

Citrate Toxicity

Patients at risk for development of citrate toxicity or a calcium deficit are those who receive infusions of plasma, whole blood, or platelets at rates >100 mL/minute, or lower rates in patients who have liver disease. The liver, unable to keep up with the rapid administration, cannot metabolize the citrate, which chelates calcium, reducing the ionized calcium concentration. Hypocalcemia may induce cardiac arrhythmia. This adverse effect occurs infrequently, but may be encountered in emergency departments and operating rooms when large amounts of blood (1 unit every 5 minutes) and components have been administered. Symptoms of hypocalcemia include tingling of the fingers, muscular cramps, convulsions, tetanus, hyperactive reflexes, carpopedal spasm, laryngeal spasm, hypotension, and cardiopulmonary arrest (AABB, 2002a). Treatment consists of slowing the rate of infusion and the administration of calcium chloride or calcium gluconate solution. However, the calcium must never be added to any IV administration set infusing blood.

Hypothermia

Hypothermia occurs when large volumes of cold blood or blood components are infused rapidly. Rapid infusions may cause chills, hypothermia, peripheral vasoconstriction, ventricular arrhythmias, and cardiac arrest. Clinically, it is important to be certain that central catheters, if placed, are not positioned in the right atrium, a situation that can stimulate arrhythmias if rapid infusions are given. In many situations, warming blood to 37°C with automatic blood warmers during rapid, massive replacement prevents hypothermia. However, time does not always permit the equipment to be set up.

Electrolyte Disturbances

Electrolyte disturbances may occur in patients as a result of chronic infusions or the infusion of multiple units over a short time, exemplified by the hypocalcemia of citrate toxicity mentioned earlier in this section.

Hyperkalemia is a rare complication of blood transfusion. It can occur in large-volume transfusions in premature infants and newborns, patients with renal disease, and patients requiring massive transfusions. The total extracellular potassium is 0.5 mEq in a fresh unit of packed RBCs and 5 to 7 mEq in a unit of packed RBCs at its expiration date (AABB, 2002b). Signs and symptoms include cardiac rhythm changes, a slow irregular heartbeat, nausea, muscle weakness, diarrhea, flaccid paralysis and paresthesia of extremities, apprehension, and cardiac arrest.

Bacterial Contamination

Bacterial contamination of blood may occur at the time of donation or in preparing the component for infusion. In addition to skin contaminants, cold-resistant gram-negative bacteria and some gram-positive bacteria may contribute to this untoward event. Organisms such as *Yersinia enterocolitica*, *Pseudomonas* species, *Citrobacter freundii*, and *Escherichia coli* are potential causes (Goodnough, 2003). These organisms, capable of proliferating at refrigerator temperatures, and those using citrate as a nutrient (AABB, 2002a), release an endotoxin that initiates this rare, potentially fatal reaction.

Inspecting the unit before administration can prevent this complication. Observation of any discoloration or abnormal color of the blood or plasma, clumping, gas bubbles, extraneous material, or obvious clots should be reported to the blood bank.

Clinical manifestations of a septic reaction include high fever, flushing of the skin, "warm" shock, hematuria, renal failure, and DIC. These signs and symptoms are similar to those of an acute hemolytic reaction, so diagnosis must be made quickly. The transfusion should be discontinued; immediate therapy, including aggressive management of shock and administration of steroids and antibiotics, is required. Cultures obtained of the patient's blood, the suspected component, and all IV solutions determine whether the blood or an IV-related infection caused the bacteremia.

Many of the reactions discussed thus far are preventable. It is thought that the incidence of bedside transfusion error (ie, those happening when blood products have left the blood bank) is underestimated because many are medically treated and not reported as transfusion reactions. Quality improvement and monitoring measures can assist in avoiding other errors, as may computerized methods of verifying necessary data.

Delayed Effects

These complications occur days, weeks, months, or years after the transfusion and usually are the result of alloimmunization or transmitted disease.

DELAYED IMMUNOLOGIC

Delayed Hemolytic Reaction

Delayed hemolytic reactions, caused by an immune antibody created in response to a foreign antigen, (eg, Rh, Kell, Duffy, Kidd), are classified as primary and secondary. The primary or initial reaction usually is mild and may occur a week or more after the transfusion. Known as *primary alloimmunization*, it rarely produces symptoms and may be clinically insignificant. The degree of hemolysis depends on the quantity of antibody produced. The secondary reaction occurs in a patient previously immunized by transfusion or pregnancy. These patients have formed a red blood cell alloantibody, but the level of this alloantibody has become so low that it is serologically undetectable. On a later occasion, when donor red blood cells possessing the corresponding antigen are infused, they provoke a rapid increase in the specific antibody. The incompatible red blood cells survive until sufficient antibody is present to initiate a rejection response. The reaction is called a *secondary* or *anamnestic* (memory) response and is caused by re-exposure to the same antigen. These reactions are rarely caused by ABO incompatibility. Manifestations of a delayed hemolytic reaction include fever, mild jaundice, hemoglobinuria, and an unexplained drop in hemoglobin. Treatment is usually not necessary, although monitoring the patient's renal function may be needed. These coated cells are removed from the body by the reticuloendothelial system (extravascular hemolysis). A direct antiglobulin test may detect the antibody, and future donor units are selected that lack the corresponding antigen to the antibody formed.

Transfusion-Associated Graft-Versus-Host Disease

Transfusion-associated graft-versus-host disease (TAGVHD) is a complex, rare, and often fatal immunologic reaction. The usual cause appears to be the transfer of immunocompetent T lymphocytes in blood components to a severely immunocompromised patient. It may also occur as a result of a transfusion from a blood relative (AABB, 2004). The donor lymphocytes engraft and multiply in a severely immunodeficient recipient. These engrafted cells react against the foreign tissue of the host recipient, causing bleeding and infectious complications (AABB, 2002b).

The onset of TAGVHD is usually 10 to 12 days after transfusion (AABB, 2002b) and begins with a high fever. Generalized erythroderma, profuse diarrhea, widespread blistering, hepatitis, bone marrow suppression, and overwhelming infections may follow. TAGVHD is associated with a mortality rate of 75% to 90% of affected patients, and bone marrow suppression and infection are the causes of death.

The only approved method to prevent or reduce the incidence of TAGVHD is gamma irradiation of all blood components containing lymphocytes. Pre-transfusion inactivation of lymphocytes by irradiating cellular components reduces the risk of TAGVHD in the following situations: (a) fetuses receiving intrauterine transfusions, (b) selected immunoincompetent or immunocompromised recipients, (c) recipients of donor units known to be from a blood relative, (d) recipients who have undergone bone marrow or peripheral blood progenitor cell transplantation, (e) neonates undergoing exchange transfusion or use of extracorporeal membrane oxygenation, and (f) patients with Hodgkin's disease (AABB, 2002b).

DELAYED NONIMMUNOLOGIC

Cytomegalovirus Infection

Recognized to be present in blood and transmitted by transfusion, CMV poses little problem to most immunologically intact transfusion recipients. CMV is in the herpes virus family, and white cells are the major reservoir of CMV transmitted by blood (AABB, 2002a). Patients most at risk for serious consequences of the infection are those who have not been previously exposed and are immunoincompetent. These include low-birth-weight neonates, patients with malignancies who are immunosuppressed as a result of therapy for their disease, patients with acquired immunodeficiency syndrome (AIDS), and recipients of bone marrow and solid organ transplants. Many of these patients have depressed cell-mediated immunity and are at risk for development of systemic CMV infections, including pneumonia, hepatitis, retinitis, and mononucleosis-like symptoms. Careful screening of donors and use of blood from CMV-seronegative donors or those with depleted leukocytes are effective steps to reduce CMV infection in specific patient populations.

Hepatitis

Hepatitis often presents clinically with self-limiting fever, fatigue, and jaundice but may lead to progressive inflammation of the liver, resulting in cirrhosis or hepatic cancer. The clinical outcome of hepatitis, manifested by elevated liver enzymes and abnormal liver function tests, results in anorexia, fatigue, malaise, dark urine, fever, nausea, and jaundice; it usually resolves within 4 to 6 weeks. Treatment of symptoms is the aim of hepatitis management. Some patients demonstrate few symptoms, whereas others may become extremely ill and die of fulminating hepatic failure.

Post-transfusion hepatitis (PTH) has been recognized since the 1940s as a complication of receiving blood and potentially can be caused by HAV, HBV, HCV, hepatitis D virus (HDV), and hepatitis E virus (HEV). HAV and HEV are exceedingly rare causes of PTH, largely because the virus is present only during the acute phase of the disease and there is no carrier state. HDV needs HBV to replicate and must be transmitted at the same time as HBV into a person already infected with HBV. HDV usually is transmitted through IV drug use or sexual contact with an infected person and, as a superinfection, may worsen the course of chronic hepatitis B infection. The viruses predominantly responsible for PTH are HBV and HCV, although the risk of these infections from transfusions has been substantially reduced. The incidence of PTH has decreased dramatically since 1995 because of the thorough screening of donors and the use of more sensitive laboratory tests to identify at-risk donors.

Hepatitis B Virus.   Hepatitis B virus accounts for only a small proportion of cases of PTH. The primary reasons for this low incidence are screening of donors for behaviors that expose them to viral hepatitis and the testing of all donations for HBsAg and anti-HBc. The prevalence of the HBsAg carrier state in blood donations in the United States is approximately 0.02% to 0.04% (AABB, 2002b). The American Red Cross estimates the risk of PTH attributed to HBV as 1 in 205,000 per unit transfused (Pamper, Wu, & Snyder, 2003).

The average incubation period for HBV infection is 90 days, with a range of 30 to 180 days. Although most patients clear the virus, a proportion of patients remains chronically infected although asymptomatic. Becoming an HBsAg carrier is age dependent, with 5% of adults infected with HBV becoming carriers, compared with more than 90% of infants infected becoming carriers prior to immunization and routine prophylactic immunoglobulin infusion (AABB, 2002b). Hepatitis B can be transmitted directly by percutaneous needle inoculation or by transfusion of infected blood. It can be transmitted indirectly by percutaneous introduction of infectious serum, saliva, or semen through minute cuts or abrasions on the skin or mucosal surfaces. Health care workers are strongly advised to be immunized with hepatitis B vaccine to reduce the risk of acquiring HBV infection.

Hepatitis C Virus.   Hepatitis C virus is the major etiologic agent of PTH. The American Red Cross estimates the risk of PTH attributed to HBC as 1 in 1,935,000 per unit transfused (Pamper et al., 2003). At least 50% of HCV carriers have evidence of chronic liver disease, but most remain asymptomatic. Screening blood donors for antibody to HCV has been in place since 1998. An enzyme immunoassay (EIA) for antibodies to HCV is used to identify blood donors who have been exposed. Donors found to be repeatedly active by EIA are deferred. A supplemental test, the recombinant immunoblot assay, may be used to determine which reactive EIA results are true positives because the EIA screening test is extremely sensitive but not completely specific for HCV.

The modes of transmission of HCV appear to be similar to those of HBV; however, the route of HCV infection in many infected people is unknown. The incubation period for HCV is approximately 50 days, with a range of 15 to 180 days. The initial and acute illness is usually milder than in HBV and is often subclinical. Approximately 75% of patients are anicteric. Liver abnormalities persisting after 1 year indicate chronic hepatitis and predispose the patient to cirrhosis and liver failure. Chronic HCV infection also predisposes patients to hepatocellular carcinoma. Clinical management of chronic HCV infections may include a combination of ribavirin, an antiviral agent, and interferon-alfa (AABB, 2002b).

Human Immunodeficiency Virus

Human immunodeficiency virus (HIV) is a retrovirus that infects and kills CD4-positive lymphocytes (helper T cells), thereby disabling the cellular immune system. It produces severe immunosuppression and renders the infected person vulnerable to opportunistic infections and other symptoms such as fever, night sweats, weight loss, and skin lesions. HIV-2 (type 2) is similar to HIV-1 (type 1), but the incubation period appears to be longer and transmission is less efficient than for HIV-1 (AABB, 2002b).

HIV-1 and HIV-2 can both be transmitted by transfusions. Their existence has necessitated aggressive work to safeguard the blood supply. The first test for HIV antibody was developed and testing initiated in 1985. Since then, very few cases of HIV transmission by transfusion have occurred. The American Red Cross estimates the risk of post-transfusion HIV in the United States at 1 in 1,215,000 per unit transfused (Pamper et al., 2003).

Donated blood is tested for antibody to the virus (anti-HIV-1 and anti-HIV-2) using an EIA (AABB, 2002b). The confirmatory test for repeatedly reactive anti-HIV EIA tests is the Western blot.

Of concern are donors who may have been recently infected with HIV and are able to transmit the disease, but have not yet seroconverted. Since 1996, donated blood has also been tested for HIV-associated antigen p24, which appears sooner than HIV antibodies. This test reduces the phase known as the *infectious window*—that is, the period of time that the donor may be infectious, but still has negative serologic test results (Pamper et al., 2003). Since 2002, more sensitive tests based on nucleic acid technologies (NATs) are being used to test for HIV-infected donors. These tests have reduced the infectious window from 16 days to 11 days (Pamper et al.). These techniques have virtually eliminated transmission of enveloped viruses such as HBV, HCV, and HIV via plasma derivatives, but rare cases continue to be reported as a result of window periods (Pamper et al., 2003). Techniques also have been developed to inactivate viruses in plasma derivatives, such as antihemophilic factor, albumin, IVIG, and others.

Human T-Cell Lymphotropic Viruses

Types I and II human T-cell lymphotropic viruses are spread through viable lymphocytes in blood. Human T-cell lymphotropic virus type I is associated with adult T-cell lymphoma/leukemia and a neurologic disorder called HTLV-associated myelopathy or tropical spastic paraparesis (AABB, 2002b). Transmission is by breast milk, sexual contact, and exposure to blood. The prevalence of this disease varies widely geographically and is most common in Japan and other Pacific regions, Central and South America, and parts of Africa. The only disease known to be associated with the retrovirus HTLV-II is HTLV-associated myelopathy, but its occurrence is less frequent than with HTLV-I (AABB, 2002b). The virus is prevalent in some Native American populations and among IV drug users in the United States.

Plasma, which contains no lymphocytes, is not infective. The lymphocytes that transmit the virus are prone to degradation, so that red cell components stored for 10 days or more are less likely to transmit the virus than are fresher units. Testing for HTLV-I has been ongoing since 1988, and seropositive donors have been removed from donor pools. Testing for antibodies to HTLV-II began in 1997. Combination HTLV-I/II testing began in 1998 and offers more sensitive detection of both anti-HTLV-I and anti-HTLV-II, further reducing the risk of transfusion-transmitted HTLV-I/II. The frequency of transfusion-transmitted HTLV is quite low in the United States, with an American Red Cross estimate at 1 in 2,993,000 units transfused (Pamper et al., 2003). The Western blot is again confirmatory when an EIA screening test is positive for anti-HTLV-I and -II.

Malaria

Nearly eradicated in the United States and Canada, malaria is still prevalent in other parts of the world. The number of cases of transfusion-transmitted malaria reported in the United States is 0.25 cases per million transfusions (AABB, 2002b). Monitoring for this complication of transfusion is ongoing because of increased travel, immigration, and the continued presence of malaria in many areas of the world. No laboratory test is used widely to screen blood donors for malaria, and diagnosis still is made routinely by identifying the organism on a blood smear. The patient may have a high fever, chills, and headache, which reflect the lysis of infected red blood cells as they release the parasites into the bloodstream (AABB, 2002b). Prevention is accomplished by excluding donors from regions of the world where malaria is prevalent.

Prospective donors who have actually had malaria are deferred for 3 years after becoming asymptomatic (AABB, 2002b). Travelers who have visited an endemic area are deferred for 1 year. Immigrants, refugees, and citizens from endemic countries may be accepted as blood donors 3 years after departure from the area if they are asymptomatic. Donors with a history of babesiosis or Chagas disease are deferred permanently.

Syphilis

Serologic testing for syphilis (STS) is required on all donations, although refrigerated storage of red blood cell components has nearly eradicated the transmission of syphilis because temperatures of 4°C (39°F) have a spirocheticidal effect. Most likely, only components stored at room temperature or those administered within 72 hours after donation could transmit the disease. Positive STS results also may denote immunologic abnormalities unrelated to syphilis or inadequately treated syphilis, a fact that may be more helpful to the donor than the recipient (AABB, 2002b). There have been no reports of transfusion-transmitted syphilis in several decades.

West Nile Virus

West Nile virus (WNV), which first appeared in the United States in 1999, is a seasonal infection transmitted by the bite of an infected mosquito. The virus is not spread by human-to-human contact but by mosquitoes and carriers such as birds, cats, horses, squirrels, and rabbits. In response to the increase in West Nile virus infections in 2003, investigational nucleic acid technologies (NATs) were deployed to test for the West Nile viral genome. These NATs are performed regionally, and positive results have been reported in volunteer blood donors. WNV is a risk to blood recipients (Pamper et al., 2003).

Iron Overload

Iron overload or hemosiderosis may occur in patients with hemoglobinopathies who are receiving chronic transfusions. Each unit of packed RBCs contains 200 mg of iron. Signs and symptoms include hepatic failure and cardiac toxicity. Treatment involves the administration of deferoxamine mesylate (Desferal) to bind ferric ions to remove iron without reducing the patient's circulating hemoglobin.

Blood Administration

The administration of blood and blood components can be a lifesaving therapy; in contrast, fatal consequences can result from error or improper technique. Nurses must be well versed in every phase of therapy as well as knowledgeable about the administration of components and monitoring of patients during and after the transfusion. The patient's safety depends on adherence to specific rules regarding safe administration. Some institutions have delegated the administration of blood and blood components to a restricted group of specially trained personnel. If so, competency must be evident in knowledge and skill demonstration for all aspects of transfusion (Box 17–4). Ultimately, it is the nurse who has the accountability to advocate for the patient, conduct appropriate assessments, prevent complications, and intervene when there are reactions. Outcomes for the patient would include safe therapy, effective treatment, and satisfaction with care.

Blood Samples

Mislabeled specimens account for approximately one third of transfusion-related deaths. The intended recipient must be identified positively at the time of blood sample collection at the patient's bedside. Labeling requirements are aimed at preventing a potentially tragic outcome in patient care and significantly decrease errors in blood grouping. Labels must be affixed to the blood tubes and contain the institution's required information related to the recipient, including the date of sample collection and identification of the person drawing the specimen. Although an institution may define the length of time samples may be used, the general ruling is that samples intended for use in crossmatch should be collected no more than 3 days before the intended transfusion. This helps ensure that the sample reflects the recipient's current immunologic status (AABB, 2004).

BOX 17–4   Responsibilities of a Transfusionist

- Verifying the presence of a written physician's order for the transfusion
- Verifying that documented informed consent has been obtained from the patient
- Verifying ABO and Rh compatibility between donor and recipient
- Performing procedures relevant to patient and blood identification
- Inspecting the unit before administration
- Explaining the procedure to the patient
- Taking pre-transfusion vital signs
- Selecting and using proper technique and equipment
- Observing the patient for 15 minutes at the beginning of the transfusion
- Monitoring the patient throughout the transfusion or notifying the primary nurse of this accountability
- Documenting the transfusion according to established policy
- Taking post-transfusion vital signs

Issue and Transfer of Blood and Blood Components

Patient and blood identification is of paramount importance in preventing reactions from incompatible blood. The risk of identification errors is reduced by the use of triplicate requisitions or an online ordering system. Such requisitions, identifying the patient and indicating the amount and kind of blood and time needed, are usually sent to the blood bank with the blood sample.

The mode of transfer of blood components to the nursing unit depends on institutional policy. It may involve a pneumatic tube system, a messenger service, hospital personnel, or the person who will administer the blood. One of the most common causes of hemolytic reaction is the accidental administration of incompatible blood to the patient. To prevent administration of incompatible blood, only 1 unit should be transported by a person at a time.

Patient and Blood Identification

ABO-incompatible transfusions kill as many as 24 patients each year because of misidentification of crossmatch samples or recipients, a higher fatality rate than from HIV transmission. Omission of any of the validation steps can allow for misidentification. Absolute and positive identification of the donor blood and the patient must be made. All personnel handling the blood should be responsible for checking patient and blood identification. The nurse makes the final check and must decide whether to administer the blood or question it. ABO and Rh compatibility identification is made by comparing the patient's previous ABO and Rh determination with patient's and donor's ABO and Rh on the compatibility tag; and also the blood identification number on the blood container with the identification number on the blood tag and the blood unit itself. Many health care facilities have incorporated computer information and validating systems to tie the patient to the blood bank for more reliable checking. Bar coding will be mandated by 2006 for all hospital setting transfusions.

Patient identification is made by checking two identifiers, and neither of the identifiers can be a room number. Each institution will have a policy naming the two identifiers. The patient must identify himself or herself by complete name. Identity should never be made by addressing the patient by name and awaiting a response. Errors can occur from faulty response of medicated patients. Patients unable to respond may be identified by the primary or attending nurse. Hospital numbers on the identification bracelet must match hospital numbers on the tag to prevent errors in cases of similar names. Any discrepancy must be investigated and corrected before the blood is administered. Blood must never be administered to a patient who has no identification bracelet.

In summary, the person performing the transfusion is responsible for the verification of information regarding the component, proper patient identification, administration, and documentation. Transfusion information is part of the patient's permanent record (see Box 17–4).

Reducing Blood Exposure and High-Risk Injuries

NEEDLELESS DEVICES

Health care workers are at risk for acquiring blood-borne infections through needle stick exposure to blood-filled hollow-bore needles commonly used for vascular access and blood sampling. Of greatest concern are HIV, HBV, and HCV. Shielded or self-blunting needles for vacuum tube phlebotomy, shielded butterfly needles, automatically retracting fingerstick/heelstick lancets, and plastic capillary tubes should be used for blood sampling. When the nurse needs to obtain IV access for the administration of the transfusion, IV catheters designed to prevent stylet injuries should be used. When connecting the transfusion to a primary line, blunted or integrated safety devices designed to reduce injury should be used.

BARRIER PROTECTION

Barrier protection must be used when exposure to blood may occur. Minimal protection consists of gloves for handling any blood component; liquid-resistant gowns and protective eyewear may be advisable in emergency and trauma settings. In addition, electronic infusion devices used to administer blood and blood components should have tight, Luer-locking connections to prevent high-pressure rupture, thus avoiding risk of blood exposure. Latex-free gloves and equipment are strongly recommended and required for any patient with a history of latex sensitivities.

Handling Blood

To prevent excessive warming, blood transfusion must be initiated within 30 minutes of the time it leaves the blood bank. If blood is not maintained at 1°C to 10°C (34°F to 50°F) while outside the control of the blood bank, it cannot be reissued. Banked blood stored at 1°C to 6°C (34°F to 43°F) will exceed 10°C (50°F) in approximately 30 minutes at room temperature; blood that cannot be administered immediately should be returned to the blood bank within this time. Blood should never be placed in the patient care unit refrigerators because they are not controlled and contain no alarms to warn of temperature fluctuation.

If warmed blood is ordered, an FDA-approved blood-warming device that maintains a controlled temperature should be used to warm the blood. Equipment should have a visible thermometer and an audible warning alarm. Temperatures must not rise above 37°C. These warming devices should be available in emergency departments, where it is common to administer blood rapidly. Patients receiving many units of cold blood rapidly (ie, 100 mL/minute) reportedly have increased incidences of cardiac arrest. Hot water and standard microwave ovens must never be used to warm blood.

Before the blood component is administered, the expiration date should be noted to avoid infusion of an outdated component. Sodium chloride injection, USP 0.9% (normal saline), may be used to initiate the infusion and flush administration sets at the completion of the transfusion of red blood cells, whole blood, platelets, or leukocytes. Hypotonic or hypertonic solutions should not be used to dilute blood. Extreme hypotonicity causes water to invade the red blood cells until they burst (ie, hemolysis). Hypertonic solutions dilute blood, resulting in reversal of this process with shrinkage of the red blood cells.

No medication or IV fluid (with the exception of 0.9% sodium chloride) should be added to blood or administered simultaneously through the same set unless it has been approved for this use by the FDA and available records show that the addition is safe and does not adversely affect the blood component.

Venipuncture

Peripheral veins with an adequate diameter should be used to ensure the flow of viscous components. The lower extremities are avoided in adults because thrombosis and blood pooling may occur. Areas of joint flexion should also be avoided. The peripheral IV site should be checked frequently during the infusion for early detection of infiltration. Red blood cells and whole blood can usually be administered through an 18- or 20-gauge catheter, although smaller gauges may be used for other components. A 22-gauge catheter may be used for pediatric patients, older adults, or those adults with fragile veins and skin. When a smaller catheter is used, infuse the blood or components slowly, over 2 to 3 hours, to reduce hemolysis of cells.

Blood and blood components may be administered through central venous catheters including short-term catheters such as a subclavian catheter and long-term access devices such as tunneled catheters or implanted ports. Increasing numbers of peripherally inserted central catheters and midline catheters are being placed in patients receiving long-term IV therapy. In most situations, components infuse in a timely manner through 20- to 22-gauge or larger peripherally inserted central catheters. If a dual-lumen catheter has been placed, the larger lumen should be reserved for transfusions. It is necessary to flush the catheter adequately with normal saline at the conclusion of the transfusion. A minimum of 10 mL normal saline should be used to flush the catheter vigorously after transfusion.

Rate of Infusion

The rate of infusion is governed by the clinical condition of the patient, the type and viscosity of the component being infused, and the catheter's internal diameter (gauge). Nurses have an important role in assessing the patient's clinical condition and ensuring proper rate of administration. Macrobore IV administrations sets should be used and changed after every unit or every 4 hours. Infusions should be set at a slow rate for the first 15 minutes to avoid infusion of a large quantity of blood in case of an immediate reaction. If venous spasm occurs from the infusion of cold blood, a warm pack applied to the vein through which the blood is being infused relieves the spasm and increases the rate of flow.

Most patients can tolerate infusions of 1 unit of red blood cells over 1 to 2 hours (AABB, 2002b). Patients in heart failure or at risk of fluid overload require infusions given over a longer time, but not to exceed 4 hours from the time the blood or component was released from the blood bank. If necessary, the blood bank can divide a unit of red blood cells into two aliquots that are given as two separate infusions. Each aliquot may be given over 3 to 4 hours to reduce fluid overload. If the infusion is lasting more than 2 hours, gently turn the bag over two or three times to keep the cells in suspension. Large-gauge catheters should be used when it is necessary to infuse blood rapidly; approved external-pressure devices may be used if necessary. Physicians need to be readily available because certain risks are inherent in rapid volume replacement. Electronic infusion devices for the administration of blood and its components are frequently required and especially important for slow rates of infusion to elderly, pediatric, and neonatal patients.

Blood Filters

A standard (usually 170 to 260 micron), sterile, pyrogen-free blood filter designed to remove debris, including clots, is acceptable for administration of most blood components. For best flow rates, the entire surface area of the filter should be filled with the component. A single filter may be used to infuse 2 to 4 units of blood, although some institutions have a policy that a new filter be used with each component. Filters need to be added to dedicated infusion pump sets. Once the blood filter contains debris, it should be discarded. Continued use of such filters may result in bacterial contamination, a slowed rate of infusion, or hemolysis of the blood at room temperature.

MICROAGGREGATE FILTERS

The demonstration of microaggregates, composed of leukocytes, platelets, and fibrin, led to the manufacture of microaggregate filters in the early 1960s. Over time, the filters evolved into depth filters with high efficiency. Pore size is 20 to 40 microns, and they are used for the administration of red blood cells. The volume required for priming is significant; thus, flushing the set with isotonic saline at completion of the

---

BOX 17–5 Critical Points to Address With the Patient

Patient Transfusion History

- Previous reactions may trigger need to pre-medicate the patient. Review patient record and interview patient to identify previous reactions and interventions.
- Goal: Lessen potential reactions, relieve anxiety.

Latex Sensitivity

- Use only latex-free equipment.
- Goal: Eliminate any progression of reaction.

Signed Transfusion Consent Form From Patient

- All patients must be informed of administration of blood or blood components. The patient or parent must sign forms, which a physician must witness. Some institutions grant privileges to nurse practitioners to witness transfusion consents.
- Goal: patient awareness and participation in course of therapy

Patient Education

- Inform the patient of the steps involved in having a transfusion; include length of time for the transfusion and expected outcomes.
- Instruct patient regarding signs and symptoms that could indicate a reaction.
- Share with the patient how important their personal report is to detect reactions early.
- Goals: early identification of potential reactions; lessen anxiety.

---

transfusion is recommended. Pediatric microaggregate filters are useful because of the small priming volume rather than the removal of debris.

LEUKOCYTE REMOVAL FILTERS

Red blood cell and platelet leukocyte removal filters are available to reduce a number of transfusion-associated complications: HLA alloimmunization and platelet refractoriness, transmission of cell-associated viruses (CMV), and febrile non-hemolytic reactions. Clinical conditions where benefit is realized include patients with cancer and those with renal disease, who may become immunocompromised and are at risk of alloimmunization. These filters, which remove approximately 98% of leukocytes, are quick and convenient to prime and are increasingly being used for filtration at the bedside. Some institutions pre-filter the transfusion before dispensing it from the blood bank, a practice that seems to be growing. The filters are efficient and effective, and provide a convenient method of removing leukocytes. Filters are designed for either red blood cells or platelets and should not be interchanged. These filters have no effect on the shelf life of the unit. Filters are not required for the infusion of albumin or immune globulin.

Patient Monitoring and Education

After initiation of the transfusion, the nurse-transfusionist should observe the patient for the initial 15 minutes of the infusion or longer based on professional judgment (AABB, 2002b). Staying with the patient or being in close observation is critical to detect a reaction and be immediately responsive. Many of the fatal incompatible transfusion reactions produce symptoms early in the course of the infusion. Primary nurses also share a responsibility for safe transfusion administration. They must be familiar with the various transfusion reactions, be able to recognize adverse reactions, and know what procedures to follow. The patient's report of his or her subjective symptoms is often the first indication of a reaction. Changes in vital signs or objective signs are other indicators. Box 17–5 outlines critical points in this process.

Documenting the Transfusion

All data relevant to the transfusion should be recorded in the patient's clinical and transfusion records. The time the transfusion was complete, the volume of fluid infused, and the condition of the patient should be noted. Observation of the patient for 1 hour after the transfusion is recommended. Post-transfusion monitoring of vital signs and laboratory values ensures that the clinical goal was achieved. Latex sensitivity or any other comments about the transfusion should be noted. Legal and safety issues are summarized in Box 17–6.

BOX 17–6   Legal and Safety Issues for Transfusion Therapy

- All healthcare institutional policies and procedures address the standards and guidelines of the American Association of Blood Banks, the Food and Drug Administration, and those of professional health care–related agencies (such as the Infusion Nurses Society, the Institute of Medicine, the National Patient Safety Foundation, and the Oncology Nursing Society) as appropriate.
  - Policies and procedures incorporate standards and guidelines for all facets of patient care across all settings as needed.
  - Policies and procedures are jointly reviewed and approved by the nurse executive and staff nurse committee, the blood bank or transfusion service, and the medical director or medical executive committee.
- Patients are identified using two methods of identification and two health care providers, one of whom is the transfusionist.
- Informed consent is obtained for blood and blood components; patient refusal would include all blood components.
- Standard precautions should specify how to draw blood samples and administer the transfusion to prevent exposure to blood-borne pathogens.
  - Latex-free equipment is available for latex-sensitive patients and personnel.
  - Policy is established and equipment is provided to prevent accidental blood exposure and needle-stick injury.
- The entire transfusion and the patient's reactions are documented according to institutional practice.
- Monitoring for quality and safety is ongoing.

Disposal of Equipment

Sharps must be disposed of in specially designed, puncture-resistant, leak-proof containers located near the area of use. All transfusion-related equipment should be placed in biohazard containers. Administration sets used to infuse blood components should be discarded within 4 hours after use. Bacterial growth may occur on the trapped proteins and debris contained in the set. Institutional guidelines for observing standard precautions should be followed.

KEY INTERVENTIONS: Administration of Whole Blood or Red Blood Cell Components

1. Obtain vital signs before blood arrives on the unit; this ensures prompt and timely administration. If patient's temperature is 38.8°C or 100°F or greater, notify the physician before requesting blood or component from the blood bank. An elevated temperature is not a contraindication to the transfusion, but it may make assessment and decisions regarding blood reactions difficult (Simmons, 2003).

   Assemble equipment: whole blood or red blood cell component; blood recipient set; blunt cannula if connecting to primary IV; alcohol prep pad; electronic infusion device, if needed; equipment for performing IV access if patient does not have an IV line.
2. Verify written order for transfusion.
3. Verify signed transfusion consent form.
4. Verify the blood component for donor/recipient ABO and Rh compatibility.
5. Confirm that blood numbers on the component match those on transfusion requisition.
6. Check expiration date of the component.
7. Use two identifiers for positive patient identification. Confirm that blood numbers on component match numbers on patient's identification band.
8. At bedside set up equipment for transfusion. Clamp-on blood recipient set should be closed.
9. Open one tab port of component bag and insert the spike of the blood recipient set into this port.
10. Invert and hang the component bag on IV pole.
11. Prime filter and fill drip chamber of blood recipient set half full. Prime entire surface of filter for best flow rates. Open clamp and flush all air from the line. Close clamp.
12. Attach appropriate blunt cannula to blood set if blood will be infusing by primary IV. Sodium chloride 0.9% should be used to flush any set that may contain a drug incompatible with red blood cells.
13. Scrub the injection site with alcohol and attach the blunt cannula into the injection site. Secure catheter tightly.
14. Regulate component to prescribed rate or set pump to desired rate. All blood must be infused within 4 hours from the time it was released from the blood bank.
15. Take vital signs before the start of the infusion, after the first 15 minutes of the infusion, and at the conclusion of the transfusion. Record date, time, and signature on blood requisition that accompanies the blood component. Place in appropriate part of patient's record. Document the patient's immediate response to initial administration of red blood cells, whole blood, or other blood component.

NOTE: This procedure can be converted for institutions using multilead blood administration sets. This procedure also may be modified for the administration of plasma and single-donor platelets.

Factor V Leiden

Factor V Leiden is a variant of the protein factor V (5), which is needed for blood clotting. People who have a factor V deficiency are more likely to bleed severely whereas people with factor V Leiden have blood that has an increased tendency to clot. Those who carry the factor V Leiden gene have a five times greater risk of developing thrombosis than the rest of the population. However, many people with the gene will never suffer from blood clots.

In Britain, 5% of the population carry one or more genes for factor V Leiden, which is far more than the number of people who will actually suffer from thrombosis. Factor V Leiden is the most common hereditary blood coagulation disorder in the United States. It is present in 5% of the White population and in 1.2% of the Black population.

Factor V Leiden increases the risk of venous thrombosis threefold to eightfold for **heterozygous** (one bad gene inherited) individuals and substantially more, 30- to 140-fold, for **homozygous** (two bad genes inherited) individuals. The prothrombin 20210 mutation is the second most common inherited clotting abnormality. It is more common than protein S and C deficiency and antithrombin deficiency combined; 2% of the general population is heterozygous. It is only a mild risk factor for clots, but together with other risk factors (such as oral contraceptives, surgery, trauma, high blood pressure, obesity, smoking, etc.) or combined with other clotting disorders (like factor V Leiden), the risk of clotting increases dramatically (Fig. 17–2).

Although patients with the factor V Leiden or the prothrombin gene G20210A mutations have an elevated risk for symptomatic thrombosis following surgery, studies (Ruggeri et al., 2002; Wahlander et al., 2002) have shown that 90% of the patients will not have such an event. Thus, the general preoperative screening for such genotypes is of questionable value (Box 17–7).

Treatment of Factor V Leiden

Treatment of a patient with factor V Leiden depends on the individual patient's risk of recurrent thromboembolic disease. When one has a venous clot, regardless of what thrombophilic state(s) one may have, that person will receive anticoagulation. This is accomplished by several different medications: heparin, warfarin, and low-molecular-weight heparins. These medications are generally used for 3 to 6 months. Further continuation is generally not indicated in factor V Leiden heterozygotes after a single thromboembolic episode, given the risk of bleeding associated with anticoagulation. Patients who have had multiple thromboembolic episodes or are at high risk of further episodes (for example, those with multiple deficiencies or factor V Leiden homozygotes) are likely started on long-term anticoagulation. The use of Lovenox may be indicated prior to long plane flights and other activities that increase risk of clotting.

Long-term anticoagulation has risks associated with it (approximately a 3% chance per year of having a major hemorrhage, of which approximately one in five are fatal). Beginning long-term anticoagulation is influenced by the patient's overall

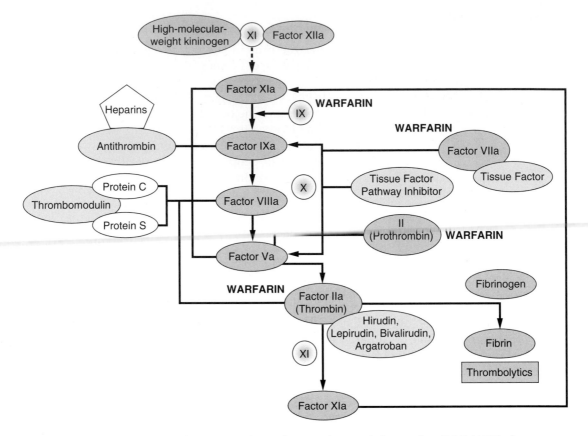

FIGURE 17–2. Clotting Cascade. Source: www-admin.med.uiuc.edu/hematology/PDF%20Files/ Medications.pdf. Accessed March 15, 2005.

BOX 17–7   Complications Associated With Factor V Leiden

- Venous thrombosis blood clots in veins, such as:
  - Deep vein thrombosis (DVT), veins in arms and legs
  - Superficial thrombophlebitis
  - Sinus vein thrombosis, veins around the brain
  - Mesenteric vein thrombosis, intestinal veins
  - Budd-Chiari syndrome, liver veins
- Pulmonary embolism (PE), blood clots in the lungs
- Arterial clots (stroke, heart attack) in selected patients (some smokers)
- Possibly with stillbirth or recurrent unexplained miscarriage
- Pre-eclampsia and/or eclampsia (toxemia while pregnant)

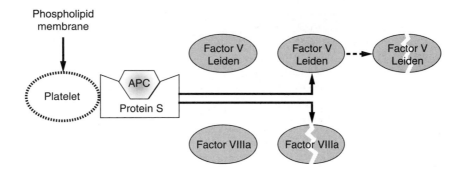

FIGURE 17–3. Effect of Factor V Leiden on activated protein C. The formation of APC is not altered by the presence of Factor V Leiden. However, the complex of APC and protein S on the platelet phospholipid's surface cannot inactivate Factor V Leiden as efficiently as it normally can (occurs about 80 times slower than is normal). It is able to inactivate Factor VIIIa normally. This is known as activated protein C resistance. Source: http://www.admin.med.uiuc.edu/hematology/PtFacV2.htm. Accessed March 30, 2005.

risk of recurrent thrombosis balanced against the risks associated with long-term anticoagulation on an individual basis.

Terminology

The terms heterozygous (*hetero*, different) and homozygous (*homo*, same) are terms used in genetics. The human genome contains two copies of the information. If the copies are the same, they are homozygous; if the copies are different, they are heterozygous. For example, take a protein called A. The normal genome would code for the protein as AA. This is homozygous for the normal protein. If there is a variation of the protein called a, there are two possible ways to get the a. The genome could be Aa, which is called heterozygous, or the genome could be aa, which is called homozygous (Fig 17–3).

References and Selected Readings

Asterisks indicate references cited in text.

*American Association of Blood Banks, America's Blood Centers, & American Red Cross. (2002a). *Circular of information for the use of human blood and blood components.* Bethesda, MD: Author.

*American Association of Blood Banks (2002b). *Technical manual* (14th ed.).Bethesda, MD: Author.

American Association of Blood Banks. (2003). *Standards for blood banks & transfusion services* (22nd ed.). Bethesda, MD: Author.

*American Association of Blood Banks (2004). *Primer of blood administration.* Bethesda, MD: Author.

*American Association of Blood Banks. (2005). *Facts about blood and blood banking.* Retrieved February 1, 2005, from http://www.aabb.org/All_About_Blood/FAQs/aabb_faqs.htm

*Brecher, M.E., & Goodnough, L.T. (2002). The rise and fall of preoperative autologous blood donation. *Transfusion,* 42(12), 1618–1622.

*Bryan, S. (2002). Hemolytic transfusion reaction: Safeguards for practice. *Journal of Perianesthesia Nursing, 17,* 399–403.

*Chan, J., Chu, R., Young, B., et al. (2004). Use of an electronic barcode system for patient identification during blood transfusion: 3-year experiences in a regional hospital. *Hong Kong Medical Journal, 10,* 166–171.

Clotting cascade. Available at http://www-admin.med.uiuc.edu/hematology/PtFacV2.htm. Accessed March 1, 2005.

*Dohnalek, L., Cusaac, L., Westcott, J., Langeberg, A., & Sandler, S. (2004). The code to safer transfusions: Bar code-enabled point-of-care systems reduce transfusion errors. *Nursing Management, 35*(6), 33–36.

*Dzik, W. (2003). Emily Cooley lecture 2002: Transfusion safety in the hospital. *Transfusion, 43,* 1190–1199.

*Galel, S.A., Malone, J.M., & Viele, M.K. (2004). Transfusion medicine. In: J. Greer, J. Foerster, J. Lukens, G. Rodgers, F. Paraskevas, & D. Glader (Eds.). *Wintrobe's clinical hematology* (pp. 832–882). Philadelphia, PA: Lippincott Williams & Wilkins.

*Gaspard, K. (2005). Hematopoietic system. In C. Porth, *Pathophysiology: Concepts of altered health states* (7th ed, pp. 279–285). Philadelphia, PA: Lippincott Williams & Wilkins.

*Goodman, C., Chan, S., Collins, P., Haught, R., & Chen Y. (2003). Ensuring blood safety and availability in the US: Technological advances, costs, and challenges to payment – final report. *Transfusion, 43*(S), 3S–46S.

*Goodnough, L.T. (2003). Risks of blood transfusion. *Critical Care Medicine, 31*(12 Suppl), S678–S686.

Goodnough, L., Shander, A., & Brecher, M. (2003). Transfusion medicine: Looking to the future. *Lancet, 361*(9352), 161–169.

*Harrod, K.S., Hanson, L., VandeVusse, L., & Heywood, P. (2003). Rh negative status and isoimmunization update: A case-based approach. *The Journal of Perinatal and Neonatal Nursing, 17*(3), 166–180.

Infusion Nurses Society. (2000). Infusion nursing Standards of Practice. Cambridge, MA: Author.

*Institute of Medicine: L. Kohn, J. Corrigna, & M. Donaldson (Eds.). (2000). *To err is human: Building a safer health system.* Washington, DC: National Academy Press.

*Institute of Medicine: A. Page (Ed.). (2004). *Keeping patients safe: Transforming the work environment of nurses.* Washington, DC: National Academies Press.

*Joint Commission on Accreditation of Healthcare Organizations. (2005). *2005 national patient safety goals.* Retrieved February 1, 2005, from http://www.jcaho.org/accredited+organizations/patient+safety/npsg.htm.

*Knezevic-Maramica, I. & Kruskall, M.S. (2003). Intravenous immune globulins: An update for clinicians. *Transfusion, 43*(10), 1460–1480.

*Kopko, P.M., Marshall, C.S., Malcom, R., Holland, P.V., & Popovskey, M.A. (2002). Transfusion-related acute lung injury – report of clinical look-back investigation. *Journal of the American Medical Association, 287*(15), 1968–1971.

*Lee, D., Mehta, M., & James, P. (2003). Differences in the perception of blood transfusion risk between laypeople and physicians. *Transfusion, 43,* 772–778.

*Massachusetts Public Health Biologic Laboratories (2004). Cytomegalovirus immune globulin intravenous (human). Boston: Author. Retrieved January 21, 2005, from http://www.rxlist.com/cgi/generic2/cytogam_ids. htm.

*McCullough, J. (2003). Transfusion medicine: Discipline with a future. *Transfusion, 43,* 823–828.

*Miller, C. (2004). Transfusion therapy. In M. Alexander & A. Corrigan (Eds.). *Core curriculum for infusion nursing* (3rd ed., pp. 299–316). Philadelphia: Lippincott, Williams, and Wilkins.

*Nichols, W.G., & Boeckh, M. (2000). Recent advances in the therapy and prevention of CMF infections. *Journal of Clinical Virology, 16*(1), 25–40.

*Pamper, G.J., Wu, Y.Y., & Snyder, E.L. (2003). Risks of transfusion transmitted infections: 2003. *Current Opinion in Hematology, 10*(6), 412–418.

*Porte, R., & Leebeek, W. (2002). Pharmacological strategies to decrease transfusion requirements in patients undergoing surgery. *Drugs, 62,* 2193–2211.

*Roberts, H.R., & Hoffman, M. (2001). Hemophilia A and hemophilia B. In: E. Beutler, M.A. Lichtman, B.S. Coller, T.J. Kipps, & U. Seligsohn (Eds.). *Williams hematology* (6th ed., pp. 1639–1657). New York: McGraw-Hill Medical Publishing Division.

*Rudnicke, C. (2003). Transfusion alternatives. *Journal of Infusion Nursing, 26,* 29–33.

*Ruggeri, M., Gisslinger, H., Tosetto, A., et al. (2002). Factor 5 Leiden mutation carriership and venous thromboembolism in polycythemia vera and essential thrombocythemia. *American Journal of Hematology, 71,* 1–6.

*Saxena, S., Ramer, L., & Shulman, I. (2004). A comprehensive assessment program to improve blood administrating practices using the FOCUSS-PDCA model. *Transfusion, 44,* 1350–1356.

*Schleis, T. (2000). The financial, operational, and clinical management of intravenous immunoglobulin administration. *Journal of IV Nursing, 23*(5S), S23–S31.

*Simmons, P. (2003). A primer for nurses who administer blood components. *MedSurg Nursing, 12,* 184–192.

*Sommer, C. (2002). Immunity and inflammation. In: C.M. Porth & M.P. Kunert (Eds.). *Pathophysiology concepts of altered health states* (6th ed., pp. 331–356). Philadelphia: Lippincott, Williams, & Wilkins.

*Tsatsoulis, D., & Amthauer, H. (2003). Finding clusters of similar events within clinical incident reports: A novel methodology combining case based reasoning and information retrieval. *Quality Safe Health Care, 12*(IIS), ii24–ii32.

*Turner, C., Casbard, A., & Murphy, M. (2003). Barcode technology: Its role in increasing the safety of blood transfusion. *Transfusion, 43,* 1200–1209.

*U.S. Department of Health and Human Services: Food and Drug Administration. (2004). *Bar code label requirement for human drug products and biological products: Final Rule.* Federal Register: February 26, 2004, 9119–9171.

*Wahlander, K., Larson, G., Lindahl, T.L., et al. (2002) Factor 5 Leiden and prothrombin gene mutations as potential risk factors for venous thromboembolism after total hip or total knee replacement surgery. *Thrombosis and Haemostasis, 87,* 580–585.

*Ward, N., & Levy, M. (2004). Blood transfusion practice today. *Critical Care Clinics, 20,* 179–186.

*Webert, K., Chan, H., Smith, J., Heddle, N., & Kelton, J. (2004). Red cell, platelet, and white cell antigens. In: J. Greer, J. Foerster, J. Lukens, G. Rodgers, F. Paraskevas, & B. Glader (Eds.). *Wintrobe's clinical hematology* (pp. 792–831). Philadelphia: Lippincott Williams & Wilkins.

Review Questions

Note: Questions below may have more than one right answer.

1. The antigen in the ABO system that denotes a person's blood group is located:
   A. On the red blood cell
   B. In the plasma
   C. In the serum
   D. On body tissue

2. Which of the following may stimulate a reaction?
   I. Antigen A combining with anti-A antibody
   II. Antigen AB combining with anti-AB antibody
   III. Antigen B combining with anti-A antibody
   IV. Antigen D combining with anti-D antibody
   A. I and II
   B. III and IV
   C. I, II, and IV
   D. All of the above

3. Methods to reduce febrile nonhemolytic transfusion reactions include:
   A. Washed red cells with a standard 80- to 170-micron filter
   B. Packed red cells with a leukocyte filter
   C. Packed red cells with a standard 80- to 170-micron filter
   D. All of the above

4. The most important intervention for patients with IVIG-associated nonallergic reactions is to:
   A. Slow the infusion rate
   B. Discontinue the infusion
   C. Continue rate because reaction will resolve
   D. Stop the infusion for 4 to 8 hours; then resume therapy

5. A patient, group O, may receive red blood cells from a donor who is:
   A. Group A only
   B. Group O only
   C. Group A or O
   D. Any group

6. A patient, group AB, may receive plasma from a donor who is:
   A. Group A, AB, or O
   B. Group AB or O
   C. Group AB only
   D. Any group

7. Intravascular hemolytic reactions are potentially caused by:
   A. ABO incompatibility
   B. Rh incompatibility
   C. ABO and Rh incompatibility
   D. None of the above

8. The primary cause of post-transfusion hepatitis is:

   A. HAV and HBV

   B. HBV and HCV

   C. HAV and HDV

   D. HBV only

9. A patient experiences the following signs and symptoms 1 hour after a unit of packed red blood cells has been infused: chills, increased pulse rate, fever, and facial flushing. Which of the following adverse reactions is suspected?

   A. Anaphylaxis

   B. Citrate toxicity

   C. Congestive heart failure

   D. Febrile nonhemolytic reaction

10. An elderly patient with a history of heart failure is most at risk for which potential adverse reaction from a unit of packed red blood cells?

    A. Circulatory overload

    B. Iron overload

    C. Acute hemolytic reaction

    D. Hypersensitivity reaction

CHAPTER 18

Pharmacology Applied to Infusion Therapy

KEY TERMS

Compartment Models
Double Decomposition
Drug Concentration
Half-life
Hydrolysis
Incompatibility
Laminar Flow
Oxidation

pH
Pharmacokinetics
Plasma Concentration
Precipitation
Receptor Site
Reduction
Therapeutic Index

Administering Drug Therapy by the Intravenous Route

The nurse whose patients receive IV drug therapy needs to be well versed in the advantages and disadvantages of drug therapy delivered by the IV route. The nurse also needs to be a skilled practitioner who can administer IV drugs safely, prevent potential hazards, and monitor the patient's response to therapy.

Advantages of the Intravenous Route

The IV route of drug administration offers pronounced advantages, particularly for patients who cannot take medications orally or for those who need medications that cannot be absorbed by any other route. The IV route allows drugs to be administered to a patient who cannot tolerate fluids and drugs by the gastrointestinal route, and the capacity for slow administration permits drug delivery to be stopped at once if sensitivity reactions occur.

In some cases, the large molecular size of certain drugs prevents absorption by the gastrointestinal route, whereas other drugs, unstable in the presence of gastric juices, are destroyed. The IV route is also appropriate for some drugs that, because of their irritating properties, cause pain and trauma when given intramuscularly or subcutaneously. The vascular system affords a means for providing rapid drug action because the drug bypasses processing in the gastrointestinal system and circulates directly in the bloodstream. Moreover, the IV route offers better control over the rate of administration of drugs; prolonged action can be provided by administering a dilute infusion intermittently or over a prolonged period.

To understand how the IV route offers rapid drug action and better control over the duration of drug action, the nurse must understand the basics of pharmacokinetics, pharmacodynamics, and pharmacotherapeutics.

Pharmacokinetics and Selected Parameters for Intravenous Drugs

The pharmacokinetic basis of therapeutics relies on various factors, such as the drug's route and frequency of administration, to achieve and maintain a proper **drug concentration** at the **receptor site**, wherever that site may be in the body. If an insufficient amount of drug reaches this site, the drug's action may appear to be ineffective, and therapy may therefore be discontinued. Conversely, what seems to be the right amount of a drug may produce toxicity, and therefore therapy may be discontinued simply because excessive amounts are in the body. An awareness of how drug **pharmacokinetics** (the way a drug is absorbed, distributed, metabolized, and eliminated by the body) affects the body is an essential part of reducing and preventing potential toxicity through excess drug dosages. Factors influencing the pharmacokinetics of drugs are presented in Box 18–1.

THERAPEUTIC INDEX

Some aspects of pharmacokinetics that are particularly relevant to IV drug administration are the therapeutic index, plasma concentration, and drug distribution. The **therapeutic index** is the margin between a drug's therapeutic and toxic concentrations

---

BOX 18–1   Factors Influencing the Pharmacokinetics of Drugs

Patient Characteristics

Age, sex, body weight, dietary habits, smoking habits, alcohol consumption, coingestion of other drugs

Disease States

Hepatic disease, renal disease, congestive heart failure, infection, fever, shock, severe burns

FIGURE 18–1. Concentration–time curves after IV injection at three different rates.

at the receptor site. Pharmacokinetic models describe and predict drug amounts and concentrations in various body fluids and the changes in these quantities over time.

PLASMA CONCENTRATIONS

Plasma concentration is a measurement representing drug that is bound to plasma protein plus drug that is unbound or free. Two factors determine the degree of plasma protein binding. The first is the binding affinity of the drug for the plasma proteins; the second is the number of binding sites available or the concentration of plasma protein. An acidic drug, such as salicylate or phenytoin, may be bound to albumin. A basic drug, such as lidocaine or quinidine, may be bound to serum globulins. Calculated plasma concentrations may assist the physician in evaluating the effectiveness of therapy. Figure 18–1 shows concentration–time curves after IV drug injection at three different rates.

DISTRIBUTION AND COMPARTMENT MODELS

Knowledge of **compartment models** enables the nurse to better understand pharmacokinetic distribution principles. In the one-compartment model, when a drug is introduced into the body, it is rapidly and homogeneously distributed throughout the entire space (compartment). Precise anatomic sites of drug distribution can be determined only by direct analysis of tissue concentrations, which is possible only in animal studies.

In the two-compartment model, the body can be divided into two compartments, a central compartment and a peripheral compartment. These compartments also may be given anatomic designations, such as the plasma compartment and the tissue compartment. The central compartment may correspond approximately to the vascular system, together with rapidly perfused lean tissues such as heart, liver, lung, kidneys, brain, and endocrine organs. The peripheral compartment corresponds to body fat, together with poorly perfused lean tissues (ie, skin and muscle). The drug concentration levels we monitor are assessed through the central compartment (ie, blood). Drug behavior in the body depends on both distribution and elimination. (American Society of Health-System Pharmacists [ASHP], 1998)

THERAPEUTIC CONCENTRATION AND LOADING DOSE

The drug concentration level may be calculated after the dosage regimen is initiated to ensure that the selected dosage produces the drug concentration desired. It may also be measured periodically to ensure that the dosage continues to produce the desired target concentration or to determine if the therapeutic regimen is failing. Table 18–1 highlights therapeutic drug concentrations and toxic values.

The loading dose is the initial dose of drug ordered. Designed to produce an immediate target concentration, this dose is not always practical or safe. An initial dose of lidocaine, calculated to achieve an average target concentration, may produce toxicity after administration as a bolus because it reaches high concentrations in the heart and brain (toxic sites of action) before it is diluted by distribution elsewhere in the body.

DRUG HALF-LIFE

The term **half-life** denotes the time required for the plasma concentration of a drug or the total amount of drug in the body to decline by one half. The half-life of a drug depends on its volume of distribution (the distribution between the plasma and the various other fluids and tissues, and the actual nature of distribution and clearance). During drug administration, it takes one half-life to reach 50% of steady state, two half-lives to reach 75%, three half-lives to reach 87.5%, and four half-lives to reach 93.75%. On discontinuation of a drug or after a drug dose,

TABLE 18–1   Selected Therapeutic Drug Concentrations and Toxic Values

Drug	Therapeutic Concentration	Toxic Value
Amikacin (Amikin)	25–35 μg/mL (peak level) or 43–60 μmol/L	>35–40 μg/mL or >60–68 μmol/L
Nitroprusside (Nipride)	0.5–1.5 μg/mL or 2.7–4.1 μmol/L	>10 μg/mL or >27.0 μmol/L
Procainamide (Pronestyl)	4–10 μg/mL or 17–42 μmol/L	10–12 μg/mL or >42–51 μmol/L
Theophylline (Slo-Phyllin)	9–20 μg/mL or 44–111 μmol/L	>20 μg/mL or >111 μmol/L
Tobramycin (Nebcin)	8–10 μg/mL (peak level) or 17–21 μmol/L	>10 μg/mL or 21–26 μmol/L
Vancomycin (Vancoled)	20–40 μg/mL (peak level) or 14–28 μmol/L	>80–100 μg/mL or 55–69 μmol/L

one half-life is required for the plasma concentration to fall to 50% of its initial level.

Disadvantages of the Intravenous Route

Despite the advantages of the IV route, there are certain actual or potential hazards. They include the following:

- Incompatibilities when one or more drugs are added to the IV solution
- Speed shock (an adverse systemic reaction to a substance rapidly injected into the bloodstream)
- Vascular irritations and subsequent problems
- Rapid onset of action, with inability to recall a drug once it enters the bloodstream
- Precipitate formation, which may occur when one or more drugs are added to a parenteral solution. The precipitate does not always form when the solution is prepared, which increases the challenge of IV administration. Some drugs, which are stable for a limited time, degrade and may or may not precipitate as they become less therapeutically active. If administered IV, fluids containing insoluble matter carry the potential danger of embolism, myocardial damage, and harmful effects on other organs such as the liver and the kidneys.
- Medication errors. Medication systems in hospitals are complex and multilayered, involving many steps and many people. According to the Institute for Safe Medication Practices, this complexity increases the probability of problems (American Hospital Association, 1999; Cohen, 1999). Errors may occur at any stage—prescribing, ordering, dispensing, administering, or monitoring the effects of medication. Common sources of medication errors in health systems are presented in Box 18–2. Table 18–2 identifies the collaborative responsibilities of health care personnel involved in IV drug therapy.

Incompatibilities

The number of possible drug combinations is overwhelming, as is the potential for **incompatibility.** Manufacturers provide an ever-increasing number of new drug products for the treatment of disease processes. Compounding drugs for IV administration is usually performed by an IV admixture service as a component of a hospital-based or home infusion pharmacy. Today, admixture programs have expanded their service base to provide compounding services for extended care, ambulatory care, and any clinical setting in which infusion therapies are delivered.

All people responsible for mixing and compounding IV drugs must be alert to the hazards involved. Compatibility charts are provided through admixture services to alert the nurse to potential problems, particularly when additions to infusions in progress are made on a nursing unit or added in a patient's residence.

A factor related to compatibility is the composition of the solution container. Box 18–3 lists drugs affected by increased *adsorption* (adhesion to the surfaces of

BOX 18–2   Common Sources of Medication Errors

Unavailable Patient Information

The patient's clinical record lacks critical patient information (laboratory values, allergies).

Unavailable Drug Information

Clinical pharmacy expertise is not provided on site.

Miscommunication

Failed communication owing to illegible handwriting, confusion of drugs with similar names, confusion of metric and apothecary systems, ambiguous or incomplete orders is a common cause of error.

Problems With Labeling, Packaging, and Nomenclature

Unit dose medications may not be available throughout the health care institution, and drug administration procedures do not ensure that medications remain labeled until they reach the patient.

Poor Storage Procedures

Stocking multiple concentrations or storing drugs in look-alike containers may contribute to error.

Inconsistent Standards

Drug device acquisition, use, and monitoring may be inadequately standardized, leading to use of unsafe equipment or errors.

Workplace Stress

Excessive interruptions and *excessive workload* may lead to error.

Limited Staff Education

In-service training should alert staff to potential for errors and serve as a reminder.

Insufficient Patient Education

Patient education is essential to good patient outcomes. Patient engagement and participation in care promotes good care and helps prevent errors.

Flawed Quality Improvement Processes and Risk Management

Quality systems should include methods for identifying, reporting, analyzing, and correcting errors as well as measurement systems for tracking the effect of system changes.

TABLE 18–2 Responsibilities for Intravenous Drug Administration

Institution	Nurse	Pharmacist	Physician
Provide written policies	Adhere to five "rights" of drug administration	Maintain a drug incompatibility profile	Provide written drug order
Issue approved drug list			
Offer continuing education	Assess and monitor patient during drug administration	Implement admixture process	Act as overall gatekeeper
Provide institutional review board approval of investigational drugs	Participate in continuing education	Perform safe compounding	Administer drugs not on approved list
	Keep current knowledge base of drug delivery systems	Act in clinical pharmacy role	Participate in continuing medical education
		Participate in continuing education	
	Educate patients		
	Update knowledge of antidotes		

substances with which they are in contact) when infused in polyvinyl chloride containers (Trissel, 1998). Factors affecting the compatibility of drugs include order of mixing, quantity of the drug and solution, room temperature, and light. Incompatibilities are not always obvious to the naked eye. They may be classified as physical, chemical, or therapeutic, and are described in Box 18–4.

CHEMICAL

The most common incompatibilities are the result of certain chemical reactions (Baldwin, 1995)—for example, **hydrolysis** is the process in which water absorption causes decomposition of a compound. In preparing solutions of salt, the nurse should understand that certain salts, when placed in water, hydrolyze, forming a strong acid and a weak base or a weak acid and a strong base. Because pH is a significant factor in the solubility of drugs, the increased acidity or alkalinity from hydrolysis of a salt

---

BOX 18–3 Drugs With Increased Adsorption When Infused Using Polyvinyl Chloride Containers

Hydralazine (Apresoline)
Insulin
Nitroglycerin
Phenothiazine tranquilizers (Thorazine, Compazine)
Vitamin A acetate (nonpalmitate form)
Warfarin (Coumadin)

BOX 18–4   Types of Incompatibilities

Physical—Those in which an undesirable change is physically observed, such as sodium bicarbonate and calcium chloride forming an insoluble precipitate (Baldwin, 1995)
Chemical—Those occurring in the molecular structure or pharmacologic properties of a substance (note: They may or may not be physically observed), such as penicillin and ascorbic acid lowering the pH
Therapeutic—Those in which an undesirable reaction results from the overlapping effects of two drugs given together or closely together, such as penicillin and tetracycline inhibiting the bactericidal effect of penicillin

---

may result in an incompatibility if another drug is added. For example, the acid salt sodium bicarbonate when placed in water hydrolyzes to form a strong alkali (sodium hydroxide) and a weak and unstable acid (carbonic acid). Many organic acids are known as weak acids because they ionize only slightly.

Reduction is the process whereby one or more atoms gain electrons at the expense of some other part of the system (ASHP, 1998).

Oxidation is the corresponding loss of electrons occurring when reduction takes place. Antioxidants are often used as preservatives to prevent oxidation of a compound.

Double decomposition is the chemical reaction in which ions of two compounds change places and two new compounds are thus formed (ASHP, 1998). A great many salts act by double decomposition to form other salts, and this process accounts for a large number of incompatibilities. For example, calcium chloride is incompatible with sodium bicarbonate; the double decomposition results in the formation of the insoluble salt, calcium carbonate.

PHYSICAL

Precipitation may occur in some parenteral solutions; some commonly prescribed drugs precipitate when added to IV solutions. Differences in the physical and chemical properties of each of these solutions may affect the stability of any drug introduced.

Moreover, a compound that is soluble in one solution may precipitate in another. Sodium ampicillin deteriorates in acid solutions. This drug, when added to isotonic sodium chloride at a concentration of 30 mg/mL, loses <10% activity in 8 hours. However, when it is added to 5% dextrose in water, usually a more acid solution, its stability is reduced to a 4-hour period.

pH and Stability

Because pH plays an important role in drug, solubility, stability, and compatibility, a definition is in order. The term **pH** stands for the degree of concentration of hydrogen ions or the acidity of the solution. The weight of hydrogen ions in 1 L pure water is 0.0000001 g, which is numerically equal to 10^{-7}. For convenience, the negative logarithm is used. Because it is at this concentration that the hydrogen ions balance the hydroxyl ions, a pH of 7 is neutral. Each unit decrease in pH represents a 10-fold increase in hydrogen ions.

The greatest number of drug incompatibilities may be produced by changes in pH (ASHP, 1998). For example, precipitation occurs when a compound is insoluble in solution. The degree of solubility often varies with the pH. A drastic change in the pH of a drug when added to an IV solution suggests an incompatibility or a decrease in stability.

Solutions with a high pH appear to be incompatible with solutions with a low pH and may form insoluble free acids or free bases. A chart denoting the pH of certain drugs and certain solutions to be used as a vehicle is helpful in warning of potential incompatibilities. A broad pH range (3.5 to 6.5) of dextrose solutions is allowed by the *United States Pharmacopeia*. A drug may be stable in one bottle of dextrose 5% in water and not in another (Baldwin, 1995).

Again, whereas one drug may be compatible in a solution, a second additive may alter the established pH to such an extent as to make the drugs unstable (Box 18–5). Buffers or antioxidants in a drug may cause two drugs, however compatible, to precipitate. For example, ascorbic acid, the buffering component of tetracycline, lowers the pH of the product and therefore may accelerate the decomposition of a drug susceptible to an acid environment.

Preservatives in the diluent may lead to problems as well. Sterile diluents for reconstitution of drugs are available with or without a bacteriostatic agent. The bacteriostatic agents usually consist of parabens or phenol preservatives.

Dilution and Solubility

Solubility often varies with the volume of solution in which a drug is introduced. For example, tetracycline hydrochloride, mixed in a small volume of fluid, maintains its pH range over 24 hours. However, when added to a large volume (1 L), it degrades after 12 hours, becoming less therapeutically active.

OTHER FACTORS

- The order in which drugs are added to infusions often determines their compatibility.
- Light may provide energy for chemical reactions to occur. Certain drugs, such as amphotericin B and nitrofurantoin, once diluted, must be protected from light.
- Room temperature may effect incompatibility. Heat provides energy for reactions, which is why reconstituted or diluted drugs are refrigerated to prolong stability.

Vascular Irritation

Vascular irritation is a significant hazard of drugs administered IV. Any irritation that inflames and roughens the endothelial cells of the venous wall allows platelets to adhere to the wall and promote the formation of a thrombus. Thrombophlebitis is

BOX 18–5   Factors Affecting Stability of Intravenous Drugs and Solutions

Precipitation of Parenteral Solution

- Some commonly prescribed drugs precipitate when added to IV solutions.
- Differences in the physical and chemical properties of each of these solutions may affect the stability of any drug introduced.
- A compound soluble in one solution may precipitate in another. Sodium ampicillin deteriorates in acid solutions. This drug, when added to isotonic sodium chloride at a concentration of 30 mg/mL, loses <10% activity in 8 h. However, when it is added to dextrose 5% in water, usually a more acid solution, its stability is reduced to a 4-h period.

pH

- A broad pH range (3.5–6.5) of dextrose solutions is allowed by the United States Pharmacopeia (USP). A drug may be stable in one bottle of dextrose 5% in water and not in another.

Additional Drugs

- One drug may be compatible in a solution, but a second additive may alter the established pH to such an extent as to make the drugs unstable.

Buffering Agents in Drugs

- Presence of buffers or antioxidants, which may cause two drugs, however compatible, to precipitate. For example, ascorbic acid, the buffering component of tetracycline, lowers the pH of the product and therefore may accelerate the decomposition of a drug susceptible to an acid environment.

Preservatives in the Diluent

- Sterile diluents for reconstitution of drugs are available with or without a bacteriostatic agent.
- The bacteriostatic agents usually consist of parabens or phenol preservatives.
- Certain drugs, including nitrofurantoin, amphotericin B, and erythromycin, are incompatible with these preservatives and should be reconstituted with sterile water for injection.

Degree of Dilution

- Solubility often varies with the volume of solution in which a drug is introduced. For example, tetracycline hydrochloride, mixed in a small volume of fluid, maintains its pH range over 24 h. However, when added to a large volume (1 L), it degrades after 12 h, becoming less therapeutically active.

Length of Time Solution Stands

- Decomposition of substances in solution is proportional to the length of time they stand. For example, sodium ampicillin with the high pH of 8–10 becomes unstable when maintained in an acid environment over time.

Order of Mixing

- The order in which drugs are added to infusions often determines their compatibility.

BOX 18–5   Factors Affecting Stability of Intravenous Drugs and Solutions   *(Continued)*

Light

- Light may provide energy for chemical reactions to occur.
- Certain drugs, such as amphotericin B and nitrofurantoin, once diluted must be protected from light.

Room Temperature

- Heat provides energy for reactions.
- After reconstitution or initial dilution, refrigeration prolongs the stability of many drugs.

---

the result of the sterile inflammation. When a thrombus occurs, the inherent danger of embolism is always present.

If aseptic technique is not strictly followed, septic thrombophlebitis may result from bacteria that is introduced through the infusion catheter and then trapped within the thrombus. This is much more serious because of the potential dangers of septicemia and acute bacterial endocarditis. Strategies for avoiding vascular irritation are presented in Box 18–6.

BOX 18–6   Strategies for Preventing Vascular Irritation

Select Most Appropriate Site

- Use veins with ample blood volume.
- Avoid veins in lower extremities.
- Start at most distal location.

Select Most Appropriate Catheter

- Select a catheter that is appreciably smaller than the lumen of the vein so that smooth blood flow can provide adequate hemodilution.

Infuse Drug Carefully

- Administer isotonic solutions after administering hypertonic solutions to flush irritating substances.
- Infuse slowly; slow administration provides greater dilution of the drug in a large vein.
- Adhere to recommendations for the following: use of filters, inspection of solution for clarity, proper reconstitution, and dilution of additives.

Monitor Regularly

- Change insertion site at designated intervals and as needed because prolonged catheter insertion increases risk of phlebitis.

Safeguards to Minimize Hazards of Administering Intravenous Drugs

Various safeguards are in place to diminish the potential hazards of IV drug administration. They include lists of drugs approved for IV use by an institution's pharmacy, laws regulating the use and availability of potentially dangerous drugs (controlled substances), standards and protocols for admixture preparation, safety improvements in drug delivery systems, standards for monitoring and documenting patient responses to drugs, resources for accurate dosage calculation, drug expiration dates, regulation of investigational drugs, patient education programs, and so forth.

Approved Drug Lists

Lists of drugs approved for administration by nurses in all clinical care settings must be readily available. In the inpatient setting, the institution's pharmacy and therapeutics committee is the group that usually approves such lists. IV nursing professionals are often members of this committee, and protocols are brought to this group for approval before a drug is added to the list. Ideally, the committee provides a list of approved drugs for administration by nurses, a list of drugs approved for addition to infusions in progress, and a list of investigational agents approved for administration (ASHP, 1998; Spath, 2000). In the alternative care environment, home health agencies and clinics may also develop lists that are subsequently approved by their medical directors before acceptance by the nursing community.

Controlled Substances Act

This act established five categories of controlled substances, known as *schedules*, based on their potential for abuse, the medical indications, and the potential for dependence on the drug. Many of the drugs administered for pain control are Schedule II drugs. Their safe use is regulated by specific prescription and record-keeping requirements.

Safe Admixture Preparation

Intravenous additives and solutions are best prepared in an IV additive station of the institution's pharmacy. Aseptic technique is observed and enhanced by a clean-room approach. A laminar-flow hood, proper illumination, and hand-washing facilities are readily available in such a setting.

USE OF LAMINAR-FLOW HOOD

Laminar flow confines airflow to a specific area. The entire body of air within that area moves with uniform velocity along parallel flow lines (ASHP, 1998). Laminar-flow hoods play a vital role in eliminating the hazard of airborne contamination of

IV solutions and admixtures. Nurses should be familiar with the general operating guidelines of the hood. Vertical and horizontal hoods are available. Laminar-flow hoods should be used according to state and federal guidelines as well as the recommendations of the ASHP.

ADMIXTURE PREPARATION POLICIES AND PROCEDURES

The IV policies and procedures addressing admixing should define potential hazards, compatibility, stability requirements, and the types of admixtures in the scope of practice. The following are some safeguards that may be implemented to protect both patients and health care personnel from potential health hazards associated with the admixing of medications:

- Aseptic technique is imperative. Bacterial and fungal contamination of drug products and parenteral solutions must be avoided.
- Proper dilution of lyophilized drugs is essential. Two special cautions to ensure complete solubility in the reconstitution of drugs must be observed: the specific diluent recommended by the manufacturer should be used, and the drug should be initially diluted in the volume recommended.
- Introduction of extraneous particles into parenteral solutions must be avoided. Fragments of rubber stoppers are frequently cut out by the needles used and accidentally injected into solutions. Large-bore (15-gauge) needles are practical for use in the nurses' station and appear to have fewer disadvantages than smaller needles, for several reasons. Smaller needles may deposit particles that may be difficult to see on inspection of the solution. The particles may be so small that they can advance through the indwelling catheter. Using filtered aspiration needles when preparing admixtures can remove extraneous particles.
- Any solution that contains visible fragments of rubber must be discarded.

See the accompanying Key Intervention for more information on compounding and administering medications in parenteral solutions.

Improved Drug Delivery Systems

Manufacturers have kept pace with demands for improved drug delivery systems for use in all clinical settings in which infusion therapy is administered. Standard methods of drug delivery and terminology still apply (see Chap. 11).

Intermittent infusion allows drugs to be administered on an intermittent basis through a slow, keep-vein-open infusion using a secondary container, single-dose additive, or multidose admixture connected to a controlled-volume set. The intermittent infusion may also be given through a self-contained administration system such as an elastomeric pump. Intermittent infusions are typically given through an intermittent infusion device (heparin lock) to conserve veins, allow freedom of motion between infusions, and provide a minimal amount of infusate for the patient whose intake may be restricted.

KEY INTERVENTIONS: Compounding and Administering Parenteral Medication

Preparations

1. Check and recheck the order with the drug label.
2. Inscribe order for drug additive directly from original order to medication label or submit electronically to pharmacy.
3. Substantiate drug orders with the drug product and the parenteral solution.
4. Inspect solution for extraneous particles.
5. Check drug product:
   - Expiration date—do not use outdated drugs, which may have lost potency or stability. Check the expiration dates of the drug and of the diluent.
   - Method of administration—intramuscular (IM) preparations are seldom used for IV administration because they may contain components, such as anesthetics or preservatives, not meant for administration by the vascular route. In addition, some are packaged in multidose vials, which may contribute to contamination, and the dosage recommended for IM administration may be inappropriate for IV administration.
   - Clarify any questions or doubts with the patient's physician.
6. Clean injection site of both the drug product and the diluent with an accepted antiseptic.
7. Use sterile syringe and needle.
8. Reconstitute medication according to manufacturer's recommendation.
9. Make sure diluted drug is completely dissolved before adding to parenteral solution.
10. After adding to solution, invert solution container to mix the additive completely.
11. Clearly and properly label solution container with the following:
    - Name of patient
    - Drug and dosage
    - Date and time of compounding
    - Expiration date
    - Preparer's signature
12. As an added precaution to prevent errors, recheck label with used drug ampules before discarding ampules.

Administering

1. Inspect solution for precipitates. If any precipitates are present, discard the solution.
2. Make sure that the drug is compatible with the IV solution if it is administered through a primary line. If incompatible, clamp the set and flush the injection port with compatible fluid. Do not use sterile water. (Note: Electronic infusion devices may be set to flush the line automatically following medication administration.)
3. Also make sure the drug is compatible with heparin when a heparinized lock is used. If incompatible, flush the lock with a compatible fluid before and after the IV injection.
4. Substantiate identity of patient with solution prepared.
5. Wear gloves when preparing medications and administering IV therapy. (If latex allergy is a concern, keep in mind that glove manufacturers have developed alternative materials to lessen this concern.)
6. Perform venipuncture consistent with institutional policy and standards of the Infusion Nurses Society (INS, 1998, 2000).
7. Ensure placement within lumen of the vessel.
8. Ensure first-dose delivery of drug in a clinically monitored environment and administer the medication at an evenly divided rate over the length of time recommended by the manufacturer, using a watch with a second hand.

9. Observe patient for a few minutes after the initial IV administration of any drug that may cause anaphylaxis.
10. Use added caution in administering any drug whose fast action could produce untoward reactions.

Peripheral and central IV catheters are adaptable as intermittent infusion devices by the addition of a catheter plug or resealable adapter. Patency of these lines is maintained by administering an amount of flush solution sufficient to fill the internal diameter of the line in use. Dilute heparin solution (hence, heparin lock) is most often used. Saline solution is being used more frequently today, and use of antibiotic flush solutions in the immunocompromised patient continues to increase.

Intravenous push is the direct injection of a medication into the vein. It may be administered through the distal Y site of an administration set, through the intermittent infusion device, or by catheter. The terms *IV push* and *bolus* may be confusing. Substances such as radiopaque dye (contrast media) used to visualize the cardiac chamber must be injected as a bolus (defined as a discrete mass). Most medications ordered for IV push or bolus administration must be administered slowly (up to 30 minutes), depending on the drug itself. Rapid injection increases the drug concentration in the plasma, which may reach toxic proportions, flooding the organs rich in blood—the heart and the brain—and resulting in shock and cardiac arrest. The rate of administration, included with the order for the medication, can reduce any misconceptions and prevent the potential risk of a life-threatening reaction from too-rapid administration of the drug.

Because delivery of drugs by IV push instantly increases the drug levels in the blood, IV push offers immediate relief to the patient. Nurses in many special care units are trained and authorized to administer specific IV pushes. In the past, the IV push was restricted to the intensive care unit, where the patient was monitored and where a potential crisis might arise requiring its immediate use in the absence of a physician. Today, nurses frequently administer IV push injections.

Many drugs given as IV injections can be potentially dangerous to the patient. The nurse must understand the action of the drug and assess the patient's condition before administering the medication (see Box 18–7 and the next section, Monitoring Response to Treatment).

Continuous administration is the term applied to medications mixed in a large volume of infusate and infused over a time in excess of 2 hours (Baldwin, 1995). Decreased tolerance to the drug can result from various factors in the patient's condition:

- Decreased cardiac output
- Reduced renal flow or poor glomerular filtration
- Diminished urinary output
- Pulmonary congestion
- Systemic edema

Greater dilution of the drug and a longer injection time can prevent drug accumulation, reduce venous irritation caused by a low pH, and allow time to assess the

---

BOX 18–7   Important Checkpoints in Intravenous Drug Administration

The Drug

- Understand the expected therapeutic effect of the medication.
- Know the recommended dosage range and the length of time required for administration.
- Understand the side effects and toxic symptoms that can occur.
- Be skilled in using proper antidotes and have appropriate antidotes readily available.

The Patient

- Ensure positive identification of the patient (check identification band). Do not rely on the patient's verbal identification of himself or herself.
- Ascertain allergy history (food and drug).
- Assess the patient's condition and be aware of any factors that can affect the drug action.
- Know what other medications the patient is receiving; be aware of therapeutic incompatibilities that may occur between any other medication the patient is receiving and the IV medication.
- Watch for the patient's response during and after injection of medication.

---

patient's response and detect early reactions. Use of the manufacturer's recommended diluent is most important because different drugs require different diluents.

Monitoring Response to Treatment

Knowing the expected therapeutic effects of the medication, the recommended dosage range, the side effects, and symptoms of toxic reactions is essential. Side effects may be manifest as gastrointestinal distress, including nausea, vomiting, and diarrhea; as allergic skin reactions; and as central nervous system dysfunction (Karch, 2000).

Major reactions may consist of respiratory distress, anaphylaxis, cardiac dysrhythmias, and convulsions. Reactions must be detected and reported at once so that proper treatment can be administered. Untoward responses are described in Box 18–8.

Nurses who administer IV medications should be knowledgeable about various antidotes and their use. Emergency supplies of antidotes should be readily available. Many are prepared in prefilled syringes for emergency use. Sterile cartridge needle units, with accurately machine-measured doses, provide a closed-injection system ready for instant use.

Accurate Calculations

An integral component of IV nursing practice is the ability to perform the mathematical calculations required to administer correct doses of medication and solution to patients. Accuracy is a priority when medications are administered IV. Guidelines to ensure safety in calculating doses are presented in Box 18–9.

BOX 18–8   Untoward Drug Responses

Accumulation—Increased concentrations of drug in circulation when the rate of administration is greater than rate of drug metabolism

Dependence—The need for continued drug administration to prevent withdrawal symptoms

Allergic reaction—Hypersensitivity resulting from previous exposure to a drug and manifested by symptoms as mild as itching or hives or as serious as life-threatening anaphylaxis

Idiosyncratic reaction—Unpredictable response not attributed to hypersensitivity

Tachyphylaxis—Rapidly developing drug tolerance

FLOW RATE CALCULATIONS

Flow rate calculations require the following basic information:

- Amount of solution to be infused
- Duration of the administration
- Drop factor of the set to be used

First, the amount of solution to be administered is determined, and then that number is divided by the delivery time:

$$\frac{1{,}000\ \text{mL}}{8\ \text{h}} = 125\ \text{mL/h}$$

Next, the drop factor of the set being used is noted. A macrodrip set takes 10, 15, or 20 drops to deliver 1 mL of solution:

$$\frac{\text{No. drops/mL of set}}{60\ (\text{minutes in an hour})} \times \text{total hourly volume} = \text{no. drops/min}$$

$$\frac{\text{mL/h} \times \text{drop factor of set}}{60} = \text{drops/min}$$

BOX 18–9   Dosage Calculation

When to calculate base dose:

- At the start of your shift
- When titrated medications are started and when a transferred patient is receiving titrated medications

Consider patient's fluid replacement and duration of infusion.
Stronger concentrations may be needed to avoid fluid overload.
Titrate the drug to the patient's condition and note the response.
Use an electronic infusion device to ensure delivery of the prescribed dose.

For microdrip or pediatric systems, the equation is:

$$\frac{mL/h \times \text{drop factor}}{60} = \text{drops/min}$$

DRUG DOSAGE CALCULATIONS

Ratio and proportion or "desired over have" (D/H) may be easily applied to calculation of drug dosages for infusion therapy. The rate of administration of IV drugs may be calculated in units per hour. For example, there are 12,500 U heparin sodium in 250 mL IV solution. The dose ordered is 800 U/hour:

$$X = \frac{250}{12,500}$$

$$X = 0.02$$

Then, calculate the rate of the prescribed dosage:

$$0.02 \text{ mL} \times 800 \text{ U} = 16 \text{ mL/h}$$

In this example, the nurse has 200 mg drug in 500 mL of dextrose 5% in water and wants to know the number of milligrams of drug the patient is receiving per hour. The amount of drug per milliliter of solution is determined by D/H, or:

$$\frac{500}{20} = 25$$

$$\frac{200}{25} = 8 \text{ mg/h}$$

PERCENT SOLUTIONS

The relationship between the amount of solute and the total quantity of solution is expressed as a percentage or ratio. Percentage strength of solution may be calculated in one of three ways:

- Percent weight in weight (w/w)—the weight of the solute (drug) compared with the weight of the solution (g drug/100 g solution)
- Percent weight in volume (w/v)—the weight of the solute compared with the volume of the total solution (g drug/100 mL solution)
- Percent volume in volume (v/v)—the volume of the solute compared with the volume of the total solution (mL drug/100 mL solution)

Expiration Dates

To ensure safe and effective drug therapy, drug containers are labeled with expiration dates that identify when a medication or product is no longer acceptable for use. Institutional policy and procedure should state that medications must not be

---

BOX 18–10   Elements of Informed Consent Regarding Investigational Therapy

- Written by the investigator
- Approved by the institution's review board or ethics committee
- Signed by the subject (patient or volunteer) or authorized representative
- Witnessed

---

administered beyond their expiration dates. Expiration dates should be verified by the nurse before drugs and infusates are given to patients.

Regulation of Investigational Drugs

Administration of investigational agents is governed by state and federal regulations. Signed informed consent is required before patients can participate in the investigation (Box 18–10). An informed consent must be written by the investigator, approved by the institutional review board, signed by the subject, and witnessed. Before approval by the U.S. Food and Drug Administration, drug studies are conducted in four phases (Box 18–11). Policies and procedures should be developed pertaining to the administration of investigational agents, regardless of the clinical setting in which care is provided.

BOX 18–11   Phases of Clinical Drug Trials

Phase I: Clinical Pharmacology and Therapeutics

- Evaluate drug safety.
- Determine an acceptable single dosage or levels of patient tolerance for acute multiple dosing of drug.

Phase II: Initial Clinical Investigation for Therapeutic Effect

- Evaluate drug efficacy.
- Conduct pilot study.

Phase III: Full-Scale Evaluation of Treatment

- Evaluate the patient population for which drug is intended.

Phase IV: Postmarketing Survelllance

- Provide additional information about the efficacy or safety profile.

TABLE 18–3   Resources for Patients and Education Programs

Brochure	Source	Website
Your Role in Safe Medication Use: A Guide for Patients and Families	Massachusetts Hospital Association	www.mhalink.org (accessed 8/23/2005)
Partners in Quality: Taking an Active Role in Your Health Care	Hospital and Health System Association of Pennsylvania	www.haponline.org
How to Take Your Medications Safely	Institute for Safe Medication Practice	www.ismp.org (accessed 8/23/2005)
Just Ask!	U.S. Pharmacopeia	www.usp.org (accessed 8/23/2005)

Patient Education

Not to be overlooked is the responsibility for patient education. A number of patient information resources are available to facilitate this process (Table 18–3). Education is a primary nursing responsibility in the acute care as well as other clinical settings. Moreover, education helps prevent hazards associated with IV drug administration.

References and Selected Readings

Asterisks indicate references cited in text.

Ahmed, D.S., & Hamran, P.M. (1999). Similar name, different diagnosis. *American Journal of Nursing, 99*(5), 11–12.

*American Hospital Association. (1999). *Quality advisory: Improving medication safety.* Chicago: Author.

*American Society of Health-System Pharmacists. (1998). *American hospital formulary service.* Bethesda, MD: Author.

*Baldwin, D. (1995). Pharmacology. In: J. Terry (Ed.). *Intravenous therapy: Clinical principles and practice* (p. 191). Philadelphia: W.B. Saunders.

*Cohen, M.R. (Ed.). (1999). *Medication errors.* Washington, DC: American Pharmaceutical Association.

Corrigan, J. (1999). *To err is human: Building a safer health system.* Washington, DC: National Academies Press.

*Infusion Nurses Society. (2000). Revised standards of practice. *Journal of Infusion Nursing. 23*(Suppl. 1).

*Infusion Nurses Society. (2005). Revised standards of practice. *Journal of Infusion Nursing. 28*(Suppl. 1).

*Intravenous Nurses Society. (1998). Revised intravenous nursing standards of practice. *Journal of Intravenous Nursing, 21*(Suppl. 1).

*Intravenous Nurses Society. (2005). Revised intravenous nursing standards of practice. *Journal of Intravenous Nursing, 21*(Suppl. 39), 40.

*Karch, A.M. (2000). *Lippincott's nursing drug guide.* Philadelphia: Lippincott Williams & Wilkins.

Leape, L. (1998). *Reducing adverse drug events.* Boston: Institute for Healthcare Improvement.

Richards, J.F., & Creamer, L. (1999). Med errors: Solving the microgram/kilogram puzzle. *American Journal of Nursing, 99*(10): 11–12.

*Spath, P.L. (2000). *Error reduction in health care.* Chicago: Health Forum, Inc.

*Trissel, L.A. (1998). *Handbook on injectable drugs* (9th ed.). Bethesda, MD: American Society of Health-System Pharmacists.

U.S. Pharmacist. Interactions Based on Case Reports (Table 2). Available at www.uspharmacist.com/oldformat.asp?url=newlook/files/comp/aug00alt.htm. (Accessed 8/24/2005.)

Review Questions

Note: Questions below may have more than one right answer.

1. Responsibilities for drug administration are shared by which of the following?

   A. Nurse and pharmacist

   B. Institution and physician

   C. A only

   D. A and B

2. Common sources of error in drug administration include all of the following *except:*

   A. Packaging

   B. Workplace stress

   C. Readily available drug information

   D. Miscommunication

3. Which of the following disease states influences pharmacokinetics of drugs?

   A. Hepatic and renal failure

   B. Congestive heart failure

   C. Presence of infection

   D. Burns

4. Potential hazards of vascular irritation can be minimized by all of the following *except:*

   A. Using veins with ample blood volume

   B. Selecting a large catheter

   C. Slowing administration

   D. Changing insertion site

5. Before preparing medication, the nurse should implement which of the following measures?

   A. Question patient regarding sensitivity.

   B. Check and recheck order with drug label.

   C. Use manufacturer's diluent.

   D. Clarify order with the pharmacist.

6. Untoward drug responses include which of the following?

   A. Dependence

   B. Allergic reaction

   C. Accumulation

   D. All of the above

7. Drugs with increased adsorption when infused via polyvinyl chloride containers include:

   A. Insulin and hydralazine

   B. Vitamin A acetate and warfarin

   C. A only

   D. A and B

8. The term *half-life* refers to which of the following?

   A. Time of initial dose of drug administered

   B. Target concentration of drug divided by two

   C. Time for plasma concentration of drug to decline by one half

   D. Time for distribution to occur

9. Quality improvement processes in drug administration include which of the following?

   A. Identifying

   B. Reporting

   C. Analyzing and correcting measurement systems

   D. All of the above

10. Which of the following is true of the Controlled Substances Act?

    A. It classifies drugs based on potential for abuse.

    B. It classifies drugs according to medical indications and potential for dependence.

    C. A only

    D. A and B

CHAPTER
19

Antineoplastic Therapy

KEY TERMS

Adjuvant

Alkylating Agents

Alopecia

Anticancer

Antimetabolite

Antineoplastic

Biotherapy

Bolus

Cell Cycle

Cytoprotectant

Cytotoxic

Extravasation

Interferons

Interleukins

Investigational Protocol

Monoclonal Antibodies

Nadir

Neoadjuvant

Plant Alkaloids

Toxicity

Vesicant

Role of the Intravenous Nurse in Chemotherapy/Biotherapy Education

Antineoplastics, which include both chemotherapeutic and biologic agents used in cancer treatment, present a real challenge to nurses responsible for their administration. Many nurses point to the reputation of antineoplastics as intimidating and express anxiety about administering them. Success with these substances usually is ensured, however, for nurses with refined IV skills, sensitive patient preparation practices, and keen awareness of how and why chemotherapy and biotherapy work.

Approximately 85% of all patients with cancer will receive antineoplastic therapy that may include either chemotherapy or biotherapy or a combination of both in the course of treatment. Successful administration of an IV cancer treatment regimen depends on adequate patient preparation and education, the competence and skill of the nurse, mutual understanding of patient and nurse on the current goal of therapy (cure, control, or palliation), and finally, the nurse's broad knowledge of indications, administration, and side effects of the cancer treatment. The nurse is critical to the experience of the patient when receiving chemotherapy/biotherapy. Nurses who are committed to the care of patients undergoing cancer treatment can make a difference in the lives of these patients.

Education for Nurses Administering Antineoplastic Drugs

The privilege of administering antineoplastic agents is preceded by extensive exposure to standardized educational preparation and practical experience. To provide consistently safe, appropriate, and high-quality patient care, many centers mandate comprehensive training programs leading to credentialing in chemotherapy administration.

To ensure consistency in practice, the Oncology Nursing Society (ONS) has developed a chemotherapy/biotherapy course that is presented nationwide. ONS members who become trainers for the course are selected based on criteria that include experience in administering chemotherapy and presenting educational content. The book, *Chemotherapy and Biotherapy: Guidelines and Recommendations for Practice* (Polovich, White, Kelleher, et al., 2005), provides a standardized framework for the didactic education to handle **cytotoxic** (cell-killing) agents and for the care of the patient undergoing cancer treatment. The instructional component is comprehensive and includes content covering the disease, drug treatment and administration, and side effects. An outline of the ONS chemotherapy/biotherapy major subject areas needed to prepare for chemotherapy administration is included in Box 19–1 (ONS, 2002).

The participant in the course must also achieve a passing score on a test in order to substantiate requisite knowledge and receive a Chemotherapy/Biotherapy Provider card. Individual employers determine clinical competence. Course information is applied during a practicum phase at an institutional level where clinical skills are exercised and evaluated. Within the *ONS Guidelines*, the clinical practicum is described and an evaluation tool is included. The clinical practicum emphasizes clinical skills and allows the nurse to demonstrate competence in the safe administration of chemotherapy and biotherapy (Polovich et al., 2005).

Safe delivery of IV antineoplastic agents is only one part of caring for patients receiving chemotherapy/biotherapy. A nurse who specializes in oncology needs a solid foundation of specialized knowledge. See Box 19–2 for a list of suggested areas of emphasis in a basic oncology education program for nurses (ONS, 2005). With specialty knowledge plus clinical experience, the oncology nurse can prepare for professional certification through the ONS.

BOX 19–1   **Preparation of the Professional Nurse to Care for Patients Receiving Chemotherapy/Biotherapy**

Major subject areas to be mastered by nurses who administer chemotherapy/biotherapy are based on *Oncology Nursing Society Position Statement on Education of the Professional RN Who Administers and Cares for the Individual Receiving Chemotherapy and Biotherapy* (11/2002)

I. Didactic Component
  A. Cancer review covering tumor cell kinetics and angiogenesis
  B. The drug development process
  C. Principles of cancer chemotherapy, biotherapy, and immunotherapy
  D. Pharmacology of cytotoxic agents
  E. Drug administration, as well as administration schedules, dose determinations, drug response, and drug delivery systems
  F. Administration procedures
  G. Safe practice considerations
  H. Mixing, storage, and labeling of chemotherapeutic agents
  I. Side effects, as well as principles of management and patient education

II. Clinical Practicum (Completed under the auspices of the nurses' institution)
  A. Drug calculation
  B. Drug preparation and handling
  C. Drug storage and transport
  D. Drug administration techniques
  E. Extravasation and hypersensitivity management
  F. Acute drug side effect management
  G. Appropriate documentation
  H. Patient and family teaching and follow-up

CLINICAL CHALLENGES

The remarkable progress of antineoplastic agents as a major treatment modality poses a growing series of challenges to infusion nurses. Ongoing and vigorous clinical investigations from cooperative groups are dedicated to drug development and discovering new therapeutic methods of delivering cytotoxic drugs. Nurses who specialize in oncology have a responsibility to maintain up-to-date expertise through study of current professional literature along with continuing education programs.

Certification is an excellent demonstration of one's knowledge in antineoplastic therapy. The Infusion Nurses Society supports certification in infusion nursing through the Infusion Nurses Certification Corporation. This certification includes content on antineoplastic therapy. Nurses successful in the test receive the designation of CRNI (Certified Registered Nurse Infusion). This may be renewed every 3 years through testing or recertification units. The ONS Chemotherapy/Biotherapy Provider card is renewed every 2 years through completion of online self-study and testing. The Oncology Nursing Certification Corporation (ONCC) offers general oncology nursing certification resulting in the Oncology Certified Nurse (OCN) designation. In 2005, ONS will offer for the first time two national certifications for advanced practice oncology nurses: one for Advanced Oncology Clinical Nurse

---

BOX 19–2   Basic Education for Oncology Nurses

Comprehensive Understanding of Cancer
- Disease statistics
- Carcinogenesis, including cell structure and cell cycle
- Primary and secondary prevention of cancer
- Seven warning signs of cancer

Current Treatment of Cancer
- Diagnostic evaluation and staging of cancer
- Treatment goals: cure, control, and palliation
- Treatment modalities: indications and side effects:
  - Radiation therapy
  - Chemotherapy
  - Biotherapy
  - Molecular targeted therapy

Patient Care Management and Treatment–Related Symptoms
- Patient assessment and evaluation
- Performance status
- Nutritional status
- Hematologic assessment
- Psychosocial assessment (coping skills and support systems)
- Systems review (cardiac, renal, hepatic, pulmonary, GI), comorbidities

Complications and Toxicities
- Short-term side effects: alopecia, GI reactions, bone marrow suppression, dermatologic and cutaneous disturbances, allergic reactions, phlebitis and extravasation, psychosocial changes
- Long-term side effects: genetic, oncogenetic, immunosuppression, reproductive alterations, psychosocial changes
- Specific organ toxicities: cardiac, renal, pulmonary, hepatic, GI, neurologic, dermatologic, reproductive

Nursing Care
- Early detection and prevention of complications
- Delivery of expert care
- Patient and family education
- Psychosocial support throughout the continuum of care (newly diagnosed, remission, recurrence, terminal)
- Follow-up support needs: complete remission, disease control, hospice

---

Specialists (AOCNS) and the other for Advanced Oncology Nurse Practitioners (AONP). Certification is renewed every 4 years by exam or by accumulating a minimum number of points (ONCC, 2005).

Patient Education

The nurse caring for an oncology patient can make all the difference in the patient's experience with treatment. The nurse acts as the coordinator of care, collaborating with all providers to ensure the highest quality of care. It is critical that patients are actively involved and informed of all aspects of their care to ensure patient satisfaction and a sense of control during treatment. The nurse's role is to advocate for and empower patients and family members to seek information and to ensure informed consent and understanding of their treatment plans. The nurse needs to evaluate whether the patient and significant other have a clear understanding of the treatment goals. Is the goal of treatment to cure, control, or offer palliative relief of symptoms? The patient and significant other should be educated in all aspects of the disease process and treatment methods. When administering antineoplastic agents, the nurse should establish open communication with the patient in all phases of care, even to the extent of actively soliciting patient assistance in clinical functions such as assessing vein status. The wise nurse listens to, and is guided by, patient statements like, "The nurse tried that vein two times last week, and it didn't work." In addition to providing a sense of patient involvement and control, the nurse can capitalize on a patient's intimate knowledge of his or her own body.

It is important to inform a patient that, as IV solutions are infused, it is normal to detect a sense of coolness along the venous pathway. Likewise, it is prudent to alert a patient to early signs of **extravasation** (pain, burning, stinging, a feeling of tightness, tingling, numbness, and any other unusual sensations) when **vesicant** (tissue-damaging) agents are infused because patients can usually detect them before they are apparent to the nurse.

Some antineoplastic and biotherapy drugs are associated with localized and generalized anaphylactic reactions. When signs and symptoms are reported early and treated properly, their course can be reversed or minimized. Particularly with these agents, patients should be encouraged to report unusual symptoms of generalized tingling, chest pains or sensations, shortness of breath, or light-headedness. Education must be tailored to the individual patient based on the patient's learning needs. It is important that the patient understands some side effects can occur once treatment is completed, or anytime during the course of their specific treatment, such as alopecia, bone marrow suppression, diarrhea, fatigue, mucositis, nausea and vomiting, depression, reproductive and sexual side effects, and changes in taste sensations. It is critical that patients are educated on side effects before treatment begins. This allows the patient not only to make an informed decision on the treatment plan, but also reduces fear and anxiety when delayed reactions occur. Education needs to be ongoing with each interaction with your patient and to be multifaceted in delivery.

As patient participation and understanding of the treatment plan increases, there is always the risk that some patients will aggressively seek to direct their own care. Patient statements like these are not uncommon: "This is the vein we'll use today," or "I'll give you one try, but then you'll have to find someone else." The professional nurse knows that such patient behaviors can be traced to understandable anxiety. They do not allow it to undermine their self-confidence. Several minutes spent explaining the rationale and process of vein selection may eliminate the problem. Patients with a cancer diagnosis experience dramatic life changes and loss of control. It is therapeutic for the nurse to allow the patient to be in control when appropriate.

Once a relationship is established, the nurse usually finds that patient behavior shifts to implicit trust in the skill and judgment of the nurse with whom he or she is most familiar. In fact, personal attachment to a particular nurse often begins during the patient education phase of treatment, even before drugs are administered.

During the active treatment phase, the staff and nurses become very important to patients and their extended families. During these uncertain times in their lives, you as a nurse can offer security, hope, and stability. It is important to connect with your patients at a personal level, while maintaining a balanced professional relationship.

Patients are best served when encouraged to tap their own resources and empowered to endure therapy without inordinate focus on the personality of the treatment provider. Ideally, a healthy partnership develops in which the patient is a valued contributor to the nurse's plan of care.

Nurses administering chemotherapy and biotherapy have a tremendous opportunity to minimize treatment-related morbidity (and thus to enhance their patients' quality of life) through competent patient education. Patient, family, and caregiver education is as integral to the cancer treatment regimen as is optimum selection of veins for drug infusion.

The primary focus of this chapter is, of course, chemotherapy and biotherapy administration. At the same time, it is important to recognize that safe and competent delivery of antineoplastics is only half the job of contemporary IV therapy nursing professionals. The more sensitive (and sometimes more influential) part of the art revolves around intuitive patient and family education, fashioned to address a particular patient's situation. Nurses need to adhere to the scope of practice and standards of care established by the Oncology Nursing Society. Key components to be included in patient/family education include the following:

- The patient is able to describe his or her understanding of extent of disease and current treatment at a level consistent with cultural and educational background and emotional state.
- The nurse and patient (and family) agree on learning outcomes based on the patient's needs.
- The patient participates in decision making regarding plan of care and life activities if desired or possible.
- The nurse selects educational methods and materials consistent with the patient's and family's learning needs and abilities.
- The nurse considers how, when, and by whom teaching will be done.
- The nurse continuously evaluates the patient's and family's comprehension, with reference to original learning outcomes.
- The nurse conscientiously documents all components of the education process. An organized and systematic form in the medical record is an efficient and effective way to ensure that this phase of therapy is up to date and critical components are not missed.

Multiple psychosocial, emotional, and physiologic barriers come into play because of the nature of the disease and public perceptions of cancer and cancer therapy. A nurse's primary concern is that the patient not only has adequate information but has absorbed sufficient information to provide legitimate informed consent. When assessing your patients, it is important to address their psychosocial status. How are they and their family members coping? Do they feel they have an adequate support system in place? Patients should be encouraged to communicate their feelings on coping with a cancer diagnosis and referred to appropriate community resources.

Some barriers to patient learning (Table 19–1) can be overcome by methods as simple as teaching in a physical environment that reduces anxiety, including the family in the educational process, and providing patient-appropriate materials. Often it is wise to allow a span of time between a scheduled teaching session and treatment itself so that the patient has time to assimilate important information and form questions concerning areas that are unclear. Certainly patient education is an ongoing process, from the outset and for the duration of therapy. The process may sort itself into a natural division of three phases, with the common outcome of all phases an increased patient understanding of antineoplastic therapy. Table 19–2 summarizes the essential components of the education process. The following guidelines are for nurses involved in patient education. They can be used to evaluate teaching content and technique by assessing the degree to which expected patient outcomes are achieved:

1. Patient demonstrates knowledge related to diagnosis and disease process
   - States diagnosis and explains disease process
   - Describes previous experience with cancer and treatments
   - Acknowledges need for treatment
   - States alternatives to prescribed treatment

(text continues on p. 494)

TABLE 19–1   Potential Barriers to Successful Patient Learning

Type of Barrier	Examples
Emotional	Anxiety related to cancer diagnosis, anticipation of cancer therapy, concern over cost issues
	Depression related to disease process and treatment
	Denial, used as coping mechanism
	External locus of control—learned helplessness and powerlessness
Physiologic	Biochemical imbalances causing nausea and vomiting, fatigue, restlessness, irritability
Psychosocial	Altered consciousness caused by disease process or medications
	Cultural attitudes, beliefs, roles, or values contributing to unwillingness to learn ("My wife/husband takes care of this kind of thing").
	Refusal to claim ownership of self-care; attention to self perceived as selfish and culturally unacceptable
	Lack of inquisitiveness in effort to be perceived as a "good patient"
Functional	Compromised literacy level or language differences
	Being overwhelmed by new information, names of drugs, disease jargon, personnel names, schedules, sequence, and so forth
	Age, undeveloped or decreased data retention or memory
Environmental	Busy, rushed, and distracting
	Unusual or foreign, high-tech, frightening or threatening surroundings
	Restrictive and depersonalized surroundings in close proximity to personnel and other patients

TABLE 19–2   Educational Essentials for Patients Receiving Chemotherapy

Outcomes	Nursing Interventions
Pretreatment Phase • Presentation of sufficient information for the patient to give valid informed consent • Provision of a nonthreatening environment conducive to learning and to accepting chemotherapy confidently	• Provide written, patient-appropriate educational materials explaining specific chemotherapeutic agents and their effects before treatment begins. Allow for extended learning period, if necessary. • Thoroughly discuss expectations of therapy. • Discuss anticipated procedures and administration technique, including need for central venous access, potential side effects, and planned interventions for symptom management. • Encourage patient involvement in decision making regarding care and treatment plan. Have patient bring pretreatment question list to clinic or office. • Conduct patient teaching in a quiet, comfortable, and private environment. • Offer opportunity for the patient and family to tour treatment area. • If possible, introduce patient to IV nurse assigned to patient. • Provide nutritional counseling. • Encourage patient to express fears, concerns, and comprehension of situation. • Emphasize variability and reversibility of side effects such as alopecia and offer patient assistance and alternatives. • Be absolutely honest with patient. • Review drug and food allergy history (document this before first treatment).
Treatment Phase • Provision of sufficient and enabling information, allowing the patient to cope effectively with immediate effects of chemotherapy • Enhancement of the patient's sense of participation in and control over care	• Explain how chemotherapy works (eg, cytotoxic effect of drugs). • Instruct patient to report immediately any discomfort, pain, or burning during the administration of chemotherapy. • Review antiemetic schedule, foods to avoid, and hydration requirements. • Identify known side effects of each drug in use. • Discuss precautions to take against potential adverse effects. • Assess potential for multiple drug therapy complications/incompatibilities, and caution patient to take only medications ordered by physician. • Instruct patient in oral hygiene and use of non–alcohol-based mouth rinses. • Provide calendar with schedule of treatments, appointments with physicians, laboratory tests, and expected time line for neutropenia or thrombocytopenia. • Assist patient in energy conservation program and in setting realistic goals for work and social activities. • As appropriate, discuss contraceptive measures, potential for infertility, and sperm banking.
Post-treatment or Ongoing Treatment Phase • Provision of sufficient information to allow patient to demonstrate self-management	• Explain self-care measures to use in managing side effects of each drug treatment. • Explain reasons for follow-up studies to evaluate disease response.

(Continued)

TABLE 19–2   Educational Essentials for Patients Receiving Chemotherapy   *(Continued)*

Outcomes	Nursing Interventions
strategies to control side effects and to promote functioning at maximum realistic potential	• Remind patient not to travel alone immediately after treatment in most cases. • Instruct patient to report temperature >101.0°F (38°C) and other signs and symptoms of complications, such as increased bruising, blood in urine or stool, bleeding gums, rashes, fatigue, shortness of breath, sore throat, oral lesions, change in bowel habits, numbness or tingling in fingers or toes. • Stress importance of good personal hygiene and hand washing; and avoidance of rectal thermometers, enemas, anal sex, and people with known communicable diseases. • Encourage patient to call for assistance with any new or unusual signs or symptoms. • Provide information on how to reach appropriate health care personnel 24 hours a day. • Confirm return appointments and assist with patient transport services, if needed or possible. • Phone patient after first and subsequent treatments when there is a potential for problems. • Solicit questions from patient and caregivers. • Review and reinforce previous information related to diagnosis, disease, and treatment.

2. Patient demonstrates knowledge related to rationale for chemotherapy and/or biotherapy:
   • Verbalizes need for chemotherapy/biotherapy
   • Expresses attitude toward and expectations about cancer treatment
   • States understanding of use of chemotherapy or biotherapy alone or with other treatment modalities, if applicable
   • Identifies treatment protocol
3. Patient demonstrates knowledge related to potential therapeutic side effects of chemotherapy/biotherapy:
   • States diagnosis and expected response to treatment
   • Identifies specific effect of treatment with antineoplastic agents
4. Patient demonstrates knowledge of treatment plan and schedule:
   • Identifies drugs to be given
   • States frequency and duration of treatment
   • Identifies studies, tests, and procedures required before treatment
   • Identifies follow-up tests, studies, and procedures needed to evaluate treatment results
5. Patient demonstrates knowledge of potential drug side effects:
   • States mechanism of drug action
   • Defines reason for side effects
   • Identifies specific side effects that may occur with each drug
   • States self-management interventions to control side effects
   • Verbalizes signs and symptoms reportable to health care professionals
   • Identifies procedures for reporting signs and symptoms

6. Patient demonstrates knowledge of techniques to manage antineoplastic treatment:
   - Maintains nutritional status to best of ability
   - Follows oral, body, and environmental hygiene measures
   - Maintains optimal rest and activity pattern
   - Uses safety precautions to prevent injury
   - Seeks and uses resources as necessary
   - Verbalizes reduced anxiety related to treatment
   - States intention to comply with treatment plan
7. Patient demonstrates knowledge relative to various access devices, if applicable.

Oncology nurses are encouraged to refer to and follow the ONS *Statement on the Scope and Standards of Oncology Nursing Practice* (Brant & Wickham, 2004). Additionally, adhering to the ONS *Standards of Oncology Education: Patient/Significant Other and Public* (Blecher, 2004) will ensure thorough patient and family education in the disease process, treatment, toxicities, and symptom management.

Legal Considerations Related to Education

A thorough understanding of legal responsibilities and implications is an essential element of professional education for the nurse administering antineoplastic agents. Nurses need to know the specific regulations related to chemotherapy administration in their own state's Nurse Practice Act.

LEGAL ISSUES: Legal Considerations Pertinent to Cancer Chemotherapy

- *Clinical education:* Before treating any patient, the nurse's successful training in IV fluid and drug administration should be documented and available in personnel files.
- *Lines of supervision:* The nurse should have a clear, written statement of the lines of supervision.
- *Standards of care:* The nurse should have a clear, written statement of the employing facility's standards of care, including a definition of reasonable care in each pertinent area of practice. Facility-specific policies and procedures should be based on nationally established standards from professional organizations, including but not limited to the Infusion Nurses Society (INS, 2005), ONS, and American Nurses Association (ANA).
- *Patient and family education:* The nurse should initiate and complete patient and family education regarding treatment goals, all medications in the treatment regimen, side effects, length of therapy, and follow-up restaging. Evaluation of the patient's understanding and response to teaching should be documented.
- *Informed consent:* Patients who are participating in clinical drug trials must sign an informed consent form before administration of the **investigational** (experimental) **protocol.** Specific regulations regarding written informed consent for noninvestigational protocols vary from state to state. Although obtaining informed consent is a physician's responsibility in most states, a nurse should make sure that consent has been granted before administering chemotherapy. The hospital or institution may be held liable if treatment is administered without the informed consent of the patient or responsible parties. Failure to obtain a patient's consent may constitute battery, defined as any physical contact of a patient without his or her permission.

It is in a nurse's best interest to request a written definition of the institution's scope of practice and to explore details of medical liability insurance covering the practice. Many employers provide adequate coverage for care administered when the nurse is on duty. All nurses—especially independent practitioners, instructors, or those working in physicians' offices—may opt for personal malpractice coverage. Nurses who assume greater responsibility in administering cancer chemotherapy are at greater risk for litigation.

Meticulous adherence to the details of defined statutes and standards of care may minimize that risk. The ANA, individual departments of professional regulation for the state's Nurse Practice Act, INS, and ONS can provide more details on legal statutes that govern nursing practice pertaining to administration of chemotherapeutic agents.

Because a patient's clinical record is a legal document that can be used as evidence in a lawsuit, it is a crucial nursing responsibility to ensure that documentation is accurate, comprehensive, and current. The essentials of adequate documentation include time of a significant incident, a thorough and objective description of the care provided, the patient's status, and the exact nature of physician involvement.

The expert oncology nurse frequently practices more autonomously than nursing colleagues in other specialties, which implies increased legal vulnerability. For example, because extensive telephone contact is common with patients with cancer, the nurse should therefore be mindful of the accepted scope of practice when responding to patient needs. Telephone protocols related to symptom management may serve as guidelines for the nurse in responding to calls from patients.

The nurse commonly is a key clinician involved in clinical trials that call for take-home investigational drugs. By law, only a pharmacist or physician may dispense medication. Therefore, packaging and delivering investigational drugs are not usually legal functions for nurses. Finally, knowledge of common dosing and scheduling of each common chemotherapeutic agent is the best protection (for patient and nurse) from delivering an incorrect and possibly lethal drug dose.

Safe Preparation, Handling, and Disposal of Chemotherapeutic and Biologic Agents

In 2004, the U.S. National Institute for Occupational Safety and Health (NIOSH) issued an alert entitled "Preventing Occupational Exposures to Antineoplastic and Other Hazardous Drugs in Health Care Settings." Drugs are classified as *hazardous* if animal or human studies indicate that exposure to them has the potential for causing cancer, developmental or reproductive toxicity, or harm to organs (NIOSH, 2004). Antineoplastic drugs are among the agents considered hazardous. Personnel who prepare, handle, administer, and dispose of chemotherapy and biotherapy drugs risk exposure to hazardous agents. Although the therapeutic benefits outweigh the risks of side effects for ill patients, health care workers who are exposed to hazardous drugs risk these same side effects without the therapeutic benefit. Guidelines have been established since 1986 for handling antineoplastics safely (Occupational Safety and Health Administration [OSHA], 1986). The 2004 NIOSH alert summarized the health effects associated with hazardous drugs and provided recommendations for safe handling.

Adherence to recommendations for safe handling of these agents minimizes potential routes of exposure through skin or mucous membrane contact, absorption, inhalation, ingestion or accidental needlestick (Polovich, 2003), as well as contact with body fluids of the patient who has received antineoplastic agents within the past 48 hours. Occupational exposures to hazardous drugs can result in skin rashes, skin and mucous membrane irritation, blurred vision, light-headedness, allergic reactions, headache, nausea, and **alopecia** (hair loss). Long-term exposure results in liver dysfunction, chromosomal abnormalities, reproductive risks, and increased risk of cancer (Itano & Taoka, 2005). These manifestations appear in direct relationship to the time, amount, and method of exposure to specific classes of antineoplastics. Health care professionals can minimize their potential health risks by strict adherence to safe handling guidelines embedded in antineoplastic policies and procedures, along with cautions during drug preparation and administration. Employees who are pregnant, planning pregnancy, or breast-feeding should be allowed to refrain from preparation and administration of hazardous agents or from caring for the patient during treatment with them (NIOSH, 2004; OSHA, 1986).

OSHA recommends that workers handling hazardous drugs be monitored through a medical surveillance program that includes medical and exposure history, physical examination, and some laboratory tests (NIOSH, 2004). A list of all employees who are exposed to hazardous drugs should be maintained with careful documentation of spills, spill cleanup, and accidental exposures. Periodic review of drug preparation and administration practices can ensure that all staff have the necessary training to handle hazardous agents in the workplace (Polovich, 2003). Successful administration of chemotherapy and biotherapy calls for expert judgment based on scientific evidence. Expert technical skills aside, the safe administration of these agents requires knowledge of preparation, administration, and disposal of hazardous drugs (Box 19–3). A basic understanding of the indications for use and mechanisms of action of antineoplastic drugs is pivotal to the quality of patient care an IV nurse provides.

Overview of Antineoplastic Therapy

Before the discovery of chemical and biologic agents to treat cancer, surgery and radiation therapy were the primary cancer treatment techniques. These modalities remain useful in treating localized tumors that can be surgically removed or destroyed by radiating the genetic material in the cancer cells.

In many cases, cancer is a systemic disease that requires systemic therapy. By nature, cancer cells deviate from normal cells in structure, function, and production; therefore, a characteristic of cancer is the cell's ability to invade surrounding tissue, blood, and lymphatic vessels and spread beyond the localized region of the primary disease site (DeVita, Hellman, & Rosenberg, 2004). The ability of these aberrant cells to metastasize forms the basis for systemic antineoplastic therapy. Antineoplastic

(text continues on p. 501)

BOX 19–3   Administration of Antineoplastic Agents: Safe Handling, Preparation, Administration, and Disposal

Drug Preparation

All antineoplastic drugs should be prepared by specially trained personnel in a centralized area to minimize interruptions and risks of contamination.

- Prepare drugs in a Class II type B or Class III vertical airflow biologic safety cabinet (BSC) Air is exhausted to the outside through HEPA filters. The blower remains on at all times. The hood is serviced and certified by a qualified technician at least every 6 months (Polovich, 2003) according to the manufacturer's recommendations.
- Never eat, drink, smoke, chew gum, apply cosmetics, or store food in the drug preparation area (OSHA, 1986).
- Cover the work surface with a plastic backed absorbent pad to minimize contamination. Change the pad immediately in the event of contamination and at the completion of drug preparation each day or shift (Itano &Taoka, 2005).
- Use aseptic preparation technique and mix according to the physician's order, other pharmaceutical resources, or both.
- Use unpowdered, disposable, good quality gloves made of latex, nitrile, polyurethane, neoprene, or other materials that have been tested with hazardous drugs. Inspect gloves for visible defects. Double glove when preparing hazardous drugs. Tuck inner glove under the gown sleeve; the cuff of the outer glove extends over the gown sleeve. Change gloves after each use, immediately if torn, punctured, or contaminated with drug or after 30 minutes of wear (Polovich, 2003; NIOSH, 2004).
- Wear a disposable long-sleeved gown made of lint-free fabric with knitted cuffs and a closed front during drug preparation. Laboratory coats and other cloth fabrics absorb fluids, so they are an inadequate barrier to hazardous drugs and are not recommended (Polovich, 2003). Discard gown after drug preparation, after handling cytotoxic drugs, and if visibly contaminated. Gowns should not be reused (NIOSH, 2004)
- Wear a plastic face shield (protect eye, mouth, and nasal opening) or goggles (only protect eyes) when the possibility of splashing is evident. Use a powered air-purifying respirator or National Institute for Occupational Safety and Health (NIOSH)–approved face mask when cleaning up cytotoxic spills. Surgical masks do not provide respiratory protection from aerosolized powders or liquids (Polovich, 2003).
- Use needles, syringes, tubing, and connectors with Luer-lock connections (Polovich, 2003).
- Guard against potential chemical contamination by priming all IV tubing under the protection of the laminar airflow hood with nondrug solution before adding hazardous drugs (Polovich, 2003). This prevents chemical exposure when connecting IV tubing.
- Guard against drug leakage during drug preparation; use special care when reconstituting agents packaged in the following:
  - **Ampules:** Clear drug from neck of ampule; break top of the ampule away from body; withdraw drug through filter needle with ampule upright on flat surface; change needle before administration.
  - **Vials:** Use multiuse dispensing pin or 18- to19-gauge needle with dispensing pin; Aspirate air slightly larger than diluent volume to create negative pressure in vial; add diluent slowly down the side of vial; withdraw dose into syringe; remove needle when pressure between vial and syringe is equalized (Itano & Taoka, 2005). Use of a closed system (such as PhaSeal [Baxa Corp., Englewood, CO.]) limits aerosolization of drug and worker exposure to sharps when withdrawing hazardous drugs from vials (NIOSH, 2004).
- Avoid overfilling syringes. Fill syringes no more than three-fourths full (Polovich, 2003) Expel air from a syringe slowly into a sterile gauze pad contained in a sealable plastic bag (Itano & Taoka, 2005).

BOX 19–3   Administration of Antineoplastic Agents: Safe Handling, Preparation, Administration, and Disposal   *(Continued)*

- After reconstituting the drug, label it according to institutional policies and procedures. Include the drug's vesicant properties and hazardous drug warning on the label.
- Transport antineoplastic drugs in an impervious packing material, such as a zippered bag, and mark the bag with a distinctive warning label stating "Hazardous Drug: Handle with Gloves, Dispose of Properly" (Polovich, 2003).
- Dispose of gowns, gloves, and preparation equipment in appropriately labeled puncture-proof containers.
- Be informed on procedures to follow in the event of drug spillage.

Drug Administration

Chemotherapeutic agents are administered by registered professional nurses who have been specially trained and designated as qualified according to specific institutional policies and procedures.

- Ensure that informed consent has been given before administering any chemotherapeutic agent; also clarify any misconceptions the patient may have regarding the drugs and their side effects.
- Review laboratory test results (eg, complete blood count, renal and liver function values) for acceptable levels. Drug dosages may need to be adjusted by the physician according to laboratory values. Cardiac (ECG or MUGA scan) and pulmonary function tests (PFTs) may need to be evaluated based on the drug's side effect profile (Alexander & Corrigan, 2004).
- Determine the vesicant/irritant potential of drugs(s) and implement measures to minimize acute side effects of the drugs before drug administration.
- Assess orders for completeness, eg, hydration and premedications such as antiemetics, antianxiety, antihypersensitivity agents (Polovich et al. 2005).
- Have available a chemotherapy spill kit, extravasation management information and antidotes and equipment, and emergency drugs and equipment in case of adverse reactions, such as anaphylaxis (Polovich et al., 2005).
- Review the physician's order. Compare with formal drug protocol or reference source; check for completeness (schedule, route, admixture solution, etc.; Itano & Taoka, 2005).
- Determine drug dose. Verify actual height and weight. Calculate body surface area (BSA) or appropriate dose calculations, eg, mg/kg or area under the curve (AUC).
- Perform *independent* double check on dosage calculations (pharmacist and chemotherapy-credentialed nurse and/or two chemotherapy credentialed nurses) and verify dose against physician's order. Verify that the dose is appropriate for the patient, diagnosis, and treatment plan (Polovich et al., 2005).
- Check the syringe, IV bag or bottle against the original physician's order to verify medication, dose, route, time, and patient identification.(use two different patient identifiers). Perform double check with two chemotherapy-credentialed nurses (Polovich et al., 2005).
- Wear personal protective equipment (PPE), including nonpowdered surgical latex, nitrile, polyurethane, or neoprene disposable gloves and a disposable gown made of a lint-free, low-permeability fabric with a closed front, long sleeves, and elastic or knit closed cuffs. Double gloving is recommended (NIOSH, 2004). Change gloves after each use, tear, puncture, or contamination or after 30 minutes of wear (Polovich et al., 2005).
- Wear PPE for biologic agents, such as interferon, classified as hazardous (NIOSH, 2004). Because of limited occupational exposure data, use PPE when handling other biotherapy agents, eg, interleukin-2 or monoclonal antibodies, to maintain consistency of nursing practice (Itano & Taoka, 2005) Use gloves when handling oral antineoplastic agents. Use face shield if there is risk of splashing, eg, intravesical instillation (Polovich, 2003).

(Continued)

BOX 19–3   Administration of Antineoplastic Agents: Safe Handling, Preparation, Administration, and Disposal   *(Continued)*

- Gather all supplies needed for drug administration. Protect the work surface with a disposable absorbent pad. Perform all work below eye level. Don PPE, inspect drug container within delivery bag for leaks prior to removing the hazardous drug from the delivery bag. Do not prime or expel air of intravenous (IV), intramuscular (IM), or subcutaneous (SQ) injection syringes (Polovich, 2003).
- Administer the drug or drugs according to established institutional policies and procedures and physician's order, using safe handling precautions.
- Flush IV tubing with 100 mL appropriate flush solution, eg, normal saline, to patient through distal port to remove chemotherapeutic agent before disconnection.
- Document drug administration, including any adverse reaction, in the medical record.
- Establish a mechanism for identifying the patient receiving antineoplastic agents for the 48-hour period after drug administration.
- Implement standard precautions when handling body secretions such as urine, stool, blood, or emesis of patients who received hazardous drugs within the prior 48 hours.. Wear a disposable gown if potential splash contamination is a concern. NIOSH specifies use of two pairs of appropriate gloves and a gown whenever handling linens, feces, or urine from patients who have received hazardous drugs within the last 48 hours (NIOSH, 2004). Dispose of PPE after each use or when it becomes contaminated.
- In the event of accidental exposure, remove contaminated gloves or gown immediately and discard according to institutional procedures.
- Wash the contaminated skin with soap (nongermicidal) and copious amounts of water (OSHA, 1986). Refer to MSDS for agent-specific interventions.
- For accidental eye exposure, flood the eye immediately with water or isotonic eyewash for at least 15 minutes. Areas where hazardous drugs are routinely handled should be equipped with an eye wash station (Polovich, 2003).
- Obtain a medical evaluation as soon as possible after exposure and document the incident according to institutional policies and procedures.

Drug Disposal

Regardless of the setting (hospital, ambulatory care, physician's office, or home), all equipment and unused drugs are treated as hazardous and disposed of according to the institution's policies and procedures.

- Hazardous drug waste containers should be available in all areas where hazardous drugs are prepared and administered. Any item that comes is contact with a hazardous drug during preparation or administration is considered potentially contaminated and must be disposed of as hazardous waste (Polovich, 2003).
- Discard all contaminated equipment, including needles, intact to prevent aerosolization, leaks, and spills. Dispose of contaminated sharps in puncture-proof hazardous waste container.
- Place contaminated materials including PPE in a sealable 4-mm polyethylene or 2-mm polypropylene bag and dispose of in a leakproof, punctureproof container with a distinctive warning label identifying "Hazardous Waste" (NIOSH, 2004; Polovich, 2003).
- Put linen contaminated with bodily secretions of patients who have received chemotherapy/biotherapy within the previous 48 hours in a specially marked laundry bag and place the bag in an impervious bag marked with a distinctive biohazard warning label.

BOX 19–3   Administration of Antineoplastic Agents: Safe Handling, Preparation, Administration, and Disposal   *(Continued)*

- Follow established institutional policies and procedures for management of spills. The size of the spill might dictate who is to conduct the cleanup and decontamination and how the cleanup is managed. A small spill is one that is <5 mL or 5 g. outside of BSC. A large spill is >5 mL or 5 g.
- Obtain a spill kit, which is readily available in areas where preparation and administration of hazardous drugs occur (Polovich et al., 2005). The spill kit includes the following: PPE (disposable low-permeability gown, two pairs of disposable gloves, shoe covers, splash goggles or safety goggles, and NIOSH-approved respirator.) and additional equipment for cleanup (plastic waste bags, plastic-backed spill pads, 250 mL and 1 L spill-control pillows, small scoops to collect broken glass pieces, disposable toweling, puncture-resistant containers, plastic scraper, two disposal bags, hazardous waste labels.
- For large spills, limit access to area of spill. Post warning sign.
- Put on a double pair of nonpowdered gloves, face shield, and tightly closing disposable gown to dispose of a large spill >5 mL. Wear NIOSH-approved respirator mask.
- Clean up small amounts of liquids with gauze pads; for large spills >5 mL, contain spill with spill-control pillows or absorb liquids with absorbent toweling (Polovich, 2003).
- Clean up small amounts of solids or powder with a damp absorbent gauze pad or soft toweling.
- Clean the spill area from the least contaminated to the most contaminated area with a detergent followed by a clean water rinse.
- Collect broken glassware with scoop and place in a punctureproof container. Dispose of all contaminated material in a sealable 4-mm polyethylene or 2-mm polypropylene bag marked with a distinctive biohazard warning label.
- Remove PPE and place in waste bag; seal bag and place in a punctureproof container.
- Keep in mind that contaminated reusable items are washed by specially trained personnel wearing double unpowdered latex gloves.
- Document spills according to established institutional policies and procedures.

(Adapted from Polovich, M., White, J.M., Kelleher, L.O., et al. [Eds.]. [2005]. *Chemotherapy and biotherapy: Guidelines and recommendations for practice* [2nd Ed.]. Pittsburgh, PA: Oncology Nursing Society.)

---

therapy includes chemotherapy and biotherapy. These systemic modalities are indicated for hematologic malignancies or for solid tumors that have either the potential to spread or have already metastasized.

Chemotherapy

Chemotherapy agents work by disrupting cellular events occurring within the cell cycle of both cancer cells and normal cells. Chemotherapy controls cancer with **cytotoxic** (cell-killing). chemical agents designed to kill rapidly dividing cancer cells with minimal impact on cells with normal, healthy mitotic characteristics. Because of the effect on normal cells as well as cancer cells, the side effects that are experienced are related to the rapidly proliferating normal cells.

Nitrogen mustard was the first modern chemical used therapeutically to treat the uncontrolled cellular proliferation that characterizes cancer. This lucky discovery resulted from scientific observation that bone marrow depletion (hypoplasia) occurred in soldiers exposed to mustard gases during World War II. In the 1960s and 1970s, drug development focused on screening natural and plant sources for antitumor agents, for example, cisplatin. The 1980s and 1990s saw the development of new chemotherapy agents, such as paclitaxel; various analogues of previous agents, such as ifosfamide; or modifications to chemotherapy drugs, including Abraxane to minimize the toxic side effects to normal tissues.

Chemotherapy drugs are grouped according to their specific effect on cancer cell chemistry and the cell cycle phase in which they interfere. The **cell cycle** refers to a series of phases in normal cell and cancer cell growth. Cell cycle time is the length of time needed for a cell to replicate.

Chemotherapy agents fall into two categories: cell cycle phase-specific agents are active only during a particular phase in the cell proliferation cycle; cell cycle phase-nonspecific agents are active at any point of the cell proliferation cycle. Regardless of whether the chemotherapy is cell cycle specific or cell cycle nonspecific, the basic mechanism of antineoplastic action is the same: to disrupt DNA synthesis. This disables cell reproduction, so the cancer cells die. Chemotherapy generally is most effective when the cell is actively dividing.

Chemotherapeutic agents are further categorized into major groups such as **alkylating agents,** nitrosoureas, **antimetabolites, plant alkaloids**, antitumor antibiotics, taxanes, topoisomerase I inhibitors, and miscellaneous. Within each of these categories is a spectrum of agents with various toxicities, all of which relate to their antineoplastic properties.

Chemotherapy drug toxicities can be appreciated by understanding that these agents are designed to destroy rapidly dividing cells; therefore, the toxicities that are seen occur in cells that divide rapidly, such as bone marrow, hair follicles, gastrointestinal mucosa, and reproductive tissues. Thus, the most frequent side effects of these drugs include cytopenias, alopecia, mucositis, nausea, vomiting, and infertility.

Table 19–3 provides a quick reference chemotherapy guide for drug handling, dosing, administration, side effects, and major toxicities. Comprehensive tables are available and should be used for more detailed information on indications for use, drug preparation, pharmacokinetics, and protocols.

Biotherapy

Biotherapy, previously called immunotherapy, refers to systemic treatment with agents from biologic sources or those agents that affect biologic responses. As a class, these agents are known as biologic response modifiers because of their ability to influence and change the relationship of the tumor and the host, resulting in therapeutic effects. Biologic agents are classified by their action: agents that augment, modulate, or restore the immune response of the host; agents that have direct **anticancer** activity (antiproliferation or cytotoxic effect on cancer cells); and agents that have other biologic effects such as differentiation and maturation of

(text continues on p. 521)

TABLE 19-3 Quick Reference to Commonly Administered Parenteral Chemotherapeutic Agents

Drug	Usual Dose	Usual Administration Technique	Comments and Major Toxicities
Amifostine (Ethyl) Chemoprotectant	740–910 mg/m² for reduction of bone marrow, kidney, or nerve toxicity 200–340 mg/m² for reduction of xerostomia	IVPB over 15 min 15–30 min prior to chemotherapy agents IVP over 3–5 min prior to radiation SQ	Transient hypotension (dose limiting) Nausea, vomiting, and somnolence (common) Sneezing, flushing, hypocalcemia
Arsenic trioxide (Trisenox) Novel arsenical differentiation agent	Induction: 0.15 mg/kg until bone marrow remission (up to 60 doses) Consolidation: 0.15 mg/kg × 25 doses over a period up to 5 wk	IVP (100–250 mL of D₅W) over 2 h	"Differentiation syndrome" characterized as leukocytosis, fever, dyspnea, chest pain, tachycardia, hypoxia, and sometimes death. Corticosteroids seem to benefit this syndrome (dose limiting) QT prolongation (common) Avoid other drugs that prolong QT interval Rash, pruritus, headache, arthralgias, anxiety, bleeding, nausea, vomting (common) Liver and renal toxicity (uncommon)
Asparaginase (Elspar) Enzyme Non-chemotherapeutic agent	15–25,000 IU/kg as a single dose 200 IU/kg/d for 28 d	IVP 30 min IVPB (D₅W, NS) ≤1,000 mL IM	Hypersensitivity (life threatening, requiring anaphylaxis precautions and a 2-unit test dose) IM reduces incidence of anaphylaxis Coagulopathy is common and requires monitoring Nausea, vomiting, abdominal cramps, anorexia, elevated liver function tests, transient renal insufficiency (common) Depression, lethargy, drowsiness, fatigue, confusion Fever, pancreatitis
Azacytidine (Vidaza) Antimetabolite	Initial cycle: 75 mg/m² SQ daily for 7 d. Every 4 wk. Subsequent cycles: 100 mg/m² daily for 7 d	SQ Gently roll syringe between palms to mix medication immediately prior to administration. Divide dose >4 mL into 2 syringes and inject into 2 sites. Rotate sites.	Myelosuppression (dose limiting) Prolonged leucopenia Nausea, vomiting, diarrhea (common) Mucositis (rare) Liver enzymes elevated and liver function compromised (common) Transient azotemia Lethargy, confusion, coma have been reported

(Continued)

503

TABLE 19–3 Quick Reference to Commonly Administered Parenteral Chemotherapeutic Agents *(Continued)*

Drug	Usual Dose	Usual Administration Technique	Comments and Major Toxicities
Bleomycin (Blenoxane) Antitumor Antibiotic	10–20 U/m² q wk or twice weekly IM, IV, or SQ Constant infusions over 3–7 d at 20 U/m²/d Cumulative lifetime dose should not exceed 400 units	IVP, IM, or SQ, IVPB (rare)	Reversible or irreversible pulmonary fibrosis (dose limiting) Hypersensitivity (administer test dose) Fever and chills (premedicate with acetaminophen) Pruritic erythema, hyperpigmentation, photosensitivity (common) Alopecia, nausea, and vomiting Renal or hepatic toxicity Mucositis, myelosuppression (rare)
Bortezomib (Velcade) Proteasome inhibitor	1.3 mg/m² IV twice weekly for 2 wk followed by 10-d rest period	IVP over 3–5 s	Myelosuppression Nausea, vomiting, diarrhea, constipation, anorexia Peripheral neuropathy (dose limiting) Hepatic and renal toxicity Rash, flulike symptoms, fever, fatigue Orthostatic hypotension
Busulfan (Busulfex) Alkylating agent	Induction: 4–12 mg/d Maintenance doses are usually 1–3 mg/d, but can range from 2 mg/wk to 4 mg/d	Oral, or IV infusion over 2 h	Nadir: 11–30 recovery 24–57 Prolonged myelosuppression with slow recovery (dose limiting) Severe thrombocytopenia, anemia, electrolyte imbalances Nausea, vomiting, anorexia, mucositis, hyperpigmentation, elevated liver function tests (common) HTN, tachycardia, thrombosis, vasodilatation Interstitial lung disease
Carboplatin (Paraplatin) Alkylating agent	360–400 mg/m² q4wk *Dose is commonly based on a desired area under the curve (AUC) using a specific formula	IV infusion (D₅W, NS) May dilute to as low as 0.5 mg/mL Can be given intraperitoneally and intra-arterially	Nadir at d 21; recovery by d 28–30 Myelosuppression, especially thrombocytopenia (dose limiting) Nausea, vomiting, anorexia Ototoxicity

Drug / Classification	Dosage	Administration	Side Effects / Nursing Considerations
Carmustine (BCNU) Alkylating agent Nitrosourea Irritant	150–200 mg/m² q6wk as a single dose or divided over a period of 2 d	IVPB (D$_5$W, NS) Infuse in 100–250 mL over 1–2 h (max 2 h) Carmustine wafers implanted during surgical resection of glioblastoma multiforme	Increase in creatinine and blood urea nitrogen *Do not use aluminum needles.* Delayed nadir 4–5 wk after administration and may last 60 d Myelosuppression (slow at onset, cumulative, dose limiting) Severe nausea and vomiting Alopecia, painful/burning venous irritation during administration Hypotension Infiltrates and/or pulmonary fibrosis Azotemia, decreased kidney size, renal failure Impotence, testicular damage causing infertility, facial flushing
Cisplatin (Platinol) Alkylating agent Vesicant if concentrated	20–40 mg/m² d × 3–5 d q3–4wk 20–120 mg/m² given as a single dose q3–4wk Closely monitor creatinine clearance (may require dose adjustments) 100–200 mg/m² for IP ovarian cancer	IV infusion (D$_5$W, NS) 250–1,000 mL Infuse over 30 min–8 h Prehydrate 1–2 L NS with 20 mEqK + 8 mEq MgSO$_4$ (commonly given) Posthydration 1–2 L is also common Intraperitoneal (IP) Intra-arterially	Hydration should be adequate to maintain an I/O of 100 to 150 mL/h before administration of the drug Severe nausea and vomiting—lasting 24–96 h Aggressive antiemetic tx. is required Peripheral neuropathy (dose limiting for cumulative doses) Nephrotoxicity (dose limiting for individual doses) Ototoxicity Nadir on d 18–23 and recovery by d 39 (mild) Alopecia Electrolyte imbalances, especially K or Mg wasting *Use 5µ-em filter for solutions containing mannitol* *Do not use aluminum needles*
Cladribine (Leustatin) 2-CdA Antimetabolite	0.09 mg/kg/d × 7 d (for hairy cell leukemia) Other malignancies 0.1–0, 3 mg/kg/d × 7 d repeated q4–5wk	24 h continuous infusion for 7 d A second cycle of tx has been given to some nonresponding patients	Unstable in D$_5$W Thrombocytopenia, neutropenia with nadir at 7–14 d Universal lymphopenia Cellulitis at catheter site, rash, asthenia, fever, chills, fatigue

(Continued)

TABLE 19–3 Quick Reference to Commonly Administered Parenteral Chemotherapeutic Agents *(Continued)*

Drug	Usual Dose	Usual Administration Technique	Comments and Major Toxicities
		Can be given as 2-h infusion and by SQ injection	Renal toxicty (dose limiting)
Cyclophosphamide (Cytoxan) Alkylating agent	May be given as single dose or in several divided doses, common doses of 500–1,500 mg/m² q3wk	IVP over 5–10 min (doses <750 mg)	Leukocyte nadir 8–14 d and recovery in 18–25 d
			Myelosuppression (dose limiting)
	50 to 200 mg/m²/d orally for 14 d of a 28-d tx cycle	IVPB (D₅W, D₅NS) infuse in 100–150 mL over 15–30 min	Nausea and vomiting 6–10 h after treatment
	400 mg/m²/d for 4 d every 4–6 wk	Higher doses require hydration of 500 mL or more of NS	Alopecia, nail and skin hyperpigmentation
			Nasal congestion and burning, metallic taste during infusion
			Hypersensitivity reactions
			Testicular atrophy and amenorrhea
			Acute hemorrhagic cystitis (give dose in AM)
			Frequent voiding; hydrate to prevent cystitis
			Mesna (uroprotectant) for high doses
			Cardiac necrosis and/or acute myopericarditis with high dose (rare)
			Secondary malignancies
Cytarabine (Ara-C) Antimetabolite	60 to 200 mg/m² IV for 5–10 d	IVP (low dose) over 1–2 min, IV in 50 mL or more approximately over 30 min	Nadir in 5–7 d, leucopenia, thrombocytopenia, anemia (dose limiting)
	100 mg/m² IV or SQ BID for 5 d every 28 d	For high dose, IV (D₅W, NS) in 250–500 mL over 1–3 h	Nausea, vomiting, anorexia, diarrhea (common)
	High dose: 1–3 g/m² q12h for 3–6 d		Metallic taste, mucositis (common)
	10 mg/m² SQ q12h for 15–21 d	Cytarabine liposome administered only intrathecally or intraventricular over 1–5 min	Rare syndrome of sudden respiratory distress, rapid progression to pulmonary edema
	10–30 mg/m² intrathecally up to 3 times per wk		Keratoconjunctivitis with high doses (use dexamethasone eyedrops for prevention)
			Cerebellar toxicity (lethargy, confusion, slurred speech)
			Most cases resolve, but in some cases irreversible and/or even fatal
			Flulike symptoms, bone/muscle pain, skin rash, alopecia (common)
			Concurrent tx with Decadron is recommended for IT or intraventricular route

Drug/Classification	Dose	Administration	Side Effects/Comments
Dacarbazine (DTIC) Alkylating agent Irritant	375 mg/m² on d 1 and 15 (as part of the ABDV regimen for Hodgkin's disease) 5-d course of 150–250 mg/m²d repeated q3–4wk 650–1,450 mg/m² as a single dose q3–4wk 400–500 mg/m² By IVP on days 1 and 2 q3–4wk 200 mg/m² daily continuous 96-h infusion repeated q3–4wk	IV (D$_5$W, NS) in 100 mL or more Infuse over 30–60 min Can be given IVP or by rapid infusion over 15 min, but may increase venous irritation	Nadir at 2–4 weeks after treatment, leucopenia, thrombocytopenia, anemia (dose limiting) Severe nausea and vomiting; prevent with aggressive antiemetic support Fever, anorexia, metallic taste (common) Flulike symptoms with high doses Facial flushing *Irritant: Avoid extravasation. Local pain at injection site. Slow rate of infusion to decrease pain from venous spasm.* *Protect from light. Pink solution indicates decomposition.*
Dactinomycin (Cosmegen) Antitumor antibiotic Vesicant	*Adults* 1–2 mg/m² q3wk 0.25–0.6 mg/m²/d × 5 d q3–4wk 12 µg/kg/d × 5 d for gestational trophoblastic neoplasia 15 µg/kg/d × 5 d *Children* 0.25–0.5 mg/m²/d × 5 d; not to exceed 0.5 mg/d	IVP slowly over 2–3 min IVPB (D$_5$W, NS) in 50 mL over 20–30 min As an isolated perfusion for solid tumors, this can be administered at doses of 50 µg/kg (lower extremity) and 35 µ/kg (upper extremity)	Leukopenia, thrombocytopenia 1–2 wk after tx. Nadir at 3 wk (dose limiting) Severe nausea and vomiting (occur 1 h after dose and may last several hours) Erythema, actiniform lesions, hyperpigmentation, alopecia (common) Mucositis, anorexia, diarrhea (uncommon) Skin irritation, erythema, or necrosis in previously irradiated areas ("radiation recall")
Daunorubicin (Cerubidine) Antitumor antibiotic Vesicant	30–60 mg/m²/d q3–4wk 45 mg/m²/d × 3 d (tx of acute leukemia) Pediatric doses will vary; patients >60 y may need lesser dosing. Specific dosing will also depend on the tx plan	Single IV injection or split into 3–5-d schedule running IV over 2–5 min	Nadir between 1–2 wk, recovery in 2–3 wk Grade 3–4 neutropenia with higher dosing (dose-limiting) Nausea and vomiting 1 hr after dose and lasting for several hours (prevented by antiemetics) Alopecia, mucositis (common) Rash, diarrhea, elevated liver enzymes (uncommon)

(Continued)

Drug	Usual Dose	Usual Administration Technique	Comments and Major Toxicities
	Liposomal daunorubicin 40 mg q2wk	IVPB over 60 minutes	Cumulative cardiotoxicity at max. lifetime dose of 500–600 mg/m² (aggravated by concurrent radiation) Arrhythmias, usually asymptomatic/transient, congestive cardiomyopathy Fever, chills, hyperuricemia Red urine—advise patient
Dexrazoxane (Zinecard) Cardioprotectant	Dosage ratio of 10 mg/m² of dexrazoxane for every 1 mg/m² of doxorubicin (10:1 ratio)	Slow IVP or rapid IV infusion (NS, D₅W) over 15–30 min In final concentration of 1.3–5 mg/mL	This medication is to be given 30 min before administration of doxorubicin Dexrazoxane may add to myelosuppression Mild nausea, vomiting, anorexia (common) Fever, mucositis, fatigue, anorexia (uncommon) Hypotension, DVTs, liver toxicity
Docetaxel (Taxotere) Antimicrotubule agent	60–100 mg/m² q1–3wk 40 mg/m²/wk for 6 wk followed by 2-wk rest 75 mg/m² q3wk *Other doses have been evaluated	IV over 1–3 hours Final concentration of 0.3–0.74 mg diluted in 250 mL D₅ or NS Avoid PVC tubing or bags to administer docetaxel	Severe neutropenia (dose limiting) Total alopecia (universal) Edema, fluid retention, ascites, pleural effusions are common (dose limiting) *Recommended premedication:* dexamethasone 8 mg BID 1 d prior to docetaxel for a total of 3 d to reduce fluid accumulation Capillary leak syndrome in patients after cumulative dose of 400 mg/m² Hypersensitivity or anaphylaxis (uncommon when premedicated with steroids and antihistamines) Peripheral neuropathy, mucositis, diarrhea (mild, common) Rash, hand-foot syndrome, elevated liver functions (uncommon)
Doxorubicin (Adriamycin) Antitumor	Usual dose of 60–75 mg/m² as a bolus injection or a continuous infusion	Bolus (extravasation precautions) over 2–5 min	Nadir at 10–14 d and recovery in 21 d Myelosuppression (universal, dose limiting with individual dose)

Drug/Classification	Administration	Dose	Side Effects/Comments
Antibiotic Vesicant	IVPB (D5W, NS) in 50–100 mL over 20–30 min via central line Has also been given intra-arterially to liver, intravesicularly, and intraperitoneally	over 2–4 d q3–4wk (higher bolus doses of 80–90 mg/m² have also been used) 20–30 mg/m² daily for 3 d q3–4wk	Alopecia, hyperpigmentation of nail beds and dermal creases, facial swelling (common) Nausea and vomiting, anorexia, mucositis—especially with daily schedule Radiation recall (irritation of previously irradiated areas) Cardiotoxicity: CHF, ECG changes, monitoring of LVEF (dose limiting) Lifetime cumulative dose 550 mg/m² May enhance cyclophosphamide cystitis Red urine up to 24 h after administration Erythematous streak up the vein ("Adria flare") Incompatible with heparin and 5-FU
Doxorubic n (Doxil) Liposomal doxorulticin Anthracycline	Liposomal doxorubicin is *not a vesicant*. Doses of 20 mg/m² are given over 30 min, larger doses are given over 1 h in 250 mL of D₅W	20 mg/m² q3wk (Kaposi's sarcoma) 50 mg/m² q4wk (ovarian cancer)	Same toxicities as doxorubicin HCl Mild nausea, mucositis (common) Severe hand-foot syndrome (can be dose limiting) Acute infusion reaction: rate related: flushing, shortness of breath, facial swelling, chest tightness, hypotension—decrease rate or stop infusion. Alopecia (uncommon)
Epirubicin (Ellence) Anthracycline Antitumor Antibiotic Vesicart	Bolus (extravasation precautions) free-flowing line over 2–5 min Continuous infusion through a central line	100 mg/m²/d on day 1, repeated q21d or 60 mg/m²/d on day 1 and day 8 repeated q28d	Epirubicin of ≥90 mg/m² produces a degree of myelosuppression equivalent to doxorubicin 60 mg/m² (dose limiting) Leukopenia, expected nadir 10–14 d (dose limiting) Thrombocytopenia, anemia Hyperpigmentation of nail beds and dermal creases, dermatitis, radiation recall Alopecia (expected) Nausea, vomiting, mucositis, fatigue (common) CHF increased risk with higher doses Red urine, fevers, anaphylactic reactions, parenthesis, headache *If extravasated, will cause local tissue damage, flush along vein, facial flush, urticaria, phlebitis

(Continued)

TABLE 19–3 Quick Reference to Commonly Administered Parenteral Chemotherapeutic Agents *(Continued)*

Drug	Usual Dose	Usual Administration Technique	Comments and Major Toxicities
Etoposide (VP-16) Plant alkaloid	50–120 mg/m²/d × 3–5 d 100 mg/m²/d × 5 d q3wk (tx of testicular in combination with cisplatin) Oral doses are generally twice the IV dose	Slow IVBP infusion as 0.2–0.4 mg/mL in (D₅W, NS) *only* in 250 mL over at least 30 min–1 h Etoposide phosphate IVBP over 5 min or longer	Leukopenia; nadir within 7–14 d and recovery within 20 d; (dose limiting) Thrombocytopenia/anemia uncommon Mild alopecia Nausea and vomiting: mild; anorexia (common) Elevated bilirubin and transaminase levels Peripheral neuropathy *Transient hypotension associated with rapid administration: Infuse over 30 min–1 h* Discontinue infusion if hypersensitivity/bronchospasm occurs
Fludarabine (Fludara) Antimetabolite	25–30 mg/m²/d for 5 consecutive d q4wk	IVPB, IV infusion (NS, D₅W) Infuse in 50–150 mL, in a glass container or PVC bag	Leukopenia; nadir 13 d, thrombocytopenia nadir 16 d (dose related may be cumulative, and dose limiting) Lymphopenia (common and clinically important) Central nervous system toxicity—delayed blindness, coma, death—can occur up to 21–60 d after the last dose (rare, occurs in extreme high doses and is dose limiting) Somnolence, confusion, weakness, fatigue Nausea, vomiting (rare), diarrhea, anorexia Tumor lysis syndrome associated with large tumor burdens Cough, pneumonia, dyspnea chills, fever, malaise
Fluorouracil (5-FU) Antimetabolite	Numerous regimens used, including: 300–450 mg/m²/d IVP × 5 d q28d 600–750 mg/m² IVP every wk or every other wk	IVP, IVPB in 50 mL or more (NS, D₅W) Continuous infusion (D₅W, NS) CADD pumps over 5 d (see deltec.com) Intraocular 1 mg/0.1 mL in preservative-free NS	Nadir at 9–14 d, with recovery in 21–25 d; less common with continuous infusion Dermatitis, nail hyperpigmentation, alopecia, and chemical phlebitis with long-term infusion Nausea, vomiting, and anorexia Severe diarrhea associated with prolonged infusions (dose limiting)

Drug/Class	Dosage	Administration	Side Effects
	1,000 mg/m² infused over 24 h × 4–5 d 300 mg/m²/d infused indefinitely	Also may be given by arterial infusion, intracavitary, intraperitoneally, topically, or orally mixed in liquids	Mucositis (more common with 5-d infusion and bolus dosing) Cerebellar ataxia and headache (rare, with higher doses) *Toxicities are more common and more severe in patients with dihydropyrimidine dehydrogenase deficiency.
Gemcitabine (Gemzar) Antimetabolite	1,000 mg/m² every wk × 7 wk, then 1-wk break, then repeat cycle Combination with cisplatin: 1,000 mg/m²/d on days 1, 8, 15 of a 28-d cycle 1,250 mg/m²/d on day 1 and 8 of a 21-d cycle	IV over at least 30 min Use with NS only.	Mild to moderate neutropenia, myelosuppression with anemia, recovery within 1 wk (dose limiting) Mild nausea and vomiting, diarrhea, mucositis, flulike symptoms Fever during administration Rash with pruritus Elevations of hepatic transaminase level, hyperbilirubinemia Peripheral edema Proteinuria, hematuria, elevated BUN (uncommon)
Idarubicin (Idamycin) Antitumor Antibiotic Vesicant	12 mg/m²/d for 3 d 8–15 mg/m² as a single dose q3wk	IVP over 1–5 min (extravasation precautions)	Myelosuppression (dose limiting for each individual dose) Nausea, vomiting, (common) Diarrhea and mucositis (occasional) Alopecia (partial), extravasation reactions, and rash Transient arrhythmias, decreased left ventricular ejection fraction, and CHF increased risk with higher doses (cumulative dose-limiting toxicity)
Ifosfamide (Ifex) Alkylating agent	1,000–1,200 mg/m² over 5 consecutive d q3–4wk Higher doses (2,500–4000 mg/m²/d) have been given over 2–3 d	IVPB only (D₅W, NS) in 250–1,000 mL over 30 min or longer	Leukopenia, thrombocytopenia (dose limiting); anemia Nausea, vomiting, anorexia, constipation and diarrhea, mucositis Alopecia, rash, urticaria, nail ridging Increased ALT, AST, and bilirubin Hemorrhagic cystitis and hematuria (dose limiting) *Hydration of >2 L/d to maintain urinary output, frequent voiding. Mesna recommended.*
Mesna (see p. 513)		Recommended aggressive hydration to reduce risk of hemorrhagic cystitis. Mesna must be given with ifosfamide.	CNS toxicity: somnolence, lethargy, disorientation, confusion, dizziness, malaise, myoclonus, seizures: reversible (dose limiting) Electrolyte imbalance

(Continued)

TABLE 19–3 Quick Reference to Commonly Administered Parenteral Chemotherapeutic Agents *(Continued)*

Drug	Usual Dose	Usual Administration Technique	Comments and Major Toxicities
Irinotecan (Camptosar, CPT-11) Topoisomerase I inhibitor Irritant	125 mg/m² every wk × 4, then 2-wk rest and repeat cycle 350 mg/m² q28d If combined with cisplatin: 80 mg/m² on day 1 q4wk 60 mg/m² every wk × 3 wk	IV in 500ml (D₅W preferred) over 60–90 min or longer	Myelosuppression, especially neutropenia and diarrhea (common and dose limiting) Consult manufacturer's recommendations for guidelines Diarrhea, "acute cholinergic" along with cramping, nausea, vomiting during or immediately following drug administration, or for several days after drug administration; treated with anticholinergics and antidiarrheal agents Moderate to severe nausea, anorexia Alopecia, flushing, rash (common) Elevated liver enzymes
Leucovorin, Calcium Tetrahydrofolic acid derivative Non-chemotherapeutic agent	Methotrexate rescue: 10–25 mg/m² q6h × 6–8 doses starting up to 24 h after the methotrexate To potentate the cytotoxic effect of 5-FU: 20–500 mg/m² dose	IVP at any convenient rate IM Oral IVPB (D₅W, NS) 50–250 mL over 15 min	Fatigue, fevers, salivation, lacrimation Increased PT times of patients taking Coumadin Advise patients not to take St. John's wort Interactions with metroclopramide and prochlorperazine Rare hypersensitivity reactions Thrombocytosis, nausea, diarrhea, rash, headache Dose adjustments are made based on MTX serum levels and serum creatinine levels
Mechlorethamine (Nitrogen Mustard) Alkylating agent Vesicant	Hodgkin's disease: 6 mg/m² on days 1 and 8 (MOPP regimen) Up to 0.4 mg/kg as a single agent monthly	IVP over 1–5 min (extravasation precautions) into the tubing of a rapidly running IV May be given intracavitary injection; usually painful—patients should be given appropriate analgesia Intraperitoneal should be avoided	Leukopenia and thrombocytopenia within 24 h, with a nadir at 6–8 d to 3 wk (dose limiting) Severe nausea and vomiting beginning 1–3 h after treatment (dose limiting); aggressive antiemetic premedication is mandatory Discoloration of infused vein and phlebitis Alopecia and mucositis Vesicant antidote is sodium thiosulfate if extravasation occurs

Drug / Classification	Dosage	Administration	Side Effects / Comments
Melphalan (Alkeran) Alkylating agent Vesicant	16 mg/m² IV (60-min stability) Multiple myeloma: 0.1 mg/kg/d for 2–3 wk or up to 6 mg/m² for 5 d q6wk	IVPB over 15–30 min	Metallic taste Amenorrhea and impaired spermatogenesis, sterility (common) Diarrhea, anorexia, jaundice, tinnitus, skin rash (topical application) Secondary malignancy and hearing loss (rare) Incompatible with other antineoplastic agents Short stability Myelosuppression, prolonged recovery, effects cumulative (dose limiting)
Mesna Uroprotective agent (non-chemotherapeutic)	20% of iphosphamide dose given just before and at 4 and 8 h after iphosphamide	IVPB (D$_5$W, NS) 50–100 mL IVP (<100 mg) IVPB (D$_5$W, NS) in 50 mL (up to 500 mL) over 30 min to 1 h Can also be given as 24-h continuous infusions	Nausea, vomiting Vein reactions, scarring Diarrhea, mucositis (uncommon) Pulmonary fibrosis, alopecia, vasculitis, infertility, secondary leukemia (uncommon) Nausea, vomiting, diarrhea, abdominal pain, altered taste Rash and urticaria Lethargy, headache, joint or limb pain, fatigue
Methotrexate Antimetabolite	Solid tumors: 20–40 mg/m² 1–2 wk Leukemias and lymphomas: 200–500 mg/m² q2–4wk Low dose: <100 mg/m² Moderate dose: 100 mg/m²–1,000 mg/m² High dose: >1,000mg/m² Intrathecal: usually 10–15 mg in preservative-free NS	Intrathecally IM	Myelosuppression expected (dose limiting) Mucositis, sore throat, and pruritus with high dose Hematemesis Nausea and vomiting (uncommon) Diarrhea (common) Renal toxicity, dose related and more likely to occur in patients with compromised renal function; reversible Hepatotoxicity, pulmonary dysfunction (rare) Encephalopathy with multiple intrathecal doses Confusion, ataxia, tremors, irritability, seizures, and coma Hypersensitivity reactions associated with fever, chills, and rash Skin erythema, depigmentation or hyperpigmentation, alopecia, and photosensitivity Doses >80 mg/wk should be accompanied by leucovorin rescue

(Continued)

Drug	Usual Dose	Usual Administration Technique	Comments and Major Toxicities
Mitomycin C (Mutamycin) Antitumor Antibiotic Vesicant	10–20 mg/m² q6–8wk It is recommended that total cumulative doses not exceed 50 mg/m² to avoid excessive toxicity. Can be given intravesically, intraperitoneally, intraocularly, and intra-arterially	IVP over 2–5 min Use vesicant precautions IVPB (D₅W, NS) in up to 250 mL over 30 min	Leukopenia and thrombocytopenia: delayed, cumulative, and dose limiting; anemia Nadir at 4–5 wk, recovery 2–3 wk later Alopecia (4%), dermatitis, and pruritus Nausea, vomiting, anorexia, fatigue (common) Diarrhea, mucositis, fever (uncommon) Hepatotoxicity; veno-occlusive disease (rare) Parenthesis, lethargy, weakness, and blurred vision Interstitial pneumonitis infrequent toxicity but can be severe Bronchospasm, acute SOB when given with a vinca alkaloid Hemolytic-uremic syndrome (rare) Nephrotoxicity at doses >50 mg/m²
Mitoxantrone (Novantrone) Antitumor Antibiotic Irritant	12 mg/m²/d × 3 d (in combination with cytarabine) for induction therapy for ANLL Acute leukemia 10–12 mg/m² Other: 12 mg/m² q3–4wk Can be given IM, intraperitoneally, and by intravesical instillation	IVP has been used (over ≥3 min, dilute in at least 50 mL), but IVPB preferred route IVPB (D₅W, NS) in at least 50 mL 15–30 min or longer	Pain on injection and phlebitis Leukopenia expected, nadir at 10–12 d, with recovery on day 21 Alopecia (mild), pruritus, and dry skin Nausea, vomiting, diarrhea, and mucositis (mild) Cumulative cardiomyopathy: max. lifetime dose is 140–160 mg/m² Hypersensitivity: hypotension, urticaria, and rash Blue-green urine, stool, and sclera for 24–48 h after treatment; ve n may be discolored.
Oxaliplatin (Eloxatin) Alkylating agent	85 mg/m² on day 1 q2wk in combination with 5FU protocol	IVPB in 250–500 mL of D₅W over 2–6 h	Fever, conjunctivitis, phlebitis, and amenorrhea Myelosuppression mild, occasionally dose limiting; risk of grade 3 and 4 neutropenia is significantly increased with combination of 5FU

Drug	Dose/Schedule	Administration	Side Effects/Toxicities
	130 mg/m² q3wk in combination with 5FU protocol Numerous regimens refer to chemotherapy text for doses/schedules of protocols	Should be administered *prior to* 5-FU	Nausea, vomiting, diarrhea, dehydration, hypokalemia, metabolic acidosis Hand-foot syndrome Elevations of transaminase enzymes, hyperbilirubinemia Tachycardia supraventricular arrhythmia, HTN, phlebitis, thromboembolism Acute/chronic neurologic symptoms, aggravated with exposure to cold (dose limiting) Hypersensitivity Fatigue, back pain, arthralgia
Paclitaxel (Taxol) Plant alkaloid Taxane Irritant/Potential Vesicant	Variety of doses/schedules including: Ovarian: 135–175 mg/m² over 3 h q3wk or 135 mg/m² over 24 h repeated q3wk Breast: 175 mg/m² over 3 h q3wk (doses up to 200–250 mg/m² have been administered) Non-small cell lung cancer: 135 mg/m² as CI over 24 h (higher doses have been given in combination with carboplatin)	IV infusion (NS, D₅W, D₅NS, D₅ Ringer's) Over 1, 3, or 24 h Concentration of 0.3–1.2 mg/mL in glass, polypropylene, or polyolefin containers Avoid contact of the undiluted Taxol with plasticized polyvinyl chloride equipment Use in-line filter of 0.22 μm or less, and non-PVC-containing infusion set	Pancytopenia (dose limiting), shorter infusions produce less neutropenia; mild anemia, infection Premedicate to avoid hypersensitivity reaction, with dexamethasone, diphenhydramine, and ranitidine (or cimetidine) Hypersensitivity: urticaria, wheezing, chest pain, dyspnea, and hypotension (common) Cardiovascular: hypertension, hypotension, premature contractures, bradycardia—monitor vital signs during 1st h; ECG abnormalities (common) Peripheral neuropathy (increases with cumulative doses) Nausea, vomiting, diarrhea Mucositis (with longer infusions) Alopecia—complete, rash, flushing, nail changes, arthralgia/myalgia Liver toxicity, interstitial pneumonitis (uncommon)
Paclitaxel protein-bound (Abraxane) Taxane Vesicant	260 mg/m² IV q3wk	IV over 30 min Extravasation precautions Do not use in-line filter.	Contains human albumin which may be prohibited in certain religious/cultural beliefs. Myelosuppression, primarily neutropenia (dose limiting) Thrombocytopenia (uncommon); anemia (common) Sensory neuropathy (common) Hypersensitivity reactions: dyspnea, flushing, hypotension, chest pain, arrhythmia (uncommon)

(Continued)

515

TABLE 19–3 Quick Reference to Commonly Administered Parenteral Chemotherapeutic Agents *(Continued)*

Drug	Usual Dose	Usual Administration Technique	Comments and Major Toxicities
			No premeds needed for hypersensitivity prevention
			Hypotension and bradycardia during 30-min infusion (uncommon)
			Nausea, vomiting, diarrhea, mucositis (common)
			ECG abnormalities (common)
			Dyspnea and cough
			Ocular/visual disturbances, eg. keratitis, blurred vision; severe, reversible
			Arthralgia/myalgia; transient, resolved within a few days. Interstitial pneumonia, lung fibrosis, and PE (rare)
Pegaspargase (Oncaspar) Pegylated form of asparaginase	2,500 IU/m² q14d with other agents for induction and maintenance	IM	Acute liver dysfunction, hypercholesterolemia
			Coagulopathy
			Hypersensitivity and anaphylaxis can still occur (used when patient is allergic to asparaginase)
			Pancreatitis, hyperglycemia, fever, chills, anorexia, lethargy, confusion, headache, seizures, azotemia (same as asparaginase)
Pemetrexed (Alimta) Antimetabolite	500 mg/m² q21d with cisplatin (75 mg/m² over 2 h) to follow 30 min later	IV infusion over 10 min	Myelosuppression, especially neutropenia, thrombocytopenia
			Fatigue, nausea, vomiting, dyspnea
			Side effects reduced with vitamin supplementation: Administer folic acid 350–1,000 μg daily starting 1–3 wk prior to the first cycle and daily for 1–3 wk after the final cycle. Vitamin B₁₂ injection 1,000 μg IM given 1–3 wk before the first cycle and repeat q9wk until treatment is completed
			Dexamethasone 4 mg BID for 3 d starting the day before treatment decreases incidence of skin rash
Pentostatin (Nipent) Antimetabolite	4 mg/m² q2wk	IV bolus over 5 min or further diluted in 25–50	Severe leucopenia, lymphopenia common, can lead to serious infection (dose limiting)
			Thrombocytopenia, anemia

Drug	Dosage	Administration	Toxicity
	Dose reduction may be necessary for renal dysfunction exhibited by creatinine clearance <60 mL/min	mL (NS, D$_5$W), IVPB over 20 min or longer. Recommended hydration of 1–2 L of D$_5$ .45NS before and after each treatment	Nausea, vomiting, fever fatigue (common). Anorexia, diarrhea, mucositis, rashes, dry skin, headache (uncommon). Elevated hepatic transaminase levels, nephrotoxicity (uncommon). Keratoconjunctivitis, photophobia, arthralgia, cough. Neurotoxicities rare with standard dose, increased with higher dosing. Acute tubular necrosis, hepatitis (rare)
Streptozocin (Zanosar) Alkylating agent Irritant	500–1,000 × 5 d q4–6wk; 1,000–1,500 mg/m^2/wk. Doses >1,500 mg/m^2/d should not be exceeded owing to increased risk of nephrotoxicity. Doses should be adjusted for creatinine clearance <50 mL/min	IVPB (D$_5$W, NS) in 100 mL or more over 30–60 min. Continuous infusion × 5 d. Can be given IVP, recommended slow administration	Cumulative myelosuppression, anemia, leukopenia, and thrombocytopenia. Eosinophilia. Nausea and vomiting (severe), anorexia, diarrhea, abdominal cramps (potentially dose limiting). Nephrotoxicity (renal tubular damage) with proteinuria (common and potentially dose limiting). Vein irritation during administration; slow infusion to minimize pain. Transient increases in ALT, AST, alkaline phosphatase, and LDH. Glucose intolerance and glycosuria. Fever, delirium, depression (rare)
Teniposide (VM-26) Plant alkaloid	165 mg/m^2 2 times/wk for 8–9 doses (with cytarabine protocol). Maintenance dose of 250 mg/m^2 weekly for 4–8 wk. Several other regimens have been used: 100 mg/m^2 1–2qwk	IV infusion (NS, D$_5$W). Infuse in concentration of 0.1–0.4 mg/mL over 30–60 min or longer. Can be given as continuous IV infusion and intraperitoneally. Administer via non-DEHP PVC containers or glass	Leukopenia; nadir 10–14 days (dose-limiting). Anaphylaxis may occur. Mucositis, nausea, vomiting, diarrhea, anorexia (uncommon). Alopecia (mild). Hypotension (rapid IV infusion). Fatigue, seizures, somnolence, fever, renal insufficiency, and secondary malignancies (rare)

TABLE 19–3 Quick Reference to Commonly Administered Parenteral Chemotherapeutic Agents *(Continued)*

Drug	Usual Dose	Usual Administration Technique	Comments and Major Toxicities
Thiotepa Alkylating agent	20–60 mg/m^2/d × 5 d 80–90 mg/m^2/d × 5 d Nontransplant: 12–16 mg/m^2 q1–4wk Transplant: 900 mg/m^2 Intrathecal: 1–10 mg/m^2 1–2 times weekly Bladder instillation: 30–60 mg every wk × 4 wk Numerous routes of administration	IVPB (D$_5$W, NS) in 50–100 mL over 10 min or longer	Leukopenia: nadir at 14 d and recovery after 2–4 wk (dose limiting) Anemia, thrombocytopenia Alopecia Hypersensitivity reactions: angioedema, hives, rash, and pruritus Nausea, vomiting, anorexia, mucositis, diarrhea, fever (uncommon) Headache, dizziness, and weakness of lower extremities Paresthesias associated with intrathecal administration Impaired fertility—azoospermia and amenorrhea
Topotecan (Hycamtin) Topoisomerase 1 inhibitor	1.5 mg/m^2/d × 5 consecutive days q21d for the first four courses of tx Subsequent tx.should be administered at a dose of 1.25 mg/m^2/d × 5 d Numerous other doses have been evaluated.	IV over 30 min	Dose-limiting neutropenia grade 4 with nadir on day 10–12 Mild thrombocytopenia, anemia (common) Total alopecia Nausea, vomting, diarrhea (common) Headache, fever, fatigue, anorexia, malaise, elevated liver enzymes (common) Hypertension tachycardia, urticaria, renal insufficiency, hematuria, dizziness, peripheral neuropathy, homer's syndrome, mucositis (uncommon) Dyspnea Patients with moderate renal compromise require a dose adjustment

Drug	Dose	Administration	Toxicities/Comments
Trimetrexate (Neutrexin) Antimetabolite	45 mg/m² × 21 d with concomitant leucovorin. Leucovorin must also be given 3 d after cessation of tx. with trimetrexate	May be given by IV push, but is more often administered by infusion diluted in 50 mL D₅W over 60–90 min or as a continuous infusion	Inhibits parasitic infective agents that cause *Pneumocystis carinii* pneumonia and toxoplasmosis; Flush line with D₅W to clear line prior to NS.; Patients with hypoalbuminemia are more likely to experience severe anemia, mucositis, thrombocytopenia; Myelosuppression dose related (leucovorin greatly reduces these toxicities); Fever, shaking, chills, malaise; Transient elevations of liver enzymes
Vinblastine (Velban) Plant alkaloid Vesicant	Has also been given 110 mg/m² in combination with 5FU every wk × 6 wks followed by 2 wk of rest; 6–10 mg/m² q2–4wk; Also given every wk and as a continuous infusion in a dose of 1.7–2 mg/m²/d for 96 h through a central line	IVP over 1–5 min; Extravasation precautions; IVPB not recommended	Dose-limiting leukopenia with early nadirs; Thrombocytopenia and anemia (uncommon); Extravasation: Treat with application of heat.; Rash and photosensitivity; Nausea, vomiting, and constipation; abdominal cramping, anorexia; Peripheral neuropathy, myalgias, headache, seizures, depression, dizziness, and malaise; Acute bronchospasm, dyspnea, chest pain, tumor pain, fever, especially when administered with mitomycin C; Severe jaw pain, pharynx, bones, back; Phlebitis and vein discoloration; SIADH and angina pectoris (rare)
Vincristine (Oncovin) Plant alkaloid Vesicant	0.5–1.4 mg/m² q1–4wk; Usually the maximum dose is 2 mg.; 0.5 mg/d to 0.5 mg/m²/d over 96 h via a central line	IVP over 1 min; Occasionally given as a continuous infusion (D₅W, NS)	Leukopenia (mild and rare); thrombocytopenia (rare); Alopecia; If extravasated, treat with application of heat.; Nausea, vomiting (rare); constipation; abdominal pain, anorexia; *Intrathecal administration is fatal.*; Peripheral neuropathy, paresthesias, paralytic ileus, and myalgias (cumulative, dose limiting); Acute bronchospasm, dyspnea when administered with mitomycin C; Diplopia, ptosis, photophobia, cortical blindness; Azoospermia and amenorrhea

(Continued)

TABLE 19–3 Quick Reference to Commonly Administered Parenteral Chemotherapeutic Agents *(Continued)*

Drug	Usual Dose	Usual Administration Technique	Comments and Major Toxicities
Vinorelbine (Navelbine) Vinca alkaloid Vesicant	30 mg/m²/wk	IV syringe (NS, D₅W), IV bag (0.45 NS, NS, D₅W, D₅ 0.45 NS, Ringer's, lactated Ringer's) Infuse over 6–10 min into side port of a free-flowing IV, flush with 100–200 mL of solution to reduce risk of phlebitis	Myelosuppression, mostly leucopenia (dose limiting) Acute reversible dyspnea, chest pain, wheezing after IV administration; prevented by premedication with steroids. Injection site erythema, pain, phlebitis Fatigue, tumor pain, jaw pain Mild nausea, constipation, diarrhea, stomatitis Hepatic: transient elevated LFTs Chest pain with or without ECG changes

*Pfizer drug literature.

ALT, alanine aminotransferase; ANLL, acute nonlymphocytic leukemia; AST, aspartate aminotransferase; CHF, congestive heart failure; D₅W, 5% dextrose in water; HTN, hypertension; IM, intramuscular; I/O, intake/output; IVP, intravenous push; IVPB, intravenous piggyback; LDH, lactate dehydrogenase; LFT, liver function tests; LVEF, left ventricular ejection fraction; MTX, methotrexate; NS, normal saline; PE, pulmonary embolism; SOB, shortness of breath; SQ, subcutaneous.

The information here is provided as guidance only. Nurses should always consult the manufacturer's current prescribing information before administering drugs. A pharmacist should be consulted for information on compatibilities, concentrations, and stability.

(From Fischer, D.S., Knobf, T.M., Durivage, H.J., Beaulieu, N.J. [2003]. *The cancer chemotherapy handbook* [6th ed., pp. 48–239]. Chicago: Mosby; Perry, C., Anderson, C.M., Donehower, R.C. (2004). Chemotherapy. In M. Abeloff, J. Armitage, J. Niederhuber, & M. Keaton, *Clinical oncology* (3rd ed.). Elsevier.

cells, or alter the ability of the tumor cells to metastasize or survive (Itano & Taoka, 2005).

Biologic agents are proteins derived from and/or copied from proteins that exist naturally in the human body. These agents fall into several categories: cytokines (interferons, interleukins, and hematopoietic growth factors) and monoclonal antibodies. Promising new therapies target cancer cells at a molecular level, and hence are called molecular targeted therapy. These agents aim their antineoplastic activity at cell membrane receptors, signaling pathways and proteins, enzymatic activity, and regulatory cell growth controls that are more aberrant and abundant in cancer cells than normal cells. Because of this specificity, the therapeutic efficacy is enhanced while the toxicity to normal cells is decreased (DeVita, Hellman, & Rosenberg, 2004; Itano & Taoka, 2005).

Cytokines are hormonelike messenger molecules that cells use to communicate. T lymphocytes produce interferon when in contact with viruses and tumors. The **interferons** (IFNs) are cytokines that initiate immune responses that are antiviral, antitumor (prevent malignant transformation of cells, down-regulate cell division, communicate with other cytotoxic immune cells) and immunomodulatory (enhance natural killer ([NK] cell activity).

Interleukins do not possess cytotoxic activity. Their effectiveness is through their influence on the cells of the immune system. Interleukins stimulate the production of cytokines and the migration of active immune cells (T-helper cells, monocytes/macrophages, cytotoxic T cells and NK cells) to the tumor. Table 19–4 provides an overview of interleukin and interferon dosing, administration, and side effects and major toxicities.

Hematopoietic growth factors represent a milestone in cancer treatment. Because of recombinant DNA technology, these agents are able to mimic the activity of colony-stimulating factors (CSFs). The use of these growth factors has enabled rapid recovery of bone marrow activity; thus allowing patients to receive frequent, dose-dense therapy. Table 19–5 lists the most common hematopoietic growth factors used with chemotherapy/biotherapy.

Monoclonal Antibodies

Monoclonal antibodies (mAb) are defined by the Food and Drug Administration as intact immunoglobulins produced by hybridomas, immunoconjugates, immunoglobulin fragments or recombinant proteins derived from immunoglobulins. The philosophy behind the monoclonal antibodies used in oncology is to facilitate antitumor effects directly on a specific target associated with cancer cells. The antitumor effect can be demonstrated by apoptosis, antibody-dependent cell cytotoxicity, complement-mediated cytolysis, or by delivery of radiation or cellular toxins. This target specificity facilitates more direct attack on the cancer cells and less toxicity.

The specific targets are usually expressed on the cell surface of cancer cells. Targets identified in current FDA-approved monoclonal antibodies include cluster of differentiation (CD) markers and growth factor receptors (epidermal growth factors, vascular endothelial growth factors, etc.). When the antibodies bind to

(text continues on p. 524)

TABLE 19–4 Biotherapy Agents

Drug	Usual Dose	Administration/Precautions	Common and Major Toxicities
Aldesleukin (Interleukin-2, Proleukin) Biologic response modifier: cytokine production, proliferation of lymphocytes enhanced cell cytotoxicity	**High dose:** 600,000–720,000 units/kg q8h for 5 consecutive days for 2 cycles, separated by 7–10 d Low dose: 6 million units/m^2 for 4 d weekly for 4 wk	IV infusion over 15 min Do not use in-line filters 24-h infusion, SQ Do not mix with NS or bacteriostatic water Do not mix with other meds	**Capillary leak syndrome:** hypotension, edema, pulmonary congestion, renal insufficiency, arrhythmias, diarrhea, and possibly CNS and hepatic toxicity (dose limiting) Transient myelosuppression, prolonged anemia, transient hyperbilirubinemia, elevated transaminase, electrolyte imbalances. Fever, chills, malaise, headache, nasal stuffiness, myalgia, arthralgia, erythroedema, nausea, vomiting (common) Lethargy, delirium, angina pectoris, CHF, frank respiratory failure, infections (uncommon)
Interferon-α-2A (Roferon)	Dependent on type of interferon and cancer being treated	Roferan: SQ, IM	Constitutional symptoms (dose limiting) **Acute:** fever, chills, nasal congestion, diarrhea, malaise
Interferon-α-2B (Intron-A) Biologic response modifier, antiviral, immunostimulant	2 million units/m^2 to 30 million units/m^2 from 3 times per wk to daily. Adjustments made based on patient tolerance and lab values	Intron-A: SQ, IM, IVP, IV Infusion over 20 min	**Chronic:** fatigue, anorexia, weight loss, depression, anemia Neutropenia, thrombocytopenia: transient (can be dose limiting at higher doses) Cardiovascular toxicity: CHF, arrhythmias: reversible (rare) CNS toxicity: delirium, psychosis, peripheral neuropathy reversible (rare) Hyperglycemia, hypocalcemia (rare)

TABLE 19–5   Hemopoietic Growth Factors

Drug	Usual Dose	Administration/Precautions	Common & Major Toxicities
Epoetin alfa (Procrit, Epogen)	**Chemotherapy-induced anemia:** EPO 20,000–40,000 units weekly	EPO: SQ	Pain at injection site, hypertension, especially in renal failure patients (common)
Darbepoet n (Aranesp)	Darbepoetin: 2.25 μg weekly	Darbepoetin: SQ, IV	Nausea, vomiting, diarrhea, headache, edema, fever (rare)
	Renal Failure or HIV disease: Initial: 50–100 units/kg 3 times wk Maintenance: 25 units/kg 3 times wk		Allergic reactions, thrombotic vascular events in patient with vascular disease (rare)
Filgrastim (Neupogen)	5 μg/kg/d no earlier than 24 h after administration of last dose of chemotherapy	SQ, IV Discontinue when ANC >7,000/mm^2	Transient bone pain (20%), splenomegaly, local inflammation of injection site, mild LFTs elevation
Pegfilgrast m (Neulasta)	6 mg administered once per chemotherapy cycle	SQ; do not administer in the period from 14 d prior and 24 h after chemotherapy	Splenic rupture, acute respiratory distress syndrome (ARDS), precipitation of sickle cell crises (rare)
Sargramostim (Leukine)	250 μg/kg/d	2-h IV infusion	Fever, flulike symptoms (common) Hypersensitivity reactions > G-CSF
	Acute leukemia: start 11 d after induction chemotherapy when marrow is hypoplastic		Diarrhea, asthenia, rash, malaise, fluid retention (peripheral edema, effusions; occasional)
	Mobilization of progenitor cells: immediately after infusion of progenitor cells		With transplant doses: capillary leak syndrome
	Bone marrow transplant: given 2–4 h after infusion of bone marrow infusion		
Oprelvekin (Neumega)	50 μg/kg/d beginning 6–24 h after chemotherapy	SQ Administer until platelet count is ≥50,000.	Mild to moderate fluid retention with dilutional anemia (responds to diuretics) Transient atrial arrhythmias, visual blurring

G-CSF, granulocyte colony-stimulating factor (Filgrastim [Neupogen]) these targets, it activates the immune system and mediates the process of cell destruction.

A hybridoma technique can be used to produce mAbs. Within the process, murine immunization with a selected antigen stimulates antibody-forming immune cells to produce antibodies with various specificities. These cells are fused with a tumor cell to produce immortalized hybridoma cells. To select the desired antigen specificity, the hybridoma cells are screened in vitro and the specific mAb is grown by clonal expansion. Sometimes antigenicity against these murine hybridomas limits the therapeutic effect of the mAb. To prevent these immune responses, the mAb is fused with a humanized component. Further technology has also enabled the production of a fully humanized mAb; although this still does not eliminate the risk of immune responses. Efforts are still being made to produce a mAb free of antigenicity.

The future of mAbs is promising as discoveries are made to develop more potential targets and pathways. The mAb is a good option when treating patients who are intolerant of or would like to delay treatment with chemotherapy. Also, combination treatments with mAbs are attractive owing to the potential enhancement of antitumor responses without increases in toxicities. As we continue to research the unknown, the approach to and strategy for treating cancer with mAbs is becoming more defined (Nabel, 2004; Ross, Schenkein, Pietrusko, et al., 2004; USDHHS, FDA, 1997). Table 19–6 identifies the currently approved monoclonal antibodies, their indications, dosing, method of administration, side effects, and nursing considerations.

Goals of Antineoplastic Therapy

The goal of all anticancer therapy is the eradication of all cancer cells. A *cure* is described as a prolonged absence of detectable disease. When cure is unrealistic, *control* (therapy that extends life) can be the goal of therapy. *Palliation* is a legitimate goal for patients with advanced or incurable disease. Even when there is no real hope of complete cure, cancer cells often remain somewhat sensitive to antineoplastic agents, so disease progression can be slowed. Agents often can control pain caused by tumor pressure, ease fluid obstruction and edema, and control hypercalcemia and other organic carcinoid processes (Polovich et al., 2005). Tumors vary in their responsiveness to chemotherapy. While great strides have been made in childhood cancers in terms of cure, other tumors have responded to chemotherapy and patients have experienced longer survival times (Box 19–4). In some tumor types, chemotherapy has afforded patients improved quality of life through palliation. Remaining cancers are less responsive to chemotherapeutic intervention (Casciato, 2004). Biotherapy agents (interferons and interleukins) are commonly used in advanced cancers where other treatment methods do not offer positive outcomes. Generally, they have been found to provide longer survival times, longer times to disease progression, and higher response rates than more traditional chemotherapy given for the same malignancy, for example, melanoma and renal cell carcinoma. Although not currently approved as antitumor therapy, hematopoietic growth factors are often used for alleviation of both the symptoms

(text continues on p. 530)

TABLE 19–6 Monoclonal Antibodies

Drug	Dose	Method of Administration	Complications	Considerations
Rituximab (Rituxan) Nonvesicant *Drug specificity:* targets CD20 positive B lymphocytes *Indications:* Non-Hodgkin's lymphoma	375 mg/m² weekly × 4–8 doses	IV infusion through recommended infusion guidelines Do not administer as an IV push or bolus. For first infusions, initiate at 50 mg/h. If no symptoms, increase rate in 50 mg/h increments every 30 min to maximum of 400 mg/h as tolerated. For second infusion, initiate at 100 mg/h. If no symptoms, increase rate in 100 mg/h increments every 30 min to maximum of 400 mg/h as tolerated.	*Common:* Infusion-related reactions or hypersensitivity reactions. Symptoms include hypotension, angioedema, hypoxia, and bronchospasm. Fatal reactions have been reported, especially with the first infusions. Symptoms have included hypoxia, pulmonary infiltrates, acute respiratory distress syndrome, myocardial infarction, ventricular fibrillation, or cardiogenic shock. *System-specific:* Tumor lysis syndrome and severe mucocutaneous reactions (eg, paraneoplastic pemphigus, Stevens-Johnson syndrome, lichenoid dermatitis, vesiculobullous dermatitis, and toxic epidermal necrolysis)	Monitor patient closely for infusion-related reactions. If symptoms occur, slow or stop infusion and administer medical treatment as indicated (ie, acetaminophen, diphenhydramine, bronchodilators, or IV saline). When symptoms are completely resolved, resuming infusion at 50% of rate (eg, from 100 mg/h to 50 mg/h) can be considered. Premedications such as diphenhydramine and acetaminophen can be considered to prevent infusion-related reactions. Hypersensitivity/anaphylactic medications such as epinephrine, antihistamines, and corticosteroids should be available during infusion. Antihypertensive medications may need to be held at least 12 hours prior to rituximab administration owing to the potential rituximab infusion-related hypotension. Gently invert bag to mix.

(Continued)

TABLE 19-6 Monoclonal Antibodies *(Continued)*

Drug	Dose	Method of Administration	Complications	Considerations
Trastuzumab (Herceptin) *Drug specificity:* targets overexpressed HER2 positive cells Nonvesicant *Indications:* metastatic breast cancer and overexpression of the HER2 protein	Loading dose (LD) 4 mg/kg over 90 min Maintenance dose (MD) 2 mg/kg over 30 min weekly (experimental dosing: LD 8 mg/kg, MD 6 mg/kg q3wk).	Do not administer as an IV push or bolus. Loading dose given over 90 min. If tolerated well, may infuse maintenance dose over 30 min. Dextrose solutions should not be used with trastuzumab.	*Common and system-specific:* Cardiotoxicity including congestive heart failure, disabling cardiac failure, death, and mural thrombosis leading to stroke. Symptoms include dyspnea, increased cough, paroxysmal nocturnal dyspnea, peripheral edema, S_3 gallop, or reduced ejection fraction.	Obtain baseline cardiac assessment including history and physical exam and one or more of the following: ECG, echocardiogram, and MUGA scan. Extreme caution should be practiced in patients with pre-existing cardiac dysfunction. Monitor patient closely for infusion-related reactions such as chills and fever. This was observed in about 40% of patients in clinical trials. Treatment can consist of acetaminophen, diphenhydramine, and meperidine, with or without reduction in trastuzumab infusion rate. Hypersensitivity/anaphylactic medications such as epinephrine, antihistamines and corticosteroids should be available during infusion. If known hypersensitivity to benzyl alcohol, reconstitute with sterile water for injection instead of supplied diluent, which contains 1.1% benzyl alcohol. Gently invert bag to mix.

Gemtuzumab (Mylotarg) Monoclonal antibody + calicheamicin (cytotoxic antitumor antibiotic) *Drug specificity:* targets CD33 positive cells Nonvesicant *Indications:* acute myelogenous leukemia	9 mg/m^2 over 2 h Repeat dose after 2 wk. Hematologic recovery is not required prior to the second dose.	IV infusion Chemotherapy precautions should be exercised owing to the chemotherapy component of gemtuzumab. Do not administer as an IV push or bolus. Premedicate with acetaminophen 650–1,000 mg orally and diphenhydramine 50 mg orally; thereafter, continue prophylaxis with two additional doses of acetaminophen 650–1,000 mg orally, one q4h as needed. Premedication with methylprednisolone may also be considered. Vital signs should be monitored during infusion and for the 4 h following infusion.	*Common:* Myelosuppression and severe infections may result. Can occur at recommended doses. *System-specific:* Fatal hepatotoxicity has been reported such as hepatic veno-occlusive disease (VOD). Symptoms include rapid weight gain, right upper quadrant pain, hepatomegaly, ascites, elevations in bilirubin and/or liver enzymes. Use with extra caution if bilirubin >2 mg/dL. System specific: Patients with WBC counts ≥30,000 cells per microliter or symptomatic intrinsic lung disease may be at increased risk for pulmonary events such as dyspnea, pulmonary infiltrates, pleural effusions, noncardiogenic pulmonary edema, pulmonary insufficiency and hypoxia, and acute respiratory distress syndrome.	Monitor patient closely for infusion-related reactions such as dyspnea or clinically significant hypotension. Consider discontinuation if anaphylaxis, pulmonary edema, or acute respiratory distress syndrome occurs. Most symptoms occurred after the end of the 2-h infusion and resolved after 2–4 h with supportive treatment with acetaminophen, diphenhydramine, and IV fluids. Fewer infusion-related reactions occurred with the second dose. Hypersensitivity/anaphylactic medications should be available during infusion. Preparation should be done within a biologic safety hood with the fluorescent light turned off. Use immediately. Use chemotherapy checking, handling and disposal procedures. Use low protein-binding 1.2-micron filter. Gently invert bag to mix and protect from light.

(Continued)

TABLE 19–6 Monoclonal Antibodies *(Continued)*

Drug	Dose	Method of Administration	Complications	Considerations
Alemtuzumab (Campath) *Drug specificity:* targets CD52 positive B and T cells Nonvesicant *Indications:* B-cell chronic lymphocytic leukemia	Usual initial dose: 3 mg over 2 h daily. If tolerated, slowly escalate daily to a maintenance dose of 30 mg 3 times per wk (ie, Monday, Wednesday, Friday) for ≤12 wk. Requires maintenance dose. Do not exceed recommended maintenance dose of 30 mg 3 times per wk.	Do not administer as an IV push or bolus. Use 5-micron filter. Premedicate with acetaminophen 650 mg orally and diphenhydramine 50 mg orally.	*Common:* Severe pancytopenia/marrow hypoplasia, autoimmune idiopathic thrombocytopenia, and autoimmune hemolytic anemia. Can result in opportunistic infections. *Dose-limiting effects:* Single doses >30 mg or cumulative doses >90 mg per wk have been associated with higher incidence of pancytopenia.	Dose escalation to the recommended maintenance dose of 30 mg 3 times per wk is required. If alemtuzumab is withheld for ≥7 days, dose escalation must begin at 3 mg again. Monitor patient closely for infusion-related reactions. Hypersensitivity/anaphylactic medications should be available during infusion. Anti-infective prophylaxis (ie, trimethoprim/sulfamethoxazole DS, famciclovir) should be initiated with alemtuzumab and continue until CD4 + count is ≥200 cells/µL or 2 mo after completion of alemtuzumab, whichever occurs later. Gently invert bag to mix.
Cetuximab (Erbitux) *Drug specificity:* targets epidermal growth factor receptors (EGFR) Nonvesicant *Indications:* colorectal cancer with EGFR expression	Loading dose: 400 mg/m² over 120 min, maintenance dose 250 mg/m² over 60 min weekly Maximum rate: 5 mL/min	IV infusion Do not administer as an IV push or bolus. Loading dose given over 120 min. If tolerated well, may infuse maintenance dose over 60 min. Use 0.22-micron filter. Premedication with diphenhydramine 50 mg IV is recommended.	*Common:* Acneform rash seen in about 90% of patients. Described as skin drying and fissuring, multiple follicular- or pustular-appearing lesions. Most commonly located on the face, upper chest, and back, but could also be located on the extremities. Occurs within the first 2 wk of therapy, and most cases resolved with cessation of cetuximab. Events did continue beyond 28 d in nearly half of the cases.	Monitor patient closely for infusion-related reactions. Hypersensitivity/anaphylactic medications should be available during infusion. Gently invert bag to mix. Instruct patient to wear sunscreen and hats and limit sun exposure.

	Dose	Administration	Toxicities	Nursing Considerations
			Other: Severe infusion reactions in 3% of patients; about 90% of these were with the first infusion. Symptoms included rapid onset of airway obstruction (bronchospasm, stridor, hoarseness), urticaria, and hypotension.	1 h observation period is recommended.
Bevacizumab (Avastin) *Drug specificity:* targets vascular endothelial growth factor (VEGF) receptors Nonvesicant *Indications:* colorectal cancer (has been studied in other malignancies at various doses)	Loading dose: 5 mg/m² over 10 min every 14 d	IV infusion Do not administer as an IV push or bolus. Loading dose given over 120 min. If tolerated well, may infuse maintenance dose over 60 min. Use 0.22-micron filter.	*Common:* Gastrointestinal perforations/wound healing complications. Can be serious or fatal. Symptoms included abdominal pain, which has been seen with constipation and vomiting. *System-specific:* Proteinuria, nephrotic syndrome, congestive heart failure, and hypertensive crises *Other:* Hemorrhage. Fatal or serious hemoptysis in patients with non–small cell lung cancer. If recent hemoptysis, patient should not receive bevacizumab.	Bevacizumab should not be administered at least 28 d following major surgery, and surgical incision should be fully healed. The bevacizumab half-life of 20 d should be considered when determining the length that bevacizumab should be suspended prior to elective surgery. Monitor patient closely for infusion-related reactions. Premedications can be considered for infusion-related reactions. Hypersensitivity/anaphylactic medications should be available during infusion. Do not mix with dextrose solutions. Gently invert bag to mix.

BOX 19–4   Tumor Responsiveness to Chemotherapy

Curable
- Childhood cancers (50% or more): acute lymphocytic leukemia, non-Hodgkin lymphoma, Wilms' tumor, Ewing's sarcoma, retinoblastoma, rhabdomyosarcoma
- Hodgkin lymphoma and certain aggressive lymphomas (50% or more)
- Carcinoma of the testis (75% or more)
- Choriocarcinoma in women (90% or more)
- Adult acute leukemia, ovarian carcinoma (15% to 20%)

Improved survival (Substantial improvement in survival but rarely curative)
- Neuroblastoma (in childhood)
- Aggressive non-Hodgkin lymphomas
- Small cell lung cancer
- Carcinoma of the breast
- Osteogenic sarcoma

Palliation (Chemotherapy may substantially palliate symptoms, even though the effects of treatment on survival are unknown or negligible)
- Non-Hodgkin lymphoma (low or intermediate grade)
- Chronic leukemias
- Multiple myeloma
- Carcinoma of the prostate
- Endocrine gland cancers

Occasional responses (Chemotherapy occasionally produces responses and, in some cases, modest improvement in survival at the expense of moderate to severe toxicity)
- Brain cancers
- Carcinoma of the head and neck
- Malignant melanoma (with skin or lymph node involvement)
- Non–oat cell lung carcinoma
- Soft tissue sarcomas
- Transitional cell carcinomas (of the urinary bladder)

(From Casciato, D. [Ed.]. [2004]. *Manual of clinical oncology* [5th ed.]. Philadelphia: Lippincott Williams & Wilkins.)

---

related to malignancy and the side effects of chemotherapy. Their antitumor effects are still under investigation.

Combined Modality Therapy

Although any treatment modality can be used alone, usually antineoplastic regimens rely on drug combinations. In addition, combining the available treatment modalities aims to optimize cancer cell kill while minimizing associated toxicities. One of the important roles of chemotherapy is as **adjuvant** treatment, following surgery and/or radiation therapy, to reduce the incidence of both local and systemic recurrence and to improve the overall survival of patients. A good example of this is in women with breast cancer, where adjuvant chemotherapy is particularly

---

BOX 19–5   Anticancer Drug Combinations

ABVD	doxorubicin + bleomycin + vinblastine + dacarbazine
AC-T	doxorubicin + cyclophosphamide followed by paclitaxel
CHOP-Rituximab	cyclophosphamide + doxorubicin + vincristine + prednisone + rituximab
CAF	cyclophosphamide + doxorubicin + fluorouracil
CVD	cisplatin + vinblastine + dacarbazine
EC	etoposide + carboplatin
FEC	fluorouracil + epirubicin + cyclophosphamide
FAM	fluorouracil + doxorubicin + mitomycin
ICE	ifosfamide + carboplatin + etoposide
IFN+DTIC	interferon-α-2b + dacarbazine
MOPP	mechlorethamine + vincristine + procarbazine + prednisone
MP	melphalan + prednisone
MVAC	methotrexate + vinblastine + doxorubicin + cisplatin
PEB	cisplatin + etoposide + bleomycin
TIP	paclitaxel + ifosfamide + cisplatin
XELOX	capecitabine + oxaliplatin

---

effective in decreasing the rate of recurrence following surgery and radiation therapy. **Neoadjuvant** chemotherapy is the use of chemotherapy prior to treatment for localized cancer when the local therapy is less than completely effective. In this case, vital normal organs are spared, while the tumor is reduced in size and rendered easier to treat by local therapy, that is, surgery. This has led to less extensive surgery and sparing of the larynx, the anal sphincter, and the bladder and better quality of life for patients.

With the exception of oral alkylating agents used for chronic leukemias, single-agent chemotherapy regimens are rare in contemporary practice. *Combination chemotherapy* involves simultaneous multiagent use that capitalizes on synergistic drug actions on the cell cycle to maximize their antitumor effects. Chemotherapy drugs can also be combined with biotherapy agents. Combining agents also modifies dose-limiting toxicities. Box 19–5 lists common combinations of antineoplastics agents. A classic example of combination chemotherapy is the MOPP regimen—mechlorethamine (Mustargen), vincristine (Oncovin), procarbazine, and prednisone—used to treat Hodgkin's disease. The CHOP-Rituxan protocol is an example of combination chemotherapy with a monoclonal antibody to treat non-Hodgkin's lymphoma. The use of chemotherapy combined with biotherapy is well illustrated in the IFN-DTIC regime to treat metastatic melanoma.

The specific and fixed sequence in which drugs are administered yields specific and predictable toxicities. Figure 19–1 illustrates a chemotherapy regimen's depletion of bone marrow, which results in neutropenia. The **nadir** refers to the lowest drop of the blood count between chemotherapy cycles. Chemotherapy regimens are usually repeated every 21 to 28 days, depending on the protocol. This allows for recovery of the bone marrow.

Combining antineoplastic agents potentially provides the greatest collective benefit of each therapy and thus the greatest likelihood of cure. A combination of therapies, either for cure or control, may expose a patient to significant **toxicity.** Most patients (especially those who have been cured) report that the discomfort caused by these toxicities was well worthwhile (DeVita et al., 2004).

The importance of the nurse's own positive attitude when educating patients about the dramatic potential benefits of chemotherapy and biotherapy in balance with its toxicities and side effects cannot be overemphasized. The nurse offers hope to patients and their families and helps to relieve anxiety related to therapy by reassuring the patient that every effort will be made to control side effects.

Systemic Drug Delivery Technique

Proper pretreatment evaluation can have an enormous impact on the efficacy of the nurse's care plan and on the patient's chemotherapy experience. This evaluation includes a nursing assessment and a review of the treatment plan and the physician's orders. The nurse should ascertain answers to the following questions before proceeding with treatment:

- Does the patient understand enough to provide fully informed consent?
- Is the patient being treated with chemotherapy for the first time? If not, is the record complete regarding previous chemotherapy experience, physical and emotional response, experience with and management of side effects, and successful intervention?
- Is assessment of the patient's and family's ability to manage at home complete? Is the patient familiar with resources to assist with sequelae of chemotherapy?
- Has the nurse assessed and reviewed the patient's physical history before administering treatment? Have all compromised organ systems been considered in dose calculation, especially liver and kidneys, which metabolize and clear the agents?
- Has the patient mobilized available coping mechanisms? Is the patient ready for therapy?
- Is the patient prepared for potential hair loss?
- Has an antiemetic regimen, both medical and dietary strategies, been explained and initiated, and does it include both immediate and delayed nausea and vomiting?
- Does the patient have special premedications for the drugs that he or she is to receive, for example, cimetidine, diphenhydramine, and dexamethasone prior to paclitaxel to prevent hypersensitivity reactions?
- Does the patient have special hydration and electrolyte replacement needs? Have replacements been ordered? Does the patient understand the need to continue supplementing fluids after treatment? Is the patient capable of fulfilling this requirement?
- In the past 48 hours, have laboratory values been obtained to include appropriate studies of complete blood counts, platelets, blood urea nitrogen, creatinine, and liver function studies? Are they within normal limits? Has there been any dose adjustment based on toxicity?

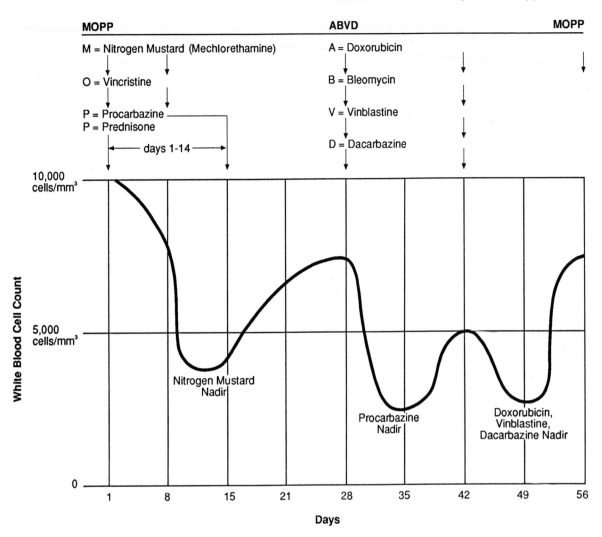

FIGURE 19–1. MOPP/ABV ± D administration schedule and corresponding white blood cell count nadirs (From Goodman, M.S. [1986]. *Cancer: Chemotherapy and care.* Evansville, IN: Bristol-Myers).

- Does the nurse have a therapy protocol and a written and signed physician order that specifies patient name, drug name(s), dosage per square meter of body surface area, total dose, and rate, frequency, and route of administration?
- Is the patient as physically comfortable as possible, with easy access to a nurse call light?
- Are all necessary treatment supplies at hand, such as safe handling equipment, IV therapy materials, and hazardous waste containment? Is light adequate to facilitate venipuncture and patient observation? Is the environment conducive to privacy, especially in the event of emesis?

- Is the nurse prepared for anaphylaxis or extravasation? Is proper emergency equipment readily available? Are necessary professional staff and supplies available in the event of patient emergency?
- Does the patient have adequate venous access?

Successful chemotherapy treatment relies on proper preparation in these areas. Individual patients often require extended pretreatment evaluations for special needs, such as those who are exceptionally anxious, lack family or social support, are cognitively challenged, or are scheduled to receive investigational antineoplastic agents. When chemotherapeutic protocols change, any or all of these steps must be repeated or modified to update patient education. When the nurse and patient have combined their resources to satisfy these questions, administration of chemotherapy may begin.

Routes and Modes of Administration

Although chemotherapy can be administered through a variety of routes (Table 19–7), the oral and IV continue to be most common. Antineoplastic agents are delivered orally (Box 19–6) if they can be tolerated and absorbed by the gastrointestinal tract. Although it is anticipated that 25% of all new antineoplastic agents will be oral, IV administration is far more common. Successful IV administration demands careful vein selection and venipuncture.

VEIN SELECTION

Vein selection depends on the purpose and length of infusion and the vesicant and irritant properties of the drugs. Peripheral veins may be used for bolus or short-term infusion. Central venous access is preferred for patients scheduled for long-term infusions or those at risk of extravasation caused by vein fragility or inaccessibility. Most patients receive chemotherapy for a minimum of 4 to 6 months, with most

---

BOX 19–6   Oral Antineoplastic Agents

Altretamine (Hexalen)
Bexarotene (Targretin)
Busulfan (Myleran, Busulfex)
Capecitabine (Xeloda)
Chlorambucil (Leukeran)
Cyclophosphamide (Cytoxan)
Estramustine (Emcyt)
Etoposide (VePesid, Etopophos)
Gefitinib (Iressa)
Hydroxyurea (Hydrea, Mylocel)
Imatinib (Gleevec)

Levamisole (Ergamisol)
Lomustine (CeeNU)
Melphalan (Alkeran)
Mercaptopurine (6-MP, Purinethol)
Mitotane (Lysodren)
Procarbazine (Matulane)
Temozolomide (Temodar)
Thalidomide (Thalomid)
Thioguanine (TG, Tabloid)
Tretinoin (Vesanoid)

regimens repeated anywhere from weekly to every 4 to 6 weeks. Patients with widespread metastatic disease may require years of chemotherapy, and therefore a central line placement should be considered early in the treatment plan.

For peripheral venous access, patients should be positioned comfortably in a chair with extended armrests and hand and arm stabilizers. Successful IV nurses allow ample and unhurried time to assess both arms and hands to avoid areas of sclerosis, thrombosis, hematoma, or phlebitis. The examination of both arms also gives the nurse a baseline reference should changes occur during treatment.

If veins are obscure, comfortably warm, moist compresses may be applied to the patient's hands and forearms. Clothing can be loosened to allow full view of the IV site. Watches and tight jewelry should be removed if they constrict the venous pathway or impede the smooth flow of drugs along the venous network.

Alternating arms from treatment to treatment may help minimize vascular irritation and phlebitis associated with IV administration of chemotherapy drugs; it also allows time for healing. Documentation should specify which arm and location was used for each treatment. If not informed of this procedure, and if treated by various nurses, a patient may unwittingly prefer to have all treatments in one arm, increasing the risk of phlebitis.

⚠ **SAFE PRACTICE ALERT** Aseptic techniques, including sterile venipuncture procedures, standard precautions, and safe handling of antineoplastics, require a nurse's constant vigilance, especially because of the susceptibility of these patients to systemic infection resulting from neutropenia.

A nurse should follow a pattern for venipunctures, using the most distal veins first and moving proximally For example, if a forearm venipuncture was unsuccessful, or if blood was drawn earlier, cytotoxic agents administered to the same arm might leak into tissue surrounding the recent proximal puncture. With vesicant therapy, necrosis could result. Thus, if the first venipuncture is unsuccessful, the opposite arm should be used for the next attempt (Polovich et al., 2005).

Large veins along the distal forearm (cephalic, median, and basilic) are easy to access and may provide safe, convenient venipuncture sites. Using these larger veins diminishes the risk of chemical phlebitis from the irritant/vesicant properties of antineoplastic drugs, especially with **bolus** (IV push) administration (DeVita et al., 2005). In the event of extravasation, this area also offers a greater mass of soft tissue than the hand and may be more easily grafted, thereby avoiding functional impairment.

Because IV solutions often contain admixtures incompatible with cytotoxic drugs (for example, heparin sodium combined with doxorubicin), there is a potential for precipitates to develop, which can result in vein irritation and phlebitis. Compatibility issues are imperative to consider, not only with antineoplastics but with adjunctive drug therapies, such as those involving antiemetics or corticosteroids.

Vesicant chemotherapy should not be administered using previous IV sites. Ideally, vesicants should be administered through a central line. The following precautions

(text continues on p. 538)

TABLE 19–7   Routes of Administration of Antineoplastic Agents

Route	Advantages	Disadvantages	Complications	Nursing Implications
Oral	Ease of administration Increased patient independence	Inconsistency of absorption Potential drug/herb/diet interactions	Drug-specific complications Swallowing difficulties	Teach compliance with medication schedule.
Subcutaneous/Intramuscular	Ease of administration Decreased side effects	Requires adequate muscle mass and tissue for absorption Inconsistent absorption	Infection Bleeding Pain/discomfort	Evaluate platelet count before administration. Use smallest gauge needle possible. Prepare injection site with an antiseptic solution. Assess injection site for signs and symptoms of infection.
Intravenous	Consistent absorption Required for vesicants	Sclerosing of veins over time	Infection Phlebitis	Check for blood return before, during, and after drug administration.
Intra-arterial	Increased doses to tumor with decreased systemic side effects Local treatment	Requires surgical procedure or special radiography for catheter and/or port placement	Bleeding Embolism Pain Arterial injury Arterial catheter leak, break migration Pump malfunction	Monitor for signs and symptoms of bleeding. Monitor prothrombin time, activated partial thromboplastin time (aPTT). Monitor catheter site.
Intrathecal/Intraventricular	More consistent drug levels in cerebrospinal fluid Bypasses blood–brain barrier	Requires lumbar puncture or surgical placement of reservoir or implanted pump Pump occlusion/malfunction Requires additional education for nurse, patient, family	Increased intracranial pressure Headaches Confusion Lethargy Nausea/vomiting Seizures Infection	Observe for signs of infection. Monitor reservoir or pump functioning. Monitor patient for headache or signs of increased intracranial pressure.

Route	Mechanism	Requirements	Adverse Effects	Nursing Interventions
Intraperitoneal	Direct exposure of intra-abdominal surfaces to drug	Requires placement of peritoneal catheter or intraperitoneal port	Abdominal pain Abdominal distention Bleeding Paralytic ileus Intestinal perforation Infection Nausea	Warm chemotherapy solution to body temperature. Check patency of catheter or port. Instill drug/solution according to protocol—infuse, dwell, and drain or continuous infusion. Reposition patient according to protocol to allow for intraperitoneal distribution.
Intrapleural	Sclerosing of pleural lining	Requires insertion of a thoracotomy tube Physicians must administer intrapleural agents	Pain Infection	Monitor for complete drainage from pleural space before instillation of drug. Following instillation, clamp tubing and reposition patient every 10–15 min for 2 h for adequate distribution of the drug. Attach tubing to suction according to protocol. Assess client for pain, provide analgesia. Assess client for anxiety; provide emotional support.
Intravesicular	Direct exposure of bladder surfaces to drug	Requires insertion of indwelling catheter	Urinary tract infection Cystitis Bladder contracture Urinary urgency Allergic drug reactions	Maintain sterile technique when inserting indwelling catheter. Instill solution, clamp catheter for specified time, and unclamp to drain according to protocol.

(From Polovich, M., White, J.M., Kelleher, L.O., et al. [Eds.] [2005]. *Chemotherapy and biotherapy guidelines and recommendations for practice.* Pittsburgh, PA: Oncology Nursing Society; Temple, S.V., & Poniatowski, B.C. Nursing implications of antineoplastic therapy. In: J.K. Itano & K.N. Taoka [Eds.] [2005]. *Core curriculum for oncology nursing* (pp. 793–794). St. Louis, MO: Elsevier Saunders.)

must be considered if an existing IV line is the only available site for chemotherapy administration:

- Ensure venous patency before treatment and use transparent dressings that allow the site to be seen without disturbing the dressing.
- Flush the line before and after treatment.
- When establishing a new IV line, avoid joint flexion areas, the wrist or antecubital fossa, whenever possible. The chosen vein should feel smooth and resilient, not hard or cordlike.

Several factors contraindicate the use of the antecubital fossa. This area includes the important anatomic structures of the median nerve and brachial artery. Serious complications—tissue damage, and later, necrosis may occur. Extensive tissue necrosis could require complicated, costly, and psychologically difficult reconstructive efforts.

In addition, phlebotomists favor antecubital fossa veins for drawing blood specimens. If repeated needle insertions and infusions trigger tissue fibrosis, future blood sampling may become difficult. Moreover, prolonged infusions restrict arm mobility because elbow function is limited during infusion and the area's fat and tissue volume make it difficult to visualize and detect early subcutaneous infiltration.

Despite the nurse's technical competence, usable veins sometimes are difficult to locate and access. A limit of two unsuccessful venipunctures is suggested before a nurse seeks assistance from a coworker. Repeated venipunctures increase anxiety levels for both patient and nurse and may decrease the likelihood of successful vein catheterization.

The lower extremities or an arm with impaired circulation or lymphedema should not be used for infusing cytotoxic agents. Stagnant or sluggish blood flow delays the agent's flow into the general circulation, and the agent also can potentiate any local reaction. Impaired circulation in the extremities can result from an invading neoplasm, existing phlebitis, varicosities, axillary node dissection on the side of a mastectomy, an immobilized fracture, or even extensive hematomas or inflamed areas.

SAFE PRACTICE ALERT Perform a thorough examination of the extremity before inserting the catheter into the vein. Avoid using phlebitic, bruised, inflamed, or sclerotic areas. A useful and often overlooked peripheral infusion site is the basilic vein on the medial aspect of the forearm.

ADMINISTRATION TECHNIQUES

Most chemotherapeutic and biotherapy regimens can be administered on an outpatient basis. Many regimes once given in the inpatient setting have been modified and are given in the outpatient setting. Hence, some patients may have outpatient stays from 1 hour to 8 hours duration. When treating an outpatient using a peripheral site, an angiocatheter is preferred, given its stability in the vein. The gauge of the angiocatheter may vary, dependent on the size of the cannulated vein and the length of treatment. Select the smallest gauge and the shortest length catheter to accommodate the prescribed therapy (Polovich et al., 2005).

Tape should be applied so that the needle insertion site and immediate surrounding area are clearly visible. A common extravasation site is just above the insertion site. If obscured, subtle infiltration evidence may go unnoticed. Tubing should be taped independently, then looped so that blood return can be checked during administration. When the IV catheter is securely in place, the remainder of the IV set should be arranged to remain intact and functional, even in the event of sudden movements like vomiting.

Before cytotoxic drug administration, an IV fluid flush should be given to test and ensure venous patency. If a fragile vein bursts, or if an IV catheter has perforated its wall, conventional IV fluids are absorbed without damaging surrounding tissue. A patient with a capped peripheral IV catheter or a permanent central venous catheter requires a flush solution infusion before chemotherapy/biotherapy administration to avoid drug incompatibilities. At least 10 mL IV of fluid between drugs avoids inopportune chemical interactions. Likewise, a final flush clears the line and vein after antineoplastic administration is complete.

Bolus (IV push) administration calls for slow, even pressure. Small-gauge IV catheters offer greater resistance than larger IV catheters. Any unusual resistance calls for cessation of infusion to investigate the cause. If the bevel of the IV catheter is resting against the vein wall, careful repositioning may resolve the problem. If the nurse applies too much force, the patient may experience pain or venous spasm. A fast, forceful infusion may even cause nausea or exaggerated hypersensitivity sensations (such as nasal congestion with Cytoxan). Most adverse reactions can be avoided when there is even push pressure and constant supervision of all administration processes.

Short-term chemotherapy may also be delivered with a conventional mini-infusion piggyback approach. When injecting vesicants, IV catheter stability and adequate blood return must be checked approximately every 2 to 5 mL. Do not pinch the IV tubing to determine blood return and patency. Instead use either a suction check (gently aspirate the line using a syringe at the Y site closest to the patient while clamping off the fluid from the IV bag) or the gravity check (free the IV bag and tubing and gently lower it to a point below the patient's IV site; Polovich et al., 2005). Immediate cessation of drug administration is required if there is any doubt about venous patency. With vesicants, the compromised site should be treated as an extravasation; with nonvesicants, treatment can be resumed with a new catheter site.

After chemotherapy/biotherapy, the catheter tubing is flushed with appropriate, compatible flush solution to remove all drug from the system and the catheter is removed with a dry sterile sponge. The extremity is elevated and pressure applied until bleeding stops. A dressing is applied to the site. Because thrombocytopenia is a common sequel of chemotherapy, blood leakage into subcutaneous tissues can result in hematomas that are painful and unsightly, and, until reabsorbed, preclude use of the site. Patients also should be cautioned not to handle heavy items with the treated extremity immediately after chemotherapy.

Venous Access Devices

A central venous access device (VAD) may be required for patients with a vesicant in their treatment programs or with impaired peripheral venous vasculature. Tunneled, nontunneled, or implanted subcutaneous devices can be used for either long- or short-term treatment plans. They can be percutaneously inserted, either centrally or peripherally, eventually to dwell in the superior vena cava or above the junction of the right atrium. They have become the state of the art in antineoplastic administration because of their ease of placement, convenience, and safety benefits. Central VADs eliminate peripheral venipuncture for drawing blood specimens and dramatically enhance patient security and comfort. Some of the other advantages of a central line are that it:

- Preserves the peripheral venous system
- Serves as a line for blood and nutritional products, antibiotics, analgesics, and antiemetics, as well as antineoplastic agents
- Allows home infusion of vesicants and multiple-drug therapies that otherwise can be administered safely only in acute care settings
- Is cost effective

Potential disadvantages include costs of insertion and maintenance, thrombus owing to improper or inadequate irrigation, infection or sepsis, air embolism, and catheter severance or migration. Before discharge, patients and families need training in meticulous device maintenance and should receive written instructions for later reference.

Vascular access devices afford dramatic quality-of-life advantages, but they demand extraordinary patient and/or caregiver responsibility with maintenance activities. It is imperative that the nurse ensures that the patient and caregiver have learned the proper handling and maintenance of his or her central line. Proper instruction can prevent catheter occlusions caused by inadequate irrigation, infections, or catheter breakage, or air embolism caused by line mismanagement, poorly stabilized or improper connections, or mishandled clamps. If the patient or caregiver cannot properly care for the access device, the device may be compromised and may need to be removed. Alternative support for home maintenance of these devices may need to be sought and arranged.

Box 19–7 lists various devices for long-term venous access. Device selection depends on frequency of access, treatment, duration, administration mode, venous integrity, and patient preference (Murphy, Lawrence, & Lenhard, 2000). Criteria for patient assessment are featured in Box 19–8. Common placement sites are discussed in Chapter 14.

In fact, these venous access devices are so simple and reliable that there is a real risk of complacency for nurses treating these patients. Individual manufacturer recommendations for care and maintenance should be followed strictly, particularly because specific diameters, volumes, lumen sizes, and clamping procedures vary among models. Although IV therapy is the primary use of these devices, these or similar ones can also be placed intra-arterially for organ profusion or intraperitoneally for chemotherapy administration into the abdominal cavity.

Implanted ports offer an alternative to percutaneously inserted central venous catheters. Advantages include reduced infection risk, no care requirements for external catheters, and diminished risk of drug infiltration or vein sclerosis from irritating drugs administered peripherally. Implantable devices are available from a variety of manufacturers.

Implanted ports carry a risk of needle dislodgment and consequent extravasation when long-term infusions of vesicant drugs such as doxorubicin (Adriamycin),

---

BOX 19–7   Selected Venous Access Devices and Their Uses

Tunneled Central Venous Catheters
Frequent venous access for blood sampling, delivery of blood products, and therapy
Bone marrow transplantation
Multiple transfusions, such as for treating patients with leukemia
Single bolus injections of chemotherapy
Infusion of total parenteral nutrition, fluids, pain management, and antibiotic therapy
Short- or long-term, inpatient or outpatient chemotherapy infusions, vesicant or nonvesicant
Note: Patient or responsible caregiver must be capable of caring for this device.

Small-Gauge, Peripherally Inserted Central Venous Catheters
Short-term infusion of chemotherapy or vesicant or nonvesicant chemotherapy, total parenteral nutrition, blood, fluids, pain management, and antibiotic therapy
Inpatient or outpatient infusion therapy
Single bolus injections of chemotherapy
Frequent venous access needed for chemotherapy
Frequent blood sampling
Brief life expectancy
Note: Patient or responsible caregiver must be capable of caring for this device.

Implanted Ports
Infrequent venous access
Single bolus injections of chemotherapy
Inpatient or outpatient infusion of chemotherapeutic agents
Short- or long-term chemotherapy
Total parenteral nutrition, blood sampling, blood transfusions, fluid replacement, antibiotic therapy, pain management
Alternative for patients physically unable to care for other access device
Young children (when frequent venous access is not required)
Cosmesis or patient preference

---

or vincristine (Oncovin) are administered through implanted devices. Proper needle placement must be assessed and documented at least every 8 hours with these vesicants. A patient with an implanted device receiving a continuous infusion of a vesicant requires inpatient care. This is not the case with vesicant administration through indwelling central venous catheters, such as the Hickman catheter. Complications are rare and usually avoidable when professional standards and chemotherapy administration practices are observed. When complications do occur, however, they are severe and often life threatening.

Infusion Systems

Venous access devices provide another key benefit to patients requiring continuous or intermittent chemotherapy; they allow treatment at home. External ambulatory infusion systems for antineoplastics reduce inpatient admissions and costs and allow patient autonomy in familiar home surroundings.

BOX 19–8   Patient Assessment Criteria for a Central Vascular Access Device

General assessment guidelines for assessing whether a central vascular access device (VAD) is appropriate for the patient include the frequency of venous access, longevity of treatment, mode of drug administration, venous integrity, and the patient's preferences. Priorities for central VAD placement are compared below.

Low Priority	High Priority
Infrequent venous access	Frequent venous access
Short-term therapy	Long-term, indefinite treatment period
Intermittent single injections	Continuous infusion of chemotherapy
Administration of nonvesicant, nonirritating drugs	Administration of vesicant, irritating drugs
No previous IV therapy	Venous thrombosis or sclerosis from previous IV therapy
Both extremities available	Venous access limited to one extremity
Venous access with two or fewer venipunctures	More than two venipunctures to secure venous access
Patient does not prefer central VAD	Patient prefers central VAD
	Home infusion of chemotherapy
	Prior tissue damage owing to extravasation

All external ambulatory infusion systems are self-powered independent of household electrical current. They are battery powered, lightweight, and reusable. They infuse either through a piston valve (Autosyringe) or a peristaltic mechanism. The administration rate is controllable. Mechanically powered pumps feature alarm systems that detect any back pressure that might occur with occlusion or infiltration. These pumps also detect air in the line, and an alarm sounds when the fluid reservoir is empty.

The list of ambulatory infusion system products and technologies continually changes as new improvements are made. IV nurses are better served to keep abreast of manufacturer-provided instructional materials, patient education information, and troubleshooting support services of the devices currently favored in their own clinical setting. Nurses also must be intimately familiar with system operations to educate patients and families in early detection of complications, including line occlusion, thrombosis, infiltration or extravasation, and system failure.

Following is a list of assessment factors to consider when recommending use of an ambulatory infusion system:

- Level of patient and family understanding of pump and alarm features and functions; degree of patient and family compliance, reliability, dexterity, and comfort with the device; patient or family visual acuity keen enough to see pump function clearly

- 24-hour availability or proximity to health care provider in the event of pump failure or occlusion
- Drug regimen that matches device capacities and features
- Insurance coverage of unit rental

Infusion systems can be attached by belt or shoulder strap to ease patient movement. Mechanical systems usually call for hands-on programming and reprogramming, requiring an on-site visit from a nurse when changes are needed. The same is true for replenishing fluid and drug reservoirs. Developments to ease ambulatory infusions (such as pump reprogramming by computer or over phone lines, without hands-on human intervention) are promised for the near future.

Regional Drug Delivery

Although systemic IV administration of chemotherapy is most common, some tumors respond better to local exposure to antineoplastics. Alternative methods of drug administration have been established to deliver high concentrations of chemotherapeutic agents locally, into a body cavity or into the organ site of the tumor. A drug can be directed into the area of known disease, such as intraperitoneally to treat malignant ascites or metastatic seeding of peritoneum from ovarian cancer. Intravesical administration of chemotherapy and biologic response modifiers is frequently used to treat bladder cancer. Intrathecal or intraventricular administration is used for cancers known to have invaded the central nervous system; intrapleural is beneficial for malignant effusions and sclerosing purposes; topical application can be used for early malignancies of the integumentary system. Intra-arterial administration provides higher concentrations for the regional delivery of chemotherapy. Regional delivery of these infusions results in increased exposure of the tumor to the drug, whereas less systemic circulation and exposure to the antineoplastic agent decreases the risk of systemic side effects (Camp-Sorrell, 2004).

INTRA-ARTERIAL DELIVERY

Intra-arterial administration delivers antineoplastic drugs directly into the organ or tumor via the main artery supply. Although metastatic hepatic disease is the most common indication for intra-arterial chemotherapy, other organs, such as the brain, head and neck region, and pelvic area can also be perfusion sites for arterial delivery of chemotherapy (Camp-Sorrell, 2004).

The most likely alternative route of antineoplastic administration involving the IV nurse is the intra-arterial infusion, which may use either an arterial catheter or an arterial port. Arterial catheters are percutaneously inserted and can be used for short-term and long-term therapy. A totally implanted infusion pump can also be used to deliver chemotherapy via the arterial circulation.

The IsoMed Pump (Medtronic Neurological, Minneapolis, MN) is the most common totally implantable drug delivery system. The IsoMed pump is designed to deliver a constant flow of drug for hepatic arterial infusion therapy. The FDA has approved the following drugs for intra-arterial infusion: 5-fluorouracil, floxuridine, doxorubicin, methotrexate, bleomycin, cisplatin, amikacin, heparin, and glycerin.

The arterial catheter and implanted pump are surgically placed. The pump's reservoir is filled and the catheter access port is flushed after assembly in the OR. The catheter tip position and perfusion of the intended region is confirmed postoperatively before drug therapy is started. The drug is placed in the pump reservoir and is subsequently forced through a flow-restrictive tubing by pressurized gas. The pump flow rate can be altered by fluctuations in pump temperature. Patients must agree to report any fever so that pump refill schedules can be assessed and adjusted. Because infection and thrombosis are the most common complications, patients also are instructed to report edema, fever, erythema, or pain at the site (Camp-Sorrell, 2004).

About every 1 to 4 weeks, the pump is refilled by percutaneous injection with either active antineoplastics or a heparin solution to maintain constant perfusion to the area and patency of the catheter. The device's side port may be used for direct intra-arterial access. The nurse must be intimately familiar with techniques and risks of this route of drug delivery, adhere strictly to details available from manufacturer data, and demonstrate competency accessing and filling the pump. An implantable pump can also support effective pain management when used to infuse low-dose narcotics through the intrathecal delivery mode.

INTRATHECAL DELIVERY

Intrathecal therapy is another alternative route of cancer chemotherapy that might call for IV nurse involvement. A cerebrospinal access device, such as the Ommaya reservoir, is subcutaneously implanted into the lateral ventricle of the brain to avoid repeated lumbar punctures in treating meningeal carcinomatosis, the infiltration by cancer of the cerebral leptomeninges. The reservoir provides access to the cerebrospinal fluid through a burr hole in the skull.

First, the reservoir is pumped several times to fill the device with cerebrospinal fluid (CSF). Then, the skin is prepared and the reservoir is punctured at a 45-degree angle, using sterile technique, with a 25- to 27-gauge scalp vein needle. Sufficient CSF is removed for laboratory studies and to keep exchanges isovolumetric; that is, enough CSF is withdrawn to equal the amount of the drugs to be infused while reserving 3 mL to use as flush following the procedure. Then, a chemotherapeutic agent, such as methotrexate or cytarabine, which is admixed with a preservative-free solution, is injected slowly over 5 to 10 minutes through a scalp vein needle into the reservoir. Following the drug, flush with the reserved CSF. Remove the needle, and pump the reservoir to distribute the drugs into the intraventricular space. Preservative-free morphine sulfate also can be administered into an Ommaya reservoir for prolonged pain relief (Camp-Sorrell, 2004).

Complications of Chemotherapy

Regardless of the nurse's skills and standards, sometimes patients experience problems unique to the administration of cytotoxic agents. A common reason for the problems is the condition of the veins. Elderly, poorly nourished, and debilitated patients often have fragile veins. Unskilled nurses may unwittingly cause painful and unsightly hematomas that eliminate use of the treatment area until reabsorption is complete. Nurses should attempt to catheterize fragile veins with a loose tourniquet or with no tourniquet because distention and rapid engorgement may cause the vein wall to rupture when the tourniquet is released.

A second nurse may apply gentle hand pressure directly above the venipuncture site to distend it. Other distention techniques include application of moderate heat or asking the patient to clench or pump the fist. Gravity flow may be maximized if the patient dangles the extremity. The nurse may lightly finger-tap the site to distend the vein. Catheter gauge and length should be part of the decision process. A central line should also be a consideration. Regardless of the chosen technique, fragile veins require a cautious approach and allowance of ample time to prepare for successful venipuncture on the first attempt.

Localized Acute Allergic Reactions

The nurse should be prepared for allergic reactions whenever any antineoplastic agent is administered IV. A localized allergic reaction, known as a *flare*, often is associated with administration of doxorubicin hydrochloride and mechlorethamine. The first manifestation may be erythema along the venous pathways. Blotchiness, hivelike urticaria, or the rapid appearance of welts also may occur. The patient may report itchiness, stinging, or an increasing sensation of heat in the area. This localized venous reaction is felt to be an inflammatory response with histamine release (Polovich et al. 2005). Nursing assessment parameters to differentiate among a flare, local irritation, and extravasation are outlined (Table 19–8). Preventive measures include additional drug dilution, either by adding the drug to 100 to 200 mL solution or by administering the drug slowly. The nurse should always consult and follow the manufacturer's recommendations.

At the beginning of symptoms of a flare reaction, it is critical to distinguish a flare reaction from a drug extravasation. If an extravasation is suspected, stop the drug and follow extravasation procedures. If a flare reaction seems evident, stop the drug, flush the line with saline, and watch for flare resolution. A flare reaction lasts <45 minutes. In the case of an unresolved flare reaction, a physician's order can be obtained to administer the following medications to treat the localized sensitivity reaction:

- Hydrocortisone sodium succinate (Solu-Cortef), slow IV push, 25 to 50 mg; anti-inflammatory agent
- Diphenhydramine (Benadryl) IV push, 25 to 50 mg; antihistamine

Follow medications with a saline flush until the flare has resolved. Resume infusion of the drug. Document the reaction and treatment in the medical record. Premedication with an antihistamine and steroid may prevent another episode when the drug is administered again (Polovich et al., 2005).

Venous Spasm

Some antineoplastic agents are known to produce pain or spasm along the venous pathway. Carmustine (BCNU) is diluted with absolute alcohol, which may be the

TABLE 19–8   Nursing Assessment of Extravasation Versus Other Reactions

| Assessment Parameter | Extravasation | | Irritation of the Vein | Flare Reaction |
	Intermediate Manifestations of Extravasation	Delayed Manifestations of Extravasation		
Pain	Severe pain or burning lasting minutes or hours, eventually subsiding; usually occurs while the drug is given and around needle site	Usually occurs within 48 h	Aching and tightness along the vein	No pain
Redness	Blotchy redness around needle site, not always present at time of extravasation	Later occurrence	The full length of the vein may be reddened or darkened	Immediate blotches or streaks along vein, usually subsides within 30 min with or without treatment
Ulceration	Develops insidiously, usually 48–96 h later	Later occurrence	Not usually	Not usually
Swelling	Severe swelling usually occurs immediately	Usually occurs within 48 h	Unlikely	Unlikely; wheals may appear along vein line
Blood return	Inability to obtain blood return	Good blood return during drug administration	Usually	Usually
Other	Change in the quality of infusion	Local tingling, sensory deficits	—	Urticaria

(From Polovich, M., White, J.M., Kelleher, L.O., et al. [2005]. *Chemotherapy and biotherapy: Guidelines and recommendation for practice* [p. 82]. Pittsburgh, PA: Oncology Nursing Society.)

offending agent. The breakdown products from the photodegradation of dacarbazine (DTIC) may be responsible for acute local burning associated with the drug's use. Mechlorethamine hydrochloride (Mustargen) also can cause pain, especially in patients who have been treated chemotherapeutically over extended times.

> **⚠ SAFE PRACTICE ALERT** Although there are many special cautions for special drugs, it is important to remember that any agent can cause venous pain, in any patient, at any time.

Venous pain and spasm is generally felt to be from administration of irritating medication or solutions. Venous pain and spasm can be alleviated with these measures:

- Slowing the drug infusion rate
- Diluting the antineoplastic agent
- Applying warm or cool arm compresses above the catheter insertion site during infusion. Some patients respond better to cool compresses, some to warm. Care must be taken to avoid second-degree burns.
- Administering lidocaine 1% (0.25 mL, 3 mL total), as needed to relieve the pain associated with venous spasms. Obtain patient's allergy history and physician order prior to administration (Alexander & Corrigan, 2004).

Phlebitis

The risk for *chemical phlebitis* (inflammation of the vein owing to irritating drug or solution) exists with most IV anticancer agents, but the risk increases when two or more antineoplastics are combined. Contributing factors to chemical phlebitis are high acid pH, hyperosmolar solutions, rapid infusion rates, drug–drug interactions where precipitate is formed, and incomplete dissolution of medication particles (Alexander & Corrigan, 2004). Chemotherapeutic drugs associated with phlebitis include actinomycin, carmustine, cisplatin, dacarbazine, daunorubicin, doxorubicin hydrochloride, mechlorethamine hydrochloride, mitomycin C, streptozocin, vinblastine, vincristine, and vinorelbine.

Early phlebitis can be associated with pain, erythema, occasional limb edema, and a sensation of warmth in the affected extremity. As acute symptoms subside, venous pathways may retain dark-bluish to brown discoloration for some time while arm use is restricted. Acute phlebitis reactions are diagnosed by palpating the tip of the IV catheter along the vein course, using slight pressure to detect tenderness. The best indicator of phlebitis is a feeling of warmth at the IV catheter site associated with inflammatory swelling.

Nurses must exercise utmost caution to prevent phlebitis because treatment may be jeopardized owing to compromised peripheral venous access. Occasionally a patient with a history of phlebitic treatment sites manifests reactions to any IV drug administration. Evaluate the patient to determine if he or she is a candidate for a central line. To diminish the threat of phlebitis, the nurse may implement various preventive measures, including the following:

- Use a filter when admixing medication to eliminate particulates.
- Use recommended solutions when mixing drugs.
- Reduce the concentration of the cytotoxic agent with further dilution.
- Administer medications at the prescribed rate.
- Rotate peripheral IV catheter sites.
- Access large veins and use the smallest IV catheter gauge that will deliver the drug infusion to promote hemodilution.
- Administer hydrocortisone sodium succinate (Solu-Cortef), 25 to 50 mg, slow IV push. A physician's order is required before this drug can be administered. After ensuring vein patency, the nurse may administer half the dose before antineoplastic administration and the other half after the final flush, immediately before the needle is removed.

Repetitive needle insertions for blood sampling and antineoplastic administrations increase the likelihood of both phlebitis and thrombosis. In fact, phlebitis develops in some patients despite the most meticulous clinical efforts to avoid it. Once phlebitis has occurred, elevation of the affected extremity, application of topical heat, and administration of systemic analgesics may be indicated.

A patient's venous status should be assessed carefully before the start of a course of treatment. If veins are deep and difficult to visualize and palpate with tourniquet distention, if peripheral veins are extraordinarily small, or if the proposed treatment plan is long, a central venous access device (VAD) should be considered.

Generalized Anaphylactic Reaction

A nurse should be prepared for *anaphylactic reaction* (systemic hypersensitivity reaction) at any time, with any drug, in any patient. Anaphylaxis is a medical emergency that results in respiratory failure, cardiovascular collapse, and possibly death. Anaphylactic reactions are unpredictable. Before initiating any treatment, the nurse should be aware of the institution's policies regarding emergencies arising from administration of antineoplastic agents and the location of emergency supplies and equipment.

Taxanes (paclitaxel, Taxotere), platinum compounds (cisplatin, carboplatin, oxaliplatin), asparaginase, bleomycin, and epipodophyllotoxins (etoposide, venoposide) are chemotherapy agents that can provoke a hypersensitivity reaction (Itano & Taoka, 2005). Because of the nature of monoclonal antibodies (highly specific antibodies produced from a single clone of cells, mouse, human, and combinations), hypersensitivity reactions are common. They usually occur with the first infusion.

To prepare for the possibility of anaphylaxis, the nurse should be vigilant for any signs of flushing, sudden agitation or anxiety, headache, nausea, vomiting, cramping abdominal pain, urticaria, generalized pruritus, chest tightness or pain, respiratory distress, wheezing, coughing, shortness of breath, or asthma-type reaction. Failure to respond appropriately can result in a generalized anaphylactic reaction, seizures, or cardiopulmonary arrest.

Before therapy begins, the nurse should position the patient in a reclining position that eases management of an anaphylactic event. If the patient is seated at a table not adjacent to a bed, anaphylaxis is more difficult to handle. An emergency cart with all appropriate medications, equipment, and blood pressure monitoring equipment also should be available (Table 19–9).

The procedures of some facilities call for a standing order sheet for hypersensitivity management to be signed by the responsible physician before antineoplastic treatment. This time-saving and prudent procedure allows the nurse to begin emergency treatment even before the physician arrives. In addition, the nurse needs to record baseline vital signs before treatment. If a patient normally is hypotensive or tachycardic, the baseline blood pressure reading or pulse rate is useful in case shock symptoms occur. The same is true for a baseline reference point of the patient's mental status. Particularly with metastatic brain disease or other mental alterations, early symptoms of anaphylaxis—agitation, anxiety, speech disorders, and mental confusion—can be misleading without a clear picture of the patient's pretreatment mental state. The nurse should solicit the patient's allergy history and instruct the patient on hypersensitivity symptoms to report.

Regardless of whether a patient displays a mild reaction, generalized pruritus, or complete cardiovascular collapse, the nurse should be prepared to do the following:

- Discontinue the antineoplastic administration.
- Recline the patient smoothly, safely, and quickly.
- Administer basic cardiopulmonary resuscitative measures.
- Maintain a patent IV line for emergency drug administration.
- Provide calm reassurance.
- Administer appropriate drugs, as ordered.
- Monitor the patient until the reaction subsides.

The nurse must be aware of which agents are associated with anaphylaxis and be prepared to administer those agents recommended by the manufacturer. When

TABLE 19–9 Emergency Drugs for Hypersensitivity or Anaphylaxis

Drugs	Strength	Volume
Epinephrine	1:1,000 (1 mg/mL)	10 mL
	1:10,000	
Anhydrous theophylline	400 mg	100 mL
Diphenhydramine	50 mg	1 mL
Hydrocortisone	2 mL	100 mL
Dopamine	(200 mg) 800 mg	250 mL
Levarterenol bitartrate	2 mg	500 mL
Sodium bicarbonate	8.4%	50 mEq/50 mL
Furosemide	40 mg	4 mL
Diazepam	10 mg	2 mL
Lidocaine	100 mg	5 mL
Naloxone hydrochloride	0.1–0.4 mg	5 mL
Nitroglycerin	0.15 mg	Sublingual

the potential exists for an anaphylactic reaction, these precautionary measures might be useful:

- Test dosing (bleomycin, asparaginase)
- Pretreatment with antihistamines, steroids, anti-inflammatory or antipyretic agents (taxanes, monoclonal antibodies)
- Uninterrupted dosing to preclude significant reactive antibody buildup.

Any hypersensitivity reaction and its treatment should be documented so the offending drug can be avoided, the patient can be premedicated, or medication desensitization can be considered (Polovich et al., 2005).

Extravasation

Controversy surrounds appropriate treatment of *extravasation* (local infiltration of vesicant chemotherapy agents). Animal studies have provided data on a few effective antidotes for extravasation, but applicability to humans is limited. Currently, only sodium thiosulfate is a recommended antidote for mechlorethamine hydrochloride and concentrated solution of cisplatin (0.5 mg/mL) extravasation (Polovich et al., 2005). In fact, it often is difficult to ascertain that an infiltration actually has occurred. Table 19–8 outlined venous reactions compared with actual extravasations. It is important for the nurse to identify risk factors for peripheral extravasation: small fragile veins, superior vena cava syndrome (SVCS), peripheral neuropathy, altered mental status, excessive patient movement, venipuncture technique, site of venous access, and drug administration technique (Polovich et al., 2005). Extravasation of vesicant drugs can also occur with central venous access devices (VADs): backflow from fibrin sheath or thrombosis, dislodged Huber needle from port, catheter damage, and migration and dislodgement of the catheter from the vein (Polovich et al. 2005).

PREVENTION

Of course, years of experience in treating patients with antineoplastic drugs perfects the nurse's technique and is a good patient safeguard. It is important to keep in mind, however, that extravasation of vesicant agents can occur despite the nurse's skill. The nurse's focus should be on perfecting safe IV technique, being prepared (Table 19–10), preventing extravasation (Table 19–11), and implementing prudent preparatory measures should an extravasation occur. Although there are no guarantees, the nurse can be reasonably confident that the impact of extravasation can be minimized with early detection and treatment.

PATIENT EDUCATION

The patient must be informed of possible consequences when chemotherapeutic agents are administered so that informed consent is comprehensive and legitimate. A sensitive nurse conveys the risks in such a way that the patient can react to the information appropriately and without unnecessary fear.

TABLE 19–10   Extravasation Kit: Items and Quantities

Needles	19 gauge (4)
	25 gauge (4)
	Filter needle (1)
Tape	1-in. paper
Telfa pads	4 × 4 in. (4)
Sterile gauze dressing	4 × 4 in. (2)
Alcohol wipes	(4)
Syringes	Tuberculin: 3 mL, 5 mL, 10 mL, 20 mL
Diluent	Sterile saline solution: 10 mL (1)
	Sterile water: 10 mL (1)
Steroid cream	1% Topical lotion (optional)
Antidotes	Sodium thiosulfate (for mechlorethamine and concentrated cisplatin)
Latex or nitrile gloves	Several
Hot pack/ Cold pack	
Policy and procedure for extravasation management	
Extravasation record	
Camera	(1)

Note: *Restock kit after each use.* Kit should be available wherever vesicant drugs are being administered.

Constant surveillance by the nurse is required for patients who are confused, unconscious, or in some way unable to perceive or report early signs of extravasation. Alert and cooperative patients may report stinging, burning, and pain or an unusual sensation at the catheter insertion site. Nevertheless, extravasation can occur even without perceptible symptoms.

Being Prepared for Extravasation

Before any treatment, the nurse should be familiar with the agents known to produce tissue damage (Table 19–12) and anticipate the possibility of extravasation. When administering any antineoplastic drug, nurses should be prepared for potential extravasation, have antidotes available, ensure venous patency, anticipate insidious infiltration, and monitor the patient. A chart of vesicants and irritants, recommended antidotes, and use of hot or cold compresses should be posted in a convenient place. Antidotes should be kept readily available for administration. A delay in antidote administration increases the severity of the local tissue reaction. If standing emergency orders are available, they should be signed by the responsible physician and placed in the patient's chart.

Confirming Venous Patency

A flush of at least 5 to 10 mL normal saline solution may be infused to test venous patency and peripheral IV catheter placement before administering any antineoplastic

(text continues on p. 560)

TABLE 19–11 Extravasation of Vesicant Antineoplastic Agents: Preventive Strategies

Risk Factor	Preventive Strategy	Rationale
Skill of the Practitioner	Chemotherapy administration is done only by registered nurses who are specifically trained and supervised.	Procedures for management of extravasation vary according to the drug infiltrated.
		Certain drugs (streptozocin or BCNU) may cause a burning sensation during infusion, which is normal. However, it is abnormal and indicative of a problem if burning occurs during infusion of drugs such as doxorubicin and mitomycin.
	No attempts are made by practitioner to do procedures beyond his or her expertise.	Procedures change rapidly. Techniques need to be learned and mastered before assuming responsibility for administration of chemotherapy.
	Practitioners are skillful in venipuncture.	
	Practitioners are knowledgeable of the signs and symptoms of extravasation and drug therapy.	
	Practice is based on institutional policies and procedures that are routinely updated to meet the changing standards and methods of practice.	The definition of customary care in the community helps dictate standard of practice.
Condition of the Veins		
Small fragile veins	Use conventional methods for venous distention, such as heat and percussion.	Risk of vesicant drug seepage exists with repeated venipuncture.
Access limited owing to axillary surgery, vein thrombosis, prior extravasation	Assess all available arm veins. Assess veins in a methodical fashion, taking time to select the most appropriate vein.	
Long-term drug therapy Multiple vein punctures	If practitioners do not feel confident in their ability to catheterize a person's veins successfully, they should seek the assistance of a colleague.	
	After attempting one or two injections without success, the practitioner should seek the assistance of a colleague before trying again.	Multiple vein injections lead to thrombosis and limited availability.
	A patient who consistently needs two or more attempts to secure venous access should be considered a candidate for a venous access device (VAD). The time to place a VAD is before an extravasation, not after.	Treatment should be delayed until a VAD can be placed. Most VADs can be used immediately or within 24–48 h, so delay in drug therapy is not usually an issue.

Drug Administration Technique

Vesicant agents are never given as continuous infusions into a peripheral vein.

Use a central VAD to administer any vesicant infusing for longer than 30–60 min.

If peripheral line is on an infusion pump, disconnect pump before administration of chemotherapy. Administer short infusion vesicants by gravity.

When a vesicant is to be given as a continuous infusion, the drug should be infused through an external-based central venous catheter whenever possible.

Vesicant agents are most commonly administered through the side port of a free-flowing peripheral IV line or through a VAD.

Side-arm Technique

Ensure proper venous access site. The IV fluid should be additive free.

Catheter used to access the vein should be at least a 20 gauge to ensure an adequate blood return and fluid flow.

Secure catheter, but do not obstruct entrance site.

Assess for blood return.

Test the vein with 50–100 mL to ensure an adequate and swift drip of infusion.

With IV fluid continuing to drip, slowly inject vesicant into IV line.

The risk of infiltration of a vesicant from a peripheral vein infusion is great owing to the following:

Blood return is not assessed frequently.

The longer the infusion, the greater the possibility of IV catheter dislodgment.

The patient can move the extremity, which could dislodge the IV catheter.

Even a small amount of vesicant can cause tissue damage.

Infiltration can be subtle and difficult to detect until a large volume has infiltrated.

The patient may be sedated from an antiemetic and be unable to report sensations associated with extravasation.

The pump forces drug into tissues.

When an implanted port already exists, the Huber needle should be secured in place and checked at least three times a day to ensure placement during continuous infusion of a vesicant.

The incidence of vesicant drug extravasation from ports used for continuous infusion is well documented and presents a risk to be avoided, if possible.

The rationale for the side-arm technique is the added dilution of the drug by the continuous drip of the IV fluid.

Common pitfalls:

Not using a large enough catheter for a brisk infusion of infusate.

Vesicant backs up into IV line.

IV line has to be pinched off to inject vesicant, which defeats the purpose.

(Continued)

TABLE 19–11 Extravasation of Vesicant Antineoplastic Agents: Preventive Strategies *(Continued)*

Risk Factor	Preventive Strategy	Rationale
	Do not allow vesicant to flow backward.	
	Do not pinch off tubing except to assess for blood return.	
	Assess for blood return every 2–5 mL injection.	
	Flush IV catheter with saline at the completion of injection.	
Site of Venous Access: Choosing the Best Vein	VADs, including tunneled catheters, implanted ports, and nontunneled central venous catheters, are indicated when patients have small, frail veins and are in need of long-term indefinite chemotherapy, continuous infusion of vesicant drugs, or both.	VADs are important options for patients with poor venous access. Externally based catheters are ideal for continuous infusion of vesicant chemotherapeutic agents because the risk of extravasation is very minimal.
	Although a VAD is a good way to prevent extravasation, it is not indicated just because someone is receiving a vesicant drug.	Expert technique and a knowledgeable clinician are the most cost-effective and safe means of administering vesicant drug.
	Peripheral access is optimal in the large veins of the forearm, especially the posterior basilic vein. The veins in the hand and over the wrist are risky because of potential damage to tendons and nerves should extravasation occur.	Veins in the forearm are large and adequately supporting by surrounding tissue. Adequate tissue exists around veins to provide coverage and promote healing should a problem occur.
	Note: A large, straight vein over the dorsum of the hand is preferable to a smaller vein of the forearm.	
	The antecubital fossa is to be avoided for vesicant drug administration.	The area is dense with tendons and nerves. Seepage of a vesicant can be subtle and go unnoticed. Damage here can result in loss of structure and function.
	If the antecubital fossa appears to be the only vein available for access, the patient needs an access device.	
	Hold chemotherapy—insert VAD.	Risking extravasation and subsequent tissue damage is not worth the temptation to give "just one more treatment" before considering other options. There is no evidence that delayed chemotherapy for 24 h in selected cases is detrimental to the overall outcome.
	Avoid administering chemotherapy in lower extremities.	Risk for thrombosis is increased when chemotherapy is given in lower extremities.

Using a Pre-existing IV Line	Do not use a pre-existing peripheral IV line if any of the following are true:	It is unreasonable to disregard the potential for a perfectly adequate venous access line because it was not started by the person administering the vesicant drug. Our ability to assess the vein and evidence of blood return should be adequate to ensure the practitioner of an adequate and safe venous access.
	The IV catheter was placed >24 h earlier.	
	The site is reddened, swollen, or sore, or there is evidence of infiltration.	
	The site is over or around the wrist.	
	Evidence of blood return is sluggish or absent.	
	IV fluid runs erratically, and the IV seems positional.	
	Consider the patient's stents.	
	If the IV fluid runs freely; the blood return is brisk and consistent; and the site is without redness, pain, or swelling; then there is no reason to inflict unnecessary pain by injecting the patient again.	
	Prior dressings must be carefully removed over the catheter insertion site to fully visualize the vein during injection of the vesicant agent.	Dressings and tape can severely impede, both visually and tactilely, an assessment for an extravasation.

(Adapted from McCorkle, R., Grant, M., Frank-Stromborg, M., & Baird, S.B. [1996]. *Cancer nursing: A comprehensive textbook* [2nd ed.]. Philadelphia: W.B. Saunders.)

TABLE 19–12 Vesicant and Irritant Drugs

Chemotherapeutic Agent	Vesicant/Irritant	Pharmacologic	Nonpharmacologic	Nursing Considerations
Mechlorethamine, nitrogen mustard (Mustargen)	Vesicant	Isotonic sodium thiosulfate as antidote Prepare a 1/6 molar solution: • Mix 4 mL 10% Na thiosulfate with 6 mL sterile water for injection. • If using Na thiosulfate 25%, mix 1.6 mL with 8.4 mL sterile water. Aspirate residual drug.	Heat and cold have not proven effective.	Sodium thiosulfate neutralizes nitrogen mustard, which is excreted through the kidneys. Time is critical to successful treatment of extravasation.
Cisplatin (Platinol)	Irritant/Vesicant Potential	Use 2 mL of antidote for every 1 mg of drug extravasated. Remove needle. Inject antidote into SQ tissue. Isotonic sodium thiosulfate as antidote Prepare a 1/6 molar solution: • Mix 4 mL 10% Na thiosulfate with 6 mL sterile water for injection. • If using Na thiosulfate 25%, mix 1.6 mL with 8.4 mL sterile water. Aspirate residual drug. Use 2 mL of 10% sodium thiosulfate for every 100 mg of cisplatin extravasated. Remove needle. Inject antidote into SQ tissue.		Vesicant potential when concentration of >20 mL of 0.5 mg/mL extravasates If less than this concentration, the drug is an irritant; no treatment is recommended.

Drug	Classification	Treatment	Comments
Doxorubicin (Adriamycin)	Vesicant	Apply cold pad with circulating ice water, ice pack, or cryogel pack for 15–20 min al least 4 times/d for the first 24–48 h. Elevate site for 48 h, then resume normal activity.	Extravasations of <1–2 mL often heal spontaneously. If >3 mL, ulceration often results. Protect extravasation site from heat and sunlight. Studies on the use of DSMO have been mixed in the results.
Daunorubicin (Cerubidine)	Vesicant	—	Little information is known In mouse experiments, topical DMSO afforded some benefit.
Mitomycin (Mutamycin)	Vesicant	—	Delayed skin reactions have occurred in areas far from the original IV site. Protect extravasation site from sunlight.
Dactinomycin (actinomycin-D, Cosmegen)	Vesicant	Apply ice to increase comfort at the site. Elevate site for 48 h, then resume normal activity.	Heat application may exacerbate tissue damage.
Mitoxantrone (Novantrone)	Vesicant		Local measures are unknown. Ulceration is rare unless a concentrated dose infiltrates.
Epirubicin (Ellence)	Vesicant		Local care measures are unknown.
Idarubicin (Idamycin)	Vesicant		Cold, DMSO, and steroids were shown to be ineffective in mouse experiments.
Vincristine (Oncovin)	Vesicant	Warm compresses for 15–20 min at least 4 times/d for the first 23–48 h and elevate	Heat is a very effective treatment for rapid absorption of drug.
Vinblastine (Velban)	Vesicant		
Vindesine	Vesicant		
Vinorelbine (Navelbine)	Vesicant		

(Continued)

TABLE 19–12 Vesicant and Irritant Drugs *(Continued)*

Chemotherapeutic Agent	Vesicant/Irritant	Pharmacologic	Nonpharmacologic	Nursing Considerations
Taxane	Vesicant		Apply ice pack for 15–20 min at least 4 times/d for the first 24 h.	Its vesicant potential has been documented.
				Paclitaxel has rare vesicant potential (probably because of dilution in 500 mL)
				May be a mild vesicant
				Ice decreases local tissue damage in a mouse model.
Carboplatin (Paraplatin)	Irritant			May cause phlebitis
				Local measures unknown
Dacarbazine (DTIC)	Irritant			May cause phlebitis
				Protect dacarbazine from sunlight.
Ifosfamide (Ifex)	Irritant			May cause phlebitis
				Local care measures are unknown
Oxaliplatin (Eloxatin)				Vesicant properties have been reported; the agent is at least an irritant.
				Extravasation of moderate to high dose has led to pronounced symptoms of inflammation but without subsequent necrosis. High-dose dexamethasone should be considered as therapeutic intervention.

Drug	Classification	Treatment	Comments
Carmustine (BCNU)	Irritant		May cause phlebitis Local care measures are unknown.
Daunorubicin citrate liposomal (DaunoXome)	Irritant		May cause pain or burning at IV site Little information is known.
Doxorubicin liposomal (Doxil)	Irritant		May produce redness and tissue edema Low ulceration potential If ulceration begins or if pain, redness, or swelling persists, treat like doxorubicin.
Bleomycin (Blenoxane)	Irritant		May cause tissue irritation Little information is know
Etoposide (VP-16, Etopophos, VePesid)	Irritant	Apply warm packs	Treatment is necessary only if large amount of a concentrated solution extravasates. In this case, treat like vincristine or vinblastine.
Teniposide (VM-26, Vumon)			Same as above

(From Polovich, M., et al. [2005]. *Chemothereapy and biotherapy: Guidelines and recommendations for practice* [2nd ed., pp. 79–81]. Pittsburgh, PA: Oncology Nursing Society.)

agents. Do not pinch the IV catheter to determine blood return because of the resulting dramatic change in pressure within the vein (Polovich et al. 2005). Administration should be postponed until the nurse confirms that fluids are flowing unimpeded into the vein. If an immediate second venipuncture is difficult or ill advised, the nurse may choose to infuse additional normal saline solution into the original site to substantiate the vein competency beyond doubt. Two methods can be used to verify blood return and IV patency prior to hanging an infusion: Using a syringe inserted at the injection port closest to the patient, gently aspirate the line while pinching off fluid from the bag; or, using a gravity check by removing the bag from the pump, lower it below the patient's IV site and watch for blood return (Polovich et al., 2005). Only then should the cytotoxic agent be administered. During drug administration, if the nurse suspects the agent is not infusing properly, administration should be interrupted and further assessment of blood return and venous patency should be undertaken. When in doubt, the infusion should be stopped. The severity of the local tissue damage is in proportion to the volume of the drug extravasated.

Anticipating Infiltration

The nurse always must be alert to signs of slow leak or insidious infiltration. If the IV catheter punctures the vein's posterior wall, chemotherapeutic agents can leak into deep subcutaneous tissues. If small-gauge IV catheters are used, particularly where there is a large volume of subcutaneous fat, infiltration is more difficult to detect. This risk underscores the need for early comparison and assessment of the venipuncture site and immediate surrounding skin. It is important to monitor the site for signs of infiltration every 5 to 10 minutes for infusions <30 minutes. If the infusion is >30 minutes, check blood return every 10 to 20 minutes (Polovich et al., 2005).

Maintaining Vigilant Monitoring

Drug and blood flow rates should be monitored frequently. When administering agents using the bolus (IV push) technique, the nurse should pull back on the syringe's plunger approximately every 2 to 5 mL to check blood backflow. Although a good blood return does not always guarantee that extravasation has not occurred, any changes in blood backflow should be investigated promptly. It may be necessary to adjust and reposition the IV catheter if the bevel is resting against the vein wall.

Because infiltration is the most frequent complication of IV therapy, when a short-term vesicant infusion is needed, constant nursing attendance is required and the infusion should infuse by gravity. If the vesicant is going to be infused over >30 to 60 minutes, a central line for venous access and a mechanical infusion pump to regulate flow rate should be used.

Ensuring Safe Treatment and Care

During chemotherapy infusion, a patient should remain in the treatment area. Nurses in inpatient units should ensure that no diagnostic studies or therapies are scheduled to take a patient with cancer off the unit during infusion of antineoplastic drugs. If it is essential that the patient leave the treatment area, a saline solution should be substituted while the infusion of the cytotoxic agent is temporarily discontinued. Alternatively, the nurse may accompany the patient to supervise drug infusion while diagnostic or therapeutic interventions are conducted off the treatment unit.

Managing Extravasation

Some extravasations are difficult to detect in early stages. It bears repeating: If vesicant extravasation is suspected, it should be treated as a presumed extravasation. Although medical opinions and experiences differ regarding management of extravasation, most agree that ice should be applied 15 to 30 minutes four times daily for most antineoplastic extravasations; the exceptions are the vinca alkaloids, which call for local heat application according to manufacturer's recommendations.

Nurses should keep in mind that detailed charting of an extravasation should be completed as soon as possible after the patient's emergency needs have been met. This is important not only for medical and legal purposes; comprehensive documentation is important for any incident review activities. Litigation rarely reaches a court until several years after an event. Because a nurse-witness is permitted to review medical documents before testimony, records should be as complete and precise as possible. Documentation should include a note in the patient progress notes or nursing notes, completion of an extravasation record, and an adverse event report. Elements of nursing documentation should include the following:

- Date and time
- Type and size of venous access catheter used
- Insertion site
- Number and location of venipuncture attempts
- Drug(s) and drug administration sequence and administration technique
- Approximate volume of drug (in mL) extravasated or suspected of extravasation
- Patient's statements, complaints, reports
- Nursing management of extravasation
- Photographic documentation
- Description of site
- Time and physician notified
- Plastic surgery consultation/notification, if indicated
- Follow-up instructions to patient and date for return visit
- Nurse's signature

KEY INTERVENTIONS:	Treating Extravasation Associated With Chemotherapy Vesicants

Equipment

Infusion apparatus	Sodium thiosulfate
Normal saline solution	Cold packs and heat packs as appropriate

Procedure	*Rationale*
Stop the administration of vesicant drug and IV infusion.	To prevent further drug and fluid leakage into the subcutaneous tissues
Disconnect the IV tubing from the IV device.	
Do not remove. In the case of an implanted port, assess the needle site.	To determine if the Huber needle is properly placed

(Continued)

KEY INTERVENTIONS:	Treating Extravasation Associated With Chemotherapy Vesicants *(Continued)*
Aspirate remaining drug in the IV access device by drawing back on the (1–3 mL) syringe.	To remove drug from tissue if possible
Notify physician.	To obtain advice and direction
Initiate standing orders, if applicable.	To standardize treatment and prevent delay in extravasation management
If indicated, administer sodium thiosulfate subcutaneously with multiple punctures into the suspected extravasation site.	Direct infiltration of the antidote into the area of greatest concentration.
Remove the IV catheter or Huber needle from port.	The site can no longer be used as an IV access.
Elevate extremity before applying cooling or heat pack and topical antidotes.	To minimize swelling, surface (skin) inflammation, and erythematous reactions
Obtain a plastic surgery consult if a large volume is extravasated, patient experiences severe pain after initial injur, or if minimal healing is evident 1–3 weeks after initial injury.	Early plastic surgery evaluation and treatment may decrease wound severity.
Document extravasation in official patient record and institutional incident report.	To enhance later recall and for legal purposes
Obtain photograph of site and repeat weekly if appropriate.	To document extravasation and serial objective evaluations
Provide patient with written instructions for self-care.	To know what symptoms to report immediately, local care of site and pain management. No medications should be given distal to the extravasation injury.
Arrange for patient follow-up at appropriate intervals.	To follow symptomatology and ensure that appropriate interventions are initiated
In the case of central venous access, collaborate with physician to evaluate need for radiographic flow study to determine the cause of extravasation and need for future IV access.	To determine the cause of extravasation and need for future IV access

Management of Side Effects

Almost all therapies cause some side effects. Certain drugs or combinations of drugs affect the patient in predictable ways (Polovich et al., 2005). Chemotherapy and biotherapy have known systemic side effects. The oncology nurse can anticipate that the patient who receives multiple therapies such as chemotherapy plus radiation therapy will experience more side effects than if he or she receives either therapy alone. Patient factors, such as physiologic deficits and comorbidities can enhance the side effects.

Cytotoxic therapy affects the most rapidly growing cells in the body: bone marrow, gastrointestinal (GI) tract, hair follicles, and reproductive organs. The incidence and severity of the side effects of chemotherapy are related to the drug's dose, administration schedule, specific mechanism of action, and specific measures implemented to prevent or minimize side effects. Side effects can be acute, seen in days after drug administration; intermediate, seen in weeks following drug delivery; or chronic, extending from acute into months and years following treatment. Because the number of cancer cells killed is in direct relationship to the dose of the drug, monitoring and minimizing damage to normal cells is critical to the patient receiving the cytotoxic therapy. Some side effects, such as those that affect organ function, can be dose limiting (having side effects that limit or delay treatment).

Biotherapy, like chemotherapy, is dose dependent. The side effects of biotherapy vary based on the specific drug and its action in the body. Management of biotherapy's toxicities is similar or the same as chemotherapy side effect management (Polovich et al., 2005).

Caring for the patient receiving cytotoxic therapy presents many challenges. The focus of interventions is to prevent or minimize side effects to preserve the patient's quality of life. Advances in symptom management have made it easier for the patient undergoing chemotherapy or biotherapy. The key to providing nursing care for the patient undergoing cytotoxic therapy is to assess the patient's status prior to therapy, identify the patient's risk factors, monitor the patient for side effects, noting deviations from baseline, and last, to evaluate the effectiveness of interventions implemented. Patient education is a vital part of this process. Sharing the findings, plan, and potential interventions with the patient involves the patient in decision making, assists the patient in planning activities, and prepares the patient for self-care and monitoring (Box 19–9).

Myelosuppression

Myelosuppression (suppression of bone marrow activity) is the most common dose-limiting side effect and can affect the intensity of therapy and the quality of life. All chemotherapy affects blood counts, producing a reduction in circulating platelets, white blood cells (WBCs), and red blood cells (RBCs). Myelosuppression that causes infection or bleeding can be life threatening.

Patient education is a critical component in managing myelosuppression. The patient needs to understand that monitoring weekly blood counts is important in determining response to treatment at **nadir** (the point at which the lowest blood count is reached following therapy) and detecting problems early so that appropriate interventions can be instituted. Risk factors for myelosuppression include increasing age; patients with aplastic marrow, malignant bone marrow involvement, prior radiation to flat bones, prior dose-intensive chemotherapy, nutritional deficiencies, drug therapies, or concomitant diseases (Itano & Taoka, 2005).

Neutropenia

Neutropenia (an abnormal decrease in the neutrophil fraction of the WBCs) predisposes the patient to infection. Chemotherapy decreases the neutrophil count as mature

BOX 19–9   Patient Education: Strategies for Managing Side Effects of Chemotherapy

Infection Prevention
- Maintain meticulous hygiene:
  - Wash hands frequently, especially after using the toilet.
  - Observe good personal hygiene. Bathe daily. Cleanse perineal area after voiding or bowel movements.
  - Practice good oral hygiene before and after meals.
- Avoid injury to skin or mucous membranes:
  - Use electric razor to shave.
  - Wear gloves when working in the garden.
  - Use water-soluble lubricant during sexual intercourse. If severely neutropenic, refrain from vaginal intercourse. Avoid anal intercourse.
- Avoid sources of infection:
  - Avoid crowds or people with contagious illnesses.
  - Do not receive live vaccinations. Avoid those vaccinated with a live vaccine within the past 30 days.
  - Do not provide direct care for pets, eg, emptying kitty litter box or cleaning birdcages.
  - Avoid use of tampons, enemas, or rectal suppositories.
- Teach self-administration of hemapoietic growth factors.
- Monitor temperature. Contact physician for signs (fever >38°C or 100.4°F) and symptoms of infection (chills, productive cough, painful urination, sore throat).

Bleeding Precautions
- Be cautious with drugs. Avoid drugs known to effect platelets, eg, aspirin, or increase bleeding; consult your health care provider before taking any unprescribed, herbal, or over-the-counter preparations.
- Avoid injury/trauma to skin and mucous membranes:
  - Avoid shaving with blade razors; use an electric razor.
  - Use a soft toothbrush and rinse the mouth with mild saltwater solution. Avoid dental floss.
  - Use caution near sharp objects.
  - Avoid restrictive clothing, tampons.
  - Use water-based lubricant before sexual intercourse; if platelets are <50,00/mm^3, avoid vaginal or anal intercourse.
  - Avoid physically hazardous activity and contact sports. Avoid falls.
- Contact physician for symptoms of bleeding (easy bruising, nosebleeds, bleeding gums, blood in urine or stool, bloody sputum, change in level of consciousness).

Fatigue Reduction
- Take short, frequent rest periods.
- Plan activities around times of increased energy.
- Engage in regular exercise. Avoid strenuous activities.
- Allow family and friends to assist with tasks.
- Energize self using such activities as meditation, yoga, visualization, listening to music, or relaxing outdoors.
- Eat a balanced diet. Maintain a regular sleep schedule.
- Report symptoms of fatigue to physician to allow diagnosis of causes.

Strategies to Reduce Constipation
- Make sure to increase fluid intake to include 2 to 3 L daily.
- Encourage fruits, vegetables, and high-fiber foods.
- Avoid constipating foods.
- Have regular bowel routine.
- Obtain order for stool softener, laxative, or cathartic.

BOX 19–9   Patient Education: Strategies for Managing Side Effects of Chemotherapy *(Continued)*

Strategies to Relieve Mucositis
- Practice good oral hygiene. Keep lips moist. Avoid oral irrigators.
- Drink adequate fluids.
- Choose bland, soft foods with smooth consistency.
- Avoid irritants: chemical (citrus, spicy, mouthwashes, tobacco, alcohol) and physical (hot or cold temperatures, poor-fitting dentures).
- Rinse mouth with baking soda or saline solution or antimicrobial solutions as ordered.
- Use topical protective agents or topical analgesics.

---

neutrophils die and are not replaced. Biotherapy modulates the immune system, so the potential exists for neutropenia (Itano & Taoka, 2005). An absolute neutrophil count (ANC) of $500/mm^3$ or less places the patient at severe risk for infection, and neutropenic precautions should be instituted to prevent trauma and infections (Box 19–10).

A fever (>38.1°C or 100.4°F) is often the only reliable sign of infection in the neutropenic patient. Assess the patient for chills (rigors), sore throat, cough, dyspnea, frequency or urgency of voiding, edema, or purulent drainage at sites of skin breaks. A chest radiograph and cultures are obtained. Antipyretics should be avoided as they can mask infection. Colony-stimulating factors are used to manage neutropenia by shortening the duration and/or severity of neutropenia; this facilitates timely chemotherapy treatments with fewer dose reductions. Broad–spectrum antibiotics may be initially ordered to combat infection until a specific organism is isolated from collected cultures.

Thrombocytopenia

Thrombocytopenia (decreased platelet count) is a hematologic complication of chemotherapy. The normal platelet count ranges from 150,000 to $400,000/mm^3$. Bleeding precautions are instituted when the platelet count drops below $50,000/mm^3$.

BOX 19–10   Chemotherapy Nadir

The nadir, which is the lowest point of the white blood cell count (WBC), usually occurs 7 to 10 days from day 1 of chemotherapy. When the marrow starts to recover, there is an increase in the bands, which are immature segmented neutrophils. The absolute neutrophil count (ANC) consists of both mature and immature neutrophils. The WBC includes all the white blood cells (eosinophils, basophils, and lymphocytes). The following equation is used to calculate the ANC:

$$(\text{Segs [}segmented\ neutrophils\text{]} + \text{bands [}banded\ neutrophils\text{]}) \times \text{WBC} \times 10^1 = \text{ANC}$$

$$\text{Example: ([segs] 45} + \text{[bands] 29)} \times \text{(WBC) (1.1} \times 10^1) = 814\ \text{ANC}$$

Severe risk of frank bleeding occurs most frequently when the count is $<15,000/mm^3$. Below a platelet count of $10,000/mm^3$, bleeding can be life threatening and daily counts with platelet transfusion support are needed.

The nurse must be alert for thrombocytopenia, signaled by bleeding gums, nosebleeds, petechiae, multiple bruises, presence of blood in the urine and stools, prolonged menstruation, and a headache or change in mentation, which may indicate central nervous system bleeding. Clinical signs of thrombocytopenia are hypotension, tachycardia, and enlarged liver/spleen.

Anemia

Anemia (decrease in the number and oxygen-carrying capacity of the red blood cells) in the patient with cancer should be investigated to determine the cause: associated with chronic illness, induced by chemotherapy, as a result of malignant bone marrow involvement, or as a consequence of bleeding. The RBC count, hemoglobin (Hgb), and hematocrit (Hct) results provide evidence of anemia and are used to monitor the return of marrow function and the effectiveness of medical treatment. The management of anemia involves iron supplements for iron-deficiency anemia if indicated, transfusion of packed red blood cells, and the administration of recombinant erythropoietin. In the absence of acute bleeding, many physicians will wait to order a transfusion unless the patient is symptomatic or the hemoglobin value is 8 g/dL or lower. Erythropoietin can be effective in stimulating red blood cell production, with elevation in the Hgb and Hct realized in 6 to 8 weeks of therapy.

Signs and symptoms of anemia arise from the diminished oxygen supply to tissues and the compensation of the cardiovascular system. Anemic patients present with fatigue, dyspnea, pallor, tinnitus, tachycardia, palpitations, fainting, headaches, and irritability. Patients with anemia are frequently fatigued and should be encouraged to plan frequent rest periods balanced against time for activities to maximize energy. A significant role for nurses is administration of blood products and erythropoietin and monitoring the patient's response. It is important to teach the patient self-care strategies.

Alopecia

Not all chemotherapy causes alopecia (hair loss). Chemotherapy causes damage to the hair at the root resulting in complete hair loss or at the shaft associated with hair thinning. Many patients, especially women, have difficulty dealing with this side effect. The hair loss from chemotherapy is temporary, but for patients receiving radiation to the head, the hair loss may be permanent. Hair loss usually occurs approximately 2 weeks after the administration of the drugs. Hair regrowth can take up to 3 to 5 months after cytotoxic treatment is completed.

The patient needs to learn how to minimize trauma to the hair. Mild shampoo and gentle combing and brushing decrease breakage. Short hair is easier to manage and avoids a pulling effect present with long hair. Harsh chemicals, such as hair dyes, and devices, such as curling irons and hair dryers, should be avoided.

Once the hair falls out, lotion or moisturizer can be used on the scalp unless the patient is also receiving radiation to the area of the head. The scalp needs to be protected to avoid burns from the sun and to prevent heat loss in cold weather. Wigs, scarves, and turbans can be worn.

Psychologic reassurance and emotional support are important as patients verbalize their feelings about hair loss. Community resources, such as the *Look Good, Feel Better* program, offered by the American Cancer Society, can be especially beneficial as patients cope with alterations in appearance.

Anorexia and Taste Alterations

It is well documented that both cancer and chemotherapeutic agents can cause *anorexia* (loss of appetite resulting in decreased food intake) and changes in taste. This poses a problem for maintaining adequate nutrition. Familiar foods may taste entirely different and in some circumstances may even be perceived as unpleasant. Many patients complain of a metallic or bitter taste, particularly associated with red meats. The patient may be advised to experiment with different spices and flavorings to stimulate the taste buds that have been affected by the chemotherapy. Many patients report smells aggravate anorexia. Patients may minimize odors by cooking away from the dining area. As a general rule, most patients find that cold, rather than hot, foods taste better. Eating small meals frequently may help the patient take in more total calories rather than eating larger but fewer meals. Appetite stimulants (eg, megestrol acetate) may be ordered.

Dealing with anorexia and taste alterations is an area in which patient and family education can have a positive impact on patient outcomes. Suggestions should include serving food on glass dishes rather than plastic to help control odors. The use of plastic utensils is helpful for patients who report a metallic taste sensation from silverware. Good oral hygiene and rinsing with nonirritating mouthwash are helpful, especially before meals.

Xerostomia may occur in patients who are taking antiemetics or who have had radiation to the head and neck. For these patients, frequent mouth washing and chewing gum or hard candy can be helpful, and soft, moist foods are more pleasing to the palate.

When all of the usual interventions are unsuccessful, nutritional needs are usually met with supplements, such as liquid protein drinks or protein powder added to food; depending on the severity of symptoms, enteral or parenteral nutrition may be added to the treatment plan.

Cardiotoxicity

Cardiotoxicity can be seen with anthracycline therapy, especially doxorubicin (Adriamycin). Paclitaxel (Taxol), mitoxantrone (Novantrone), idarubicin (Idamycin), cyclophosphamide (Cytoxan), 5-FU, and FUDR are also associated with cardiotoxicity. When doxorubicin is given before cyclophosphamide, the potential for cardiotoxicity tends to increase, particularly in bone marrow or stem cell transplant patients receiving high-dose cyclophosphamide. Cardiac changes can be categorized as acute (occurs within 24 hours), subacute (occurs 4 to 5 weeks following therapy), and chronic (occurs weeks or months following therapy).

Patients receiving potentially cardiotoxic drugs should have a baseline multiple-gated acquisition (MUGA) scan or echocardiogram and periodic follow-up testing so the ejection fraction can be tracked. Serial electrocardiograms are also helpful. Early electrocardiographic changes may show a decrease in voltage of the QRS complex or nonspecific ST segment and T-wave changes. The damage to the cardiac muscle results in decreased cardiac output with shortness of breath, nonproductive cough, and progression to congestive heart failure.

Patients at greatest risk for development of cardiotoxicity are older adults with a history of hypertension, arteriosclerotic heart disease, or other coronary artery disease. Other contributing factors include prior radiation to the mediastinum or chest wall and a lifetime cumulative dose of doxorubicin >550 mg/m^2. Studies have shown that cardiac damage can be decreased by administering doxorubicin by infusion rather than IV push.

Zinecard (Dexrazozane) is a drug that acts as a cardioprotective agent for anthracycline-induced cardiotoxicity. This drug was originally developed as an antiproliferative agent but was recognized for its cardioprotective properties. Zinecard, an intercellular chelating agent chemically related to ethylenediamine tetra-acetic acid (EDTA), binds to iron before doxorubicin can and in turn prevents the formation of free oxygen radicals, thereby preventing cardiotoxicity. Zinecard is indicated for patients who have prior doxorubicin exposure of at least 300 mg/m^2 and who need to continue with doxorubicin therapy.

Constipation

A patient is considered constipated when evacuation does not occur for 96 hours or when hard, dry stool causes difficulty in defecation. Because individual bowel patterns vary, it is helpful to know the patient's usual habits. Medications (including chemotherapy), anxiety, depression, hypercalcemia, immobility, dehydration, and tumor involvement resulting in intrinsic or extrinsic compression can contribute to constipation.

Intervention depends on the underlying cause. Prophylactic laxatives, lubricants, and cathartics may help move waste through the intestinal system by increasing motility and may be needed if vinca alkaloids are administered. Rectal exams, suppositories, and rectal enemas should be avoided in patients with neutropenia and thrombocytopenia because they can be irritating to mucous membranes and cause microscopic tears, raising the risk of bleeding and infection. Impaction is best handled with an oil retention or phosphate enema to hydrate the stool.

Teaching patients to adopt various dietary habits, such as increasing intake of fresh fruits and vegetables and fiber, may help treat and prevent constipation. Adequate fluid intake of 2 to 3 L daily is recommended. It is wise to avoid constipating foods such as cheeses, eggs, and refined starches. Physical activity and exercise also help stimulate peristalsis.

Diarrhea

It is the function of the colon to absorb fluid. When this does not happen, diarrhea is the result. Diarrhea in the oncology patient can have a number of causes. Surgical procedures, such as gastric or intestinal resection, can result in a shortened GI tract or a malabsorption syndrome. Inflammatory bowel syndrome or *Clostridium difficile* and other intestinal infections can also cause diarrhea, as can cancer-related chemotherapy, radiation therapy, and biologic treatments.

The nurse needs to know the degree of diarrhea so that fluid and electrolyte imbalances can be prevented or treated. Accurate intake and output measurement, weight, and the number and character of the stools provide valuable information for fluid replacement strategies. The major electrolyte lost with diarrhea is potassium. Therefore, potassium-rich foods should be encouraged and fluid intake should consist of at least 2 L daily. In cases of severe diarrhea, IV therapy may be initiated. Pharmacologic intervention should be started as soon as possible.

Fatigue

Fatigue is defined as an overwhelming sense of exhaustion and inability to perform physical or mental work that is not relieved by rest (Itano & Taoka, 2005). Chemotherapy-induced fatigue generally peaks in 3 to 4 days following the nadir and can reappear with each cycle. For the biotherapy drugs, like interferon, interleukin-2, and the monoclonal antibodies, fatigue is common and can be dose limiting. Fatigue can easily be a consequence of anemia or infection. Dehydration, electrolyte imbalances, and compromised nutrition can affect the individual's perception of fatigue. Medications can also contribute to a sense of fatigue, especially if sedation is a side effect. Fatigue is a symptom that can accompany anxiety, depression, stress, pain, or insomnia.

Gonadal Dysfunction

Chemotherapeutic agents, especially the alkylating agents, may affect the function of the ovaries and testicles. The impact of chemotherapy can be felt in three areas: fertility, body image, and sexual functioning. Reduction in the male sperm count can result in temporary or permanent infertility. All men who wish to have children should be counseled on sperm banking prior to the start of chemotherapy. Changes in the menstrual cycle are observed within 6 months of starting antineoplastic therapy. Women can experience amenorrhea and symptoms of medical menopause. When a woman is close to or older than age 40, the chances of permanent menopause and loss of fertility following chemotherapy are more likely than for women in their 20s and 30s. Sometimes the regime of drugs can be altered in an attempt to preserve ovarian function and ability to bear children, or egg retrieval and storage can be pursued.

Roughly 40% to 100% of patients will experience some sexual dysfunction following chemotherapy. The prevalence of sexual dysfunction is unknown as it is often under-reported by patients and under-assessed by health care providers. Both men and women experience sexual effects of cancer therapy: changes in body and/or appearance, changes in self-image, decreased libido, and difficulty reaching orgasm. For men, erectile dysfunction and premature ejaculation add to sexual changes. For women, menopausal symptoms of sleep disturbances, hot flashes, irritability, and dyspareunia are common. Strategies to improve sexual function may involve pharmaceutical management and counseling, with referral to a specialist if needed.

There is limited information concerning fetal effects of chemotherapy, and therefore it is recommended that birth control should be practiced during chemotherapy and for 1 to 2 months postchemotherapy. Chemotherapy administered to women in the first trimester of pregnancy has resulted in miscarriage. Chemotherapy affects rapidly growing cells, and treatment in the second or third trimester is likely to result in birth anomalies. However, the literature has documented healthy live births without increased birth defects after antineoplastic therapy.

Mucositis

Mucositis (inflammation of the mucosal lining of the gastrointestinal tract, including the oral cavity) is a common side effect of cytotoxic therapy. The mucous membranes of the GI tract become red, irritated, and inflamed owing to either the direct effect of the drugs, for example antimetabolites, or the indirect result of the myelosuppressive effects of the drugs. Chemotherapy-induced mucositis usually begins 4 to 5 days after treatment and lasts for approximately 10 days. The patient may experience mild irritation and sensitivity to acidic or spicy foods or painful lesions and difficulty swallowing. The specific drug, dose, and patient risk factors determine the degree of mucositis. The nurse should be concerned about patients who have had head and neck radiation or who are receiving steroidal therapy. Patients who are nutritionally compromised and those with high oral flora owing to poor dental hygiene are also at an increased risk.

Preventive measures start with a thorough pretreatment dental evaluation. Assessment of oral cavity for bleeding, erythema, ulceration, and white or yellow plaques is critical to early detection of mucositis. Meticulous attention to the oral cavity with a soft toothbrush or soft swab prevents irritating delicate tissue. Irritating agents such as commercial mouthwashes containing alcohol, tobacco, alcohol, and elective dental surgery should be avoided. Application of balm, aloe vera, or a petroleum-based gel to lips prevents cracking and drying. Mouth rinses mixed with baking soda and water or saline solution may soothe the irritated mucous membranes. In addition, several mucositis cocktail formulas are available. Most contain diphenhydramine (Benadryl), an antacid, and a local anesthetic. Cultures of mouth sores may reveal a need to treat the patient with antifungal and/or antiviral agents. Soft foods with a smooth consistency and cold, wet foods are more soothing to irritated mucous membranes (see Box 19–9).

Nausea and Vomiting

Nausea and vomiting (emesis) are among the most common side effects of chemotherapy. For the patient, these distressing symptoms can significantly interfere with quality of life, leading to poor compliance with further chemotherapy treatment. Approximately 70% to 80% of all cancer patients receiving chemotherapy experience vomiting, whereas 10% to 44% experience anticipatory emesis (NCCN, 2005). Chemotherapy-induced nausea and vomiting is classified as acute, delayed, and anticipatory. Acute symptoms occur minutes to hours following chemotherapy and can last 24 to 48 hours. Many chemotherapeutic agents have the potential for delayed nausea and vomiting with onset after 24 hours and lasting for several days. Anticipatory nausea and vomiting occurs before chemotherapy and is a result of inadequately controlled symptoms over several cycles of chemotherapy. Uncontrolled nausea and vomiting can be life threatening. It can result in nutritional deficits, fluid and electrolyte imbalances, impaired wound healing, and deterioration of self-care and functional ability. As a general rule, it is easier to control nausea than to stop vomiting.

Predisposing factors for nausea or vomiting include gender (females > males), age (young > old), non–drug user, and a prior history of poor emetic control such as motion sickness, morning sickness, or prior exposure to chemotherapy. Obtaining a history may reveal other causes for nausea and vomiting such as anxiety, pain, or constipation. The frequency of chemotherapy-induced emesis depends on the emetic potential of the specific chemotherapeutic agents used. Emetic risk of drugs/regimes is identified as high, moderate, low, and minimal. Successful management of nausea and vomiting depends on keen assessment of the patient's risk factors, knowledge of the expected level of emetogenicity of the drugs administered, and a plan for prevention and early treatment to ensure nausea and vomiting control.

The ideal plan to ameliorate nausea and vomiting is an approach that combines pharmacologic interventions with nonpharmacologic strategies. Antiemetics should be initiated prior to chemotherapy and continued throughout the duration of the emetic activity of the chemotherapy drug used. The best antiemetic regime is one that uses the lowest, maximally effective dose via an appropriate route. The oral and IV antiemetics are equally effective. The 5-HT3 receptor antagonists combined with steroids and the new NK-1 receptor antagonist have demonstrated effectiveness (NCCN, 2005). Practice guidelines from national oncology groups have provided direction for antiemetic use. Although studies and guidelines provide recommendations for practice in preventing and treating nausea and vomiting, drug options must be tailored to what is most effective for the patient.

Nonpharmacologic interventions provide nurses with some latitude and an opportunity for creativity while giving the patient a sense of control. Regulating the environment to eliminate strong food, perfume, and other odors helps reduce nausea. Soft music, low lights, a quiet atmosphere, and relaxation tapes help reduce anxiety and hence nausea. Diversional activities such as cards, movies, or crafts provide distraction from chemotherapy. Some behavioral strategies include hypnosis, progressive muscle relaxation, guided imagery, biofeedback, and acupressure or acupuncture.

Suggestions for dietary manipulation include serving foods cold or at room temperature, and bland foods rather than spicy, fried and fatty, strong-flavored, sour, or tart foods. Clear liquids, gelatin, juice, ginger ale or other carbonated drinks, herbal teas, and sport drinks may help settle the stomach, provide hydration, and furnish electrolytes. It is advisable to avoid foods with strong odors.

Neurotoxicity

Some chemotherapeutic drugs, such as plant alkaloids and taxanes, are neurotoxic. They affect the central nervous system (CNS), peripheral nervous system, and/or cranial nerves. Central nervous system toxicity can be manifest as acute or chronic encephalopathies. Biotherapies, such as interferon and aldesleukin can result in changes in mentation. Peripheral nerve toxicity can affect sensory or motor function. Cranial nerve impairment depends on which nerve is involved. The signs and symptoms of peripheral neuropathy are indicated by patient complaints of numbness and tingling of hands and feet, muscle pain, weakness, and disturbances in position sense, particularly with ambulation. Clinically, deep tendon reflexes disappear. The decreased perception and sensation that the patient experiences can result in accidents. Constipation with or without a paralytic ileus is another problem related to autonomic neurotoxicity, especially from the vinca alkaloids.

Risk factors associated with neurotoxicity are the following: age (the elderly and pediatric populations), chemotherapy regimes that contain neurotoxic drugs or involve high-dose therapy, chemotherapy that crosses the blood–brain barrier, intrathecal chemotherapy, cranial irradiation, renal impairment, diabetes with existing neuropathy, excessive alcohol consumption, and concomitant drug therapy such as mood-altering drugs.

The first signs of neurotoxicity can be seen as early as during drug administration, in the case of oxaliplatin (Eloxatin) or as late as after five or more treatments with a neurotoxic drug like cisplatin (Platinol). Paclitaxel (Taxol), however, can produce paresthesia within 5 days of administration. When cisplatin is used concurrently with paclitaxel, the potential for neurotoxicity increases. It is recommended that paclitaxel be administered before cisplatin to reduce the potential of toxicity.

Amifostine (Ethyol), a **cytoprotectant** (drug to minimize toxicities of chemotherapy without compromising the cytotoxic effects of drugs on cancer cells), has been found to confer protection from the effects of ionizing radiation in patients with head and neck cancer. Amifostine is considered protective against bone marrow toxicity from the alkylating agents, nephrotoxicity from cisplatin, and hemorrhagic cystitis from cyclophosphamide. Amifostine is labeled for platinum neurotoxicity, but has also been used with paclitaxel- and carboplatin-containing treatment plans. The major side effect of amifostine is transient hypotension. Nausea and vomiting may be severe, and premedication with antiemetics is needed.

Pulmonary Toxicity

The pulmonary effects of chemotherapy/biotherapy are related to the direct damage to the alveoli and the capillary endothelium. The most common types of pulmonary toxicity are pulmonary edema, fibrosis, and pneumonitis. Patients receiving bleomycin in doses >250 units/m^2 or 400 units/m^2 total dose, or carmustine in a total dose of 1,400 mg/m^2, are at risk for development of pulmonary toxicity. Patients at a higher risk for this complication are the elderly and those with a smoking history or a pre-existing pulmonary condition. In addition to the two previously mentioned drugs, several other drugs can cause pulmonary toxicity, including cyclophosphamide, mitomycin , methotrexate, cytarabine, busulfan, and interleukin-2 (IL-2).

A baseline pulmonary function test (PFT) and ongoing monitoring are helpful in detecting early changes, such as abnormal breath sounds, dry hacking cough, and dyspnea. Steroids may play a role in prevention and have provided symptomatic relief of cough and dyspnea. With increasing symptoms, the chemotherapy/biotherapy is postponed Antibiotics and oxygen administration may be helpful in combating infection and maintaining adequate tissue perfusion.

Renal Toxicity

Baseline renal function tests (BUN, creatinine and creatinine clearance, urinalysis, and uric acid) should be done before administering chemotherapeutic agents known to affect renal function. The drugs most frequently associated with renal toxicity are cisplatin, methotrexate, iphosphamide, mitomycin, and, to a lesser degree, carboplatin. When the patient demonstrates renal insufficiency (elevated blood urea nitrogen and creatinine levels associated with oliguria, proteinuria, and hematuria), consideration needs to be given to reducing the dose to protect the kidneys from further damage and compensate for the longer half-life of the drug—a consequence of poor renal function.

Strategies used to protect the kidneys include vigorous hydration, hypertonic saline solutions, mannitol, and furosemide (Lasix). The patient needs to be monitored for renal compromise. Early intervention can avert the need for dialysis. The patient's urine pH is monitored during high-dose methotrexate to maintain an alkaline environment and to prevent precipitation of the drug in the renal tubules with renal damage.

Tumor lysis syndrome (TLS) is another disorder that can cause renal damage. In patients with a large tumor burden who are receiving chemotherapy where a rapid cell kill is expected, TLS should be anticipated and prevented using allopurinol to reduce uric acid. Additionally, the use of concurrent nephrotoxic drugs increases the patient's risk for renal toxicity. General nursing strategies are to monitor renal function by assessing intake/output and weight, to administer hydration, force diuresis, and administer chemoprotectants including amifostine, mesna, allopurinol, and leucovorin rescue to prevent renal toxicity.

References and Selected Readings

Asterisks indicate references cited in text.

*Abeloff, M., Armitage, J., Niederhuber, J., Kastan M. (Eds.). (2004). *Clinical oncology* (3rd ed.). New York: Churchill Livingstone.

*Alexander, M., & Corrigan, A. (Eds.). (2004). *Core curriculum for infusion nursing: Infusion Nurses Society* (3rd ed.). Philadelphia: Lippincott Williams & Wilkins.

*Blecher, C.S. (Ed.). (2004). *Standards of oncology education: Patient/significant other and public* (3rd ed.). Pittsburgh, PA: Oncology Nursing Society.

*Brant, J.M., & Wickham, R.S. (Eds.). (2004). *Statement on the scope and standards of oncology nursing practice.* Pittsburgh, PA: Oncology Nursing Society.

*Camp-Sorrell, D. (Ed.). (2004). *Access device guidelines: Recommendations for nursing practice and education.* Pittsburgh, PA: Oncology Nursing Society.

*Casciato, D. (Ed.). (2004). *Manual of clinical oncology* (5th ed.). Phildelphia: Lippincott Williams & Wilkins.

*DeVita, V.T., Hellman, S., & Rosenberg, S.A (Eds.). (2004). *Cancer: Principles and practice of oncology* (7th ed.). Philadelphia: Lippincott Williams & Wilkins.

*Fischer, D.S., Knobf, T.M., Durivage, H.J., Beaulieu, N.J. (2003). *The cancer chemotherapy handbook* (6th ed., pp. 48–239). St. Louis.

Goodman, M.S. (1986). *Cancer: Chemotherapy and care.* Evansville, IN: Bristol-Myers.

*Hickey, M., & Newton, S. (2005). *Telephone triage for oncology nurses.* Pittsburgh, PA: Oncology Nursing Society.

*Itano, J.K., & Taoka, K.N. (Eds.). (2005). *Core curriculum for oncology nursing* (4th ed.). St. Louis, MO: Elsevier Saunders.

*Intravenous Nurses Society. (2000). Intravenous nursing standards of practice. *Journal of Intravenous Nursing.* 23(Suppl. 6), S1–S88.

Jacobs, L.A. (Ed.). (2002). *Standards of oncology nursing education: Generalist and advanced levels* (3rd ed.). Pittsburgh, PA: Oncology Nursing Society.

*McCorkle, R., Grant, M., Frank-Stromberg, M., & Baird, S.B (1996) *Cancer nursing: A comprehensive textbook* (2nd ed.). Philadelphia: W.B. Saunders.

*Murphy, G.P., Lawrence, W., Jr., & Lenhard, R.E., Jr. (Eds.). (2000). *American Cancer Society textbook of clinical oncology.* Atlanta: American Cancer Society.

*Nabel, G.J. (2004). Genetic, cellular and immune approaches to disease therapy: Past and future. *Nature Medicine,* 10(2), 135–141.

*National Comprehensive Cancer Network (NCCN). (2005). *NCCN practice guidelines in oncology: Antiemesis.* www.nccn.org accessed February 4, 2006.

NIOSH. (1997). *Preventing allergic reaction to natural rubber latex in the workplace.* Publication No. 97-135. Washington, DC: Department of Health and Human Services, National Institute for Occupational Safety and Health (NIOSH).

*NIOSH. (2004). *Preventing occupational exposures to antineoplastic and other hazardous drugs in health care settings.* Publication No. 2004-165. Washington, DC: Department of Health and Human Services (DHHS). Center for Disease Control and Prevention, National Institute for Occupational Safety and Health, (NIOSH)

*Occupational Safety and Health Administration (OSHA). (1986). *Guidelines for cytotoxic (antineoplastic) drugs.* Publication No. 8-1.1. Washington, DC: Department of Labor, Occupational Safety and Health Administration, Office of Occupational Medicine.

*Oncology Nursing Certification Corporation (ONCC). (2005). *Oncology nursing certification bulletin.* Pittsburgh, PA: Author.

*Oncology Nursing Society (ONS). (2002). *Education of the professional RN who administers and cares for the individual receiving chemotherapy and biotherapy.* Pittsburgh, PA: Author.

*Oncology Nursing Society (ONS). (2005). *Cancer basics.* Pittsburgh, PA: Author.

*Polovich, M (Ed.). (2003). *Safe handling of hazardous drugs.* Pittsburgh, PA: Oncology Nursing Society.

*.Polovich, M., White, J.M., Kelleher, L.O., et al (Eds.). (2005). *Chemotherapy and biotherapy: Guidelines and recommendations for practice* (2nd ed.). Pittsburgh, PA: Oncology Nursing Society.

*Ross, J.S., Schenkein, D.P., Pietrusko, R, et al. (2004). Targeted therapies for cancer. *American Journal of Clinical Pathology,* 122(4), 598–609.

*U.S. Department of Health and Human Services, Food and Drug Administration (USDHHS, FDA). *Points to consider in the manufacture and testing of monoclonal antibody products for human use.* Available at www.fda.gov. March 23, 2005.

Review Questions

Note: Questions below may have more than one right answer.

1. If a second venipuncture site is needed, and the patient's other arm is not an option, the second site should be located:
   A. Distal to the original site
   B. Proximal to the original site
   C. In the lower extremity
   D. Alongside the original site

2. All of the following drugs are classified as vesicants *except:*
   A. Dactinomycin
   B. Daunorubicin hydrochloride
   C. Doxorubicin
   D. Dacarbazine

3. The risk of allergic reactions occurs when administering which one of the following biotherapy agents:
   A. Hematopoietic growth factors
   B. Monoclonal antibodies
   C. Interferons
   D. Interleukins

4. All of the following elements of documentation of an extravasation are essential *except:*
   A. Mentation of the patient
   B. Date and time of the treatment
   C. Antineoplastic agents given and their sequence
   D. Approximate quantity of drug extravasated

5. Patient education and understanding of antineoplastic treatment is enhanced when:
   A. The environment is new
   B. The patient has received sedation for anxiety
   C. The patient is ready to learn
   D. The patient is bilingual

6. Precautions taken when preparing and handling antineoplastic agents include all of the following *except*:
   A. Wear personal protective equipment consistent with Occupational Safety and Health Administration (OSHA) guidelines.
   B. Prepare drugs under a Class II biologic safety cabinet.
   C. Use a nonaerosol needle.
   D. Clip or recap all needles after reconstitution of drugs.

7. After chemotherapy administration, body fluids are considered to be contaminated for:
   A. 12 hours
   B. 24 hours
   C. 48 hours
   D. 72 hours

8. The maximum lifetime dose of doxorubicin is usually considered to be:
   A. 150 to 175 mg/m^2
   B. 550 mg
   C. 4,500 to 5,500 mg
   D. 450 mg/m^2

9. The side effect most likely to affect body image is:
   A. Diarrhea
   B. Red-tinged urine
   C. Alopecia
   D. Fatigue

10. A reversible side effect of chemotherapy is:
    A. Pulmonary fibrosis
    B. Amenorrhea
    C. Myelosuppression
    D. Sterility

CHAPTER
20

Pain Management

KEY TERMS

Dermatomes

Epidural

Intrathecal

Opioid

Titration to Effect

Role of Nurses in Pain Management

Nurses and physicians are accountable for responding to and managing a patient's pain level. In 1999, the Joint Commission on Accreditation of Healthcare Organizations (JCAHO) wrote criteria for hospitals, nursing care, and long-term care facilities regarding their management of pain. Later, the JCAHO developed six standards for pain management. These standards reflect the consensus of an expert panel of physicians, nurses, pharmacists, therapists, and representatives of other health care organizations. The standards, effective since January 2001, emphasize a collaborative and interdisciplinary approach, individualized pain control plans, assessment and frequent reassessment of pain, use of pharmacologic and nonpharmacologic strategies, and establishment of a formalized approach to pain management. The standards address rights and ethics, assessment of people with pain, care of people with pain, education of people with pain, continuum of care, and improvement of organization performance (Phillips, 2000).

Nurses in any facility must recognize that proper pain management is a patient's right, as defined in each institution's mission statement. Documentation of protocols, educational requirements, and evaluation are significant components of the quality improvement process. More precisely, the policies and procedures need to support safe medication prescription or ordering including scheduled prescriptions and patient-controlled analgesia. Intraspinal administration of medications and pain management technologies used in the care of patients with pain must be supported by protocols and educational requirements as well as evaluation of quality improvement processes. The patient must be monitored during the postprocedure period for pain intensity, duration, location, character, and responses of treatment. The nurse must ensure that patients are educated about pain and managing pain as part of their treatment. The patient's discharge planning process needs to provide for continuing care based on the patient's assessed needs at the time of discharge (St. Marie, 2002).

Creating institutional commitment requires administrative backing. Whatever the level of administrative support, the plan must be well thought out and defined and must incorporate all levels of care. It should not exclude any individual or discipline. Ideally, the institution appoints a project leader who is skilled in managing change and has knowledge of current pain management, good communication skills, and tenacity.

Initiating a Pain Management Project

The first step in developing a pain management project is to examine what is occurring in an organization in a well-defined time frame. A search of the current literature defines the basis for evidence-based practice (see Chap. 10). The literature is replete with documents that demonstrate how inadequately health care professionals have been able to control patients' pain. Many health care professionals, however, find it difficult to believe that pain management is *that* bad in their own institutions.

Data should be collected in a nonbiased, objective manner. Helpful information is gained through measuring the knowledge and attitudes about pain at all levels of nursing staff and medical staff. This information provides a baseline of comparison for measuring outcomes against educational offerings and changes in clinical intervention. Measurement tools are available through the Internet, or an institution can develop its own. An Internet site that offers measurement tools is maydaypain@smtplink. coh.org.

The institution needs to develop a time frame for completion of measures to monitor outcomes. A team of data collectors can gather information about how pain is documented, what percentage of patients' charts have pain ratings documented, and what percentage of patients' charts have pain ratings within acceptable ranges (as predetermined by the lead group). The team also can gather data through interviews of care providers about what they view as barriers to effective pain management. Patient satisfaction surveys have been viewed as having little value because patients tend to rate their pain management higher than do other measurement modalities. The survey, however, may still provide insight when used in consort with other measurements This information should be disseminated throughout the institution at multiple levels, using newsletters, magazines, staff meetings (interdisciplinary), flyers, and posters.

Motivating Change

If the results from the aforementioned measurement tools are not as desired, then change needs to occur. Three places to start are as follows:

- Staff education
- Routine pain orders
- Documentation

STAFF EDUCATION

Staff education encompasses both nursing and physician education. A common mistake of institutions is that they educate only nursing staff, which leads to frustration among nurses who are unable to initiate change without challenging physicians about how they write orders. Such conflicts can become unpleasant. Education is an expensive process for institutions that have limited resources. Developing self-learning packets for nursing review and access may be necessary. Physician education usually is best done through lecture and physician-directed newsletters.

To move pain management forward in professions, dispelling myths and misconceptions is essential. Post evaluation of the knowledge and attitudes of both disciplines should be monitored within a given time frame. Patient education could coincide with staff education; all patients should be well informed as to the options available.

ROUTINE PAIN ORDERS

Routine pain orders need to be rewritten. Administrative support once again is paramount for this task. Routine orders or written pain orders should be available from admission to discharge and need to continue if the patient is referred to an extended care facility or for home care. The pain orders should follow three principles:

- Decrease the use of meperidine HCl (Demerol).
- Decrease the use of intramuscular (IM) injections.
- Decrease the use of prn (as-needed) medications.

The use of Demerol has been well documented as problematic in American Pain Society publications (American Pain Society, 2003) and in the U.S. Agency for Health Care Policy and Research (AHCPR) Acute Pain Guidelines. When a patient receives meperidine, the body creates a metabolite called normeperidine. As the administration of meperidine continues, the normeperidine accumulates, creating toxicity resulting in seizures. (Beaule, Smith, & Nguyen, 2004; Ezri, Lurie, Stein, Evron, & Geva, 2002; Latta, Ginsberg, & Barkin, 2002). The intramuscular injections are painful, making it necessary for the patient to endure pain before receiving relief. When possible, the oral or IV routes should be used. A common misconception is that opioid dosing by the IV route is equal to the IM route (American Pain Society, 2003). Routine pain orders should not reflect this mistaken belief. Analgesia delivered on a PRN or as-needed basis results in the patient experiencing pain before receiving relief, once again. It is preferable to administer analgesia on schedule when pain is a steady state, such as after surgery or a procedure, or for persistent or end-of-life pain.

Routine standing orders for postoperative pain control should facilitate performance of up-to-date pain control measures. The goal of pain management is to keep the patient's pain score low enough to allow for deep breathing and coughing, early ambulation, decreased complication rates, and improved overall quality of life. Recently, a critical review of range orders or "as-needed" orders for opioid analgesics was done by the American Pain Society and the American Society for Pain Management Nursing. A consensus statement was developed to clarify protocol and enhance safety and effectiveness of orders for opioid analgesic agents. This consensus statement recommends that institutions allow PRN range opioid orders to meet safe and effective pain management. The prescriber should construct orders that contain a dosage range with a fixed time interval. The dosage range should be large enough to permit appropriate and safe dose titration with the maximum dose within the range not greater than four times the minimum dose. The nurses should base decisions about the implementation of range orders following a thorough assessment of pain and knowledge of the opioid to be given. Safety and quality of pain management practices should be monitored (American Society for Pain Management Nursing [ASPMN], 2004).

DOCUMENTATION

Documentation should follow the concept that pain intensity is documented to reflect assessment, intervention, and reassessment. If blood pressure, pulse, respirations, and temperature are documented on a graphic sheet, the pain intensity rating also should be on the same graphic sheet. A single graphic facilitates documentation and ensures that all members of the health care team who view the graphic sheet see pain information. If the pain rating is poor (per the institution's definition) and pain medications are given, then pain evaluation needs to take place between 30 and 50 minutes after the intervention. Policies and procedures should define pain ratings and interventions as well as methods for providing patient-controlled analgesia (PCA) and epidural, intrathecal, and other forms of pain management. The basic requirements of effective pain control are given in Box 20–1.

Conducting Follow-Up and Continuing Education

A team of "pain experts" is crucial to an effective pain management plan. The properly trained and interested personnel can assist with patients who are difficult to manage or help rework systems that create barriers to effective pain management.

BOX 20–1   Requirements for Effective Pain Control

- Assessment
- Intervention
- Reassessment

Evaluations need to be scheduled and completed at a predetermined time after implementation of system changes. The evaluation tool used should be identical to the first tool so that appropriate comparisons can be made. Evaluations should address knowledge and attitudes, documentation of pain, pain ratings, and patient satisfaction surveys (McNeill, Sherwood, Starck, & Thompson, 1998).

Even if the outlined goals are met, education does not stop there. Continuing education needs to be established. For example, some institutions have mandatory in-service education, similar to cardiopulmonary resuscitation training, certification, and recertification. Other institutions have yearly *pain fairs* in which each department, station, or floor displays how they handle pain management. Innovative ideas are shared at these fairs and may include continuous quality improvement projects.

RESEARCH ISSUES: Patient Satisfaction and Pain Management

McNeill, J.A., Sherwood, G.D., Starck, P.L., & Thompson, C.J. (1998). Assessing clinical outcomes: Patient satisfaction with pain management. *Journal of Pain and Symptom Management, 16,* 29–40.

This study looked at patients' ($N = 157$) pain experience during hospitalization. It also examined the revised American Pain Society Patient Outcome Questionnaire (APS-POQ) for overall reliability and validity. A significant difference was found between dissatisfied patients and satisfied patients in their general level of pain in the last 24 hours, with both groups having high pain ratings. The mean pain score in the dissatisfied group was 9.2, and the mean pain score in the satisfied group was 8.07. The APS-POQ was compiled from several existing and widely used pain assessment instruments and has been used in three other studies. Comparison of these three studies consistently showed high patient pain rating, yet satisfaction in the physicians and nurses caring for them.

As readers of this chapter read forward about pain management theories, physiology, assessment, and intervention, they should consider changes they want to initiate in their institutions. A methodical approach to change of this magnitude is imperative. Pain research and innovation is quite interesting, but will not succeed if it does not move toward improvement. If improvement of the clinical practice of pain management is to take place, then nurses must (a) make it easy to do the right thing, (b) make pain management cost effective, and (c) improve patient outcome and document accordingly.

Acute Pain

Acute pain results from an illness, injury, or surgery. This type of pain gradually improves as the body heals. Acute pain affects millions of patients worldwide. If it is not managed properly, acute pain increases the cost of health care by increasing the length of hospitalization, the time spent in intensive care settings, and patient morbidity and mortality. The following factors influence the incidence, intensity, and duration of postoperative pain:

- Site, nature, and duration of surgical procedure
- Type of incision
- Degree of intraoperative trauma
- Physiologic and psychologic features of the patient
- Preoperative preparation
- Amount of preoperative pain
- Presence of complications
- Anesthetic management before, during, and after surgery
- Quality of postoperative care

The amount of postoperative pain varies among individuals. Nurses must pay attention to the needs of each patient to control pain effectively. They must be cognizant of individual variability and listen to what each patient says. Nurses cannot assume that, because a particular surgery is performed, the patient will experience an expected amount of pain. Having said that, nurses can assume that postoperative pain is more severe after intensive surgery such as upper abdominal, intrathoracic, renal, and lower abdominal surgery; extensive surgery of the spine; and surgery of the major joints and large bones. Based on that assumption, nurses can proactively work with physicians in generating and implementing standing orders for postoperative pain management.

The importance of high-quality postoperative pain control cannot be overemphasized. When a person's pain is not well controlled, the sympathetic nervous system becomes dominant, commanding the body to produce more glucocorticoids and catecholamines. This, in turn, increases the workload of the heart. Other physical stresses include a more rapid respiratory rate with shallower respirations, hyperglycemia, and decreased peristaltic action. These changes lead to postoperative complications such as hypoventilation, hypoxemia and atelectasis, cardiac arrhythmia, congestive heart failure, deep vein thrombosis, and paralytic ileus. Postoperative pain control also influences the ability to cough, breathe deeply, and ambulate after major surgery. Fortunately, much progress has been made in the field of postoperative pain management. Nurses today are fortunate to have an abundance of innovative options for postoperative pain management. Health care institutions nationwide have developed acute pain services to provide daily assessment and intervention. See Box 20–2 for available options.

BOX 20–2   Options for Pain Control

- Systemic analgesics and adjuvant medications (administered orally, rectally, transdermally, intramuscularly, IV, subcutaneously, by continuous infusion, or by patient-controlled analgesia
- Intraspinal opioids, including epidural and intrathecal
- Regional analgesia using local anesthetic agents
- Topical anesthetic agents
- Nonsteroidal anti-inflammatory drugs
- Electrical analgesia through transcutaneous electrical stimulation or electroacupuncture
- Psychologic analgesia in the form of hypnosis, relaxation techniques

Chronic Pain

Chronic pain is defined as pain that either remains at the same level of intensity or becomes more intense over time instead of healing or fading. It is associated with progressive cancer and long-term disability or illness. Chronic pain is complex and cannot be managed simply with one treatment. The IV nurse's technologic expertise and knowledge about infection control assists the team to provide patient care using technology-based means of pain control.

A patient with chronic or persistent pain admitted to the hospital creates a unique set of pain management problems. When these patients are chronic opioid consumers, acute pain management with opioids fall out of the normal expected dosing. As well, one might expect that the chronic opioid consumer will have tolerance to the side effects of further opioid administration. In fact, these patients are not immune to side effects of opioid administration such as respiratory depression. Patient safety parameters include closer monitoring of pain intensity and sedation levels. Options of regional analgesia techniques and nonopioid analgesics must be considered for this patient population. Pre-planning a postoperative analgesia regimen includes using the amount of opioid the individual consumes continuously as a baseline and predicting the postoperative analgesia requirement above this baseline opioid. These patients require close monitoring in an intensive care setting during the early postoperative period (Swenson, Davis, & Johnson, 2005).

Patients who benefit from the use of pain control technology for the treatment of chronic pain include those with central nervous system or spinal cord injuries and patients with cancer pain that is refractory to conventional methods of pain control. The use of ambulatory devices facilitates the administration of pain medications (see Chap. 11). An oncology patient who in the past would have been hospitalized for pain control can be maintained safely on an outpatient basis for an extensive period (see Chaps. 19 and 23).

Opioids

Opioid is the preferred term for opioid *analgesics*. Opioids are effective when they bind with particular opioid receptors in the body. This chapter addresses only the mu and kappa receptors. The mu is the most powerful opioid receptor and requires binding with mu agonists when pain control is necessary. Mu agonists combine with the mu receptor, such as morphine sulfate, meperidine HCl, hydromorphone, and fentanyl citrate. Other opioids combine with the kappa receptor; nalbuphine and buprenorphine HCl (Buprenex) are examples. An opioid that combines with the mu receptor used with an opioid that combines with the kappa receptor will compete with each other for the mu receptor. Clinically, when a patient is receiving a morphine sulfate infusion of 3 mg/hour and the nurse administers a moderate to high dose of nalbuphine, the morphine sulfate becomes ineffective and pain intensifies. If the patient is physically dependent on an opioid, he or she may experience physical withdrawal. Opioids that combine with the kappa receptor are weaker analgesics (Box 20–3).

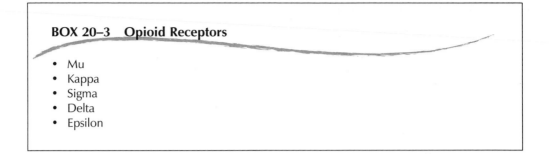

BOX 20–3   Opioid Receptors

- Mu
- Kappa
- Sigma
- Delta
- Epsilon

For lengthy procedures in which it is uncomfortable for the patient to maintain a certain position, an opioid often is given to provide analgesia. Opioids are also given during conscious sedation to provide analgesia for the injection of the local anesthetic and for tourniquet pain (Yaney, 1998). Practice criteria for IV conscious sedation have been developed by the INS (INS, 2000).

Side Effects

Side effects and complications associated with opioids include the following:

- Respiratory depression
- Mental status changes (euphoria)
- Urinary retention
- Nausea, vomiting
- Pruritus
- Constipation
- Orthostatic hypotension
- Bradycardia

Respiratory depression (six to eight respirations/minute) is caused by an accumulation of carbon dioxide in the blood, which communicates with the brain (medulla oblongata) to slow respirations until the carbon dioxide level returns to normal. A person may normally experience respiratory depression and simultaneous apnea during regular sleep patterns. Institutional protocol should address assessment of respiratory depression during sleep. Protocol also should address patients with a history of sleep apnea because patients with unrecognized or untreated sleep apnea who are given continuous opioids are at risk for developing further apnea. When patients are being treated for sleep apnea with continuous positive airway pressure (CPAP) machines, this treatment must continue while in the hospital. These patients need more extensive monitoring; some practitioners may recommend intensive care for these patients. All opioids directly depress brain stem–regulated ventilation, producing a dose-dependent reduction in respiratory rate (Yaney, 1998).

Oxygen saturation monitors are reliable indicators of the patient's oxygen level in the blood; the monitors do not measure the level of carbon dioxide, however. The oxygen saturation may remain normal for 2 to 4 minutes of apnea. More sophisticated continuous carbon dioxide monitors are needed. No machine, however, replaces thorough bedside nursing assessment of level of sedation, respiratory rate, depth, and quality.

Sedation is indicative of significant levels of opioids in the blood and impending respiratory depression. Sedation may reflect hyponatremia or infection, especially in the elderly. Good nursing assessment differentiates symptoms by considering the complete picture, such as the patient's baseline mental status, respiratory rate, blood chemistries, amount and type of opioid, and other clinical diagnoses or potential diagnoses. Currently, there are no validated or reliable sedation scales for opioid-induced sedation.

Urinary retention may be related to opioid administration and is caused by relaxation of the detrusor muscle located in the floor of the bladder. The patient may or may not feel the urge to void. Administration of bethanechol contracts the bladder, allowing it to empty. Catheterization is another option for immediate relief of urinary retention; however, risk of nosocomial infection increases.

Nausea may be reversed by either opioid antagonists, such as nalbuphine HCl (Nubain) or naloxone HCl (Narcan), or by antiemetics. If opioid antagonists are used, the doses should be kept low to prevent reversal of analgesia. If antiemetics are used, a synergistic effect with the opioid can result in sedation. When reversal of nausea is not accomplished with antiemetics or low-dose opioid antagonism, the physician should be notified and further evaluation performed.

Systemic opioids may cause histamine release and *pruritus*, which may be relieved with antihistamines and by changing the medication. When opioids are administered intraspinally (epidural or intrathecal), pruritus is related to the action of the opioid at the dorsal horn of the spinal cord and may be reversed with low-dose opioid antagonists.

Opioids slow the peristaltic action of the bowel, as does pain. Adequate pain control with close bowel monitoring and possible administration of both a stool softener and a peristaltic agent alleviates *constipation*.

Methods of Opioid Administration

Routes of administration include intravenous (IV) patient-controlled analgesia (PCA), subcutaneous analgesia, and intraspinal analgesia. Each of these routes requires specific nursing assessment, planning, implementation, and evaluation.

INTRAVENOUS PATIENT-CONTROLLED ANALGESIA

Patient-controlled analgesia allows the patient to control IV delivery of an analgesic and to maintain therapeutic serum medication levels. The physician's order for PCA should include the following:

1. Loading dose, given IV push at initiation of therapy
2. Lock-out interval, during which the PCA device cannot be activated
3. Maintenance dose
4. Bolus dose
5. Maximum amount the patient may receive within a given time

The loading dose of opioid is achieved through a technique called **titration to effect.** This technique calls for administering small doses of opioid frequently to obtain a level of analgesia. Titration to effect usually occurs within 40 minutes. The patient is monitored during this time through observation of mental status, level of pain relief, respiratory rate, and amount of opioid. The nurse should be qualified through formal education to manage this technique. For IV PCA to be effective, the loading dose must be given. Once the loading dose is given and analgesia is increasing, the IV PCA can be piggybacked into the proximal port on the IV tubing.

The *lock-out* interval is a safety system that prohibits the patient from frequently administering opioid without giving it adequate time to achieve analgesia. The usual amount of time between patient-controlled boluses is 5 to 10 minutes.

The maintenance dose is the amount of opioid that is infusing continuously. For example, an average, middle-aged, 70-kg adult would receive morphine sulfate at a rate of 1 mg/hour. This maintenance dose usually is administered for the first 12 to 24 hours, after which the rate is reduced or the infusion is stopped and analgesia is maintained through self-administered boluses. This dosage is determined by the patient's age, weight, and renal function, history of chemical use or abuse, and level of pain rating (Snell, Fothergill-Bourbonnais, & Durocher-Hendriks, 1997).

The anesthesiologist, surgeon, or primary care physician determines the maximum amount of opioid the patient may self-administer in a given time. This amount is programmed into the infusion pump and offers another safety system to protect the patient from an overdose of opioid.

SAFE PRACTICE ALERT Family members or friends of the patient (otherwise called "PCA by proxy") must not administer PCA boluses to the patient. Accidental overdose may occur if assessment is incorrect or the opioid starts to accumulate in the bloodstream. New guidelines will be available in the future on "PCA by proxy" that will enhance patient safety.

The PCA device has an integral system to activate the bolus. Various devices are available. Factors to consider in device selection include the following:

- Compatibility with currently used IV systems, poles, or conversion to ambulatory system
- Battery life
- Memory retention of pumps
- Display features
- Security and safety features
- Cost effectiveness
- Delivery mode (bolus vs. continuous infusion)
- Durability
- Ease of use

A discussion of ambulatory infusion systems is found in Chapter 11. These devices have greatly enhanced the ability to manage acute, postoperative, and

FIGURE 20–1.   Prizm ambulatory infusion pump. (Courtesy of Sims-Deltec, St. Paul, MN.)

chronic pain in the hospital or alternative care setting. Devices such as the CADD PCA (Fig. 20–1) are programmable in milligrams or milliliters for use with various medications and concentrations, appropriate for subcutaneous, IV, and epidural delivery; safe to use; and comfortable. They provide a total system of pain management and comprehensive support.

SUBCUTANEOUS OPIOID INFUSIONS

The subcutaneous infusion of opioids provides analgesia to patients when IV access is unacceptable or unavailable. The level of analgesia obtained through subcutaneous infusions of opioids is similar to that obtained through IV infusions. The selection of opioid is important to the success of subcutaneous infusions. Morphine sulfate and hydromorphone HCl are the medications of choice. The goal of a subcutaneous infusion is to offer a reduced volume of more concentrated solution with minimal chemical irritation. The quality of analgesia is limited to the amount of absorption of opioid at the subcutaneous site. The conversion from oral opioid to subcutaneous is equivalent to the conversion from oral opioid to IM. Table 20–1 shows the appropriate conversions (Watanabe, Pereira, Hanson, & Bruera, 1998).

TABLE 20–1 Conversion to Subcutaneous Opioids

Analgesic	Equianalgesic Dose (mg)	
	Oral	IM or SC
Morphine sulfate	30.0	10.0
Hydromorphone HCl	7.5	1.5

IM, intramuscular; SC, subcutaneous.

The technique for subcutaneous access is simple; however, the use of proper equipment and stabilizing methods enhances patient comfort and compliance. Supplies needed for subcutaneous access include a small-gauge scalp vein needle or catheter, transparent dressing, povidone–iodine swab stick, and an adhesive bandage. The site of choice is commonly the subclavicular area, abdomen, or anterior chest wall. The site is prepared with povidone–iodine, and the needle is inserted either at an angle or perpendicular to the skin, depending on the needle used. The needle is then stabilized using the manufacturer's recommended methods.

The most common problems with subcutaneous infusion of opioids are local irritation at the needle insertion site and subcutaneous scarring. Frequent site changes (every other day) and reducing the infusion volume can minimize these complications.

The development of transdermal fentanyl has enabled a subcutaneous deposit of opioid through diffusion from a rate-controlling membrane in the Duragesic (Janssen Pharmaceuticals, Titusville, NJ) patch. Doses of fentanyl are 25, 50, 75, and 100 μg/hour. When applied to the patient's torso, the patch takes 12 to 15 hours to reach its peak effect. The patch provides analgesia for 72 hours, with subsequent changes providing steady-state analgesia without the initial 12-hour delay to peak. If the patient's pain level increases after 48 hours, the physician should be consulted. The patient may require a fast-acting opioid through another route until the dose is adjusted to provide steady-state analgesia. The character of the skin is important with transdermal fentanyl; the skin surface must be dry and body hair clipped, not shaved. The patch does not adhere to oily skin. The skin surface should be free of abrasions to avoid bolus administration of fentanyl (INS, 1998, 2000).

INTRASPINAL ADMINISTRATION

Epidural catheter placement to deliver pain medication offers analgesia, low opioid dosages, and decreased sedation; it also facilitates earlier ambulation and enhances patient comfort. A working knowledge of relevant anatomy and physiology helps ensure a high level of care.

Epi refers to outside, and *dura* refers to the covering of the spinal cord that encloses the cerebrospinal fluid (CSF). The epidural space is a potential space that is part of the spinal canal outside the dura mater, enclosed by protective ligaments. Extending from

FIGURE 20–2. Close-up of L1 epidural catheter placement.

the base of the skull to the coccyx, the epidural space ends at approximately S1 in many patients (the spinal cord ends at approximately L1; Fig. 20–2).

The epidural space contains a network of large-bore, thin-walled veins. It also contains fat (directly proportional in amount to a person's body fat) and extensions for nerves that travel out from the spinal cord. The epidural space is also called the peridural and extradural space.

The **intrathecal** space, containing the CSF that bathes the spinal cord, runs parallel to the epidural space. The dura and arachnoid mater separate the intrathecal and epidural spaces. Other terms used to identify the intrathecal space are subarachnoid space and spinal space. The term *intraspinal* is used to describe both the epidural and intrathecal spaces.

When the epidural space is accessed, the anesthesiologist must insert the needle between the spinous processes and through the ligaments and enter the epidural space with a technique called *loss of resistance*. Loss of resistance occurs when the needle enters the epidural space, and the pressure placed on the plunger of the syringe allows the contents to empty into the space. When an anesthesiologist accesses the intrathecal space, the needle penetrates through the same route into the epidural space and continues through the epidural space until it punctures the dura mater. The intrathecal space contains CSF, which can be aspirated by the syringe attached to the accessing needle.

Elimination of opioids from the intraspinal space occurs through two mechanisms: diffusion up the neuraxis in the CSF and vascular uptake in the epidural space. The analgesic action occurs in the spinal cord at the location of the substantia gelatinosa of the dorsal horn. Opioid receptors are located at the substantia gelatinosa and bind with the intraspinal opioid, blocking the pain pathway through the dorsal horn to the brain. The lipid-solubility of the opioid determines the amount of opioid used, the volume needed, the placement of the epidural catheter tip, the time to produce analgesia, and the elimination time.

Extremely lipid-soluble opioids have a more rapid action than water-soluble opioids. Lipid-soluble opioids create analgesia in a narrow segment, following the **dermatomes** that surround the level of opioid injection. Water-soluble opioids create a wider spread of analgesia and take longer to achieve analgesia, which in turn is longer lasting because of the increased elimination time. Morphine sulfate is an example of a water-soluble opioid; fentanyl citrate is an example of a lipid-soluble opioid. The onset of epidural morphine or hydromorphone is 30 to 90 minutes, whereas the onset of epidural fentanyl is 5 minutes (Pasero, 2003).

Epidural analgesia can be administered through bolus dosing, continuous infusion through an external or implanted device, and patient-controlled epidural analgesia (PCEA) (Mann, 2000). Local anesthetics are often used to create analgesia in the epidural space. Pain transmission is blocked at the sympathetic chain ganglion, which lies on either side of and runs parallel to the spinal cord. Local anesthetic agents result in a sympathetic blockade and reduce the amount of opioid required to create analgesia. They increase the peristaltic action of the bowel, reduce workload on the heart, increase tidal volume of the lung, and increase vascular graft flow, reducing the incidence of deep vein thrombosis. Potential side effects are a significant reduction of blood pressure and numbness along the dermatomal distribution of the catheter tip placement. Commonly used local anesthetic agents are bupivacaine and ropivacaine.

SAFE PRACTICE ALERT If local anesthetics are used in the epidural infusion, caution must be used in raising the patient from a lying to sitting position and from a sitting to a standing position. Position elevation may cause the blood pressure to decrease, making the patient dizzy or even syncopal.

SAFE PRACTICE ALERT *Determine safety before ambulation.* When the patient has an epidural catheter placed in the lumbar region during infusion of local anesthetics, use caution when assisting the patient to a standing position. First, determine the strength in the patient's legs by asking him or her to lift the legs off the bed one at a time (testing for quadriceps strength). Second, determine sensation by touching the patient's thigh. If he or she can feel touch and has the ability to lift the leg off the bed, then proceed. Third, have the patient stand by the side of the bed, and ask her or him to bend the knees slightly and straighten them (again to determine quadriceps strength). If the patient is able to do this, proceed with ambulation. If not, check with the physician because adjustments can be made in the epidural solution or rate to facilitate ambulation.

RESEARCH ISSUES: Patient-Controlled Analgesia and Intramuscular Injections

Snell, C.C., Fothergill-Bourbonnais, F., & Durocher-Hendriks, S. (1997). Patient controlled analgesia and intramuscular injections: A comparison of patient pain experiences and postoperative outcomes. *Journal of Advanced Nursing, 25*, 681–690.

Outcomes of patients receiving intramuscular (IM) injections versus patient-controlled analgesia (PCA) for postoperative pain showed a slight difference in improved pain scores with PCA. No statistical difference in pain score was found. The authors state that a meta-analysis, however, showed that patient satisfaction was greater with PCA than with IM injections. Therefore, the choice of PCA should be made on the basis of patient satisfaction or financial considerations, rather than on improved analgesia.

Epidural access may be achieved through the placement of a percutaneous epidural catheter, a fully **implanted** epidural access portal system, or a fully implantable medication infusion pump. The epidural space is accessed by using a special needle (i.e., the Touhy needle), which is placed between the spinous processes and penetrates through the ligaments entering the epidural space through loss of resistance. When the needle is properly placed, the catheter is threaded through the needle. When the epidural catheter is used for temporary analgesia, the catheter is taped to the back and connected to the external infusion pump. When the epidural catheter is used for long-term analgesia, the catheter is connected to the implantable pump, port, or external catheter for connection to an external infusion pump (Bennett et al., 2000).

Before the epidural catheter is placed, the patient should be informed of the potential risks involved and informed consent should be obtained. Bleeding can occur in the epidural space and exit out the insertion site of the catheter. Patients who receive anticoagulant therapy or who have liver damage should have a bleeding time determined before catheter placement. If the bleeding time is less than 10 minutes, the catheter may be safely placed.

LEGAL ISSUES: Low-Molecular-Weight Heparin

In 1997, the U.S. Food and Drug Administration issued a warning regarding the use of low-molecular-weight heparin in conjunction with an epidural catheter. The nurse must be aware of the risk of an epidural hematoma.

Prevention of perioperative venous thromboembolism has given rise to the use of anticoagulation in patients. This creates new challenges for managing patients with neuraxial blockade. Consensus statements have been written through the American Society of Regional Anesthesia and Pain Medicine. "Patient management is based on appropriate timing of needle placement and catheter removal relative to the timing of anticoagulant drug administration." These consensus statements are available on www.asra.com/items_of_interest/consensus_statements, accessed 8/16/2005.

Sterile technique consistent with established standards of practice is used during catheter placement. The physician should be notified if a patient is febrile before placement or has a known infection. Patients may express concerns related to placement, care, and potential problems. They should be told the catheter is placed into the tissue around the spinal cord, not into the spinal cord itself. They need to know that their blood pressure may decrease because of muscle relaxation and sympathetic blockade when local anesthetic is injected. Administration of IV fluids usually remedies this problem (Box 20–4).

A spinal headache may occur if the needle enters the CSF or intrathecal space and discharges CSF into the epidural space. This leak decreases the fluid padding around the brain. Classic spinal headaches are positional; that is, the patient experiences a headache when upright but not when lying down. The location of the headache varies. Spinal headache may be relieved with a blood patch, a procedure in which the anesthesiologist realigns the needle in the epidural space close to the dural puncture site. The anesthesiologist then withdraws 10 to 15 mL of blood from

---

BOX 20–4   Points to Cover in Obtaining Informed Consent for Epidural or Intrathecal Administration

- Bleeding may occur.
- Infection is a possibility.
- An allergic reaction to the local anesthetic agents may occur.
- Injection is not into the spinal cord but into the tissue around the spinal cord.
- During the procedure, the patient may feel a tickle down the leg, which is the catheter coming into contact with the nerve. The patient needs to tell the anesthesiologist about this feeling.
- Blood pressure may decrease because the medication relaxes the muscle.
- A headache may occur if the needle enters the cerebral spinal fluid or intrathecal space.

---

the patient's arm and injects the blood into the epidural needle. He or she then removes the epidural needle and instructs the patient to avoid the Valsalva maneuver, either through lifting or bearing down, for 24 hours. The blood patch plugs the leaking dural membrane and increases pressure in the epidural space, forcing the CSF in the intrathecal space toward the brain to relieve the headache soon after the patch is performed.

Epidural Catheters

A small-lumen, temporary catheter made of nylon or Teflon is placed initially. Long-term delivery is possible through the use of a long-term epidural catheter or an epidural portal system.

The following references are classic references, and their recommendations hold true today. According to the literature (Hassenbusch et al., 1990; Patt, 1989; Waldman, 1990; Yablonski-Peretz et al., 1985), potential candidates for epidural pain management should be evaluated for the following:

- Confirmed patient response to epidural analgesia
- Appropriate coagulation studies
- Absence of active, untreated bacterial infection
- Acceptance of the therapy and understanding of potential side effects
- Adequate support systems to meet the patient's needs

Care and Management   Consistent with Intravenous Nurses Society (INS) Standards of Practice (INS, 2000), the delivery of medications and maintenance of epidural catheters should be established in IV policies and procedures specific to the Nurse Practice Act. Policies and procedures for obtaining, delivering, administering, documenting, and discarding medication should be in accordance with state and federal regulations (INS, 2005).

All medications administered by epidural catheter should be preservative free. Alcohol is contraindicated for preparing the site or accessing the catheter because of

FIGURE 20–3.   DuPen Eupucath. (Courtesy of Davol, Inc., Subsidiary CR Bard Inc., Salt Lake City, UT.)

the potential for migration of alcohol into the epidural space and possible resultant nerve destruction. Povidone–iodine may be used; however, it can irritate the nerves if it migrates into the epidural space. A 0.2-μm filter without surfactant should be used for medication administration. Before use, the catheter should be aspirated to determine the absence of CSF. Epidural catheters may be placed for short- or long-term use.

Mechanical problems may occur with the epidural catheter system, including leaking catheter hub, disconnected catheter, occluded catheter, or leaking at the skin site. Leakage at the catheter hub is common with temporary epidural catheter systems. The patient experiences breakthrough pain from leakage of medications, and bedding or clothing is wet. The nurse must tighten the hub or replace the hub if it is cracked. Clean technique is appropriate for manipulating the catheter hub (Figs. 20–3 and 20–4).

When the catheter becomes disconnected from the medication infusion, it may be in the patient's bed or on the floor. If the catheter is not grossly contaminated, sterile scissors can be used to clip the catheter one-half inch from the distal end. The new end may then be reconnected to the hub of the catheter and tightened. If the catheter is found on the floor, the epidural catheter must be removed and another form of analgesia used. No alcohol or povidone–iodine is necessary for removal of the catheter.

FIGURE 20–4.   Epidural catheter and points at which damage may occur. 1, tighten catheter; 2, leak may occur.

When the epidural catheter is occluded, the electronic infusion device should stop and the alarm should sound. Nursing interventions include ensuring that all clamps are open and checking the tubing for kinking. The hub is loosened and then retightened to secure it to the catheter, and the infusion is restarted. If this is unsuccessful, the anesthesiologist or pain management team should be called. Supplemental pain medication may be given by an alternative route.

The dressing over the catheter exit site may be damp from leaking at the skin site. The nurse needs to assess whether the patient is experiencing pain. If the patient is comfortable, no treatment is necessary other than to replace the wet dressing. If the patient is uncomfortable, the dressing should be removed to see if the catheter has pulled out of the epidural space. The physician should be notified that there is leaking and the patient is uncomfortable. Supplemental analgesia should be initiated.

Aspiration   Aspiration of the epidural catheter is required to determine if the catheter is displaced, either in an epidural vein or in the CSF. Positive aspiration of the catheter, however, does not guarantee either condition and should not be considered conclusive. The physician should be notified. If the patient is oversedated, the epidural catheter may have migrated into the intrathecal space. If the patient is receiving epidural local anesthetic and feels numbness in the toes only, the catheter may be intrathecal. Aspiration of a small amount of blood (1 to 2 mL) is also inconclusive because the pool of medication in the epidural space may have mixed with a pool of blood in the epidural space that resulted from the trauma of insertion. If the syringe fills with >3 mL blood and the patient is receiving inadequate analgesia, however, the nurse can conclude that the epidural catheter is in an epidural vein. If so, the epidural catheter needs to be pulled back out of the vein and into the epidural space. Only an anesthesiologist or trained member of a pain management team should do this. If there is >5 mL clear fluid, the nurse can assume it is CSF unless there is a high-volume infusion of medication and poor diffusion through the dura, resulting in higher pools of medications in the epidural space. The clear fluid can be tested to determine glucose level. A higher level of glucose indicates CSF, and the physician should be consulted.

LEGAL ISSUES: Dislodging the Catheter

There is always the risk of pulling the catheter out of the epidural space. The patient needs to be advised of this risk. The nurse must not allow the patient to suffer while the epidural system is being managed. An alternative form of analgesia is necessary.

LEGAL ISSUES: Fractured Catheter

When the nurse removes the epidural catheter on completion of postoperative analgesia need, the integrity of the removed catheter must be evaluated. If the catheter tip is intact, document "tip intact."

Flushing With Preservative-Free Saline Flushing is performed to determine patency of the catheter; 3 mL preservative-free saline is instilled. If resistance is met, the connector to the epidural catheter should be loosened and a second attempt to flush made. If leaking occurs, the epidural catheter connector should be tightened.

Breakthrough Pain Breakthrough pain may indicate that the pump is programmed incorrectly, the epidural catheter is disconnected and leaking, the epidural catheter is no longer epidural, the catheter has migrated into an epidural vein, or the patient is receiving too low a dose. Regardless of the reason for breakthrough pain, intervention must be initiated to provide pain control.

When an epidural catheter is not functioning adequately, breakthrough pain can be remedied by administration of 2 to 4 mg IV morphine sulfate, every 20 minutes as needed. If the patient is sensitive to morphine sulfate, 0.2 to 0.3 mg IV hydromorphone may be substituted, every 20 minutes as needed.

Epidural Port

The epidural port consists of the portal and catheter and contains a filter to remove large particulate matter. The catheter portion of the port system is positioned in the epidural space using the technique discussed earlier, and the catheter is then threaded through a percutaneous tunnel. A subcutaneous pocket is prepared for the port. The system is intended for repeated injection or infusion of preservative-free morphine sulfate into the epidural space (Fig. 20–5).

RESEARCH ISSUES: Epidural Morphine Treatment

Samuelsson, H., Malmberg, F., Eriksson, M., & Hedner, T. (1995). Outcomes of epidural morphine treatment in cancer pain: Nine years of clinical experience. *Journal of Pain and Symptom Management, 10*, 105–112.

After 9 years of clinical experience, Samuelsson, Malmberg, Eriksson, and Hedner published their outcome study of 146 cancer patients in a community hospital–based pain service. One hundred twenty-one patients stayed on lifelong or chronic epidural opioids. Mean time was 92 days, with a range of 2 to 2,040 days. Forty-nine percent of patients were managed on an outpatient basis. The authors concluded that long-term epidural morphine therapy was a beneficial alternative in the treatment of intractable cancer pain.

Implanted Pumps

In the 1980s and 1990s, advancements in medical technology facilitated convenient alternatives to conventional methods of long-term drug delivery. Systems such as the implanted pump (including pump, catheter, and optional access port) are implanted surgically and require periodic refilling. The pump releases prescribed amounts of medication into the body. A physician or nurse may use a computer during refill and checkup sessions to communicate by telemetry with the pump and to set the prescription as ordered. The pump delivers a controlled amount of medication through

FIGURE 20–5. Epidural port. (Courtesy of Sims-Deltec, St. Paul, MN.)

a catheter to the area in the body where it will be most effective. These pumps are battery operated and usually last 3 to 4 years. Potential risks include infection at the implant site, catheter plug or kinking, dislodgment, and leaking.

Patients should be cautioned to report redness, swelling, and pain near the incision and to avoid such activities as scuba diving, which results in pump under-infusion and diminished medication effect. The pump site should be avoided during diathermy and ultrasound treatments. Atmospheric pressure, body temperature, blood pressure, and concentration and viscosity of the medication may affect flow rates.

Possible complications include cessation of therapy owing to battery depletion, migration of the catheter access port, pocket seroma, complete or partial catheter occlusion, CSF leak, and drug toxicity. The use of needles larger than 22 gauge may compromise the self-sealing properties of the septum. Noncoring needles are recommended to minimize septal damage. The IV nurse is cautioned to follow procedures for the use of implanted pumps, consistent with the manufacturer's guidelines and institutional policy (Fig. 20–6).

Patient Identification Card When the pump is implanted, the surgeon should complete the patient registration and implantation record. The manufacturer issues

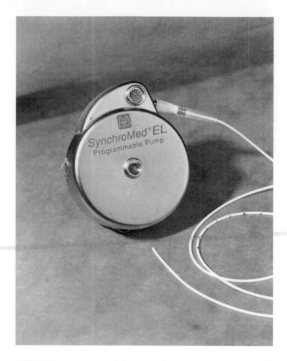

FIGURE 20–6.   SynchroMed pump. (Courtesy of Medtronic, Minneapolis, MN.)

BOX 20–5   Instructions for Patients After Implantation

Action

- Avoid traumatic physical activity.
- Avoid long, hot baths, saunas, and other activities that increase body temperature.
- Consult physician during febrile illness.
- Consult the physician before air travel or change of residence.
- Avoid deep sea or scuba diving.
- Report any unusual symptoms or complications relating to the specific medication therapy or the device.
- Return at the prescribed time for pump refill.

Result

- Prevent tissue damage around the implant site.
- Increased medication flow.
- Assess the effects of increased medication flow.
- Adjustments in medication dosage may be required to compensate for anticipated change in medication flow.
- Dosage may require modification.
- Ensure safety.
- Ensure compliance.

the patient a wallet-sized identification card containing information pertinent to the implanted pump. The physician should fill in the space provided for any medical emergency instructions. This patient should carry this card at all times.

Postimplantation Care After the implantation is complete, the pump can be filled with the medication. The 10-mL pump is filled with 6 mL, and the 18-mL pump is filled with 10 mL. The reduction is necessary only for the first infusion. Thereafter, the refills can completely fill the chamber. Patients should be monitored carefully after implantation to confirm proper pump performance, wound healing, and favorable response to therapy. Instructions for patients with implanted pumps are listed in Box 20–5.

Pump Refill Procedure The pump requires refills at specific intervals, depending on the volume of the reservoir and rate of administration. The technique used to refill the pump should be sterile.

KEY INTERVENTIONS: Refilling the Pump

1. Obtain the following equipment: sterile fenestrated drape (1), sterile extension tubing with clamp (1), sterile towel (1), sterile gloves (1 pair), 20-mL syringe with drug solution, sterile 2 × 2-inch sponge (1), sterile empty 20-mL syringe (1), povidone–iodine swabs (3), sterile 22-gauge noncoring needle (2), 0.22-μg filter, pressure monitor, template.
2. Warm 20-mL syringe with drug solution to room temperature.
3. Identify the outer perimeter of the pump by palpating the pump pocket. Locate pump septum.
4. Wash hands thoroughly and dry.
5. Using sterile technique, place all sterile items on opened sterile towel. Put on sterile gloves.
6. Disinfect pump site with povidone–iodine. Use three separate preps. Start at the center of the pump and work outward beyond the periphery of the pump.
7. Place fenestrated drape over prepared pump site. Sterile template may be aligned over septum.
8. Securely connect barrel of empty 20-mL syringe and extension tubing to the noncoring needle. Close clamp.
9. Using a perpendicular angle, insert needle into center of septum.
10. Open clamp, allowing pump to empty.
11. Close clamp. Record returned volume, adding 1 mL for amount of drug remaining in extension tubing. Disconnect and discard syringe barrel.
12. Securely attach air-purged syringe with drug solution to extension tubing. Open clamp.
13. To instill the solution into the pump, release extension tubing clamp and allow drug to return to syringe. This test confirms proper needle placement. Continue to inject and check needle placement at 5-mL increments until syringe is emptied.
14. Pull needle out quickly and apply digital pressure with sterile sponge. If necessary, apply a sterile adhesive bandage.

Stationary Infusion Devices

Abbott Laboratories' (North Chicago, IL) LifeCare PCA Classic and PCA Plus II meet the needs of the sedentary patient receiving pain management. The Classic is

FIGURE 20–7. LifeCare PCA Plus II infuser. (Courtesy of Abbott Laboratories, Inc., North Chicago, IL.)

a single-mode PCA device for low-cost PCA procedures. The Plus II has the ability to dose in micrograms or milligrams (Fig. 20–7).

Staff Education

Although information on the safe administration of epidural medication and monitoring of potential side effects is available, little has been written about preparing the registered professional nurse for administering and monitoring epidural analgesia. The initial step is to establish the rationale and criteria on which the policy and procedure for administration of epidural analgesia will be based, as outlined in Table 20–2.

Development of a care plan illustrating potential side effects and appropriate nursing interventions is an essential component of the process. A sample care plan is detailed in Figure 20–8. The clinical program should be intensive and, ideally, skills checklists will be used to identify criteria for assessing appropriate techniques.

Intravenous Conscious Sedation

Intravenous conscious sedation (IVCS) requires a physician's order and should be provided in a controlled clinical setting. Practice criteria for IVCS has been defined by the INS. Consistent with the criteria, only a qualified anesthesia

TABLE 20–2   Curriculum for Nurse Involvement With Epidural/Intrathecal Infusions

Criteria	Rationale
If epidural analgesia is already being used without proper staff education, the analgesia should be maintained by trained personnel (MDA, CRNA) until staff nurse(s) are proficient, meet preapproved criteria, and are RNs.	Ensure patient safety during learning period.
Instructions include: Epidural/intrathecal medications, including morphine, hydromorphone, fentanyl, and local anesthetics Epidural/intrathecal equipment Monitoring of mental status and respiratory rate, depth, and quality Dressing changes Medication changes Pump programming Troubleshooting catheter Managing side effects	• Nurse understands action of medication in intraspinal space. • Nurse is familiar with equipment and can differentiate epidural infusion and IV infusion. • Nurse appropriately monitors effects of opioid and local anesthetics given in the intraspinal spaces. • Temporary epidural catheters can easily fall out during dressing changes; precautions are needed during dressing changes. Nurse avoids alcohol at epidural site. • Nurse verifies that only preservative-free opioids or local anesthetics are used. • Nurse troubleshoots pump to minimize delays in pain control. • Nurse understands occlusion management and leaking of the epidural catheter when it occurs. • Nurse understands interventions for nausea, vomiting, constipation, pruritus, and other side effects.
Epidural/intrathecal administration of medications in patients with: Postsurgery pain Post-trauma pain Intractable cancer pain Refractory nonmalignant pain with appropriate psychologic/physical evaluation	Nurse understands the patient selection criteria.
The nurse notifies the anesthesiologist when there is: Pain at insertion site Inadequate analgesia Pain with administration of infusion or injection Drainage from catheter exit site that requires multiple dressing changes, especially when accompanied by inadequate analgesia Clear drainage greater than 8–10 mL when catheter is aspirated Before injection An unresolvable occlusion	These problems require assessment by an anesthesiologist or personnel from the pain management team.
Intrathecal infusions are not connected to an external pump.	The intrathecal space contains cerebrospinal fluid and is a good medium for bacterial growth, increasing the risk of infection.
The nurse removes the epidural catheter when ordered.	Nurse with special training in the technique of epidural catheter removal and documentation of this removal ensures safe patient care.

In date / Initials	NURSING DIAGNOSIS/PATIENT PROBLEM / DESIRED OUTCOME	ACTIONS/INTERVENTIONS SET & REVIEWED W/PATIENT/FAMILY [ ] YES [ ] NO	TARGET DATE	DATE OF DAILY REVIEW/INITIALS	RESOLUTION DATE / EVALUATION
	1. Knowledge deficit related to the use of epidural analgesia for post-operative pain control Patient demonstrates knowledge related to epidural catheter use for post-operative pain control and verbalizes understanding of need to report pain as soon as perceived	1. Describe the placement of the catheter, its use, who will administer pain medication and the use of an apnea monitor for immediate post-op period			
	2. Potential for injury due to catheter displacement (i.e. intrathecal space) Catheter will remain in epidural space or will be removed immediately if dislodged	1. RN will monitor: a. The patency of the catheter b. The condition of the dressing c. Observe catheter site of intactness and hash marks indicating length d. Negative aspiration before each medication administration			
	3. Potential for ineffective breathing pattern related to respiratory depression secondary to epidural analgesia Patient will exhibit effective breathing pattern: • respirations of six or greater, regular and non-labored	1. Maintain apnea monitor for first 24 hours or until a baseline dose is established to maintain patient comfort			

Initials	RN Signatures	Initials	RN Signatures
	Primary Nurse		
	Social Worker:		
	Other		

FIGURE 20–8. Patient care plan for postoperative pain control using epidural analgesia. Reprinted from *Oncology Nursing Forum* with permission from Oncology Nursing Press, Inc. (Camp-Sorrel, D., Fernandez, K., & Reardon, M.B. [1990]. Teaching oncology nurses about epidural catheters. *Oncology Nursing Forum, 17*[5], 683–689.)

INI date Initials	NURSING DIAGNOSIS/PATIENT PROBLEM DESIRED OUTCOME	ACTIONS/INTERVENTIONS SET & REVIEWED W/PATIENT/FAMILY [ ] YES [ ] NO	TARGET DATE	DATE OF DAILY REVIEW/INITIALS	RESOLUTION DATE EVALUATION
	3 Potential for ineffective breathing (Continued)	2 Have Naloxone (Narcan) 4mg available at all times while epidural narcotics are being used			
		3 Maintain IV access at all times while epidural catheter is in place			
		4 Monitor for signs of restlessness, miosis			
	4. Potential urinary retention related to atonic bladder from sacral analgesia	1 If urinary catheter not in place, measure intake and output every four hours for first 24 hours and every eight hours thereafter			
	.. Patient will demonstrate adequate urinary elimination				
	5 Potential for alteration in comfort related to displacement or dysfunction of the catheter	1 Use visual analog scale and Pain Flow Sheet to monitor patient comfort level every four hours			
	:. Patient will report adequate pain control	2 Administer medication as ordered or notify anesthesiologist of inadequate pain control. * Note: No other narcotics, tranquilizers or sedatives may be given unless ordered by anesthesiologist			

Initials	RN Signatures	Initials	RN Signatures

Primary Nurse:

Social Worker:

Other:

FIGURE 20-8. *(Continued)*

601

Init/date	NURSING DIAGNOSIS/PATIENT PROBLEM DESIRED OUTCOME	ACTIONS/INTERVENTIONS SET & REVIEWED W/PATIENT/FAMILY [ ] YES [ ] NO	TARGET DATE	DATE OF DAILY REVIEW/INITIALS	RESOLUTION DATE / EVALUATION
	6. Potential for discomfort related to pruitus secondary to release of histamine from the morphine effect.	1 Administer antipruritic as ordered by anesthesiologist PRN			
	:Patient will inform caregiver when itching begins. Patient will report relief of itching.				
	7. Potential for hypotension related to vasomotor disturbance	1 Monitor vital signs every four hours while epidural is in use			
	:Blood pressure will be maintained at adequate level	2 Maintain adequate intravenous or oral fluid intake			
		3 Elevate lower extremities			
		4 When getting OOB, allow patient to dangle at bedside first			
	8. Potential for injury related to infection secondary to epidural catheter.	1 Monitor catheter insertion site every shift for redness, edema, drainage			
	:Patient will remain infection-free as evidenced by absence of purulent drainage, redness or tenderness at catheter insertion site	2 Maintain strict sterile technique during preparation and administration of medications			
		3 Monitor temperature and WBC to detect possible infection.			

Initials	RN Signatures	Initials	RN Signatures

Primary Nurse

Social Worker:

Other

FIGURE 20-8. (*Continued*)

provider or attending physician selects and orders the medication. The patient's infusion nurse should be competent, and the institution should have an educational and competency verification system. Informed patient consent should be obtained, the patient should be monitored, and IV access should be continuously maintained (INS, 2000).

Continuous Local Anesthetics

Local anesthetics block nerve conduction and may offer excellent postoperative pain control by achieving uninterrupted pain relief, minimizing opioid requirements, and avoiding the adverse effects of opioids. Continuous local anesthetic is given through a 16-gauge introducer needle placed under the subcutaneous tissue and above the fascia or muscle adjacent to or in the wound site after surgery. After placing the introducer, the surgeon threads a 20-gauge epidural catheter through the needle. The surgeon removes the introducer and secures the site with a semipermeable transparent dressing. The patient receives a loading dose of local anesthetic before beginning the continuous infusion, via disposable infusion pump or electronic infusion device. Pain intensity is monitored and documented. Breakthrough pain may be managed with oral analgesics, such as oxycodone.

Toxic effects of continuous local anesthesia include dizziness, ringing in the ears, a metallic taste, perioral anesthesia, and slowed speech. If signs of toxicity are recognized early, decreasing the infusion rate may alleviate the problem. Elderly patients may be at a higher risk for toxicity owing to a decreased ability to clear local anesthetics. The nurse should instruct the patient and family about what to do and whom to call about unrelieved pain, symptoms of infection, determining when the infusion is complete, removing the catheter, and dressing the site (Pasero, 2000).

Documentation

Documentation should include the type of pain management provided, route of administration, methods used, IV or other access route, site care and maintenance, assessment of pain and degree of pain relief, and problems encountered in dealing with the particular type of access used. Flow sheets facilitate accuracy of documentation and provide a guideline for all areas of concern, including pain rating (intensity) and level of consciousness (Figs. 20–9 and 20–10).

When PCA systems are implemented, the nurse records the date, time, medication, patient's name and room number, physician's name, and his or her own name on an appropriate flow sheet. The continuous nature of the injection does not permit the nurse to record the exact dosage administered on the standard control sheets found in many health care institutions. Many such facilities have developed individualized flow sheets specifically for PCA control. The American Pain Society has developed quality assurance standards for pain relief (Box 20–6).

PAIN ASSESSMENT FLOW SHEET

DATE: _____

MEDICATION ORDERED: _____

CONTINUOUS RATE: _____

PCA DOSE: _____

LOCKOUT: _____

CHECK ONE:

EPIDURAL: _____

INTRATHECAL: _____

IV-PCA: _____

(Addressograph Plate)

Date	Time	1 Hour Assessment				4-HOUR ASSESSMENT					Checks Made Here - See Nurse's Notes:										
		Sed. Scale	Respir. Rate	Med. Inf. As Ordrd. Tubing Secure	Pain Scale	B.P./ Pulse Lying	B.P./ Pulse Sitting	No Loss Of Sens. Lower Extrem.	Drsg. Dry Intact, No Edema S/S of Inf.	Urinary Ret.	Pruritis	Break Through Pain	Catheter Checked For Placement	Drsg. Chg. (Kit Utlzd.)	Catheter Flushed 3cc NS.	Nausea Vomiting	Pulse Ox.	R.N.'s Initials

RN SIGNATURE / INITIALS:

_____

_____

_____

_____

N/V ECOG SCALE:
0 - No Nausea or Vomiting
1 - Nausea/Vomiting X 1/day
2 - Nausea/Vomiting Less Than X 6/day
3 - Vomiting X 6/day
4 - Dehydration - IV Therapy

PAIN SCALE:
0 - No Pain
1 - 2 - Discomfort
3 - 4 - Mild Pain
5 - 6 - Distress
7 - 8 - Severe Pain
9 - 10 - Excruciating Pain

SEDATION SCALE:
0 - No Sedation-Pt. Found Awake.
S - Normal Sleep-Easy To Awake.
1 - Mild Drowsy, Easy To Arouse.
2 - Moderate, Frequently Drowsy, Still Able To Arouse.
3 - Severely Somnolent, Unable To Arouse.

FIGURE 20–9. Pain assessment form. (Courtesy of Midwestern Regional Medical Center, Zion, IL.)

PAIN ASSESSMENT ORDERS:

_____
_____
_____
_____
_____
_____
_____
_____

NURSE'S NOTES:

_____
_____
_____
_____
_____
_____
_____
_____
_____
_____
_____
_____
_____
_____
_____
_____
_____
_____
_____
_____
_____
_____
_____
_____
_____

FIGURE 20–9. _(Continued)_

PATIENT–CONTROLLED ANALGESIA
Sample Flow Sheet

HOSPITAL I.D.

PATIENT I.D.

DATE_____
MEDICATION_____

LOADING DOSE_____
(IF APPLICABLE)

TIME	12MN	2A	4A	6A	8A	10A	12N	2P	4P	6P	8P	10P
DOSE VOLUME (ML)												
LOCK–OUT												
4 HR LIMIT (ML)												
# DOSE DEL.												
TOTAL VOL. DEL.												
SEDATION (1–5)												
PAIN (1–5)												
RESP. RATE												
NURSE'S SIG.												

ADMIN. SET CHANGE

NEW PCA UNIT

CONDITION I.V. SITE

SCALES

SEDATION
1 = WIDE AWAKE
2 = DROWSY
3 = DOZING INTERMITTENTLY
4 = MOSTLY SLEEPING
5 = AWAKENS ONLY WHEN AROUSED

PAIN
1 = COMFORTABLE
2 = IN MILD DISCOMFORT
3 = IN PAIN
4 = IN BAD PAIN
5 = IN VERY BAD PAIN

FIGURE 20–10.   Sample flow sheet for patient-controlled analgesia.

BOX 20–6 American Pain Society Quality Assurance Pain Relief Standards

- Recognize and treat pain promptly.
  - Chart and display pain and relief. (Process)
  - Define pain and relief levels to initiate review. (Process)
  - Survey patient satisfaction. (Outcome)
- Make information about analgesics readily available. (Process)
- Promise patients attentive analgesic care. (Process)
- Define explicit policies for use of advanced analgesic technologies. (Process)
- Monitor adherence to standards. (Process)

References and Selected Readings

Asterisks indicate references cited in text.

*American Pain Society. (2003). *Principles of analgesic use in the treatment of acute pain and cancer pain* (5th ed.). Glenview, IL: Author.

American Pain Society Quality of Care Committee. (1995). Quality improvement guidelines for the treatment of acute pain and cancer pain. *Journal of the American Medical Association, 274*(23), 1874–1880.

*American Society for Pain Management Nursing. (2004). *The use of "as-needed" range orders for opioid analgesics in the management of acute pain*. A consensus statement of the American Society for Pain Management Nursing and the American Pain Society. Pensacola, FL: Author.

Barnason, S., Merboth, M., Pozehl, B., & Tietjen, M.J. (1998). Utilizing an outcomes approach to improve pain management by nurses: A pilot study. *Clinical Nurse Specialist, 12*(1), 28–36.

*Beaule, P.E., Smith, M.I., Nguyen, V.N., (2004). Meperidine-induced seizure after revision hip arthroplasty. *Journal of Arthroplasty, 19*(4), 516–519.

*Bennett, G., Burchiel, K., Buchser, E., et.al. (2000). Clinical guidelines for intraspinal infusion: report of an expert panel. *Journal of Pain and Symptom Management, 20*(2), S37–43.

Clarke, E.B., French, B., Bilodeau, M.L., Capasso, V.C., Edwards, A., & Empoliti, J. (1996). Pain management knowledge, attitudes and clinical practice: The impact of nurses' characteristics and education. *Journal of Pain and Symptom Management, 11*, 18–31.

Davidson, J. (1997). The nurse's role in monitoring a patient who is consciously sedated. *Critical Care Nurse, 17*, 102–104, 106.

Davol, Inc. Subsidiary of C. R. Bard, Inc., P.O. Box 8500, Cranston, RI; ONC 60290-88810M.

Dufault, M.A., & Sullivan, M.C. (1999). Generating and testing pain management standards through collaborative research utilization. *Journal of Nursing Scholarship, 31*, 355–356.

DuPen, S.L. (1987). A new permanent exteriorized epidural catheter for narcotic self-administration to control cancer pain. *Cancer, 59*, 986–993.

Edwards, A.D. (1999). The role of systemic lidocaine in neuropathic pain management. *Journal of Intravenous Nursing, 22*(5), 273–279.

*Ezri, T, Lurie, S, Stein, A, Evron, S, Geva, D. (2002). Postoperative nausea and vomiting: Comparison of the effect of postoperative meperidine or morphine in gynecologic surgery patients. *Journal of Clinical Anesthesia, 14*(4), 262–266.

Hader, C., Guy, J. (2004). Your hand in pain management. *Nursing Management. 35*(11), 22–24.

*Hassenbusch, S.J., Pillay, P.K., Magdinec, M., et al. (1990). Constant infusion of morphine for intractable cancer pain using an implanted pump. *Journal of Neurosurgery, 73*, 405–409.

Hutchinson, R. (2004). Pain control: COX 2 selective NSAIDS. *American Journal of Nursing, 104*(3), 52–54.

*Infusion Nurses Society. (2000). Revised standards of practice. *Journal of Infusion Nursing, 23*(Suppl 1).

Infusion Nurses Society. (2004). *Core curriculum for infusion nurses*. Philadelphia: Lippincott Williams & Wilkins.

*Infusion Nurses Society. (2005). Revised standards of practice. *Journal of Infusion Nursing, 28*(Suppl 1).

*Intravenous Nurses Society. (1998). Revised intravenous nursing standards of practice. *Journal of Intravenous Nursing, 23*(Suppl.).

*Intravenous Nurses Society. (2000). *Core curriculum for intravenous nursing* (pp. 16–18, 196). Philadelphia: Lippincott Williams & Wilkins.

Janssen Pharmaceuticals. (1999). Product literature: *Duragesic*. Titusville, NJ: Author.

Krames, E.S. (1996). Intraspinal opioid therapy for chronic nonmalignant pain: Current practice and clinical guidelines. *Journal of Pain and Symptom Management, 11*, 333–352.

*Latta, K.S., Ginsberg, B., Barkin, R.L. (2002). Meperidine: A critical review. *American Journal of Therapeutics, 9*, 53–68.

*Mann, C. (2000). Comparison of intravenous or epidural patient-controlled analgesia in the elderly after major abdominal surgery. *Anesthesiology, 92*(2), 433–441.

Max, M. (1990). American Pain Society quality assurance standards for relief of acute pain and cancer pain. In: M.R. Bond, J.E. Charlton, & C.J. Woolf (Eds.). *Proceedings of the VI World Congress on Pain* (pp. 196–189). Amsterdam: Elsevier.

McCaffery, M., & Pasero, C. (1999). Pain control: Teaching patients to use a numerical pain-rating scale. *American Journal of Nursing, 99*(12), 22.

*McNeill, J.A., Sherwood, G.D., Starck, P.L., & Thompson, C.J. (1998). Assessing clinical outcomes: Patient satisfaction with pain management. *Journal of Pain and Symptom Management, 16,* 29–40.

Messinger, J.A., Hoffman, L.A., O'Donnell, J.M., & Dunworth, B.A. (1999). Getting conscious sedation right. *American Journal of Nursing, 99*(12), 44–50.

*Pasero, C. (2000). Pain control: Continuous local anesthetics. *American Journal of Nursing, 100*(8), 22.

*Pasero, C. (2003). Epidural analgesia for postoperative pain. *American Journal of Nursing, 103*(10), 62–64.

*Patt, R.B. (1989). Interventional analgesia: Epidural and subarachnoid therapy. *American Journal of Hospice Care, 6*(2), 11–14.

*Phillips, D.M. (2000). JCAHO pain management standards unveiled. *Journal of the American Medical Association, 284*(4), 428.

*St. Marie, B.J. (Ed.) (2002, 2005). *Core Curriculum for Pain Management Nursing.* Philadelphia: W.B. Saunders.

*Samuelsson, H., Malmberg, F., Eriksson, M., & Hedner, T. (1995). Outcomes of epidural morphine treatment in cancer pain: Nine years of clinical experience. *Journal of Pain and Symptom Management, 10,* 105–112.

*Snell, C.C., Fothergill-Bourbonnais, F., & Durocher-Hendriks, S. (1997). Patient controlled analgesia and intramuscular injections: A comparison of patient pain experiences and postoperative outcomes. *Journal of Advanced Nursing, 25,* 681–690.

*Swenson, J., Davis, J., Johnson, K. (2005). Postoperative care of the chronic opioid-consuming patient. *Anesthesiology Clinics of North America, 23*(1), 37–48.

*Waldman, S.D. (1990). The role of spinal opioids in the management of cancer pain. *Journal of Pain and Symptom Management, 5,* 163–168.

*Watanabe, S., Pereira, J., Hanson, J., & Bruera, E. (1998). Fentanyl by continuous subcutaneous infusion for the management of cancer pain: A retrospective study. *Journal of Pain and Symptom Management, 16,* 323–326.

*Yablonski-Peretz, T., Klin, B., Beilin, Y., et al. (1985). Continuous epidural narcotic analgesia for intractable pain due to malignancy. *Journal of Surgical Oncology, 29,* 8–10.

*Yaney, L.L. (1998). Intravenous conscious sedation: Physiologic, pharmacologic, and legal implications for nurses. *Journal of Intravenous Nursing, 21,* 9–19.

Review Questions

Note: Questions below may have more than one right answer.

1. Which pain management modality is to be avoided if at all possible?
   A. IV administration
   B. Continuous infusion of opioid
   C. Intraspinal infusion of opioid
   D. Intramuscular administration

2. When a patient experiences breakthrough pain, the first nursing intervention should be to:
   A. Believe the patient and record the level of pain
   B. Increase medication dose consistent with nursing judgment
   C. Contact the physician
   D. Verify the physician's order in the clinical record

3. Which of the following opioid agonist/antagonists may be administered to reverse nausea?
   A. Nalbuphine (Nubain)
   B. Nortriptyline
   C. Neupogen
   D. Naloxone (Narcan)

4. Epidural morphine has been associated with a high incidence of pruritus thought to be related to:
   A. An allergic reaction causing histamine release
   B. Opioid receptors binding with the opioid at the substantia gelatinosa
   C. Activity of the opioid at the chemoreceptor sites
   D. Rostral spread of the opioid in the CSF

5. Alcohol is contraindicated for site preparation or when accessing an epidural catheter because of the potential for:
   A. Migration into the intrathecal space
   B. Possible nerve damage
   C. Obliterating the catheter
   D. Damage to the Silastic

6. Temporary epidural catheters are typically used for:
   A. Postoperative pain management
   B. Trial of epidural analgesia for patients with intractable cancer pain
   C. Long-term use for patients with intractable cancer pain
   D. A and B only

7. Aspiration of 3 mL of clear fluid from an epidural catheter could mean which of the following?
   A. The aspirant is medication.
   B. The aspirant is CSF.
   C. The epidural catheter is in epidural space.
   D. All of the above

8. Presence of up to 10 mL of clear fluid in the syringe after aspiration of an epidural catheter is evidence of which of the following?
   A. Catheter patency
   B. Catheter kinking
   C. Catheter migration into the intrathecal space
   D. Catheter damage

9. Nursing standards of practice for pain management have been established by which of the following organizations?
   A. American Pain Society
   B. American Epidural Society
   C. American Academy of Pain Medicine
   D. American Society for Pain Management Nursing

10. Factors to be considered in pain assessment include:
    A. Patient's self-report of pain rating
    B. Nurses' report of patient's pain rating
    C. Physicians' report of patient's pain rating
    D. All of the above

11. When a patient is discharged to an extended care facility, pain orders should follow which of the following principles?
    A. Decrease the use of Demerol
    B. Decrease the use of intramuscular injections
    C. Decrease the use of as-needed medications
    D. All of the above

12. Options for pain control include all of the following except:
    A. Systemic analgesics
    B. Intraspinal opioids
    C. Subcutaneous opioids
    D. Topical anesthetic agents

UNIT 5

Special Applications of Intravenous Therapy

CHAPTER 21

Pediatric Intravenous Therapy

KEY TERMS

Child-Life Worker
Comfort Basket
Intraosseous

Neonate
Play Therapy

Intravenous Therapy in Infants and Children

This chapter focuses on features of IV therapy that are unique to neonatal and pediatric patients. It highlights developmental considerations, disorders, and disease processes unique to this population, IV therapies commonly used in children and adolescents, and necessary adaptations and adjustments to vascular access techniques and devices for neonatal and pediatric patients. Two ongoing considerations in the administration of pediatric IV therapy are emotional preparation of the child and initiation of IV access. This chapter examines these topics in detail, along with special nursing considerations and specific IV therapeutic modalities.

Physiologic and Psychologic Stages of Development

Physiologic Considerations

Human beings change both physically and emotionally throughout childhood, whereas parameters characteristics remain relatively constant after adulthood. For example, body circumference increases more than 3-fold in length and approximately

20-fold in weight from birth through adolescence (Batton, Maisels, & Appelbaum, 1982). The body circumference of the adult, however, changes relatively little throughout the remainder of life. Thus, the stress levels and basal metabolic rates of the child are much higher than those of the adult.

FLUID BALANCE

Although the laws regulating fluid balance are the same in all age groups, water and electrolyte distribution vary drastically from infancy to adulthood. In general, the amount of water content decreases with age and changes in areas of distribution. Body surface area (BSA) is approximately five times greater than body weight in the infant, leading to insensible water loses that can affect fluid balance (Frey, 2001). The newborn has the largest proportion of free water in the extracellular spaces. At a rate of exchange seven times greater than that of the adult, the infant exchanges approximately half of its total extracellular fluid daily. The basal metabolism rate is also twice as great in relation to body weight in the infant as it is in the adult. Table 21–1 compares body surface area, water distribution, and blood volume for infants and children. These factors, in addition to the inability of the kidneys to concentrate urine in infants, can cause dehydration, acidosis, and overhydration (Fann, 1998). From infancy to adulthood, the body surface area decreases in proportion to body weight, approaching adult parameters by the third year. Total body water gradually decreases also, from 70% to 80% of body weight as a term infant to 52% to 60% of body weight as an adolescent and adult. From puberty to adulthood, the percentage of total body water is less for females than males (Table 21–1). Because neonates have a higher level of total body water than adults, water-soluble drugs, such as theophylline, must be given at higher concentrations (Matyskiela-Frey, 1985).

As the child matures, there is a fluid shift from the extracellular fluid compartment. After the first year, total body water content decreases and distribution gradually changes to less fluid in the extracellular fluid compartments and more fluid in the intracellular fluid compartments.

BLOOD VOLUME

The major differences from neonate to adult include a gradual decrease in blood volume, maturation of the immune system with regard to blood typing, changes in blood counts, and changes in requirements. The red blood cell of the infant is nucleated at birth and has a reduced half-life (23.3 days) compared with the that of the adult (26 to 35 days; Luban & Keating, 1983). Synthesis of fetal hemoglobin (HbF) declines rapidly after birth, whereas that of adult hemoglobin (HbA) rises concomitantly. The higher affinity for oxygen of HbF facilitates transfer of oxygen from mother to fetus in utero, but persistence of HbF after birth may result in neonatal respiratory distress and tissue hypoxia because of the inability of HbF to release oxygen to the tissues (Cahill-Alsip & McDermott, 1996). Manipulations of the infant, such as suctioning and IV starts, as well as crying, can increase peripheral leukocyte counts. In the newborn, neutropenia rather than neutrophilia is a more common indicator of sepsis. Platelet counts do not differ greatly from neonate to adult, but

TABLE 21-1   Body Surface Area, Fluid Distribution, and Blood Volume for Various Ages

Age	Body Surface Area (BSA)	Total Body Water (TBW)	Extracellular Fluid (ECF)	Intracellular Fluid (ICF)	Circulating Blood Volume
Premature neonate (<37-wk gestation)	Five times greater than body weight	At 24 wk = 86% of body weight At 32 wk = 80% of body weight	The lower the gestational age, the greater the ECF	Increases as age increases	95 mL/kg
Neonate (term infant to 28 d)	Two to three times as great as that of an adult	70% to 80% of body weight	40% to 50% of TBW is contained in ECF compartment	Increases as age increases	80–90 mL/kg
Infant (1–12 mo)	Proportionately larger than that of the adult	Approximately 75% of body weight	ECF decreases from 45% to 27% in first year	Increases as age increases	75–80 mL/kg
Toddler (1–3 y)	By end of third year, approaches adult parameters	64% of body weight	30% of TBW in ECF compartments	34% of TBW in ICF compartments	70–75 mL/kg
Preschool (3–6 y)	Proportionately equal to adult	60% of body weight	24% of TBW in ECF compartments	36% of TBW in ICF compartments	70 mL/kg
School Age (6–12 y)	Proportionately equal to adult	60% of body weight	24% of TBW in ECF compartments	36% of TBW in ICF compartments	65–70 mL/kg
Adolescent (13–18 y)	Proportionately equal to adult	Males 60% Females 52%	20%–30% of TBW in ECF compartments	40%–50% of TBW in ICF compartments	65–70 mL/kg

(From Swanson, A. [2004]; Nathan, D.G., & Orkin, S.H., [1998]; Hazinski, M.F. [1988].)

thrombocytopenia may easily develop in neonates from extrinsic sources. The immune system matures during infancy. Circulating antibodies are derived from the mother during the last several prenatal weeks; therefore, premature infants have a less efficient humoral immunity. As an infant is exposed to outside antigens, antibody production begins.

Specific physical assessment areas indicative of hematologic function in children include color changes in skin, lips, conjunctivae, mucous membranes, and nails, such as blue for cyanosis, pale for anemia, or yellow for jaundice. The fingernails and toenails should be examined for clubbing, the skin for petechiae, and the mucous membranes for bleeding. Blood oozing from old venipuncture sites often is a precursor to the onset of disseminated intravascular coagulation. When a tourniquet is placed on an extremity, evidence of petechiae distal to the tourniquet may indicate idiopathic thrombocytopenic purpura (ITP) or other platelet disorders. Laboratory values as simple as the commonly done complete blood count, which includes hemoglobin, hematocrit, white cell count, platelet levels, and cell differential, can provide a very good picture of the child's hematologic status. These values vary among age groups. Clotting studies and levels of specific factors may be analyzed if a bleeding disorder is suspected.

Circulating blood volume decreases gradually in proportion to body weight from neonate to adolescent, ranging from 95 mL per kg in the premature neonate to adult levels of 60 to 75 mL per kg in the adolescent (Table 21–1). The higher proportion of blood volume to lower body weight of the neonate and infant means that blood loss percentage is much higher in this group, even with small losses. The following is an example comparing blood volume loss between a 5-kg infant and a 75-kg adult:

25 mL blood loss from 75-kg adult = <0.4% of total circulating blood volume (5,250 mL)
25 mL blood loss from 5-kg infant = 6% of total circulating blood volume (400 mL)

Owing to smaller body surface area and large circulating blood volume, the same amount of blood loss could be devastating to an infant, whereas it would not harm an adult.

Electrolytes

Infants and children are especially prone to fluid and electrolyte imbalances because their bodies are made up of more water in proportion to surface area than those of adults. Moreover, their immature body organs compromise their ability to handle imbalances.

Laboratory values to monitor in children include sodium, potassium, chloride, calcium, and glucose. In particular, plasma sodium concentration does not vary greatly from infancy to adulthood. In the premature neonate and neonate, potassium and chloride concentrations are higher than any other time, whereas magnesium and calcium levels in the infant are lower than in older children and adults. Altered calcium regulation combined with a high serum phosphate may lead to hypocalcemia-associated tetany. (Swanson, 2004) Phosphate levels remain slightly higher than adult levels until about 5 years of age, at which time electrolyte parameters are within normal adult ranges.

Gastrointestinal disturbances, such as diarrhea, most often alter potassium levels. Children usually do not experience cardiac symptoms until the serum potassium falls below 3 mEq/L. Hyperkalemia is more common, especially in premature infants. For children with renal failure, hyperkalemia does not decrease as expected during rehydration (Barnard & Hazinski, 1992). The hallmarks of hyperkalemia in children are similar to those in adults—tented T waves and prolonged P-R intervals on the electrocardiogram. Other common electrolyte imbalances in children include hypocalcemia, hyponatremia or hypernatremia (as seen with dehydration), and chloride disturbances. Infants are especially prone to hypocalcemia because more calcium is deposited in the bones when the infant is stressed and growth hormone is secreted. Other causes of hypocalcemia include transfusion of citrated blood, pancreatitis, newborn intake of cow's milk, hyperphosphatemia, hypomagnesemia, vitamin D deficiency, and malabsorption. Conversely, lower calcium can result from excessive use of diuretics, tumor breakdown when initiating chemotherapy, and immobilization (Fann, 1998).

ACID–BASE BALANCE

Acid–base balance is part of the overall picture of fluid balance. In the neonate and infant, higher BSA equals increased metabolism and more production of waste products that must be excreted. Buffering mechanisms are less mature, resulting in a deficit of bicarbonate. Combined with increased production of waste and immature renal system, metabolic acidosis is more common in this age group. As the infant matures, pH ranges approach normal parameters of 7.35 to 7.45.

When a child has diarrhea, he or she loses bicarbonate in the stool. Metabolic acidosis results. Conversely, when a child is vomiting or has a nasogastric tube, metabolic alkalosis can result from the large amount of acid lost in gastric secretions. When replacing electrolytes, frequent monitoring of laboratory values and fluid balance is necessary to prevent acid–base imbalances.

ORGAN FUNCTION

In the premature baby and term infant, renal function is immature, with inability to concentrate and excrete effectively, acidify urine, or maintain fluid and sodium balance. In the term infant, renal immaturity results in excretion of larger volumes of solute-free water than is seen in older pediatric patients [Swanson, 2004]. By the end of the second year, renal function reaches full maturity. Many drugs are excreted by the renal system. Less efficient renal function owing to immaturity in the neonate or disease process in the older child may decrease excretion of drugs, causing longer half-life and possible toxicity. In these patients, penicillins and aminoglycosides are given with longer intervals between doses (every 12 or 18 hours vs. every 6 or 8 hours). In children with cystic fibrosis, whose extrarenal clearance pathways eliminate drugs more quickly, IV aminoglycosides such as tobramycin (Nebcin) must be given at two to three times the normal dose (Matyskiela-Frey, 1985).

The immature hepatic system in the neonate and infant, owing to decreased ability to secrete bile and conjugate bilirubin, can affect intravenous medication and/or solution administration. Throughout the first year of life, the liver function remains immature. The ability to metabolize drugs is dramatically less than that of the adult, as is the formation of the plasma proteins and ketones, the storage of glycogen and vitamins, and the capacity to break down amino acids. Some drugs also may compete with binding sites on the albumin molecule, displacing bilirubin from these sites in neonates and increasing the risk of hyperbilirubinemia. Such drugs include salicylates, sulfonamides, phenytoin (Dilantin), furosemide (Lasix), and sodium benzoate (Guyon, 1989). Many commercially available medications and drug diluents contain sodium benzoate in the form of the preservative benzyl alcohol, which has been linked with toxicity and death in premature infants. Thus, care should be taken to stock only preservative-free diluents in the nursery and neonatal intensive care unit (Meyer, 1982).

Digestive and metabolic processes are usually complete by the beginning of toddlerhood (Hockenberry, 2003).

Thermoregulation, the maintenance of normal body temperature, is a challenge to the premature neonate owing to large surface area, dermal immaturity, and thin layer of subcutaneous fat. Physiologic stress and Increased metabolism in response to hypothermia results in higher oxygen and caloric requirements. This process of thermoregulation continues throughout the infant's first several months of life. Neonates do not shiver to maintain heat as adults do, and during infancy, the child's ability to shiver increases. The older infant usually has acquired the benefit of insulation by the gradual growth of adipose tissue. By early childhood, the skin is thicker and the body has a higher percentage of fat and a decreased surface area to volume ratio; these factors enable children to cope with environmental cold stresses much better than the young infant (Frey, 2001). When performing procedures such as IV insertion and dressing changes, the nurse must maintain a neutral thermal environment for the infant to prevent the possibility of cold stress, thus permitting the infant to maintain a normal core temperature with minimum oxygen consumption and calorie expenditure. The neutral thermal environment for smaller infants is 35.4°C ± 0.5°C, and for larger infants it is 32.5°C ± 1.4°C (Frey, 2001). A warm environment can be maintained using a variety of tools, including the following: warmer beds, incubators, cotton blankets, head coverings, heat lamps kept a safe distance from the skin, and hot packs for infant use; only the extremity of the IV insertion site should be exposed.

Knowledge of the condition of the integumentary system, particularly that of premature infants, is of extreme interest to the infusion therapy specialist. The skin of the premature infant requires special precautions owing to underdevelopment of the stratum corneum, with resultant thin, fragile skin. This dermal fragility can lead to dermal stripping, loss of water, and increased absorption and possible toxicity of agents, such as solvents and bonding agents that are applied to the skin. Neonatal skin care is specifically of importance to the nurse practicing IV insertion and device care in this age group. Because there is less cohesion between the dermis and epidermis, tape removal can strip epidermis, so as little tape as possible and tape padded with gauze or cotton fibers is used. For skin cleaning in premature neonates, the Association of Women's Health, Obstetric and Neonatal Nurses (AWOHNN) recommends wiping with chlorhexidine for 30 seconds twice or povidone iodine twice and allowing it to dry, removing these products with sterile water or saline after the procedure is complete, and avoiding use of isopropyl alcohol to clean skin or remove other cleaning agents (AWOHNN, 2001). Except for specific congenital or acquired skin conditions, such as dystrophic epidermolysis bullosa, eczema, and other disorders, the barrier function of the integumentary system of the full-term neonate and older child is intact.

Psychologic Stages of Development

A more subtle area of concern is the child's emotional needs, which require patience, education, and understanding from IV nurses. Psychologic age and ability as well as each child's particular developmental stage exert major influences on emotional needs. For example, when hospitalized, some children regress and exhibit behaviors more common in a younger age group (eg, a child who is toilet trained may regress to the diaper stage). These children resume developmental landmarks once treatment ends or the child's condition stabilizes. Thus, even though children of varied ages and intellectual capacities receive similar IV therapies, they require education before, during, and after IV therapy that considers their particular emotional and developmental variables.

DEVELOPMENTAL STAGES

A full understanding of each developmental stage enables the health care team to provide appropriate, nonthreatening care. It enhances the ability of staff to recognize that children's needs vary markedly, not only according to stress levels but also by growth and developmental levels.

The pediatric population can be divided by age into the following stages: **neonate** (0 to 28 days), infant (1 to 12 months), toddler (1 to 3 years), preschool (4 to 5 years), school age (6 to 12 years), and adolescent (12 to 18 years) (Hockenberry, 2003). The unique IV therapy needs of premature infants also are considered within the infant stage (Sater, 1998). The health care team should gear pre-IV and post-IV care according to these stages, including preparation for the procedure, IV site protection, and mobility and safety needs. For example, most children are not able to understand the significance of IV therapy, including the importance of not manipulating the IV site, until they reach age 3½ to 5 years, depending on the individual child. Thus, younger children and their families require appropriate adjustments. A review of growth, development, and useful approaches when working with children of different developmental stages is highlighted in Table 21–2.

Although developmental stages are important, nurses must remember to explain all procedures to the child or parent and to assess each child individually, not just according to age or physiologic maturity. In some cases, children have disease processes, such as renal disease, that can result in growth delays, causing staff to mistake the child's actual age.

MEDICAL PLAY AND COPING MECHANISMS

Medical **play therapy,** consisting of practicing IV therapy on a doll, is an ideal teaching strategy that enhances emotional preparation through acting out. When it is

TABLE 21-2 Growth, Development, and Intravenous Insertion Tips for Various Pediatric Stages

Stage (Age)	Growth	Development	IV Insertion Tips
Infancy (birth to 12 mo) (includes neonatal period from birth to 28 d)	• Physical and developmental changes are rapid. • Head and body grow very rapidly. • Major body systems undergo progressive maturation. • Birth weight usually doubles by age 6 mo and triples by age 1 y.	• Trust vs. mistrust • Child displays social affective play. • Attachment to caregivers is paramount. • Separation anxiety begins at approximately age 6 mo.	• Infants require caregivers to meet their needs consistently. • Do not feed the baby before IV placement or aspiration may occur. • Provide comfort during and after the procedure, using a pacifier and distraction, such as a mobile.
Toddler (12–36 mo)	• Growth slows down. • Birth weight quadruples by 30 mo. • Height at age 3 y is usually approximately half adult height. • Head circumference growth slows, and chest circumference is larger than head or abdomen.	• Autonomy vs. shame • Child displays cause and effect thinking. • Exploration is prominent. • Child shows imaginative play and may be reckless at times.	• Toddlers require short, concrete explanations immediately before the IV is started. • Do not give a toddler a choice, such as "Can we start your IV now?" or the answer will be "No!" • The nurse will need an assistant to position and restrain the toddler.
Preschool/early childhood (36 mo to 6 y)	• Growth stabilizes. • Average annual weight gain is approximately 2.2 kg (5 lb). • Average height increase ranges from 6.4–7.6 cm (2.5–3 in.). • Most height growth is in legs, resulting in a more slender physical appearance.	• New gross motor skills develop. • Fantasy vs. reality • Child follows simple commands. • Child fears blood loss and invasive procedures.	• Preschoolers require preparation immediately before the procedure and may be distracted with age-appropriate toys. • Play therapy using medical toys works well with this age group. • Nurse may still need help to hold the child still.

Stage	Growth and Development	Psychosocial/Cognitive	Nursing Considerations
School age (6–12 y)	• Growth and development are gradual. • Average annual weight gain is 2–3 kg (4.5–6.5 lb). • Average height increase is approximately 5 cm (2 in.).	• Play is solitary and interactive. • Child is fascinated with superheroes/monsters. • Child may fantasize about procedures based on understanding.	• School-age children can be told about the IV a short time in advance and can assist with small tasks, such as ripping pieces of tape and helping to keep a record of intake and output. • Allow for privacy. • Allow the child to cry; don't force him or her to "be brave."
Adolescence—divided into three substages: early adolescence (11–13 y), middle adolescence (13–15 y), and late adolescence (15 y and older)	• Early, little size difference between boys and girls. • Toward the end of early adolescence, a growth spurt occurs. • Girls first surpass boys in height and weight, then boys surpass girls. • Body proportions approach adult parameters by the end of adolescence.	• Industry vs. inferiority • Logic, reasoning, and concept of permanence develop. • Child develops skills and can dramatize. • Self-esteem and values emerge. • Child finds role models. • Identity vs. role confusion • Abstract and deductive reasoning emerge. • Child needs independence, yet wants to be cared for at times. Early: • Teen seeks independence from parents/guardians. • Peers are very important. Middle: • Sexual identity and body image are very important. • Teen grapples with mortality. Late: • Career plans take shape. • Teen shows high idealism and favors close, intimate relationships. • Teen looks for a significant other.	• Adolescents vacillate between dependence and independence; approach a teen using adult language. • Prepare teens for procedures in advance, allowing them a part in their care.

pragmatic, nurses certainly can use play therapy for teaching purposes, or they may seek such assistance from **child-life workers**, ancillary members of the health care team who specialize in child development.

A coping basket or **comfort basket**, filled with items for various age groups, is easy and inexpensive to put together. The basket can include a Slinky, a clear sealed acrylic "magic wand" with floating sparkles, a kaleidoscope, and a bottle of bubbles for blowing. Such items are easy to clean and small enough to keep in a hospital treatment room, pediatric care office, or equipment bag. An adolescent may find a portable stereo with headphones a useful distraction during IV insertion (Doellman, 2004).

ESTABLISHING RAPPORT

Another important aspect of IV therapy is establishing rapport with the family and child through good communication. Communication differs for all age groups and according to the child's intellectual level.

Usually it is best to tell the child that the venipuncture will hurt but only for a short time. Define the term *time* not by minutes (young children will not understand) but by comparison with other procedures. For example, say, "The actual IV start takes about the same time it takes you to say the alphabet or count to 50." Inform the child that even though this therapy may be painful initially, it should make him or her feel better, as before the illness. Always be honest with a child. Specifically, do not promise a certain number of IV attempts or "only one stick" because a child will lose trust if several attempts turn out to be necessary. Give the child the opportunity to cry, providing as much privacy as possible. Allow children who are old enough to participate in the therapy. Tearing tape, opening alcohol swabs, or holding tubing may provide distraction and a sense of involvement, particularly if the child is of school age. Nurses may be able to assuage a child's fear of needles by telling the child that once the IV is in place, the needle is no longer there, and only a small "straw" is in the vein.

An IV therapy teaching tool with pictures and large-print words in simple language can help preschoolers understand the procedure. The learning tool can be used as a hospital coloring book (Thompson, 1994). Adolescents, in particular, require a great deal of individual attention and allowance for their independent nature versus their dependent situation. Adolescents believe they are mature and desire the chance to assess their disease status; they deserve the opportunity to participate in the decision-making aspects of their care. They feel grown up, but lack the adult's experience and knowledge. Therefore, educational techniques practiced with adolescents should encompass a common-sense approach that provides them with the opportunity to deal with IV therapy to the best of their ability.

The presence of parents during a painful or invasive procedure is controversial and needs to be evaluated on a case-by-case basis. One study concluded that patients aged 1 to 7 years are likely to experience less distress during venipuncture if parents are present, and that parental presence is unlikely to affect experienced health care providers (Wolfram, Turner, & Philput, 1997). Parents/caregivers may provide emotional support and represent security during an actual procedure, but they should not be used to restrain a child unless no other assistance is available (eg,

FIGURE 21–1. Positioning for comfort prior to venipuncture. (Courtesy of A.M. Frey.)

in home care). Parents/caregivers can be instructed to use positioning for comfort techniques to hold a child still for venipuncture while still helping a child feel secure (Fig. 21–1).

If a parent chooses not to accompany a child into the treatment room for IV insertion, the IV nurse should honor this decision and not make parents feel guilty. Providing comfort and praise after an IV insert is an ideal means of parental involvement after the procedure is completed.

PAIN REDUCTION

Studies indicate that infants and children respond to noxious stimuli and experience pain. In one study, infants and children showed significant behavioral changes and toddlers demonstrated measurable increases in heart rate during venipuncture and IV insertion (Van Cleve, Johnson, & Pothier, 1996). By using pain reduction techniques, such as imagery and the coping basket, nurses can reduce the anxiety associated with IV insertion. Recent studies have shown that a pacifier, dipped in glucose solution, has been very effective in reducing pain response in infants during invasive procedures (Greenberg, 2002). In addition, local anesthetics, such as topically applied anesthetic cream or intradermal saline at the IV site, may decrease pain sensation in children (Frey, 1998b; Lal, McClellan, Taub, & Beattie, 2001). A summary of some medications for pain reduction is provided in Table 21–3. Several new products for local anesthesia are being developed and tested in pediatric centers; these are looking to provide a faster-acting topical anesthetic delivered painlessly and that does not cause vasoconstriction. In some cases, IV conscious sedation may be necessary to provide a more generalized sedation for invasive procedures such as insertion of a peripherally inserted central

TABLE 21-3 Local Numbing Methods for Pediatric Intravenous Access Procedures

Method	Administration	Advantages	Disadvantages
EMLA cream (topical)	Cream is placed on potential venipuncture sites and covered with transparent dressing 1 or more hours before procedure.	• Topical • Noninvasive • Easy to use • May be applied at home	• Takes a relatively long time to work • May cause vasoconstriction • Precautions necessary in neonates
LMX-4 cream (topical)	Cream is placed on potential venipuncture sites 30 min or more before procedure. Usually covered with transparent dressing to avoid disturbance or ingestion of cream by child	• Topical • Noninvasive • Easy to use • May be applied at home	• Takes a relatively long time to work • Precautions necessary in neonates
NUMBY Stuff (topical) Iomed, Inc., Salt Lake City, UT	Iontophoresis—a liquid solution containing anesthetics is placed on an electrode, and the electrode is pasted to the skin and stimulated with a mild current of electricity.	• Works quickly • More depth of penetration than EMLA	• Electrical stimulation may be uncomfortable for some patients • Takes 10 min to work
Lidocaine hydrochloride 0.5%, 1% without epinephrine (intradermal)	An intradermal wheal of approximately 0.05 to 0.1 mL is made near the IV insertion site by using a very tiny needle (26- or 29-gauge insulin needle).	• Works immediately and provides good level of local anesthesia • Useful for such procedures as peripherally inserted central catheter placement	• Two sticks needed • May sting if acidity not neutralized • Can inadvertently be injected IV • May cause allergic reaction
Normal saline with preservative (intradermal)	An intradermal wheal of approximately 0.05 to 0.1 mL is made near the IV insertion site by using a very tiny needle (26- or 29-gauge insulin needle).	• Works immediately and provides equivalent level of local anesthesia as lidocaine • Does not have the potential side effects of lidocaine (stinging, allergic reaction, possible IV injection)	• Two sticks needed • Limited duration of local numbing (2 min) • Cannot be used in preterm and low-birth-weight neonates

(From Frey, A.M. [1998a,b].)

catheter (PICC) and noninvasive procedures, such as diagnostic studies (Deady & Gorman, 1997).

Conditions and Disease States

Neonates and children experience some disorders that are unique to their age grouping. Some of these disorders are highlighted. Primary indications for pediatric IV therapy include fluid therapy, medication administration, antineoplastic therapy, nutritional support, and transfusion therapy. Although these topics are covered fully in other chapters, features unique to pediatric patients are highlighted in the following sections.

Alterations in Fluid Needs

The most common cause of altered fluid and caloric needs is changes in temperature. An increase in temperature by 1°C raises the child's caloric needs by 12%, thereby increasing fluid needs as well. In the neonate, use of radiant warmers and single-walled incubators may effectively maintain the newborn's temperature, but this temperature elevation in turn increases the infant's insensible fluid losses. Phototherapy, although effectively used to treat newborn hyperbilirubinemia, increases insensible fluid losses and water requirements (Frey, 2001). These various losses must be included when determining fluid replacement needs. Conversely, a child who is hypothermic experiences a 12% decrease in caloric needs for every 1°C lost, which in turn decreases fluid requirements. Other conditions that affect fluid requirements include diarrhea and presence of nasogastric tubes.

DEHYDRATION

Dehydration can occur rapidly in children who lose more water than they receive. Being alert for signs of dehydration is an important aspect of caring for pediatric patients. Physical assessment parameters for dehydration are outlined in Table 21–4.

Dehydration is characterized by type, depending on level of serum sodium, and by degree, depending on weight loss, patient history, and physical assessment. The three types of dehydration are as follows:

- Isotonic—Sodium is within normal limits and electrolyte and water deficits are equal (eg, mild vomiting and diarrhea).
- Hypertonic—Sodium is elevated and water losses are greater than electrolyte losses (eg, too concentrated formula intake).
- Hypotonic—Sodium is low and electrolyte losses are greater than water losses or water intake is large (eg, diabetes insipidus, drowning in fresh water).

To determine the degree of dehydration, nurses must calculate the percentage of weight lost. For each 1% of weight loss, the patient also has lost 10 mL/kg of fluid, which must be made up in addition to maintenance and ongoing losses. If a child presents with severe dehydration, a fluid bolus of normal saline or lactated Ringer's

TABLE 21–4   Assessment Parameters Used to Determine Degree of Dehydration

| Parameter | Degree of Dehydration | | |
	Mild	Moderate	Severe
Weight loss	3%–5%	6%–9%	≥10%
Skin turgor	Normal	Decreased	Decreased
Mucous membranes	Slightly dry	Dry	Dry
Eyes	Normal	Sunken orbits	Deeply sunken orbits
Extremities	Warm, normal capillary refill	Delayed capillary refill	Cool, mottled
Fontanelle		Sunken	Sunken
Blood pressure	Normal	Normal	Normal to reduced
Pulse quality	Normal	Normal or slightly decreased	Moderately decreased
Heart rate	Normal	Increased	Increased; bradycardia in severe cases
Mental status	Normal	Normal to listless	Normal to lethargic or comatose
Urine output	Slightly decreased	<1 mL/kg/h	<0.5–1 mL/kg/h

at a dosage of 20 to 40 mL/kg should be initiated and repeated if necessary. Oral rehydration should be initiated at a rate of 50 to 100 mL/kg if the child is mildly to moderately dehydrated. IV therapy continues if the child does not tolerate oral rehydration therapy or the type of dehydration warrants IV correction (King, Glass, Bresee, & Duggan, 2003).

FLUID OVERLOAD

Fluid overload and intoxication are less common than dehydration, but can occur more readily in infants, whose immature kidneys are unable to excrete excess fluid. A serum sodium <130 mEq/L in an infant that is not associated with dehydration is a sign of water intoxication (Fann, 1998). Causes of water intoxication include too rapid dialysis, too rapid reduction of glucose levels in diabetic ketoacidosis, and administration of overly diluted formula (Hockenberry, 2003). Treatment includes reducing fluid delivery and administering IV furosemide.

Pyloric Stenosis

The most common cause of vomiting in neonates between 2 and 4 weeks of age, and a condition seen more often in males, is pyloric stenosis. Pyloric stenosis occurs when the circular muscle of the pylorus hypertrophies, leading to obstruction of the gastric outlet resulting in gastric distention and vomiting. The cause of this disorder is unknown, but the role of genetics is one consideration. In early stages, the infant may appear normal, but later exam reveals an often palpable olivelike pyloric mass. Owing to the severe projectile vomiting, infants with pyloric stenosis can experience hypotonic fluid volume deficit, hypokalemia, and metabolic acidosis. Treatment involves correction of the fluid, electrolyte and acid–base imbalances, and surgical pyloromyotomy to relieve the obstruction (Swanson, 2004).

Hemolytic Disease of the Newborn

Two causes of hemolytic disease of the newborn (HDN) include Rh incompatibility and ABO incompatibility. In Rh incompatibility, the anti-D antibodies that an Rh^- mother developed during her first pregnancy with an Rh^+ fetus cross the placenta and destroy the red blood cells of subsequent Rh^+ fetuses. At birth, subsequent infants are anemic and have increased levels of unconjugated (indirect) bilirubin. Deposition of excess bilirubin in the brain can cause kernicterus, a type of encephalopathy. Exchange transfusion is considered when bilirubin levels increase >1 mg/dL each hour or reach 15 to 16 mg/dL in the premature neonate and 20 mg/dL in the full-term infant (Kasprisin, 1985). ABO incompatibility occurs most frequently when a type O mother carries a type A or B fetus (Nathan & Orkin, 1998). Although HDN from ABO incompatibility is more common than HDN from Rh incompatibility, it usually is mild enough to be treated with phototherapy or a single blood transfusion, until the infant's liver matures enough to clear bilirubin from the blood. For either type of HDN, red blood cells alone or with fresh frozen plasma may be used for exchange transfusion. To treat Rh HDN, type O Rh blood crossmatched with the mother should be used; for ABO HDN, Rh-compatible, type O blood should be used.

EXCHANGE TRANSFUSION

A procedure unique to the neonatal population is exchange transfusion, in which most or all of the infant's blood volume is replaced with compatible red blood cells and plasma from one or several donors. Exchange transfusion was first used in the early 1950s for management of hemolytic disease of the newborn (HDN). With the introduction of anti-D immune globulin (RhoGAM) in the 1960s, the number of infants with HDN greatly declined; however, HDN is still the most common indication for exchange transfusion. Other indications include disseminated intravascular coagulation, sepsis, respiratory distress syndrome, and polycythemia. Exchange transfusions optimally are undertaken using two IV sites or an IV and an intra-arterial site. A combination of peripheral, central, or umbilical access devices can be used.

TECHNIQUES AND SPECIAL CONSIDERATIONS

A double-volume or two-volume exchange usually is performed when exchange transfusion equals twice the patient's blood volume. This replaces approximately 85% of the newborn's blood and lowers the bilirubin level approximately 50%, but has no effect on extravascular bilirubin. Albumin may be administered before the exchange to bind bilirubin, allowing a greater amount to be removed during the procedure. Ideally, two vascular access sites are used to allow simultaneous withdrawal and infusion. Common sites include the umbilical vessels and peripheral or central veins. If only one access is available, the push-pull method is used. Calcium and dextrose levels are monitored closely during the exchange because blood preservatives may cause levels to decrease. Complications can include those related to the catheter as well as those related to transfusion therapy.

Hypoglycemia

There are multiple etiologic factors that may cause hypoglycemia in infants; however, persistent hypoglycemia in the neonate is most often caused by hyperinsulinemia. (Sperling & Menon, 2004). In infants, hypothermia and apnea may be present, and a delay in diagnosis may be associated with developmental delay. Other causes include abrupt discontinuation of IV dextrose solutions and high glucose demand that is not met, such as in a septic infant. Infants and children who are hypoglycemic display blood glucose levels of <45 mg/dL, have poor oral intake, and exhibit neurologic symptoms, such as lethargy, hypotonia, tremors or twitching, irritability, and eye rolling (Swanson, 2004). Diaphoresis and pallor may be evident. An older child may complain of headache or display hallucinations or mental confusion. The mechanisms of hypoglycemia remain incompletely understood. Treatment involves oral or IV glucose, depending on the severity of the hypoglycemia.

Salicylate Intoxication

Salicylism or salicylate intoxication can be caused by a variety of external factors such as ingestion by the child, maternal ingestion, excessive topical application of oil of wintergreen (methyl salicylate), or incorrectly administered doses of oral or topical salicylates. Salicylism is diagnosed by history and serum levels of >150 mg/kg. Symptoms include gastrointestinal irritation, hyperthermia, hypoglycemia, and hypokalemia, as well as acid–base imbalances resulting in respiratory alkalosis and metabolic acidosis, alone or combined (Swanson, 2004).

Other organ systems may also be involved, and children who are verbal may complain of ringing in the ears (tinnitus) as well as neurologic symptoms such as confusion and seizures. Ingestion protocols are started with gastric lavage, activated charcoal for absorption, and syrup of ipecac to induce vomiting. Treatment involves correction of fluid imbalance with an isotonic solution and correction of acid–base imbalances.

Cystic Fibrosis

Cystic fibrosis (CF) is caused by an inherited autosomal recessive trait that occurs in one out of every four children born to parents both having a defective gene that codes the cystic fibrosis transmembrane regulator (CFTR). This genetic defect results in abnormal transport of sodium and chloride across the epithelium, leading to an accumulation of thick, tenacious mucous and abnormal secretion of sweat and saliva. This increased viscosity of mucus affects both respiratory and digestive system function in children with CF leading to frequent lung infections, abnormal digestion, and abnormal reproductive system function (Hockenberry, 2003).

CF is diagnosed by clinical symptoms and laboratory tests. Clinical symptoms vary in type and severity from child to child; therefore, early diagnosis does not always occur. The most common symptoms include sweat abnormality that results in increased sodium and chloride concentrations in sweat; children with CF taste salty when kissed. Other symptoms are meconium ileus, failure to thrive, and large, bulky stools related to deficiency in pancreatic enzymes from blocked ducts. Chronic respiratory infections also may be sign of CF, and these symptoms, alone or together, usually warrant laboratory investigation using a quantitative sweat chloride test. A chloride concentration of >60 mEq/L is considered positive for CF; in infants <3 months, a sweat chloride concentration >40 mEq/L is considered highly suggestive of CF. Newborn screening for CF by DNA testing is also done in some areas on a routine basis and is always done once a child has a positive sweat chloride test (Hockenberry, 2003; Swanson, 2004).

Therapeutic management of CF involves antibiotic therapy to treat pulmonary exacerbations and nutritional management with supplemental enzymes. Daily routines of chest physiotherapy and nutritional planning are used to prevent pulmonary infections and digestive complications. Infusion nurses become part of the care team involved with CF patients during pulmonary exacerbations that require intravenous antibiotics in the hospital, extended care facility, or at home. The most common organisms treated in this population include *Pseudomonas aeruginosa*, *Pseudomonas cepacia*, *Staphylococcus aureus*, and *Haemophilus influenzae* (Hockenberry, 2003; Swanson, 2004). Because treatment of CF exacerbation with intravenous antibiotics typically lasts a week or longer, venous access devices such as a peripherally inserted central catheter or totally implanted port are used to deliver a combination of a penicillin or cephalosporin and aminoglycoside (Frey, 1995). The median life expectancy for CF patients has increased more than fivefold since 1966 as aggressive therapy and genetic advances have an impact.

Meningitis

Meningitis is inflammation of the meninges, the membranes surrounding the brain and spinal column (Le Roy, 1999). Bacterial meningitis is still a major cause of death and disability in children worldwide (Duke, Curtis, & Fuller, 2003). Meningitis is most frequently seen in children between the ages of 1 month and 5 years. Meningitis can be caused by bacteria, viruses, or fungi via vascular dissemination, penetrating wounds, or contamination of devices, such as ventricular shunts (Swanson, 2004).

Meningitis is diagnosed by clinical symptoms and laboratory tests. Clinical symptoms vary by causative agent and the age of the child. Infants may present with fever, diarrhea, irritability, decreased muscle tone, and altered level of consciousness. Other physical symptoms include bulging fontanels, high-pitched or poor cry, and feeding intolerance. Older children and adolescents may have a more classic clinical picture with headache, fever, photophobia, nuchal rigidity, and mental changes (LeRoy, 1999; Swanson, 2004). Other signs on clinical exam can include a petechial rash and focal neurologic symptoms such as hearing loss, hemiparesis, and so forth.

Diagnosis of meningitis is confirmed by testing of cerebrospinal fluid obtained by lumbar puncture, or via shunt tap. Tests include cell count and differential, glucose, protein, culture, and Gram stain to identify the causative organism. In some cases, the risk of complication from the lumbar puncture (suspected increased intracranial pressure, cardiorespiratory compromise, lumbar puncture site infection, and low platelet count) is greater than the benefit (LeRoy, 1999). In these cases, treatment is initiated without testing the cerebrospinal fluid. Bacterial meningitis is most commonly caused by *Haemophilus influenzae, Streptococcus pneumoniae,* or *Neisseria meningitidis.* Meningitis can also be caused by viral and fungal organisms. Administration of appropriate antibiotics intravenously is the most immediate treatment, along with acetaminophen for headache, fever, and muscle pain. Children presenting with suspected bacterial meningitis are treated intravenously with meningitic doses of ceftriaxone and vancomycin until cultures and sensitivity test results are obtained. Infants and children are usually hospitalized and isolated if bacterial meningitis is suspected, and very ill children should be managed in a pediatric tertiary care facility after initial stabilization of cardiorespiratory and neurologic status (LeRoy, 1999). The use of corticosteroids in meningitis is controversial; the evidence that they protect against neurologic complications of childhood meningitis (particularly severe hearing loss) is strongest when meningitis is caused by *H. influenzae* type b; dexamethasone is given before the first dose of antibiotics (LeRoy, 1999; Duke et al, 2003). There are few controlled clinical trials on which to base recommendations about other adjuvant therapy for meningitis. Avoidance of secondary brain injury from hypoxia, hypotension, hypo-osmolarity, and cerebral edema, hypoglycemia, or convulsions is essential for a good outcome (Duke et al, 2003).

Sickle Cell Disease

Sickle cell disease [SCD], a chronic and potentially life-threatening disorder, is caused by inheriting an autosomal recessive gene that causes a group of blood disorders. In the United States, SCD occurs primarily in those of African American, African/Hispanic, Caribbean, and South American descent. There are several types of sickle cell disease, with the most common being: sickle cell anemia, sickle-hemoglobin C disease, sickle β-plus thalassemia, and sickle β-zero thalassemia. Sickle cell trait is an inherited condition in which both hemoglobin A and S are produced in the red blood cells, always more A than S. Sickle cell trait is a genetic marker that does not cause SCD in carriers, and children with the trait are generally healthy. However, when two individuals with sickle trait have children together, the risk of a child being born with sickle cell disease is 25% (*What is sickle cell disease?*, 2005). This disorder is diagnosed by completing a hemoglobin electrophoresis on a blood specimen. A hemoglobin S of 50% or greater indicates disease, assuming there is no hemoglobin F present. During the first year of life, hemoglobin F or fetal hemoglobin, which has a greater affinity for oxygen, decreases. While hemoglobin F is present, sickling of red blood cells does not occur. SCD is characterized by the production of abnormal sickle hemoglobin S in red blood cells instead of the normal hemoglobin A. Stressful conditions, such as illness, acidosis, dehydration, and temperature elevation distort the hemoglobin S to sickle shape. As red blood cells "sickle" from a lack of oxygen, they clump and slow blood flow, resulting in hemolytic anemia and acute and chronic tissue damage secondary to vaso-occlusion. These painful episodes, which are unpredictable and vary in severity, are commonly referred to as *sickle cell crises*. Blockage of blood flow through vessels results in lung tissue damage (acute chest syndrome), pain episodes (arms, legs, chest, and abdomen), stroke and priapism (painful prolonged erection). Damage to the spleen makes sickle cell disease patients, especially young children, easily overwhelmed by certain bacterial infections. Anemia is usually present and chronic ischemia can damage liver, kidneys, bone, brain, and tissue.

Early treatment is essential to prevent worsening of pain and major complications such as progressive organ failure. Most pain episodes are treated at home with nonsteroidal anti-inflammatories, such as ibuprofen and acetaminophen with codeine, or morphine for severe pain. Increased oral fluids, a heating pad applied to the affected area, deep-breathing exercises, and distraction methods such as music, videotapes, and imagery, as well as alternative medicine treatments, may help with pain relief. If patients become febrile, many pediatric centers treating sickle cell crises provide fast-track admission and treatment with IV fluids, electrolytes, blood transfusions, antibiotics, and pain management, incorporating an age-appropriate pain assessment tool. Sickle cell centers use an effective team approach to management of the sickle cell patient, including physician, nurse practitioner, nurses, social worker, child life therapist, nutrition counselor, and pain management team. SCD is not yet curable, although erythropoietin and bone marrow transplants do offer hope in specific cases.

Necrotizing Enterocolitis

Necrotizing enterocolitis (NEC) is an inflammatory disease of the bowel that occurs primarily in preterm infants. Although the exact cause of NEC is unknown, there appear to be some common features, including intestinal ischemia, hypertonic enteric feeding/medications in the intestinal lumen, and colonization by pathogenic bacteria in the presence of immature gastrointestinal host defenses (Hockenberry, 2003; Swanson, 2004). In full-term infants, NEC almost always occurs during the first 10 days after birth; in premature infants, NEC symptoms can appear in a wider range of 4 hours to 30 days after birth (Con-Yost, 2005). Cells lining the wall of the bowel become damaged from ischemia and stop producing protective mucus. The unprotected bowel is then further damaged by proteolytic enzymes setting up an environment in which toxins cause further damage and gas-forming bacteria invade (Hockenberry, 2003).

In addition to age and feeding history, the clinical picture of NEC includes the following symptoms: distended abdomen that often appears shiny, gastric retention, blood in stools, lethargy, poor feeding, apnea, vomiting (often bile stained), decreased urine output, hypotension, and hypothermia. Abdominal radiographic studies are done when NEC is suspected to look for intestinal dilation and characteristic pneumatosis intestinalis, or portal venous gas, which are pathognomonic signs of NEC (Con-Yost, 2005). These films are also evaluated for extravasation of air into the peritoneal space, indicative of bowel perforation. Laboratory studies reveal anemia, leucopenia, leukocytosis, metabolic acidosis, and electrolyte imbalances. NEC can lead to bowel perforation (Hockenberry, 2003; Swanson, 2004).

Prevention of NEC by withholding feedings for 24 to 48 hours is a priority in the care of neonates who have suffered birth asphyxia and in low-birth-weight infants. In cases of suspected NEC, feedings are withheld, the abdomen is decompressed with nasogastric suction, abdominal girth is measured frequently, IV antibiotics are administered, and fluid, electrolyte, and acid–base imbalances are corrected intravenously. Abdominal radiographs are done in a series to follow the course of the NEC. Should the bowel perforate, then surgical intervention is done to resect and anastomose the bowel or to create an ostomy. IV nursing specialists are key players in the treatment team of neonates and infants with NEC, providing consultation and vascular access in the form of peripheral IV or PICC for intermediate-term access.

Human Immunodeficiency Virus and Acquired Immunodeficiency Syndrome

Infants and children become infected with human immunodeficiency virus (HIV) after acquiring HIV in utero, via breast-feeding, direct contact with infected blood by exposure from parent, sexual contact, drug use, or other exposure. In the United States, HIV type I is the responsible agent for causing acquired immunodeficiency syndrome (AIDS) in children (Hockenberry, 2003). HIV infects the CD4 T lymphocytes, suppressing cell-mediated immunity, and also causes dysfunction of the B lymphocytes, suppressing humoral immunity. An infant infected with maternal HIV may show symptoms in the first 18 months of life, whereas older children may take longer to exhibit symptoms after initial infection.

Common clinical signs include lymphadenopathy, hepatosplenomegaly, oral thrush, failure to thrive, diarrhea, and parotitis. Specific illnesses that define AIDS and are commonly seen in American children include opportunistic infections such as *Pneumocystis carinii* pneumonia, lymphoid interstitial pneumonitis, as well as neurologic involvement, such as developmental delay and encephalitis (Hockenberry, 2003; Swanson, 2004). Although Kaposi's sarcoma is commonly seen in adults with AIDS, children with AIDS rarely develop this disorder (Hockenberry, 2003).

Diagnosis is determined by clinical examination as well as HIV enzyme-linked immunosorbent assay (ELISA) and Western blot immunoassay for infants >18 months. Prior to that time, persistent maternal antibodies cause these tests to be positive, and other diagnostic tests are done. CD4 lymphocyte counts <200 cells/μL in a child >18 months of age is considered diagnostic (Hockenberry, 2003; Swanson, 2004).

The treatment goals are as follows:

- Slowing the viral growth using antiretroviral agents
- Promoting or restoring normal growth and development with nutritional support and other therapies
- Preventing infection by administration of intravenous gamma globulin
- Treating infections with oral and intravenous antibacterial, antiviral, and antifungal agents
- Educating patients to prevent spread of the virus, particularly in adolescents with high-risk behaviors.

As in other chronic disorders, a team approach in a pediatric center skilled at caring for infants and children with HIV and AIDS is vital.

Hemophilia

Hemophilia is the term used to describe a group of inherited coagulation disorders that occurs when one or more coagulation proteins are missing or malfunction. Deficiency of factor VIII, often called hemophilia A or classic hemophilia, is the most common factor deficiency, followed by hemophilia B (Christmas disease or factor IX deficiency), and hemophilia C, or factor XI deficiency (Swanson, 2003). Hemophilia, transmitted as an X-linked recessive disorder, commonly appears in males and is transmitted by females.

Diagnosis is often made by eliciting a history of bleeding disorders or prolonged bleeding. Laboratory testing includes tests for hemostasis as well as specific clotting factor assays. In hemophilia, platelet function tests such as platelet counts and bleeding time will be normal, whereas factor assays may be abnormal.

Malfunction or absence of these coagulation factors result in a tendency to have prolonged bleeding, especially following tooth loss, trauma or surgery, and menstruation. Bleeding can manifest itself as subcutaneous, intramuscular, hemarthrosis, hematuria, and epistaxis.

Treatment consists of local and topical therapies to the affected area, such as ice, elevation, rest, splinting, pressure bandage wrapping, and so on. The primary therapy is replacing clotting factors intravenously (recombinant factors VIII or IX), or administering drugs that stimulate release of clotting factors (desmopressin acetate) or prevent clot destruction (aminocaproic acid [Amicar]) (Hockenberry, 2003; Swanson, 2004). Patients may require long-term intravenous access, such as an implanted central port, for therapy. Parents often give therapies at home when an episode of bleeding occurs. In addition, patients will receive prophylactic treatment prior to dental work and surgical procedures. Other goals of treatment include maintaining mobility and physical fitness while preventing long-term injuries. Gene therapy holds promise for the future.

Childhood Cancers and Antineoplastic Therapy

Because of research, new drug combinations, and aggressive therapy, the mortality rate for children with cancer has decreased greatly since the 1960s. Still, cancer remains the primary cause of death from disease in children between the ages of 1 and 14 years (Bertolone, 1997). Common cancers in children include leukemias, neuroblastoma, Wilms' tumor, rhabdomyosarcoma, lymphoma, retinoblastoma, Hodgkin's disease, and brain tumors. Many of these cancers are now curable (Bertolone, 1997). The suspected causes of cancers in children are multiple, including genetic factors, environmental (toxins, chemical agents), infectious agents, chemotherapeutic agents, and myeloproliferative disorders (Swanson, 2004).

LEUKEMIAS

Leukemia occurs when immature white blood cells proliferate in the bone marrow, spleen, and lymphatic tissue, causing symptoms such as anemia, bone or joint pain, anorexia, fever, abdominal pain, hepatosplenomegaly, tachycardia, heat and exercise intolerance, ecchymosis, and other signs of abnormal clotting, general malaise, and pallor. The two most frequently seen forms of childhood leukemia are acute lymphocytic leukemia [ALL] and acute myelocytic leukemia [AML], with ALL being more common (Swanson, 2003). Subtypes of these leukemias are recognized and somewhat related to prognosis.

History and physical manifestations, along with a blood count containing immature leukocytes, are the most common suspicious hallmarks of leukemia. The child is often referred to a tertiary oncology center after these initial findings. Subsequent bone marrow aspiration or biopsy confirms diagnosis.

Treatment of leukemia involves chemotherapy intravenously and by other routes, with or without radiation therapy. Other options include bone marrow transplantation. Owing to the intense therapy requiring reliable IV access for infusion of chemotherapy and blood sampling, a central catheter, such as a tunneled central line or an implanted port, is usually inserted in patients with leukemia.

WILMS TUMOR

Wilms tumor or nephroblastoma arises from the renal parenchyma and is the most common intra-abdominal and kidney tumor of children, accounting for 6% of childhood cancers (Hockenberry, 2003; Swanson, 2004). Most patients are younger than 5 years old at diagnosis, with peak incidence of occurrence at 3 to 4 years of age (Hockenberry, 2003). Wilms tumor is associated with other congenital anomalies, such as hypospadias. This solid tumor originates from renoblast cells in the kidney's parenchyma and may be large enough to extend across the midline, causing obstruction and pressure on other abdominal organs and structures (Swanson, 2004).

Wilms tumor often presents as a firm, nontender, one-sided mass and may be found on routine physical exam or by a caregiver during routine child care. Other symptoms include pain, fever, malaise, hematuria, anemia, hypertension, and if metastases to the lungs has occurred, respiratory symptoms such as cough, shortness of breath, or chest pain may be evident. In addition to metastasizing to the lungs, Wilms tumors can also metastasize to the liver and retroperitoneal lymph nodes via the bloodstream and lymph system; therefore, the tumor is not palpated as seeding may occur.

Surgical removal of the tumor and possible nephrectomy is performed, at which time the tumor is staged to determine the treatment plan and prognosis. Chemotherapy is indicated for all stages of Wilms tumor, whereas radiation is indicated for children with large tumors, metastasis, residual disease at the primary site, unfavorable histology, or recurrence. Survival rates are one of the highest for all childhood cancers (Hockenberry, 2003).

NEUROBLASTOMA

Neuroblastomas originate from neural crest cells and are the most common solid tumors, except for cranial tumors, in children. Neuroblastomas often arise from the adrenal medulla and sympathetic nervous system and may be present wherever sympathetic nervous system tissue is found, such as the abdomen, adrenal gland, or paraspinal ganglia (Swanson, 2004). Three fourths of the cases occur in children younger than 4 years of age, with half the cases in children younger than 2 years of age (Hockenberry, 2003). Of interest is that neuroblastomas occasionally will spontaneously regress into benign form.

Presenting symptoms are often owing to metastatic invasion of retrobulbar soft tissue and include supraorbital ecchymoses, periorbital edema, and proptosis. Clinical manifestations directly related to the primary tumor include a palpable abdominal mass that crosses the midline, lymphadenopathy, edema, pain and weakness in lower extremities from vascular compression, sensory loss, and loss of sphincter control (Hockenberry, 2003; Swanson, 2004). Diagnostic tests include radiographic and nuclear scans, bone marrow biopsy, and testing for urine catecholamines.

Treatment of neuroblastoma is based on the International Neuroma Staging System and is variable depending on age and presentation. Therefore, treatment can consist of a wide range of options, from no treatment to surgical resection only, to the full gamut of surgical resection, chemotherapy, radiation therapy, bone marrow transplant, and immunotherapy. Survival rates for children with neuroblastoma range from 75% for children <1 year to 50% for children >1 year of age (Hockenberry, 2003; Swanson, 2004).

TREATMENT OF CANCERS

The health care team that works with children who have cancer includes physicians, clinical nurse specialists, staff nurses, social workers, child-life therapists, pharmacists, surgeons, and home IV and hospice to supportive care or palliative care nurses. Childhood cancer is treated with a combination of surgery, radiation, chemotherapy, and biotherapy. Children are usually randomized to be treated according to certain protocols, which are the subject of widespread, ongoing, multicenter research studies in the Children's Oncology Group (COG). Treatment in a center belonging to this group ensures access to state-of-the-art treatment protocols based on ongoing cooperative data collection.

Because of efficacious absorption, the IV route is used to administer most antineoplastic or anticancer chemotherapy drugs required for treating childhood cancers. Many more IV protocols are designed for the child with cancer compared with the adult, primarily because many types of cancer are unique to children (eg, Wilms' tumor, neuroblastoma, retinoblastoma). Precision in regulating the specific IV chemotherapy along with monitoring IV clearance is crucial because of the incremental risk of fluid overload, electrolyte imbalances, and chemotherapy side effects. The aggressive therapy usually requires adequate long-term IV access because attempts to administer a vesicant drug by peripheral IV in an agitated child can result in extravasation injury to the child and occupational exposure to a toxic drug for the nurse. Many children with cancer benefit from the flexibility of single- or double-lumen, nontunneled, tunneled, or implanted central access devices (Callahan & De La Cruz, 2004). The function of various antineoplastic agents and administration guidelines is discussed in Chapter 19; a listing of antineoplastic agents is provided in Table 21–5.

Biliary Atresia

Cells within the liver secrete bile, which is made up of cholesterol, bile salts, and waste products, including bilirubin. Biliary atresia, a progressive inflammatory

Table 21–5   Antineoplastic Agents Used for Pediatric Patients

Category	Drugs
Alkylating agent	Busulfan Carboplatin Cisplatin Ifosfamide
Nitrogen mustard	Chlorambucil Cyclophosphamide Mechlorethamine hydrochloride Melphalan
Nitrosourea	Carmustine Lomustine
Antibiotic	Bleomycin sulfate Dactinomycin Daunorubicin hydrochloride Doxorubicin hydrochloride Idarubicin hydrochloride Mithramycin Mitomycin Streptozocin
Antimetabolite	Cytarabine hydrochloride Fluorouracil Mercaptopurine Methotrexate Thioguanine
Hormone	Leuprolide acetate
Mitotic Inhibitor	Etoposide phosphate Vinblastine sulfate Vincristine sulfate
Purine	Mercaptopurine
Miscellaneous	Asparaginase Dacarbazine Hydroxyurea Pegaspargase Procarbazine hydrochloride

(Adapted from Jew, R. [2000–2001].)

process that begins very soon after birth, is the congenital absence or closure of the ducts that drain bile from the liver. In the most common form, called *extrahepatic biliary atresia*, the delicate ducts outside the liver are affected initially. Leukocytes invade the ducts, which become damaged and necrose. Bile, trapped inside the ducts, liver, and gall bladder, rapidly causes damage and scarring, progressing to the intrahepatic ducts and cells of the liver. Further scarring of the liver tissue may result in biliary cirrhosis. On average, there is one case of biliary atresia out of every 10,000 live births. Females are affected slightly more often than males (Swanson, 2004).

The cause of biliary atresia is unknown. Autoimmune mechanisms, obstruction, inflammation, intrauterine insult, or viral infection have all been theorized as being responsible for this progressive process. About 10% of cases have other associated congenital defects in the heart, blood vessels, intestine, or spleen.

Diagnosis of biliary atresia is done via history, clinical presentation, and testing. The usual history is a full-term infant who appears normal at birth but develops jaundice after the age of 2 to 3 weeks, with yellow sclera and skin, light-colored stools, and dark urine caused by the buildup of bilirubin in the blood. Adequate bile flow is needed for the digestion and absorption of dietary fats and fat-soluble vitamins, including vitamins A, D, E, and K. When bile flow is reduced, poor growth and malnutrition may result. Special formulas containing medium-chain triglycerides (an easily digested form of dietary fat), and water-soluble vitamin supplements are often prescribed to maximize the child's growth and development. The abdomen may be swollen with a firm, enlarged liver. Weight loss and irritability develop as the level of jaundice increases; ascites and pressure make it difficult to eat, and long-term IV access, such as a tunneled catheter, may be necessary to provide parenteral nutrition (Hockenberry, 2003; Swanson, 2004). Laboratory and radiographic tests that rule out other possible causes of jaundice and diagnose biliary atresia include the following:

- Liver function tests
- Bilirubin level
- Ultrasound of the gall bladder, which may show absent or abnormally small gall bladder
- Dimethyl iminodiacetic acid (HIDA) scan, a test in which dye is injected intravenously; with biliary atresia; the dye is taken up by the liver, but cannot flow through the damaged biliary system to the small intestine
- Liver biopsy, which will also require IV access for sedation
- Surgical exploration of the baby's abdomen may be necessary.

Once the diagnosis is confirmed, the preferred treatment is to surgically remove the atretic biliary ducts outside the liver and attach the small intestine directly to the liver at the spot where bile is found or expected to drain. The segment of intestine that connects to the liver also connects to the rest of the intestine and forms a Y connection called a Roux-en-Y hepatoportojejunostomy, or Kasai procedure.

Early diagnosis of this disease is very important. If surgery is performed before the baby is 2 months old, success is much more likely. Survival without treatment is <2 years (Swanson, 2004). For this reason, all infants who are jaundiced after the age of 4 weeks should be evaluated for biliary atresia. About 20% of infants will not be helped by the Kasai procedure. In these cases, the only other treatment option is a liver transplant. Liver transplantation plays an important role in the long-term treatment of biliary atresia. Pediatric liver transplantation has evolved into a highly successful therapy and now offers significant hope for all children born with biliary atresia.

Infusion Therapies for Neonates and Children

Fluid Therapy

Fluids are delivered through a peripheral or central IV device by gravity using a volume-control chamber or, for more accuracy, through an electronic infusion device. For fluid therapy that is short lived and can be advanced quickly to oral rehydration therapy, a peripheral catheter is usually the device of choice. If hypertonic solution or chronic fluid therapy is indicated, a central access device may be recommended. Accurate intake requires precision in IV administration. Delivery of a constant flow of IV fluids is paramount. Even the smallest error can cause serious problems, especially in the compromised child. If the child's fluid requirements are not met, a number of physiologic and metabolic problems may ensue, including weight loss associated with hyperosmolality, hypernatremia, and increased hematocrit, as well as evidence of metabolic acidosis, dehydration, and, frequently in infants, multiple apnea spells and increased bilirubin.

ASSESSING FLUID NEEDS

At what rate should IV fluids be administered to a child? The child's stature and metabolic rate determine the answer. The amount of fluid required for maintenance levels depends on insensible water losses from the lungs, skin, urine, and stools and from metabolic expenditures based on both internal and external stress levels. The younger the child, the greater his or her fluid requirements because he or she has a higher percentage of total body water. In general, rates for pediatric patients vary from 5 to 80 mL/hour, depending on the child's size. Requirements vary among term, low-birth-weight, and premature, high-risk infants. Adolescent fluid requirements are similar to those for adults, ranging from 100 to 175 mL/hour.

A precise record of intake and output is the most valuable assessment tool for determining fluid requirements. To ensure accuracy in judging fluid needs, intake and output, including diaper weights, are monitored strictly for children receiving IV therapy. Infants have a greater urine volume per kilogram of body weight and a smaller bladder volume capacity than older children. Expected urine output with adequate intake should be 2 to 3 mL/kg/hour for infants, 2 mL/kg/hour for toddlers, 1 to 2 mL/kg/hour for school-age children, and 0.5 to 1 mL/kg/hour for adolescents (Hockenberry, 2003). Expected urine output for children and adolescents is 1.0 mL/kg/hour.

MAINTENANCE REQUIREMENTS

Maintenance fluid requirements for neonates and children differ in terms of the volume allowed over 24 hours, but all fluid needs are calculated in milliliters per kilogram of weight (Holiday & Segar, 1957; Table 21–6). Familiarity with three different methods of assessing 24-hour maintenance fluids is crucial: namely, the meters-squared, caloric, and weight methods (Graef & Cone, 1977). These methods address only maintenance requirements for normal metabolism; they do not address

TABLE 21–6 Formula for Calculating Maintenance Fluid Requirements

Newborn	60–100 mL/kg/24 h (used up to 72 h of age)
0–10 kg	100 mL/kg/24 h for the first 10 kg
11–20 kg	100 mL/kg/24 h for the first 10 kg, PLUS 50 mL/kg/24 h for each kilogram >10 kg
21–30 kg	100 mL/kg/24 h for the second 10 kg, PLUS 50 mL/kg/24 h for each kilogram >10 kg, PLUS 20 mL/kg/24 h for each kilogram >20 kg

Examples

A 6-kg infant would receive 600 mL divided by 24 h: 6 kg × 100 mL/kg = 600 mL over 24 h

A 32-kg child would receive 1,740 mL divided by 24 h:
  10 kg × 100 mL/kg = 1,000 mL, PLUS
  10 kg × 50 mL/kg =   500 mL, PLUS
  <u>12 kg × 20 mL/kg =   240 mL</u>
  32 kg   1,740 mL over 24 h

insensible losses or additional metabolic expenditures that require further replacement therapy.

1. In the meters-squared method, the child's height and weight are plotted on a nomogram to obtain a surface area in meters squared (m^2). This method uses an arbitrary estimated requirement of 1,500 to 1,800 mL of fluid per square meter. The advantage of this method is its simplicity; its disadvantage is the need for an accessible visual nomogram.
2. In the weight method, fluid needs are estimated based on the child's weight in kilograms. The advantage of this method also is its simplicity; its disadvantage is its decreased accuracy in patients who weigh more than 10 kg.
3. In the caloric method, usual fluid expenditure is calculated at approximately 150 mL for every 100 calories metabolized. This method, too, is simple, but not totally accurate unless actual calorie requirements and energy intake are assessed continuously. This method is the most frequently used to calculate fluid requirements.

Pharmacology

Multiple-drug therapy is routine for today's highly acute pediatric patient. Drugs administered through IV therapy include antibiotics, antivirals, and antifungals for such conditions as cystic fibrosis, meningitis, osteomyelitis, Lyme disease, joint infections, prophylaxis before and after abdominal surgery, bacterial and fungal central line infections, and systemic herpes infection. The most common pediatric disorder requiring antibiotic therapy is sepsis. Length of antibiotic therapy differs according to diagnosis, so choice of IV device is based on those factors as well as the child's vein availability. For short-term therapy (1 to 2 weeks), a peripheral IV may suffice, whereas for longer than 2 weeks, a midline catheter or PICC may be indicated (Frey, 1995; Schuman, 1990).

In addition, many IV medications used in adults are used in children. These medication categories include but are not limited to the following:

- Analgesics, such as morphine sulfate
- Antiarrhythmic agents, such as adenosine (Adenocard)
- Anticoagulants, such as heparin sodium (Liquaemin)
- Anticonvulsants, such as phenytoin (Dilantin)
- Antiemetics, such as ondansetron (Zofran)
- Chelating agents, such as deferoxamine mesylate (Desferal Mesylate)
- Corticosteroids, such as dexamethasone (Decadron, Hexadrol)
- Gastric acid inhibitors, such as ranitidine hydrochloride (Zantac)
- Vasoactive drugs, such as dopamine (Intropin) and isoproterenol (Isuprel)
- Bronchodilators, such as aminophylline
- Immunosuppressant agents, such as cyclosporine (Sandimmune)

In many cases, drugs have not yet been approved for pediatric IV administration, but are used based on ongoing and published research studies, experience with adults, and the emergency status of the child. For this reason, children often are referred to as *therapeutic orphans,* indicating the lack of information about interactions between medications and children's body processes (Hockenberry, 2003; Jew, 2000–2001).

PHARMACOKINETICS

Pharmacokinetic parameters must be considered when administering IV medications to a child. These parameters include absorption, distribution, metabolism, and excretion. Each of these is affected by the patient's level of maturity and the disease process itself (Matyskiela-Frey, 1985).

Absorption depends on adequacy of IV access and length of delivery; it usually is immediate with IV medications. Distribution occurs when a drug enters the circulatory system (it takes approximately 1 minute for blood to circulate through a child's body) and is delivered to the tissues (Holiday & Segar, 1957). Most drugs are distributed by the extracellular fluid; others are distributed by binding with protein or fat molecules.

Because neonates have less subcutaneous fat, lipid-soluble medications such as diazepam (Valium) should be given in smaller doses. The liver plays a large part in drug metabolism. In neonates with immature hepatic systems or children with liver disease, decreased liver function may alter the metabolism of such drugs as phenobarbital, phenytoin, and carbamazepine (Guyon, 1989).

PEDIATRIC DOSAGES

Dosages for pediatric patients are individualized, based on the patient's weight and metabolism. Dose and volume of medications for children can differ from those used in adults, depending on the child's age and size. Drug dosages are calculated in grams, milligrams, micrograms, units, and milliequivalents. However, a full dose of a drug may amount only to tenths of 1 mL in volume. A rule of thumb is that most drugs are packaged in single adult-sized doses, so a portion of a vial is usually needed for a child's dose. If more than two vials of a drug are needed for a single pediatric dose, calculations should be rechecked.

Before and after IV administration of certain drugs, levels of medication in the blood are tested to determine the safe dosage range for therapeutic effectiveness. These levels are known as *trough level*, or the lowest drug level drawn just before giving a scheduled dose, and *peak level*, or the highest drug level, drawn 30 minutes after the drug and postflush have infused (Korth-Bradley, 1991). Monitoring these levels and the patient's clinical status, coupled with an awareness of pharmacokinetic parameters, provides a good picture of the effects of IV medication administration in the child.

TECHNIQUES FOR MEDICATION ADMINISTRATION

One of the most frequently encountered problems with administration of medications to pediatric patients is limiting the amount of fluid used to administer and flush the drug through the IV tubing. When a child receives multiple-drug therapies, the potential to exceed fluid requirements exists. Volumes can be limited by using microbore tubing and minimal dilution volumes (Ford, Drott, & Cieplinski-Robertson, 2003).

Each method of drug administration is applicable to specific drugs and desired therapeutic outcomes. Methods of IV medication administration in children include direct IV push or bolus, continuous infusion, and intermittent infusion. Direct IV push or bolus is usually defined as an IV injection given over 5 minutes or less. Examples of IV push or bolus medications include antibiotics (eg, ampicillin), anticonvulsants (eg, phenytoin), sedatives (eg, midazolam), and antineoplastic drugs (eg, vincristine). The IV push or bolus method is used when therapeutic serum levels are needed quickly to achieve the desired effect, whether it be a high serum level of an antibiotic, cessation of seizure activity, or sedation for a procedure. Not all medications can be given in this manner because of local and systemic effects, such as phlebitis, cardiac dysrhythmias, hypotension, or anaphylaxis. The nurse administering an IV push or bolus dose must administer the drug at a certain rate and dilution, which usually is specified in drug references, and monitor the child closely to avoid adverse effects.

Continuous infusions are used primarily for administration of drugs that require maintenance of a steady blood level, or of potent drugs that must be highly titrated to individual needs. Intermittent infusions are used mainly for antimicrobials. They can be administered by several different methods:

- Calibrated chamber
- Retrograde
- Syringe pump
- Individual pump

The in-line calibrated chamber is used commonly in general pediatric settings. Medication is injected into the in-line calibrated chamber and infused at a prescribed rate. Once the infusion is complete, the usual practice is to flush the chamber and tubing with a volume of IV solution compatible with the medication, such as 5% dextrose in water or 0.9% sodium chloride. Recent literature demonstrates that using two times the volume of the dead space of the IV tubing is most efficacious in delivering the full dose of medication (Ford et al., 2003). The advantage of this method is its simplicity; however, in neonates, the tubing volume may be too large for the child's fluid needs.

Retrograde infusion is practiced mainly in the neonatal intensive care units. A specific retrograde administration set, with a volume of <1 mL, is required for this purpose. A three-way stopcock or access port is at each end of the tubing. To administer medications through the system, a medication-filled syringe is attached to the port most proximal to the patient, and an empty syringe is connected to the port most distal from the patient. The clamp between the port and the child is closed, and the medication is injected distally up the tubing (away from the child). The fluid in the retrograde tubing is displaced upward in the tubing into the empty syringe. Both syringes are removed, the lower clamp is opened, and the medication is then infused into the patient at the prescribed rate. The medication volume is then automatically incorporated into the regulated amount of fluid to be infused. This method is often used in infants or children who cannot tolerate a rapid infusion rate or additional fluid volume. This method has been replaced in many neonatal and pediatric units with the syringe pump.

An increasingly popular and accurate method of IV medication administration in children is the syringe pump. The syringe pump can be connected by an extension set directly onto a heparin lock or in a piggyback fashion into the primary line. A syringe of diluted medication, prefilled by the pharmacy or by the nurse caring for the patient, is attached to microbore tubing, and the medication can then be infused at a prescribed rate.

This system of IV medication infusion is very popular in home care. Individual patient doses may be premixed by the home care pharmacy in an elastomeric infusion pump or other single-use device. After administration of the dose, the disposable pumps are either returned to the home care pharmacy or discarded. Individual dosing systems provide premixed diluted drug doses that are easy for the caregiver or patient to administer.

EMERGENCY INTRAVENOUS MEDICATION ADMINISTRATION

Of great concern to many practitioners is correct administration of IV medications given to a child during advanced life support. These medications are administered by weight, age, or both; patient length also has been used to determine weight with a high degree of accuracy (Hockenberry, 2003). Some institutions, particularly in pediatric critical care areas, use bedside charts that list the individual doses of emergency drugs for the weight of that particular child. In addition, large multidose charts listing doses of drugs and sizes of equipment used in a pediatric code may be posted in the emergency or treatment room areas. This information is extremely helpful to nursing and medical personnel who work with adult patients and are not familiar with these dosages from experience.

Although most medications are administered by peripheral or central IV, emergency medications and fluids to treat respiratory and cardiac arrest may be administered by the intraosseous (IO) route (discussed later in this chapter) if IV access cannot be obtained.

Transfusion Therapy

Although transfusion therapy is covered fully in Chapter 17, an overview of the therapeutics unique to pediatric patients is presented here. Transfusions of blood and blood components may be administered to a child through a peripheral IV for one-time or infrequent transfusion or through a central device for chronic transfusions. Because transfusion carries the risk of iron buildup, IV chelating agents are often prescribed in addition to transfusion therapy.

INDICATIONS FOR TRANSFUSION THERAPY

Indications for transfusing blood and blood products to children are similar to those described for adults in Chapter 17. In general, indications for transfusion therapy in children include acute hemorrhage, anemia, abnormal component function or component deficiency, and removal of harmful substances, such as bilirubin, during exchange transfusion. Reduction in the blood volume of a child by 30% to 40% produces clinical evidence of shock. When 20% of blood volume is lost and loss may recur, transfusion also is indicated (Nathan & Orkin, 1998). Decreased production or altered function of platelets usually results from a maternal problem or disorder (ie, prenatal aspirin intake), congenital disorder, acquired disorder (ie, idiopathic thrombocytopenic purpura [ITP]), or chemotherapy-induced thrombocytopenia.

The most common blood components given to children are packed red blood cells, platelets, and fresh frozen plasma, as well as plasma derivatives given for congenital or acquired lack or dysfunction of that component. These products are administered in milliliters per kilogram; dosages are based on the volume limits of the child and the desired therapeutic outcome. Blood products may be modified before transfusion through several methods to reduce the risk of complications in at-risk children. These modifications include irradiation, leukocyte depletion, and warming.

Irradiation reduces the ability of leukocytes to engraft in the patient and cause graft versus host disease (Cahill-Alsip & McDermott, 1996; Roth, 1997). Recipients of irradiated blood include transplant recipients, children with lymphoma or leukemia, and neonates. Leukocyte depletion, by one of several methods, reduces the risk of febrile, nonhemolytic reactions, especially in patients who have had multiple prior transfusions. Leukocyte-depleted red cells and platelets also are given to prevent alloimmunization in children who receive platelets frequently or transmission of cytomegalovirus (CMV) when CMV-negative blood products are not available. They also are given to prospective renal allograft recipients (Cahill-Alsip & McDermott, 1996). Warmed blood products, heated in a controlled system, are used in exchange transfusions, patients with cold agglutinin disease, hypothermic patients, and in those receiving large amounts of blood quickly (>1 unit every 10 minutes) (Cahill-Alsip & McDermott, 1996). Although not indicated for routine transfusion therapy, warming reduces the chance of hypothermia, dysrhythmias, and cardiac arrest in these situations.

TABLE 21–7   Blood Component Therapy for Pediatric Patients

Blood Product	Indication	Dosage/Rate
Red blood cells (packed)	Treatment of anemia without volume expansion	10 mL/kg, not to exceed 15 mL/kg at 2–5 mL/kg/h IV drip by gravity or transfusion-approved pump
Platelets	To control bleeding associated with deficiency in platelet number or function (platelet count <20,000 or <50,000 with active bleeding)	1 unit (50–70 mL)/7–10 kg body weight Run over 30 min to maximum of 4 h; IV push or drip
Fresh frozen plasma	Occasionally volume expansion in acute blood loss; to increase levels of plasma coagulation factors in children with demonstrated deficiency	Acute hemorrhage: 15–30 mL/kg as indicated Clotting deficiency: 10–15 mL/kg at 1–2 mL/min IV push or drip
Cryoprecipitate	To replace factors not present or present in inadequate amounts owing to congenital disease	1 U/5 kg not faster than 1 mL/kg/min IV push or drip
Albumin	Hypovolemia	5%: 10–20 mL/kg as fast as tolerated, usually IV push or gravity 25%: 2–4 mL/kg over 30–60 min regulated by pump

(Adapted from Cahill-Alsip, C., & McDermott, B. [1996]; National Institutes of Health. [1990].)

Indications for transfusion of platelets, plasma, and plasma components are similar to those in adults. Table 21–7 lists some parameters for blood component therapy in children.

Infusion of IV gamma globulin or IV IgG warrants specific mention because the use of this plasma derivative in children has grown substantially since the 1980s, when safe, effective IV preparations became licensed in the United States. Before that time, children with humoral immunodeficiencies were treated with intramuscular injections or infusions of plasma. The large volume of intramuscular IgG required adequate muscle mass, the procedure was uncomfortable because the injected volume was large, and IgG levels rose slowly and were maintained only for a short time before another injection was needed to help bolster infection-fighting capabilities. Larger doses of IgG can be given by the IV route, thus maintaining adequate serum levels with more convenient administration. Approved indications for IV IgG include deficiencies of the humoral immune system and ITP, and this product is being studied as a means of heightening the immune response in many other adult and pediatric disorders, such as AIDS, neonatal sepsis, and cystic fibrosis (Frey, 1991). Antibodies against specific organisms also have been developed, allowing a more specific plan of treatment, such as anti-CMV immune globulin used in transplant recipients (Stiehm, 1991).

Techniques for Pediatric Transfusion Therapy

For the first several days of life, the mother's serum is used for compatibility testing. In infants older than 1 week and those previously transfused, compatibility testing is done on the child's blood. Group O red blood cells that are Rh negative or the same Rh as the infant are used frequently. In addition, red blood cells are tested for CMV and are given to neonates only if CMV negative. The freshest cells possible are used to avoid potassium loading in infants.

Blood and blood products in children may be administered by a 24-gauge peripheral catheter in neonates and by a 24- or 22-gauge catheter in older children. As stated by Keller (1995), "A review of the literature revealed that red blood cells could safely be transfused through needles smaller than 18–20 gauge at relatively high infusion rates without increasing the risk of hemolysis." A pump capable of infusing blood is recommended for transfusion therapy in children; in neonates, blood may be prefiltered by the blood bank and then infused from a syringe on a syringe pump. Pediatricians request blood and blood products in milliliter per kilogram increments, instead of units, because a single unit of packed red blood cells may equal the entire blood volume of several infants. In children, volume and fluid balance considerations negate the simultaneous infusion of saline, particularly in neonates; instead, the peripheral or central IV device must be flushed with 1 to 3 mL saline before and after the transfusion. The rate of blood transfusion may be very slow or even staggered with boluses of dextrose in neonates. Five to 10% of red cell volume should be infused slowly over the first 15 minutes, then the rate increased to an hourly IV rate tolerated by the child (Landier, Barrell, & Styffe, 1987).

Nursing Assessment and Management

Central venous pressure is the best indicator for restoration of blood volume to normal; pulse rate is less reliable, and 24 to 36 hours may pass before hemoglobin reflects the true extent of blood loss. A red blood cell mass deficit occurs with chronic anemia; transfusion with packed cells is not indicated until the hemoglobin level drops below 6 g/dL (Nathan & Orkin, 1998). The patient's cardiopulmonary status, activity level, and hemoglobin should be assessed before transfusion because an unstressed child can tolerate hemoglobin values of 3 to 6 g/dL without showing signs of heart failure. Also, because the most common form of anemia seen in children is iron-deficiency anemia (which rarely is treated with transfusion), other treatments may be indicated, including iron therapy, folic acid, or vitamin B_{12}.

Possible Complications

As with other therapies, transfusion therapy is not without risks. Potential complications include acute hemolytic reactions, nonhemolytic reactions (eg, febrile and allergic reactions), alloimmunization, circulatory overload, citrate toxicity, infectious disease transmission, and coagulopathy (Cahill-Alsip & McDermott, 1996). The type of reaction may be difficult to ascertain initially. These reactions are discussed in more detail in Chapter 9.

Parenteral Nutrition Therapy

Parenteral nutrition (PN) is the IV administration of a balanced solution that contains all the components of a balanced diet (Bilodeau, Poons, & Mascarenhas, 1998). PN has become one of the most important therapeutic parameters in the successful management of certain pediatric diseases. PN is started earlier in children than in adults, particularly in premature neonates, in whom PN may be started at 1 to 3 days of life (Phillips, 2004). PN may be administered through a peripheral or central IV catheter depending on the strength of the solution. Indications for PN in pediatric patients include congenital or acquired gastrointestinal disorders, such as gastroschisis and Crohn's disease; respiratory diseases, such as cystic fibrosis and bronchopulmonary dysplasia; hypermetabolic states, such as major trauma and burns; and miscellaneous disorders, such as liver disease, inborn errors of metabolism, cancer, and prematurity. Although it has saved the lives of many pediatric patients, PN is not without risks. Close monitoring is necessary.

Supplemental PN, which is usually peripheral PN but may be central, does not provide all calories and nutrients. It is used as a boost to oral intake for short-term benefit. Total PN (TPN) is used for the child whose gut is not functional for congenital or acquired reasons, such as prematurity, short-bowel syndrome, Crohn's disease, acquired immunodeficiency syndrome (AIDS), or cancer. TPN is administered through some type of central access device.

Peripheral PN usually is reserved for patients who have normal nutritional status but need short-term supplemental nutrition until they can resume oral intake. Peripheral PN therapy should be limited to <2 weeks because of limitations in the amount of calories that can be delivered while still maintaining fluid balance, and difficulty in maintaining peripheral IV access (Heird, 1993). If PN is required for a longer period, central venous PN (TPN) should be prescribed.

With the addition of TPN to their therapy, affected children can be expected to gain weight normally with only parenteral nutrients. In addition, TPN supplies enough calories to maintain the positive nitrogen balance required for normal growth and development. The parameters used to determine caloric needs are age, resting energy requirements, level of physical activity, and severity of illness.

CONSTITUENTS OF PARENTERAL NUTRITION

Usually, hospital or home IV agency pharmacy staff formulate PN solutions and perform admixture of solutions under a laminar-airflow hood. The general constituents for PN are protein, carbohydrates, fat, electrolytes, minerals, trace elements, and vitamins. Pediatric requirements for IV nutrition follow general guidelines and are based on protein, calorie, and fluid needs per kilogram of body weight.

Protein is provided in the form of crystalline amino acids; in infants younger than 6 months, a special formulation of protein, based on serum aminograms of healthy 1-month-old, breast-fed, term infants, is administered (Bilodeau et al., 1998). This solution differs from adult formulations in content of amino acids. PN protein is limited in critically ill patients who have renal, liver, and protein metabolism disorders. One gram of protein should deliver at least 30 calories (Phillips, 2004).

Carbohydrates are provided as dextrose, which provides energy for body tissue function. If carbohydrate supply is inadequate, the body breaks down protein or fat to provide metabolic needs. Dextrose, administered in milligram per kilogram per minute increments, provides the main calorie source; because the dextrose in PN is in monohydrated form, it provides not 4 but 3.4 kcal/g. For example, 100 mL dextrose 5% in water solution contains 5 g dextrose, or 17 kcal; 100 mL 10% dextrose in water solution contains 10 g dextrose, or 34 kcal. The strength of dextrose that can be administered peripherally in a child is 10% to 12.5% (Bilodeau et al., 1998; Heird, 1993; Phillips, 2004). Greater concentrations given through a peripheral IV can cause sclerosis, phlebitis, and extravasation injury if infiltration occurs. Although concentrated dextrose is needed to provide calories, the volume of fluid needed to dilute very concentrated dextrose is often deleterious to fluid balance in children, especially neonates. Higher concentrations of dextrose (up to 25%) in less volume of fluid may be delivered by central catheter. Excessive carbohydrate use can result in fatty infiltration of the liver (Bilodeau et al., 1998).

The other source of nonprotein calories is lipids, delivered as a fat emulsion used to supply essential fatty acids that are needed for brain and somatic growth, immune system function, skin integrity, and wound healing. Originally, fat infusion was kept to a minimum (only 2% to 10% of daily calorie intake) because it was thought that a higher fat intake resulted in pulmonary changes. This hyperlipidemia is now thought to have been brought on by rapid infusion rates, so a slower infusion rate over a longer period is now the rule. Fat intake now comprises 30% to 40%, to a maximum of 60% of total calories required daily (Phillips, 2004). Fat emulsions come in strengths of 10%, with 1.1 kcal/mL, and 20%, with 2 kcal/mL. Both may be infused peripherally or centrally, but the 20% solution is used most often. Fats are essential for neurologic development in the infant; however, fatty acids may displace bilirubin from albumin, causing a rise in bilirubin level and an increased risk of kernicterus. In infants with hyperbilirubinemia, the lipid intake is initially 0.5 g/kg/day, increased gradually as tolerance is demonstrated (Heird, 1993).

Micronutrients, minerals, vitamins, and trace elements are added to the PN solution in amounts established for IV maintenance requirements, based on recommended dietary allowances. Because calcium, magnesium, phosphorus, and magnesium are incompletely absorbed from the gastrointestinal tract, IV dosages may exceed the recommendations for oral intake. Calcium and phosphorous may precipitate in PN solution when higher levels are prescribed; adjustment of the protein and pH level of the solution may assist in solubility. The yellow color of the TPN solution results from the addition of multivitamins. Because multivitamins limit the shelf life of TPN, patients on home TPN are taught to add vitamins and other medication additives such as heparin.

In some cases, total nutrient admixtures (TNA), in which all the nutrients are added to one bag, have been used in children. The more common practice is to infuse the dextrose/amino acid solution separately in one bag, using a 0.22-μm filter into one arm of a Y set, and to infuse the fat, unfiltered, into the other arm of the Y. If a TNA solution is used, use of a 1.5- to 5-μm in-line filter decreases the chance that an unseen precipitate will be infused. Two deaths have been reported from pulmonary emboli when TNA solutions were used (Hill, Heldman, Goo, et al., 1996).

NURSING ASSESSMENT AND MANAGEMENT

Once the child has been deemed a candidate for PN, a complete physical assessment, including height, weight, head circumference, and nutrition and laboratory evaluations, is completed. Duration and route of PN are determined, and the appropriate catheter is placed. The patient then is started on 75% to 80% of goal calories, which gradually is increased by 10% to 20% daily until the goal of the PN regimen is reached (Bilodeau et al., 1998). Infusions may run over 24 hours for the very sick hospitalized child or may be cycled down gradually by 4-hour increments daily, maintaining the same volume of infusion over less time. Cycling down to between 8 and 18 hours of daily infusion TPN allows the child far more freedom. This is particularly true for children on home TPN, who may infuse at night while asleep and still follow a fairly normal lifestyle of school and activities. Cycling the PN also may mobilize hepatic fat stores, decreasing hepatic steatosis (Bilodeau et al., 1998). Although common in adults, cycling has been shown to be safe even in infants younger than 6 months (Collier, Crouch, Hendricks, & Cacallero, 1994). Initially, when patients were cycled on and off their PN solution, it was thought that glucose would rise once the infusion began and fall once the infusion was finished. Evidence now shows that in children younger than 3 years of age receiving more than 10% dextrose solutions, PN does not need to be tapered when starting; however, when completing the cycle, the PN rate should be decreased by 50% for the last hour to prevent rebound hypoglycemia (Bendorf, Friesen, & Roberts, 1996).

The nurse frequently monitors the patient's physical status and screens, intervenes for, and reports abnormal findings: temperature spikes, inappropriate glucose spills, chills, rashes, irritability, decreased level of consciousness, and any changes in growth or clinical picture. The nurse immediately reports any observable abnormality to the nutrition team. Results of various serum chemistry and hematology tests are assessed daily for the first week and then weekly for the stable patient in the hospital or at home.

Another major area of nursing intervention in a child receiving TPN is psychologic support. Most such patients are acutely ill infants. Even though a child on central TPN may be NPO, cuddling and holding the child should assist in meeting maternal needs. Also, allowing parents and caregivers every opportunity to participate in their child's care is extremely important. First, the nurse should assess the family's level of comprehension about TPN and intervene by offering support to decrease parental anxiety. As soon as the decision is made to place a child on TPN, it is best to use the preoperative teaching methodology of explaining purpose, procedures, and potential complications. Of course, all further questions can be handled daily. Permitting this open channel of communication not only supplies parents with the knowledge they need to become involved, but also assists them in comprehending the purpose of TPN and why adherence to protocols is so important.

COMPLICATIONS

Disadvantages of TPN are its potential complications. Every nurse must fully understand the possible complications of TPN, including the specific symptoms of each. Complications are subdivided into two categories: catheter related and metabolic.

Catheter-related complications have been previously addressed. Metabolic complications include the following:

- Glucose disturbances
- Electrolyte imbalances
- Mineral disturbances
- Acid–base imbalance
- Hepatic disorders
- Metabolic bone disease
- Refeeding syndrome

Close attention to detail during the initial assessment and ongoing monitoring can treat or even prevent most of these complications. Some predisposing metabolic abnormalities, however, may require immediate medical intervention. With the incremental advances in technology and the formation of nutrition support teams, the incidences of even the more common complications have decreased to acceptable rates. See Chapter 16 for more information on nutrition support.

Intravenous Administration Equipment

Options for volume control, delivery of small doses of medication, and assurance of safety in pediatric patients include microdrip administration sets, microbore tubing, Luer-lock connections, volume-control chambers, and infusion pumps (Hockenberry, 2003). None of these devices, however, can replace close surveillance of the patient by the health care provider.

Tubing and Administration Sets

Large-bore tubing holds a great deal of volume. Attempts to deliver a small amount of medication through this type of tubing could result in delivery of too much volume to a small child. Microbore tubing is incorporated into IV administration sets and connection devices for pediatric patients.

Minimal flow rates in neonates, infants, and children necessitate proper choice of intravascular administration set. Special sets are required to avoid the possibility of medication overdose or fluid volume overload.

Microdrip administration sets for gravity infusion (60 gtt/minute) are specific for infants and children. IV tubing with an in-line calibrated volume control chamber (50-, 100-, and 150-mL sizes are available) should be used on all children whose prescribed fluid rate is less than the volume of the chamber. The calibrated chamber also is used to administer intermittent doses of medications (Hockenberry, 2003).

Because acutely ill patients often need multiple therapies, extension sets with a three-way stopcock are used frequently in critical care units. However, such stopcocks can present concerns about infection and safety. In place of stopcocks, some institutions use multiple-arm connectors with two or more arms, each with its own clamp. These connectors provide a closed system for administration of multiple infusates into one IV site. In this case, consultation with pharmacy experts regarding compatibility issues is advisable.

Containers

Plastic rather than glass solution containers should be used whenever possible to avoid breakage in case the container falls off its pole. To avoid the risk of fluid volume overload, the volume of the solution container should be based on the age and size of the child and should not contain >500 mL of fluid, unless rates exceed that limit. In premature infants and neonates, smaller solution containers should be considered (Hockenberry, 2003).

Electronic Infusion Devices

Devices that electronically control volume, rate, and, sometimes, dose, have become the norm rather than the exception in pediatric IV therapy. Electronic infusion devices with a high degree of accuracy, no free-flow capacity, ability to infuse rates from tenths of a milliliter to hundreds of milliliters, controlled pressure settings, and microbore tubing sets are available for use in neonatal and pediatric patients. Syringe pumps are often used in intensive care and medical surgical units to deliver small-volume medications accurately.

There is debate over whether the chambered IV set is required when an electronic infusion device is used. Manufacturers of electronic infusion devices claim that their product is guarded against free-flow fluid, and products that are safety tested in proven clinical trials should be chosen for neonatal and pediatric patients. In one such trial, an intensive care nursery eliminated the use of volume control chambers with electronic infusion pumps after assessing the need for this redundant volume control (Reiser, 1999).

In the home setting, single-use pressurized pumps are convenient for individual doses. Small electronic pumps that can be hidden in a backpack are often used for intermittent and continuous doses, and large-volume pumps can be used for such therapies as cycled TPN. When choosing a pump for a pediatric patient, accuracy and safety are of utmost importance. Independent consumer groups for medical devices provide excellent, unbiased reviews of these devices for the agency to consult before purchasing a pump for use in children.

Vascular Access Devices

Peripheral Intravenous Devices

Until the late 1970s, the winged infusion needle was the device of choice for short-term IV therapy and withdrawal of blood samples for laboratory analysis in pediatric patients. Then, 22-gauge catheter-over-needle devices made of plastic, then Teflon, became available and could be used for longer-lasting IV access in pediatric patients (Batton et al., 1982). Many pediatric institutions still use winged infusion

FIGURE 21–2. A 22-gauge peripheral IV safety catheter being inserted in a child prior to stylet activation. (Courtesy of A.M. Frey.)

needles for blood sampling because the vacuum withdrawal method used in adults is often too aggressive for tiny pediatric veins.

Catheter-over-needle device design has advanced to include thin-wall safety catheters (Fig. 21–2) for greater flow rates, smaller gauge (24 and 22), shorter length, and non-kinking material. Small-gauge safety catheters such as the 24 for neonates and the 24 and 22 for children and adolescents are the choice when up to 2 weeks of IV therapy is prescribed (Wickham, 1990). After 2 weeks, peripheral access sites become increasingly unavailable, and use of a longer-lasting or central device may be warranted.

Intermediate-Term Midline Intravenous Access

A midline catheter, longer than the peripheral IV of 5/8 to 2 inches, reaches the larger vessels of the upper arm, and in neonates and children the upper thigh (Lesser, Chhabra, Brion, & Suresh, 1996). These larger blood vessels are presumed to provide greater blood flow and better hemodilution of infusions. Midline catheters are available in 24- and 22-gauge sizes, with lengths of 3 to 6 inches for children. Midline catheters are still considered peripheral IV access devices and are most commonly used for 2 to 4 weeks. Their use is associated with a lower rate of complications than is the use of central lines (Kupensky, 1998).

Because the tip of a midline catheter does not extend beyond the extremity in which it is placed, radiographic confirmation of tip placement is optional and recommended only when there is difficulty in catheter insertion or flushing (INS, 2000). As with most medical equipment, adult-sized versions of these devices are tested initially, and then studies in children are undertaken. Although very few research studies or outcome data have been published regarding midlines in neonates and children, these catheters have been used to administer IV fluids, medications, and blood products. Some limited success with midline catheters has been reported. In one neonatal report, midlines lasted an average of 6.3 days, surpassing the peripheral IV duration average of 24 to 48 hours in neonates (Dawson, 2002). Complications reported in children include phlebitis, pain, erythema at the insertion site, occlusion, and dislodgment (BeVier & Rice, 1994). Varying degrees of success have been reported with use of these devices in children; more research, particularly in the pediatric population, is certainly a mission for the IV nurse. When using such catheters, manufacturers' recommendations should be followed.

Central Venous Access

When long-term or emergency IV access is desired because of unavailability of peripheral sites, or extended or even lifelong therapy is needed, central venous access is indicated. Pettit & Hughes (1999) most aptly state, "Most authors suggest that placement of a central venous catheter should be considered if parenteral therapy is needed for more than a few weeks or long-term, if PN requiring 12.5% dextrose or greater becomes necessary, if an infant requires more than two IV starts a day, or if vesicants are being infused." Many types of central IV access devices exist, including nontunneled catheters, PICCs, surgically placed cuffed tunneled catheters, totally implanted devices, and, in the neonate, umbilical venous catheters, which are considered a central access device. Umbilical venous and arterial catheters are discussed in the section on Umbilical Catheterization. Choice of device depends on the duration and type of therapy prescribed, input from the patient and family, and disease process. Although these devices are described in detail in earlier chapters, features unique to the pediatric population are outlined in the following sections.

Of concern to children and parents is catheter care, safety, cost, and body image. For instance, in toddlers, catheter dislodgment may occur easily; an infant may bite through the catheter during the teething period. A child who is extremely afraid of needles may not do well with an implanted port, which has to be accessed with a needle periodically. Conversely, an older child or adolescent may choose an implanted port over a tunneled catheter to avoid disturbance of body image. If the central device is to be used for continuous infusions or cycled daily therapies, such as TPN, a tunneled catheter, such as a Broviac, may be the best choice; if intermittent treatments are prescribed, a port might be best. Pediatric hospitals often use clinical nurse specialists who can demonstrate pros and cons of each device, assist families in their choice of venous access, introduce children with similar devices, and help decrease anxiety about insertion and care.

NONTUNNELED CENTRAL VENOUS CATHETERS

For the purposes of this chapter, nontunneled catheters include percutaneously placed femoral, jugular, and subclavian catheters. These catheters are referred to as *nontunneled* to distinguish them from longer-dwelling cuffed Silastic catheters that are surgically tunneled under the skin. In children and adults, nontunneled catheters often are used for IV access in critical situations, such as in a patient with multiple trauma or in children in the pediatric intensive care unit who need several weeks of IV access and possibly PN.

Nontunneled percutaneously placed catheters usually are short and may have from one to four lumens (Fig. 21–3). They usually are made of a stiffer material such

FIGURE 21–3. Nontunneled double-lumen catheter. (Courtesy of A.M. Frey.)

as polyurethane for easier insertion by percutaneous skin puncture. Catheter sizes range from 3 to 5 French. In children, these catheters may be inserted nonsurgically, usually by a physician, using local anesthetic and mild sedation.

Although venous anatomy is similar in all age groups, some differences in children necessitate choosing specific sites over others. The preferred sites for percutaneous placement of nontunneled central lines in children are femoral veins, internal and external jugular veins, and subclavian veins, in that order (Lavelle & Costerino, 1997). For anatomic reasons, the right side is preferred when catheterizing the internal jugular or subclavian veins.

The femoral site is the first choice in children because it has easily identifiable landmarks for catheter placement, it is easy to apply pressure to the site if needed, and its location will not hinder any cardiopulmonary resuscitation efforts (Stenzel, Green, Fuhrman, et al., 1989; Fig. 21–4). The internal and external jugular veins are chosen next. Their advantages include ease of identification of landmarks and accessibility. They also have a larger diameter, present fewer technical difficulties with catheterization, and carry fewer risks of complications than subclavian veins. The right internal jugular vein runs an almost straight course to the superior vena cava, whereas the left is more angled (Cobb, Vinocur, Wagner, & Weintraub, 1987). Use of the internal jugular vein carries a risk of carotid artery puncture; thus, it should not be used in a child with a clotting disorder. Even though it is located superficially, valves and angles in the external jugular vein make threading a catheter difficult (McGee & Mallory, 1988).

The subclavian vein is the least common site because of anatomic considerations. In infants younger than 1 year of age, higher arching of the subclavian vein causes acute angles that can obstruct placement. After 1 year of age, the subclavian arch assumes the horizontal position similar to that of the adult (Cobb et al., 1987). Curvature and softness of the chest and clavicles make landmarks difficult to identify,

FIGURE 21–4. Double-lumen nontunneled right femoral catheter in multiple-trauma patient in pediatric intensive care unit. (Courtesy of A.M. Frey.)

and the apices of the lungs are higher in children. Subclavian catheter insertion in neonates is technically difficult and can result in life-threatening complications such as pneumothorax, hydrothorax, hemothorax, and massive hemorrhage (Dolcourt & Bose, 1982).

Maintenance includes daily flushing. Dressing changes should be done weekly or more often, as needed (see Table 21–8).

Catheter stiffness, high incidence of thrombus, and easy dislodgment limit use of these catheters to a relatively short period, ranging from a few days to 4 weeks (Viall, 1990). Catheters placed in jugular and femoral locations may be occluded because infants tend to have a shortened neck and frequently adduct their legs, causing kinking in the catheter placed in the neck or groin. The femoral location is also the diaper area, and the dressing may become soiled frequently and exposed to infective organisms prevalent in this region. These factors, in addition to potential for air embolism, also limit use of this device for home infusion, particularly in younger children. Contraindications to percutaneous insertion of a nontunneled central line include vascular abnormality or disease in the involved extremity, skin compromise or injury at the proposed entry site, presence of a clotting disorder, or a treatment plan requiring a different type of device.

PERIPHERALLY INSERTED CENTRAL CATHETERS

A PICC is defined as a catheter inserted into a peripheral vein, usually of the arm or leg, with the tip residing in the superior or inferior vena cava (INS, 2000). Published reports from the 1970s and 1980s mainly described two purposes for the use of PICCs in neonates and children: provision of PN in neonates (Dolcourt & Bose, 1982; Filston & Johnson, 1971; Loeff, Matlak, Black, Overall, Dolcourt, & Johnson, 1982; Shaw, 1973; Sherman, Vitale, McLaughlin, & Goetzman, 1982) and provision of several weeks of IV antibiotics in children with cystic fibrosis (Dietrich & Lobas, 1988; Williams et al., 1988; Zanni, Shutack, Schuler, Christie, & Holsclaw, 1985). Before reports of PICC use in neonates and children, central venous access was accomplished using a medical or

TABLE 21–8 Routine Care and Maintenance of Pediatric Intravenous Access Devices

Device	Patency	Dressing	Connector Tubing/ Cap Change	Comments
Peripheral IV	• 1 mL of 10 U/mL heparinized saline q8h or after each medication infusion • Consider saline flushes for catheters 22 gauge and larger or for intervals of q4h or more often • Use benzyl alcohol–free flushes for neonates	• Transparent • Changed only with site change	• Connector tubing changed when site is changed or if compromised • Cap changed if removed or compromised	• Inexpensive • Maximum dwell: 6 d, according to latest research • May be placed for frequent blood samples (for tests requiring that samples be taken every 15 min to q4–6h)
Peripherally inserted central catheter (PICC)	• 2 mL of 10–100 U/mL heparinized saline q12–24h • For any age child with one or more medication doses daily, use 10 U/mL. • If more than one lumen, flush each lumen as needed.	• Initially: transparent dressing over gauze, changed in 48 h to transparent only • Second dressing is not changed on PICCs unless loose, soiled, wet, compromised • Steri-Strips not changed unless very soiled	• T-connector tubing considered part of catheter if placed aseptically during insertion procedure • Not changed unless compromised • Cap changed weekly, if removed, or if compromised	• Moderately inexpensive • Used for intermediate-term therapies, but no dwell limit set • Can clot, dislodge, or break if care not taken • 3 French or larger may be used for blood sampling; discard volume = 3 × that of device and attached tubings or ~2 mL.
Nontunneled catheter Jugular Subclavian Femoral	• 2 mL of 10–100 U/mL heparinized saline q12–24h • For child of any age with one or more medication doses daily, use 10 U/mL • If more than one lumen, flush each lumen as needed	• Initially: transparent dressing over gauze, changed in 48 h to transparent only, then weekly dressing change or if loose, soiled, wet, compromised	• T-connector tubing not used • Cap changed weekly, if removed, or if compromised	• Short-term catheter placed in emergencies, traumas, intensive care unit • High infection rate, especially with femoral site • May have one, two, or three lumens

(Continued)

TABLE 21-8 Routine Care and Maintenance of Pediatric Intravenous Access Devices *(Continued)*

Device	Patency	Dressing	Connector Tubing/ Cap Change	Comments
Tunneled catheter (Broviac)	• 2 mL of 10–100 U/mL heparinized saline q12–24h • For child of any age with one or more medication doses daily, use 10 U/mL	• Initially: transparent dressing over gauze, changed in 48 h to transparent only, then weekly dressing change or if loose, soiled, wet, compromised	• Connector tubing not usually used • Cap changed weekly, if removed, or if compromised	• Long-term catheter placed for months to years of therapy • Expensive to place and maintain, prone to infection, breakage, clotting • May be used for blood sampling; discard volume = 3 × that of device or ~1–4 mL
Implanted port	• 2 mL of 10 U/mL heparinized saline for child of any age with one or more medication doses daily • At discharge and monthly: use 5 mL of 100 U/mL heparinized saline flush	• Use noncoring needle in 22- to 20-gauge, ½–1½ in. • Initial septum access while child sedated during insertion of port if port is being used after • Pad under needle wings with gauze • Dressing change with needle change weekly	• Connector tubing already attached to noncoring needle set • Cap change with weekly needle change or if removed or compromised	• Long-term device placed for years of therapy, especially in larger children and adolescents needing intermittent treatments • May be used for blood sampling; discard volume = 3 × that of device or ~3 mL for small arm port, or 5–7 mL for larger chest port

FIGURE 21–5.   Two types of central venous catheters: **(left)** double-lumen tunneled catheter with fixating cuff *(arrow)*; **(right)** 3 French single-lumen PICC. (Courtesy of A.M. Frey.)

surgical procedure to place a nontunneled, tunneled, or implanted device or an umbilical catheter in neonates. The development of smaller, easier to insert, more biocompatible catheters resulted in renewed interest in the PICC as a central access device in neonates and children ensued (Frey, 1995; Weeks-Lozano, 1991).

Pediatric-sized PICCs are manufactured of polyurethane, or softer Silastic material shown to have low incidence of irritation and thrombus formation, allowing PICCs to remain in place for months to years (CDC, 2002). Catheter size should be chosen according to vein size and availability and prescribed treatment plan. Appropriate PICC sizes for children, from the smallest to largest, include:

- Single-lumen devices
- 28-gauge neonatal size
- 2 French (23 gauge)
- 3 French (20 gauge)
- 4 French (18 gauge)
- Double-lumen PICCs
- 3.5 French (18 gauge) to 5 French (16 gauge; Fig. 21–5)

Insertion can be done without general anesthesia. PICCs may be inserted in children in the hospital, outpatient, or home setting. Restraint and use of local anesthetic or conscious sedation may provide for easier insertion (Doellman, 2004). Ultrasound, once a tool used only by radiologists, now has become smaller and more portable and is being used increasingly by nurses, as well as radiologists, to locate veins suitable for PICC placement in pediatric and neonatal patients (Donaldson, 1995).

Insertion of PICCs is similar in adults and children, although a child may be more anxious and less likely to cooperate. The PICC may be inserted in neonates and children by one of four methods:

1. Winged steel needle—used as prototype for later PICCs and in neonates (Dolcourt & Bose, 1982; Loeff et al., 1982; Sherman et al., 1982).

2. Winged breakaway metal introducer needle—less popular than methods 3 and 4 below because of the potential for catheter shear (Chathas, et al., 1986; Frey, 1995).

3. Peel-away IV catheter—very popular method because of the ease of use, and most similar to insertion of a peripheral IV catheter, with which many nurses are familiar (BeVier & Rice, 1994; Frey, 1995; Thiagarajan, Ramamoorthy, Gettemann, & Bratton, 1997).

4. Modified or unmodified Seldinger technique—the latter method is becoming increasingly popular because the inserter is able to place a larger-gauge catheter using a small-gauge introducer needle or catheter (Frey, 2002).

In neonates, PICCs are inserted into the veins of the antecubital fossa, as well as the axillary, saphenous, popliteal, and external jugular veins (Chathas, 1986; Fig. 21–6). In older children, the median cubital basilic, basilic, and cephalic veins in the antecubital fossa, or slightly above or below this site, are ideal (Fig. 21–7).

Maintenance of PICC catheters in pediatric patients includes dressing care, maintenance of patency, changing of end caps, site protection, and avoidance of complications (Table 21–8). Care must be taken to avoid undue pressures when flushing these small catheters, and flush never should be forced if resistance is felt (Hadaway, 1998). In addition, rapid injectors used in radiology are avoided with PICCs because the catheter may rupture (Kaste & Young, 1996; Rivitz & Drucker, 1997; Ruess, Bulas, Riveera, & Markle, 1997).

Although PICCs are associated with fewer complications than surgically placed catheters, PICC use in neonates and children is not without complications, some of which can be severe or fatal (Clarke & Reddy, 1979). Major complications in neonates with PICCs include mechanical complications (10% to 40%), especially catheter occlusion. Catheter-related bloodstream infection was the next most frequent

FIGURE 21–6.   A 2 French (23-gauge) PICC in place, with dressing on site. Patient is receiving prostaglandin infusion through the PICC. (Courtesy of A.M. Frey.)

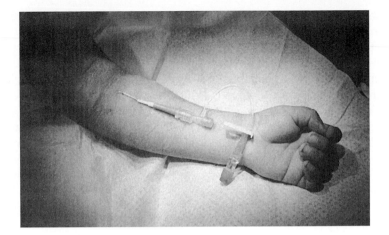

FIGURE 21–7.   A 3 French (20-gauge) Silastic PICC in place, prior to dressing application, in left median cubital basilic vein of a 3-year-old for TPN after repeat surgery for Hirschsprung's disease. (Courtesy of A.M. Frey.)

reported complication in neonates (0% to 19.1%; Chathas, Paton, & Fisher, 1990; Oellrich, Murphy, Goldberg, & Aggarwal, 1991; Trotter, 1996). In reports of mixed neonatal/pediatric and pediatric/adult PICC programs, complications, noted from most commonly reported to least, were occlusion, pain/phlebitis, dislodgment, and catheter fracture. The rate of catheter-related bloodstream infection in older children is low (0.8% to 8%) compared with neonates (Frey, 1999). Research is still lacking on the best type of PICC materials, best methods of care, duration of dwell, securement, and other practices, although more studies are being published about PICCs in children.

TUNNELED CENTRAL VENOUS CATHETERS

Tunneled catheters are most often chosen for long-term venous access, as are implanted ports, which are discussed in the next section. In the early 1970s, Broviac developed the first tunneled catheter for patients who required long-term TPN (Broviac, Cole, & Schribner, 1973). Broviac catheters have since become a popular choice when long-term central IV access is needed, such as with children who have cancer. The Groshong catheter with a valved internal tip, developed in the 1980s, also is tunneled, but is made of thinner-walled silicone than the Broviac (Wickham, 1990).

Single- and double-lumen Broviacs and single- and double-lumen Groshongs are used in children; the triple-lumen devices tend to be somewhat large for pediatric use. Both catheters contain a Dacron polyester cuff that anchors the catheter in place subcutaneously several weeks after insertion (Camp-Sorrell, 1990; Fig. 21–5). Both catheters have a Luer-locking proximal hub or hubs outside the patient; the Broviac has an open distal tip on the internal portion, whereas the distal tip of the Groshong is closed with a two-way slit valve. Other companies also manufacture pediatric-sized tunneled catheters.

If no contraindications to general anesthesia exist, tunneled catheters are often inserted in the operating room or radiology suite by a surgeon or interventional radiologist. Often, several procedures are coordinated with catheter insertion to avoid unnecessary trauma while the child is awake; for example, a patient newly diagnosed with leukemia may have one visit to the operating room for Broviac insertion, bone marrow biopsy, and lumbar puncture.

In older children, the catheter usually is inserted percutaneously into the subclavian vein. In infants and neonates, because of the small size of the subclavian vein and proximity of other structures, this approach can be extremely dangerous. Therefore, in children younger than 5 years, the catheter usually is inserted through the facial vein or the external or internal jugular vein to the superior vena cava (Fig. 21–8).

After proper placement is verified by chest radiography, subcutaneous tunneling of the catheter is done either up the parietal occipital area or down the chest wall to the fourth or fifth intercostal space, depending on the catheter type. This distal exit site from the original phlebotomy site provides a barrier against infection (Von Meyenfeldt, Stapert, De Jong, Soeters, Wesdorp, & Creep, 1980), facilitates catheter maintenance, and provides the child with full-range neck mobility.

In some children, chest access sites are not available because of many previous central lines, vein thromboses, or other surgery or complications. An alternate site for catheter placement is the femoral vein to the inferior vena cava, particularly in children younger than walking age. The proximal portion of the catheter is then tunneled under the skin of the abdomen or out onto the thigh.

FIGURE 21–8. Inserted pediatric infant-sized Broviac catheter. Note that the catheter is threaded into the external jugular to the right atrium and tunneled subcutaneously down the chest wall.

Care of tunneled catheters, detailed in Table 21–8, includes dressing changes, flushing to maintain patency, and prevention of infection, occlusion, and dislodgment. Care of tunneled catheters is continually researched, and procedures for children are based on manufacturers' guidelines, catheter volume, experience with adults, and ongoing and previously published research studies. These protocols vary among institutions and should be reviewed regularly, based on research studies and the needs of the child.

The complications most frequently reported for tunneled catheters in children include infection, with the highest risk in the first 100 days of use, and mechanical complications, such as occlusion and dislodgment. Toddlers exhibit the highest rate of complications (Wiener & Albanese, 1998).

Tunneled catheter infection rates can range from 5% to 31.6% and should be reported in terms of rate per 1,000 catheter days to maintain consistency of data (Decker & Edwards, 1988). The most common infectious organisms reported include coagulase-negative *Staphylococcus*, coagulase-positive *Staphylococcus, Pseudomonas, Escherichia coli, Candida,* and *Enterococcus* (CDC, 2000). In the past, tunneled catheters were removed when catheter-related bloodstream infection was suspected. However, more recent studies have shown promising results in treating infected tunneled catheters and implanted ports in children with a combination of antibiotics and urokinase. In a 1998 publication, Jones concluded that "catheter-related infections, including bacteremia and exit site, tunnel, and pocket infections, can be treated in many cases without removal of the device."

Occlusion may be mechanical, thrombotic, or nonthrombotic. Mechanical occlusions may be evaluated by assessing the catheter for kinking or clamping, repositioning the child, and further assessing as needed using dye studies. Thrombotic occlusions may be corrected with tissue plasminogen activator (TPA); nonthrombotic occlusions are treated with hydrochloric acid, ethanol, or sodium bicarbonate, depending on the cause and pH of the occlusion (Jacobs, 2003; Ruble, Long, & Connor, 1994). Dislodgment may be prevented by carefully looping the external "tail" of the catheter under the dressing or taping it to the chest. Children of all age groups who have tunneled catheters should wear T shirts to prevent inadvertent catheter trauma. If breakage occurs, a permanent splicing procedure can be accomplished using a manufacturer's repair kit that matches the broken segment of the tunneled catheter (Viall, 1990).

Because of the complications possible with tunneled catheters, activities such as swimming and contact sports, where exposure to organisms or catheter damage can occur, may be prohibited. Alternate activities should be planned carefully (Marcoux, Fisher, & Wong, 1990). Tunneled catheter removal is a surgical procedure, and because of adherence of the Dacron cuff to tissue in the subcutaneous tunnel, it usually is done using local anesthesia and conscious sedation.

IMPLANTED CENTRAL VENOUS ACCESS PORTS

Low-profile pediatric ports have been available for several years and are made of stainless steel, titanium, plastic, or a combination of these materials (Fig. 21–9). Ports are ideal for children who require intermittent therapy, can tolerate the needle access, and do not like the inconvenience of an external catheter, such as patients with cancer,

FIGURE 21–9. Two types of implantable central venous ports: **(left)** a smaller port intended for arm implantation; **(right)** a pediatric-sized, low-profile chest port. (Courtesy of A.M. Frey.)

short-bowel syndrome, or cystic fibrosis (Marcoux et al., 1990). Ports are a good long-term choice for children older than 1 year. Before that age, lack of subcutaneous tissue may cause the port to erode through the skin. In children with cancer, one author reports ports being used the least frequently in children younger than 3 years and most frequently in children older than 15 years of age. When advising patients and family about venous access devices, an important consideration is that the port requires access with a needle at least monthly. Ports are accessed from the top or side, depending on the design, with a noncoring needle or, in some brands, an IV catheter.

Venous access ports are implanted in the chest, upper abdomen, or forearm, with the catheter threaded into a central vein. A 22- to 20-gauge, 1/2-inch needle for a forearm port and a 22- to 20-gauge, 3/4- to 1-inch needle for a chest port are usually adequate for the viscosity and flow of pediatric infusions (Fig. 21–10).

A hospital or home IV nurse, parents, or patients themselves in some cases may access the port after return demonstration of correct technique. Of concern in patients with cystic fibrosis is use of the arm port versus the chest port. Chest physiotherapy, involving chest percussion, is a large part of the treatment plan for cystic fibrosis. A chest port may obstruct this therapy.

Needles are changed every 7 days while the port is being used; dressings over the accessed port can be changed with the needle or more frequently. When the port is not being used for infusion of medications, PN, transfusion therapy, or blood sample withdrawal, patency is maintained by flushing the port with heparinized saline (Marcoux et al., 1990). Care of implanted ports is detailed in Table 21–8. More on port description and care may be found in Chapter 14.

Complications reported with ports are similar to those identified for tunneled catheters, including infection and occlusion; in most studies, implanted ports had

FIGURE 21–10. Dressing being applied to accessed implanted central venous port in 12-year-old receiving chemotherapy for a brain tumor. (Courtesy of A.M. Frey.)

longer survival times and fewer complications than tunneled catheters (CDC, 2002). Although risk of port dislodgment is minimal, the noncoring needle may be dislodged and cause infiltration and possible tissue injury if vesicant drugs are being administered. Slight discomfort has been reported with needle access of the port, but this diminishes in time, and a high level of satisfaction also has been reported (Poole, Ross, Haase, & Odom, 1991).

Umbilical Access

UMBILICAL CATHETERIZATION

Most sites for neonatal IV therapy are similar to those discussed earlier in this chapter. A site unique to the newborn population is the umbilicus, which contains two arteries and one vein. Umbilical catheterization is common practice in many neonatal and intensive care units for treatment of acutely ill infants. This mode of therapy provides an easy route for vascular administration of transfusions, medications, fluids, PN, and blood withdrawal, although it is not without complications. Risks include thrombosis, embolism, vasospasm, vascular perforation, infection, and hemorrhage (Bryant, 1990). To prevent these complications, a specially designed umbilical catheter with the following features should be selected:

- Flexibility
- Relatively rigid walls for accurate pressure monitoring
- Smoothness of the tip to prevent perforation of the vessel wall during catheter insertion
- Radiopacity to visualize the location of the catheter tip by radiography

FIGURE 21–11. Double-lumen umbilical venous catheter in newborn. (Courtesy of A.M. Frey.)

- Small-volume capacity so that only a small amount of blood need be withdrawn to clear the catheter for blood sampling
- Size from 3.5 to 5 French, single- or double-lumen (Fig. 21–11)

Procedure

Within minutes of birth, the umbilical arteries normally constrict; delays in the process, however, occur in states of hypoxia and acidosis. Most infants are catheterized in the first day of life because umbilical catheterization is more difficult or impossible past the fourth day of life. The procedure for umbilical catheterization begins with aseptic technique, including hand washing, gloving, masking, and gowning. Equipment is set up using a cutdown tray and recommended catheter size. All IV tubing must be purged of air. The infant is restrained temporarily using leg/arm restraints and an assistant. The umbilical stump is cleaned with a povidone–iodine solution; excess should not be allowed to pool at the infant's side or skin irritation or blistering may occur (Lipton & Schafermeyer, 1997). The sterile field is set up around the umbilicus, using a fenestrated drape that exposes the umbilical area. Dissection begins at the umbilical cord approximately 1.5 cm from the skin until the umbilical vessels are identified. Two thick-walled, pinpoint-sized arteries are easily distinguishable from a large, thin-walled vein. The heparinized catheter is passed through either the umbilical artery or vein, depending on the type of therapy desired.

There are important differences between arterial and venous umbilical catheterization. Arterial catheterization accomplishes five goals: blood sampling, measurements of arterial pressures, parenteral or antibiotic therapy in the vascularly compromised child, exchange transfusions, and measurements of arterial pH and blood gases. Venous umbilical catheterization accomplishes four goals: blood sampling, parenteral or antibiotic therapy in the vascularly compromised child, direct measurement of central venous pressure, and infusion of TPN. Placements differ between the umbilical arterial and venous routes. Ideally, the umbilical arterial catheter (UAC) is positioned above the level of aortic bifurcation in good position for arterial measurements and exchange transfusions. Comparatively, the tip of the umbilical venous catheter (UVC) should be positioned in the inferior vena cava near the right atrium in good position for central venous pressure and TPN administration.

Once the catheter is placed correctly and position is confirmed radiographically, a suture may be placed superficially through the stump and tied firmly to the catheter for anchorage. The umbilical catheter is taped to the infant's abdomen using goalpost taping, often referred to as a tape bridge. The UAC usually is connected to a three-way stopcock for pressure monitoring, blood drawing, and fluid administration. In the UVC, when fluid administration is not necessary, the line may be heparinized. It is of the utmost importance to maintain patency of the indwelling catheter because blood clots can otherwise form. Flushing with heparin (1 to 10 U/mL preservative-free normal saline) should be done frequently.

Nursing Assessment and Management

Nursing care and assessment (Frey, 2001; Lipton & Schafermeyer, 1997; Stanford, 1990) should include the following:

- Examine buttocks and extremities hourly to detect blanching or color changes caused by arterial spasms or catheter malposition. If color changes are noted, apply warm soaks to opposite extremity for 15 minutes to trigger reflex vasodilation in the affected limb.
- Use Luer-lock connections to prevent disconnection of the tubing with resultant hemorrhage.
- Closely monitor peripheral edema, unequal femoral pulses, and respiratory distress, which could indicate emboli formation.
- Observe and document the quality of the arterial waveform on the monitor; change in quality or dampening of the waveform may indicate a problem with the umbilical arterial line.
- Monitor the umbilicus daily for signs of infection during treatment and for 12 hours after catheter removal; provide routine cord care daily.

Risks and Complications

Reported risks and complications associated with UACs include aortic, mesenteric, or renal artery thrombus formation resulting in visceral infarction and subsequent necrotizing enterocolitis; renal insufficiency; hypertension; congestive heart failure; lower limb ischemia; sepsis; aortoiliac aneurysms; and hypoglycemia from glucose infusion into the pancreatic circulation. Risks and complications associated with UVCs include those complications associated with other central venous lines in infants, such as sepsis, arrhythmias, vessel or heart perforation, and cardiac tamponade (Sigda, Speights, & Thigpen, 1992).

Studies of infectious complications associated with umbilical catheters indicate that incidences for catheter colonization are similar, ranging from 40% to 55% for UACs and 22% to 59% for UVCs. The documented bloodstream infection rates reported were 5% for UACs and 3% to 8% for UVCs (CDC, 2002). Neonates with very low birth weight receiving prolonged antimicrobials were at increased risk for UAC bloodstream infection; neonates with higher birth weight receiving PN were at increased risk for UVC-related infection (Landers, Moise, Fraley, Smith & Baker, 1991).

Mechanical complications include hemorrhage, occlusion, and air embolism (Lipton & Schafermeyer, 1997; Stanford, 1990). If complications arise, report them immediately to the appropriate physician/practitioner so immediate assessment and treatment can be provided. Early intervention can reduce the risk of morbidity and mortality when using umbilical access for IV therapy. Because of the risk of complications and the short dwell time when using the umbilical vessel for IV therapy, many physicians now prefer to use an alternate peripheral or central site as soon as possible.

Surgical Cutdown

Although alternative choices of access, such as the IO and central venous routes, have diminished the need for venous cutdown, this method remains a viable option for emergency vascular access in resuscitation of the pediatric patient. When acute hypovolemia and acidosis cause severe enough peripheral vasoconstriction that percutaneous placement of venous access is impossible, and if IO access cannot be achieved, venous cutdown may be warranted (Gauderer, 1992).

The most common cutdown sites are the distal saphenous vein at the ankle, the proximal saphenous vein at the groin, the basilic vein at the antecubital, and the axillary vein, which is used in newborns (Winci, 1997). Because this procedure requires venous laceration or minor surgery, a physician or surgeon usually performs it. Meticulous sterile technique is required. The size of the IV catheter placed can range from 22 to 16 gauge, depending on the size of the vessel. Complications reported with venous cutdown include local injury of contiguous structures such as an artery or nerve, hemorrhage, hematoma, extravasation, phlebitis with prolonged use, localized cellulitis, suppurative phlebitis, and catheter-related bloodstream infection (Winci).

Obtaining successful IV access is essential to provide efficacious pediatric advanced life support. In many cases, during a code situation, peripheral veins have collapsed because of cardiac arrest and poor perfusion. Time for performance of a surgical cutdown can range from 2 to 40 minutes, with a median time of 8 minutes (Kanter, Zimmerman, Straus, & Stoeckel, 1986).

Intraosseous Access

Intravenous access should be obtained within 5 minutes from the start of a resuscitation effort. After traditional routes have been attempted or often simultaneously, IO access is a realistic goal. **Intraosseous** infusion is defined as infusion of blood, fluids, or drugs through a rigid needle directly into the bone marrow cavity (Hockenberry, 2003). This technique was widely used from 1922, when first described by Drinker, Drinker, and Lund (1922), through the 1960s. As IV device technology improved, facilitating peripheral venous access, IO technique lost popularity. Since 1983, however, interest in IO therapy has increased because of a letter to the editor of *American Journal of Diseases of Children* that questioned the abandonment of this route (Turkel, 1983).

The IO technique is based on the fact that the extensive network of venous sinusoids quickly takes up fluid injected into the medullary cavity of the bone, and drugs given by the IO and central venous routes are equally effective, working faster than those administered by peripheral IV (Manley, Haley, & Dick, 1988). The tibia and femur are the preferred sites for IO administration because the limbs are readily accessible during resuscitation efforts and the marrow cavity is well developed, even in neonates (Tocantins & O'Neil, 1945).

The preferred site for IO infusion in children up to 5 or 6 years of age is the anterior medial aspect of the tibia, 1 to 3 cm below the tibial tuberosity, thus avoiding the growth plate at the end of the bone (Hockenberry, 2003; Miccolo, 1990; Fig. 21–12). The tibial sites are preferred because less subcutaneous tissue over the bone enhances ease of access, as opposed to the femur, where subcutaneous tissue may make IO access difficult. Other sites include distal medial tibia, midanterior distal femur, iliac crest, and humerus, and the sternum in children older than 3 years of age, before which the sternum is too thin to support the IO needle (Miccolo). Contraindications to IO access include site infections, fractures, burns, and bone disorders, such as osteogenesis imperfecta (brittle bone disease) and osteopetrosis (marble bone disease), in which bones may fracture easily (Manley et al., 1988; Miccolo). IO access is

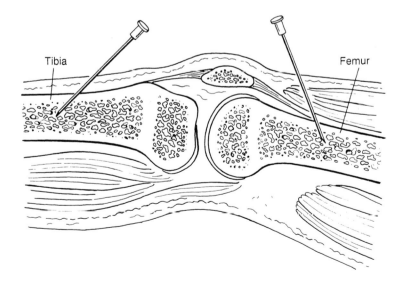

FIGURE 21–12. The anterior medial aspect of the tibia (lateral view) is the best site for intraosseous access in the child younger than 6 years of age.

FIGURE 21–13.   A 16-gauge intraosseous needle and stylet.
(Courtesy of A.M. Frey.)

indicated during emergencies, such as respiratory or cardiac resuscitation efforts or when two attempts at peripheral IV access are unsuccessful (Manley et al.).

A short, rigid needle with a stylet is used to obtain IO access (Fig. 21–13); alternatively, a lumbar puncture needle may be used for infants, although this needle can bend easily and is awkward to insert. Disposable bone marrow aspiration needles are now manufactured for IO access; 16, 18, or 20 is the recommended gauge because a small-lumen needle can become blocked with bone fragments or bend on insertion (Hockenberry, 2003).

After antimicrobial cleansing of the desired site, the IO needle is inserted perpendicular to the bone surface at a slight angle away from the epiphyseal plate. A screwing motion is used to insert the needle into the bone until decreased resistance is noted and the needle stands without support, usually at a depth of 1 cm in an infant or child (Hodge, 1997). Further advancement may cause penetration of the opposite wall of the bone and result in extravasation of infusates. Some IO needles are now manufactured with a premarked shaft to indicate depth. After insertion, the stylet is removed and bone marrow content, similar to blood, is aspirated; this sample may be used for readings of $Paco_2$ and pH, important parameters indicating success of resuscitative efforts (Manley et al., 1988).

A short connector tubing and flush solution, similar to that used with IV catheters, is connected to the hub of the IO needle, and a split sterile gauze dressing and tape are placed to secure the site. If the child is awake, intradermal anesthesia before IO needle placement is advised. The site should be observed for infiltration of infusates into surrounding tissues; the same bone should not be used for repeated access if infiltration occurs. Types of infusions given by the IO route are listed in Table 21–9. Infusates may be administered by gravity, manual pressure, or infusion pump.

Complications are relatively rare. A 0.6% incidence of osteomyelitis, the most common complication (Rosetti, et al., 1985), has been reported in the literature and is

TABLE 21–9 Intraosseous Infusions

Fluids	Medications	Blood Products
• 5%, 10%, and 50% dextrose • Saline • Lactated Ringer's solution • Parenteral nutrition	• Analgesics • Anesthetics • Antibiotics • Anticonvulsants • Antisera • Catecholamines • Contrast media • Miscellaneous (eg, atropine, calcium, dobutamine, dopamine, epinephrine, heparin, insulin, levarterenol, lidocaine, phenytoin, sodium bicarbonate)	• Albumin • Dextran • Packed red blood cells • Plasma • Whole blood

(Adapted from Arbeiter H.I. & Greengard, J. [1944]; Chameides, L. [1994]; Dieckmann R. et al., [1997]; Glaeser P.W., & Losek, J.D. [1986]; Miccolo, M.A. [1990]; Mofenson, H.C., Tascone A., Caraccio T.R. [1988].)

related to long-term use and infusion of hypertonic solutions. Other complications can include the following (Hodge, 1997; Manley et al., 1988; Simmons, Johnson, Perkin, & van Stralen, 1994):

- Cellulitis
- Compartment syndrome
- Abscess
- Local necrosis
- Fat embolism (although a possibility, this has not been reported in children, probably because of the low fat content of bone marrow in children, especially those younger than 4 years of age)
- Bilateral tibial fractures

To prevent complications, the site should be monitored closely, especially during infusion of potential vesicants. Success rates with IO therapy have been reported as high as 97% (Roth, 1997). Replacement of the IO needle with IV access is recommended as soon as conventional IV access is feasible.

Peripheral Intravenous Access

Equipment

Equipment and supplies are set up before venipuncture, usually in a treatment room, if possible, thus preserving the child's room and bed as a safe place where invasive procedures are not performed (Piercy, 1981). In an intensive care environment, supplies may be prepared away from the bedside so as not to cause undue anxiety before the actual venipuncture. In the home, supplies usually are set up in an area where lighting is maximized and a flat surface, such as a kitchen table, can be used as a work area. The nurse will need the following:

- Peripheral IV safety catheter in 24- or 22-gauge size
- Luer-locking microbore connector tubing
- Needleless cap
- 1 to 2 mL of flush solution in a syringe
- Padded arm board
- 1/2- and 1-inch tape
- Semipermeable transparent dressing
- Gauze pads
- Alcohol solution to clean the site
- Nonsterile gloves
- Latex-free tourniquet or rubber band
- Site protector (optional)
- Warm packs (optional)

IV Insertion

Peripheral IVs are used to administer fluids, medications, and PN and even to draw frequent blood samples. Although the standards of the Intravenous Nurses Society (INS, 2000) state that indwelling peripheral IV catheters should not be used routinely to acquire blood samples in children, the frequency of venous sampling for certain diagnostic tests necessitates the use of peripheral IV devices (INS). Examples include short-duration blood tests that require blood sampling every 15 minutes (eg, growth hormone) to every 4 to 6 hours (eg, clotting studies or blood glucose levels; Roulston-Betts, 1998). In such cases, the IV is used only for that purpose to avoid skewing results of the laboratory tests.

Depending on the child's age, finding a site for administering IV therapy typically is more difficult than in the adult. Both hydration status and previous IV therapy may be used as predictors of difficulties in obtaining an intact venous access. In the child, the site selected for IV therapy should involve minimal risk and allow maximum efficacy and safety.

General IV insertion techniques have been described previously and are not discussed in this chapter; however, some special techniques for achieving venous access in children are highlighted. To dilate veins in children, a smaller tourniquet may be necessary. In neonates, a latex-free rubber band with a tape tab provides an easily removable tourniquet for scalp IVs (Fig. 21–14). In some cases, especially when placing an IV in a premature neonate, no tourniquet is used. Additional aids to locate and dilate veins may include warm soaks or transillumination (Mattson & O'Connor, 1986).

Insertion of IVs in children requires stabilization of the extremity before venipuncture so that movement of the child does not dislodge the newly inserted device, necessitating subsequent sticks (Frey, 1998b). An arm board usually is an adequate restraint (Fig. 21–15) and can be taped to the treatment room table to provide passive restraint during IV insertion. Box 21–1 refers to core competencies associated with peripherally inserted central catheters. Many of those same competencies apply to standard peripheral insertion as well.

FIGURE 21–14.   Rubber band used as a tourniquet on infant's scalp. (Courtesy of A.M. Frey.)

PERIPHERAL INTRAVENOUS SITES

When selecting the optimal site for IV therapy, nurses should follow certain basic strategies. These include using veins distally to proximally and inserting the IV device in line with venous flow—for example, facing down or toward the heart in a scalp vein or facing up in an arm or leg vein. A vein in the nondominant extremity should be chosen when possible. The thumb should be left untaped or another extremity used if the child sucks his or her thumb (Frey, 1998b). In addition, the nurse always closely monitors an infusing IV, at least every 1 to 2 hours, depending on the type of infusate, size of the patient, and location of the IV access device.

FIGURE 21–15.   An arm board is used to support the area of the IV site and provide light restraint during IV insertion. (Courtesy of A.M. Frey.)

BOX 21–1   Core Competency for Peripherally Inserted Central Catheter (PICC) Insertion in Pediatric Patients

PICC Insertion Skills Checklist for: _____ Date: _____

Preceptor: _____ *(Complete one checklist for each insertion.)*

Original PICC course completed: Date _____

Initial clinical competency verification: Circle age group:

Date: _____ PICC Preceptor: _____ neonatal   pediatric
Date: _____ PICC Preceptor: _____ neonatal   pediatric
Date: _____ PICC Preceptor: _____ neonatal   pediatric
Date: _____ PICC Preceptor: _____ neonatal   pediatric
Date: _____ PICC Preceptor: _____ neonatal   pediatric

Periodic competency verification: (Concentrate on items noted from CQI report of individual's PICC insertion/outcomes.)

Date: _____ PICC Preceptor: _____ satisfactory   unsatisfactory
Review specific aspects of PICC insertion/care listed below based on CQI data:

_____

Date: _____ PICC Preceptor: _____ satisfactory   unsatisfactory
Review specific aspects of PICC insertion/care listed below based on CQI data:

_____

Date: _____ Continuing Education (describe): _____
Date: _____ Continuing Education (describe): _____
Date: _____ Continuing Education (describe): _____

Individual maintains competency according to CQI review and agency policy. Use additional forms if needed.

_____

Insertion method: Breakaway needle/Peel-away sheath/Modified Seldinger/Other

_____

COMPETENCY CRITERIA (Place a check in a column to the right.)	Met	Not Met	N/A
Consults with MD/NP as needed to plan correct catheter type for therapy ordered and for patient-specific needs/activities.			
Checks MD/NP order for placement, number of lumens, local anesthetic or conscious sedation protocol, and tip location verification.			
Applies tourniquet briefly to select appropriate vein and measures for correct catheter length (double-checking this measurement).			
Uses barrier precautions according to procedure, including hand washing, masks, gloves, goggles, sterile drapes, and powder-free sterile gloves (gown if indicated).			
Maintains sterility when setting up equipment and throughout procedure. Places all needed supplies on sterile field.			

BOX 21–1 Core Competency for Peripherally Inserted Central Catheter (PICC) Insertion in Pediatric Patients *(Continued)*

COMPETENCY CRITERIA (Place a check in a column to the right.)	Met	Not Met	N/A
Wearing sterile gloves, prepares equipment in kit for use. (Draws up flush solutions, assembles and preflushes extension set and needle-free cap, and so forth.)			
Correctly measures catheter and cuts to premeasured length appropriate for brand used.			
Positions patient appropriately to facilitate threading catheter.			
Prepares skin according to procedure guidelines.			
Positions sterile drapes to maintain sterility of site and equipment during procedure.			
Follows standard precautions to avoid contact with blood and body fluids throughout procedure.			
Injects local anesthetic if ordered.			
Applies tourniquet and positions it for ease of removal after venipuncture. Changes sterile gloves.			
Performs venipuncture using technique appropriate for brand.			
Releases tourniquet once venous access is achieved.			

COMPETENCY CRITERIA (Place a check in a column to the right.)	Met	Not Met	N/A
Follows steps specific to insertion method, using instruments/technique appropriate for brand of device.			
If using upper extremity, instructs patient to turn head toward insertion site with chin on chest.			
Threads catheter to premeasured length.			
Removes introducer using technique appropriate for brand.			
Removes guidewire (if applicable) using technique appropriate for brand.			
Attaches connector tubing and needleless cap (if applicable to brand) and verifies catheter patency with saline flush.			
Applies skin-protectant solution around periphery of dressing area.			
Secures catheter to skin using appropriate technique for procedure (sterile tape strips, hub-lock device, or sutures).			

(Continued)

BOX 21–1   Core Competency for Peripherally Inserted Central Catheter (PICC) Insertion in Pediatric Patients   *(Continued)*

COMPETENCY CRITERIA (Place a check in a column to the right)	Met	Not Met	N/A
Applies dressing. Places small pressure dressing over site using folded gauze covered with transparent dressing for first 24–48 hours.			
Labels dressing appropriately.			
Flushes catheter with heparinized saline if indicated by brand.			
Arranges for radiographic or fluoroscopic verification of catheter tip placement.			
Charts procedure, including patient teaching, catheter brand, gauge, length, local anesthetic, type of dressing, and patient's response/tolerance of procedure.			

Traditionally, the head was frequently used in the neonate and young infant because the scalp has an abundant supply of superficial veins (Fig. 21–16). The bilateral superficial temporal veins just in front of the pinna of the ear and the frontal vein, which runs down the middle of the forehead, are usually easy to find and involve minimal risk to the patient. Scalp veins are readily available until approximately 12 to 18 months of age, when hair follicles mature and superficial layers of skin thicken,

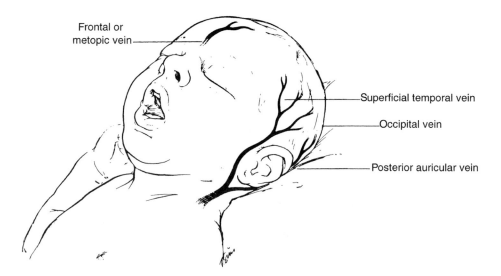

FIGURE 21–16.   Sites for scalp vein infusions.

making venous access difficult. The scalp as an IV site, however, can be distressing to parents, who may believe that the IV is in the brain. Moreover, a scalp IV can restrict mobility and be easily dislodged. With the advent of small IV catheters for peripheral access, scalp veins are no longer the first choice for IV access in infants.

If the scalp is chosen as the IV site and the head must be shaved, the smallest area possible should be shaved or clipped, saving the hair for the parents as the child's first haircut, which should help alleviate some distress at the use of this site. When inserting an IV in the scalp, the nurse should be aware of artery location, because distinguishing veins from arteries in this area is difficult. Use of an arterial IV could damage the artery and the area to which oxygenated blood is delivered. Inadvertent arterial puncture reveals bright red blood, pulsation, and blanching of the skin caused by arteriospasm when the IV device is flushed (Fay, 1983). Should arterial puncture occur, the IV device should be removed and pressure held on the site until bleeding stops.

Other favorable peripheral IV sites, moving from distal to proximal locations, include the hand, forearm, upper arm, foot, and antecubital fossa. Some unusual sites such as the axilla, abdomen, and popliteal area also have been used when chronically ill infants and children exhibit greatly diminished peripheral venous access from long use (Table 21–10).

TABLE 21–10 Peripheral Intravenous Access Sites for Pediatric Patients

Sites	Veins
Preferred Sites	
Hand	Metacarpal, digital
Forearm	Accessory cephalic, basilic, median antebrachial
Antecubital fossa	Median basilic, median cephalic, median cubital
Upper arm (below axilla)	Basilic, cephalic
Foot	Greater saphenous, lesser saphenous, median marginal
Scalp	Frontal, temporal, posterior auricular, occipital
Lower leg	Greater saphenous, lesser saphenous
Secondary Sites*	
Wrist	Superficial veins on the ventral surface: infiltration in this area may result in pressure on the radial nerve.
Knee	Popliteal vein: usually limited to neonates because of decreased mobility
Axilla	Axillary vein: usually limited to neonates; infiltration may cause pressure on structures in chest cavity
Abdomen	Superficial veins: rarely used, usually limited to chronically hospitalized patients; infiltration may result in damage to abdominal wall.

Sites listed in order of preference.
*Secondary sites should be considered only when preferred sites are not available.

Foot veins are used up to walking age and occasionally in older children when other usual sites are not available, such as in patients with burns or multiple trauma (Fig. 21–17). Depending on the regulations of the state's Board of Nursing and institutional policy, external jugular and femoral veins may be used for IV access and blood samples, although these last two sites usually are accessed by a physician, nurse practitioner, or emergency personnel.

TECHNIQUE

Intravenous insertion in children requires patience and practice until the learning curve is diminished and skill level increases. No more than two or three attempts at

FIGURE 21–17.   A 24-gauge peripheral IV in large saphenous vein of neonate. (Courtesy of A.M. Frey.)

FIGURE 21–18. Locating and palpating veins in a pediatric patient prior to IV placement. (Courtesy of A.M. Frey.)

IV access should be made. Veins should be located by anatomy and palpation prior to venipuncture (Fig. 21–18). If unsuccessful, the nurse should consult a more experienced person or consider alternate access. Limiting the number of venipuncture attempts decreases physical and emotional trauma to the child and can preserve venous integrity (Frey, 1998b). Consideration should be given to using an IV specialty nursing team for IV procedures in children because such teams have a higher rate of success when placing IVs and can be quite cost effective. One study demonstrated that using staff nurses and physicians who were not IV specialists to place IVs in children resulted in a low rate of success for IV placement and increased cost to the hospital (Frey, 1998a).

A firm but gentle insertion technique is necessary for a successful venipuncture in a child because blood return may not appear as readily as in the adult, and the nurse may not feel the characteristic pop of entering a vein (Frey, 1997). With certain brands of safety catheters, the blood return is first evidenced in the catheter immediately after the vein is punctured. Threading the IV catheter can occasionally be difficult in children (Fig. 21–19). After initial flashback of blood, but before threading the catheter into the vein, the nurse verifies that the catheter tip and the stylet have entered the vein lumen by advancing the IV device slightly. Other measures include attaching a small connector tubing with flush solution and flushing gently as the catheter is advanced. Sometimes, just waiting a few seconds until the child has calmed down can decrease the incidence of venous spasm and facilitate catheter threading.

Postinsertion Care of the Peripheral Intravenous Site

Frequent assessment of the site must be done; dressing changes usually are done only when the IV site is changed, as recommended by infection control research (CDC, 2002). Peripheral and central catheter care is summarized in Table 21–8.

FIGURE 21–19.   A 24-gauge peripheral IV safety catheter being inserted into dorsal metacarpal vein of school-aged child. (Courtesy of A.M. Frey.)

Stabilization is essential, primarily in the younger child whose comprehension of the importance of not manipulating the IV site is minimal. The nurse should tape IVs in a U-shaped chevron or H pattern and loop the extension tube so that if the child pulls on the IV, the tension affects the loop, not the IV site (Hutchinson, 1991). Sites requiring stabilization include those over joints, such as the dorsum of the hand near the wrist. The advantage of using a padded arm board for stabilization is that it restricts the child's range of movement, thereby decreasing the risk of dislodging the IV needle. The foot also demands stabilization, primarily when using the large saphenous vein (Fig. 21–17). An important aspect of IV access in the foot involves maintaining normal joint configuration by placing padding under the foot, thus preserving the natural bend at the ankle and preventing foot drop or contracture injuries. See Legal Issues: Site Monitoring for a comprehensive review of legalities associated with monitoring pediatric infusion patients.

In younger children, especially toddlers, great care must be taken to protect the IV site. Coverings such as a clear plastic IV protector, an easily removable wrap secured with Velcro, or stretch netting may keep little fingers away from the IV site, while providing easy visualization (Vallino, 1998). Stretch netting slipped over the IV can serve to protect the site as well, especially for home IV access. A roller bandage should not be used to cover an IV site because it is time consuming to unravel and makes site assessments difficult (INS, 2005). In general, children's medical centers rarely use restraints because restraints not only are confining but foster a sense of frustration and mistrust in the child. Restraints should be used only with an extremely uncooperative child or a child who may injure himself or herself or remove the IV. In those cases, alternate resources, such as parental monitoring, should be considered.

SITE ROTATION

Although 48 to 72 hours is the recommended interval for site rotation in adult patients, owing to increased risk of phlebitis, a survey indicated that most (71.9%)

children's hospitals changed peripheral IV sites only when necessary (Bossert & Beecroft, 1994). One large study done in a pediatric critical care unit demonstrated that peripheral IV sites could remain in place safely for up to 144 hours (6 days), after which the incidence of bacterial colonization increased threefold. In fact, this same study demonstrated that newer sites had an increased chance of complications over those sites left in place (Garland, Dunne, Havens, et al., 1992). New CDC guidelines and literature review recommend not rotating IV sites on a regular basis in pediatric patients unless a complication occurs (CDC, 2002; Oishi, 2001). Removal of the IV should be done carefully, without using scissors near the site (INS, 2000).

RESEARCH ISSUES: What Are Correct Flushing Techniques for Peripheral IV Devices?

Bossert & Beecroft, 1994; Crews, Gnann, Rice, & Kee, 1997; Danek & Noris, 1992; Gyr, Burroughs, Smith, Mahl, Pontius, & Swerczek, 1995; Hanrahan, Kleiber, & Fagan, 1994; Heilskov, Kleiber, Johnson, & Miller, 1998; Hockenberry, 2003; Kotter, 1996; Krueger-Paisely, Stamper, Brown, Brovan, & Ganong, 1997; LeDuc, 1997; McMullen, Fioravanti, Pollack, Rideout, & Sciera, 1993.

Flushing techniques for peripheral and central devices are a topic of controversy. Studies done in the early 1990s indicate that saline alone may be efficacious in maintaining the patency of 22-gauge catheters in children; however, the numbers of 24-gauge catheters reported was small, and one study demonstrated increased patency in 24-gauge catheters when a dilute heparin flush was used. More recently published research revealed increased patency and decreased tenderness when IVs were flushed with heparinized saline (10 U/mL), whereas several studies in neonates demonstrated no significant difference between normal and heparinized saline flush. In all the neonatal studies, 24-gauge catheters were used, and the IVs were flushed at least every 4 hours. One study evaluated flushes used for short-term IVs in patients in the emergency department, noting that saline was equivalent to heparin flush for patency. Another recent study examined intervals between heparin flushes, noting that 8 hours was optimal for flushing 22-gauge catheters in pediatric patients. Several studies also noted that positive-pressure flush technique, in which the connector tubing was clamped before syringe removal, helped to maintain patency of IV catheters. The most common practice reported in a survey of children's hospitals was irrigation of peripheral IVs with 1 mL of a solution of 10 units of heparin per milliliter of saline every 8 hours. Clearly, more research, especially with 24-gauge catheters and flush intervals longer than 4 hours, is needed to come to a scientific conclusion regarding flush solution and technique for flushing peripheral IVs in children.

MANAGING COMPLICATIONS

Complications of IV therapy in children are similar to those of adults and are described earlier in this textbook. The most common peripheral IV complication is infiltration, which can lead to an extravasation injury, depending on the infusate IV site (dorsal metacarpal veins of the foot are a high-risk site), skill of the inserter, and the child's activity. Current pediatric treatment modalities include application of cold, elevation of the extremity, and local pharmaceutical intervention with such agents as hyaluronidase, nitroglycerin ointment, and glyceryl trinitrate (Brown, Hoetzer, & Piercy, 1979; Denkler & Cohen, 1989; Flemmer & Chan, 1993).

Young children very rarely exhibit a phlebitic response to peripheral IV access, which differs from the much higher rates of phlebitis found in adults. Phlebitis rates reported in children hospitalized in intensive care units were 13%, whereas for those children on general units, phlebitis rates were 10%. In children older than 10 years, phlebitis rates reported (21%) approached those of adults (Nelson & Garland, 1987; Tully, Friedland, Baldini, & Goldman, 1981). Risk factors for development of phlebitis include catheter location, infusion of hyperalimentation fluids with continuous IV lipid emulsions, and length of intensive care stay before catheter insertion (Garland et al., 1992).

LEGAL ISSUES: Site Monitoring

Site monitoring is of the utmost importance in pediatric patients because infiltration can occur quickly and effects can be devastating if the infiltrated infusate has caustic properties. Risk factors for an infiltration injury include age younger than 1 year, catheter dwell time <72 hours, administration of anticonvulsant medications, and use of steel butterfly needles instead of catheters. IV sites in those areas with very little superficial tissue, particularly the dorsum of the foot in infants, are more prone to extravasation injury. Patients who are unable to communicate because of age, sedation, or physical condition also can be at higher risk for IV injury. Infiltration injuries can be a reason for litigation if the injury is extensive or limits function. Recommended frequency for peripheral IV site assessment, while therapies are infusing, ranges from every 1 to 2 hours, or more often if the infusate is known to be an irritant or vesicant. Peripheral IV sites used as heparin or saline locks, without an infusate running, should be assessed at least once per shift (every 8 to 12 hours). In home care as well, patients and caregivers are taught how to recognize signs of IV complications and to take corrective actions. Peripheral IV access should not be used for continuous infusions in alternative settings, such as the home, unless the site can be monitored. For this reason, central venous access is often used in the home and alternative setting.

(From Brown et al., 1979; Denkler & Cohen, 1989; Garland et al., 1992; Guhlow & Kolb, 1979; INS, 2000.)

Alternative-Site Pediatric Intravenous Therapy

Much routine and some high-acuity stable neonatal and pediatric IV therapy has moved out of the hospital and into the home, subacute care facility, or outpatient infusion center. Home infusion is estimated at one-third the costs of hospitalization (Ringel, 1995a). Disorders treated at home or other locations with IV modalities include but are not limited to cystic fibrosis; hemophilia; bone, soft tissue, and joint infections; neonatal sepsis; gastrointestinal disorders; immunologic dysfunction; and oncologic disorders and treatment sequelae (Ferris, 1990; Schuman, 1990). IV therapies administered in the home or at alternate sites include fluids, antibiotics or antifungals, PN, chemotherapy, analgesics, chelating agents, chemotherapy, pain control medications, and blood components. Even neonates and infants are sent home safely under the care and supervision of agencies skilled in neonatal and pediatric care (Cady & Yoshioka, 1991).

Pediatric patients usually receive one or more doses in a controlled environment to verify that there is no adverse reaction. With TPN, the therapy is usually cycled to infuse over several hours before discharge to home or transfer to alternative site care. Intermediate- to long-term catheters are often used for IV therapy at home to avoid the trauma and possible omitted therapy for frequent peripheral

IV site changes. Occasionally peripheral IVs, but more often, midline, PICC, and tunneled or implanted central devices are chosen for pediatric home or alternate site care.

Readiness, willingness, and ability of the patient and family and extensive teaching with demonstrated feedback should be documented before patient discharge and be ongoing during the patient's course of treatment until service is discontinued. School-age and older children can participate in their own care. Outcome data on pediatric home care, lacking in the published literature, is another opportunity for nursing research. The pediatric home infusion nurse must be an experienced IV practitioner, as might be indicated by CRNI status, as well as an expert in recognition and treatment of pediatric abnormal states. In 1995, Ringel summarized this concept, "Pediatric infusion has to be done by a company dedicated to pediatrics or that has a pediatrics division.... If children are given to a provider that does not have the expertise for high-acuity patients, they (children) can end up back in the hospital" (Ringel, 1995b). Pediatric home care is now the fastest growing portion of the home care market (see Chapter 23) (Ferris, 1990; Schuman, 1990).

References

Asterisks indicate references cited in text.

*Arbeiter, H.I., & Greengard, J. (1944). Tibial bone marrow infusions in infancy. *Journal of Pediatrics, 25,* 1.

*Association of Women's Health, Obstetric and Neonatal Nurses (AWHONN). (2001), *Neonatal skin care. Evidence-based clinical practice guideline* (pp. 3, 4, 6–8). Washington, DC: Author.

*Barnard, J., & Hazinski, M.F. (1992). Pediatric gastrointestinal disorders. In: M.F. Hazinski (Ed.). *Nursing care of the critically ill child* (pp. 715–803). St. Louis, MO: Mosby.

*Batton, D.G., Maisels, J., & Applebaum, P. (1982). Use of peripheral intravenous cannulas in premature infants: A controlled study. *Pediatrics, 70,* 488.

*Bendorf, K., Friesen, C.A., & Roberts, C.C. (1996). Glucose response to discontinuation of parenteral nutrition in pediatrics less than 3 years of age. *JPEN Journal of Parenteral and Enteral Nutrition, 20*(2), 10–22.

*Bertolone, K. (1997). Pediatric oncology: Past, present, and new modalities of treatment. *Journal of Intravenous Nursing, 20,* 136–140.

*BeVier, P.A., & Rice, C.E. (1994). Initiating a pediatric peripherally inserted central catheter and midline catheter program. *Journal of Intravenous Nursing, 17,* 201–205.

*Bilodeau, J.A., Poon, C., & Mascarenhas, M.R. (1998). Parenteral nutrition and care of central venous lines. In: S.M. Altschuler & C.A. Liacouras (Eds.). *Clinical pediatric gastroenterology* (pp. 637–652). Philadelphia: Churchill Livingstone.

*Bossert, E., & Beecroft, P.C. (1994). Peripheral intravenous lock irrigation in children: Current practice. *Pediatric Nursing, 20,* 346–355.

*Broviac, W., Cole, B., & Schribner, B.H. (1973). A silicone rubber atrial catheter for prolonged parenteral alimentation. *Surgery, Gynecology and Obstetrics, 136,* 602.

*Brown, A.S., Hoelzer, D., & Piercy, S.A. (1979). Skin necrosis from extravasation of intravenous fluids in children. *Plastic and Reconstructive Surgery, 64,* 145–150.

*Bryant, B.G. (1990). Drug, fluid, and blood products administered through the umbilical artery catheter: Complication experiences from one NICU. *Neonatal Network, 9,* 27–46.

*Cady, C., & Yoshioka, R.S. (1991). Using a learning contract to successfully discharge an infant on home total parenteral nutrition. *Pediatric Nursing, 17,* 67–74.

*Cahill-Alsip, C., & McDermott, B. (1996). Hematologic critical care problems. In: M.Q. Curley, J.B. Smith, & P.A. Moloney-Harmon (Eds.). *Critical care nursing of infants and children* (pp. 793–817). Philadelphia: W.B. Saunders.

*Callahan, C., & De La Cruz, H. (2004) Central line placement for the pediatric oncology patient: A model of advanced practice nurse collaboration. *Journal of Pediatric Oncology Nursing, 21*(1), 16–21.

*Camp-Sorrell, D. (1990). Advanced central venous access, selection, catheters, devices, and nursing management. *Journal of Intravenous Nursing, 13,* 361–370.

*Centers for Disease Control and Prevention (CDC). Guidelines for the prevention of intravascular catheter-related infections. (2002). *Morbidity and Mortality Weekly Report: Recommendations and Reports, 51*(RR10); 18:III.

*Chameides, L. (1994). *Textbook of pediatric advanced life support.* Dallas, TX: American Heart Association.

*Chathas, M.K. (1986). Percutaneous central venous catheters in neonates. *Journal of Obstetric, Gynecologic, and Neonatal Nursing, 141,* 324–332.

*Chathas, M.K., Paton, J.B., & Fisher, D.E. (1990). Percutaneous central venous catheterization: Three years' experience in a neonatal intensive care unit. *American Journal of Diseases of Children, 41,* 1243–1250.

*Clarke, T.A., & Reddy, P.G. (1979). Intravenous infusion technique in the newborn. *Clinical Pediatrics, 18,* 550–554.

*Cobb, L.M., Vinocur, C.D., Wagner, C.W., & Weintraub, W.H. (1987). The central venous anatomy in infants. *Surgery, Gynecology and Obstetrics, 165,* 230–234.

*Collier, S., Crouch, J., Hendricks, K., & Cacallero, B. (1994). Use of cyclic parenteral nutrition in infants less than 6 months of age. *Nutrition in Clinical Practice, 9,* 65–68.

*Con-Yost, C. (2005). Neonatal necrotizing enterocolitis. *Journal of Infusion Nursing, 28*(2), 130–134.

*Crews, B.E., Gnann, K.K., Rice, M.H., & Kee, C.C. (1997). Effects of varying intervals between heparin flushes on pediatric catheter longevity. *Pediatric Nursing, 23,* 87–91.

*Danek, G.D., & Noris, E.M. (1992). Pediatric IV catheters: Efficacy of saline flush. *Pediatric Nursing, 18,* 111–113.

*Dawson, D. (2002). Midline catheters in neonatal patients: Evaluating a change in practice. *JVAD, 7*(2), 17–19.

*Deady, A., & Gorman, D. (1997). Intravenous conscious sedation in children. *Journal of Intravenous Nursing, 20,* 245–252.

*Decker, M.D., & Edwards, K.M. (1988). Central venous catheter infections. *Pediatric Clinics of North America, 35,* 579–612.

*Denkler, K.A., & Cohen, B.E. (1989). Reversal of dopamine extravasation injury with topical nitroglycerin ointment. *Plastic and Reconstructive Surgery, 84,* 811–813.

*Dieckmann, R., (1997). *Pediatric emergency and critical care procedures.* St. Louis, MO: Mosby–Year Book.

*Dietrich, K.A., & Lobas, J.G. (1988). Use of a single silastic IV catheter for cystic fibrosis pulmonary exacerbations. *Pediatric Pulmonology, 4,* 181–184.

*Doellman, D. (2004). Pediatric PICC insertions: Easing the fears in infants and children. *JAVA, 9*(2), 68–71.

*Dolcourt, J.L., & Bose, C.L. (1982). Percutaneous insertion of Silastic central venous catheters in neonates. *Journal of Obstetric, Gynecologic, and Neonatal Nursing, 15,* 324–332.

*Donaldson, J.S., Morello, F.P., Junewick, J.J., O'Donovan, J.C., et al. (1995). Peripherally inserted central venous catheters: US-guided vascular access in pediatric patients. *Radiology, 197,* 499–504.

*Drinker, C.K., Drinker, K.R., & Lund, C.C. (1922). The circulation in the mammalian bone marrow. *American Journal of Physiology, 62,* 1–92.

*Duke, T., Curtis, N., & Fuller, D.G. (2003) The management of bacterial meningitis in children. *Expert Opinion on Pharmacotherapy, 4*(8):1227–1240.

*Fann, B.D. (1998). Fluid and electrolyte balance in the pediatric patient. *Journal of Intravenous Nursing, 21,* 153–159.

*Fay, M. (1983). The special challenges of pediatric IVs. *Dimensions of Critical Care Nursing, 2,* 24.

*Fein, J.A., Boardman, C.R., Stevenson, S., & Selbst, S.M. (1998). Saline with benzyl alcohol as intradermal anesthesia for intravenous line placement in children. *Pediatric Emergency Care, 14,* 119–122.

*Ferris, E.W. (1990). A neonatal home intravenous therapy program. *Journal of Intravenous Nursing, 13,* 383–387.

*Fetzer, S.J. (2001). Reducing venipuncture and intravenous insertion pain with eutectic mixture of local anesthetic: A meta-analysis. *Nursing Research, 51*(2), 119–124.

*Filston, H.C., & Johnson, D.G. (1971). Percutaneous venous cannulation in neonates and infants: A method for catheter insertion without "cutdown." *Pediatrics, 48,* 896–901.

*Flemmer, L., & Chan, S.L. (1993). A pediatric protocol for management of extravasation injuries. *Pediatric Nursing, 19,* 355–358.

*Ford, N.A., Drott, H.R., & Cieplinski-Robertson, J.A. (2003) Administration of IV medications via soluset. *Pediatric Nursing, 29*(4), 283–286, 319.

*Frey, A.M. (1991). The immune system, pt. 2. Intravenous administration of immune globulin. *Journal of Intravenous Nursing, 14,* 397–405.

*Frey, A.M. (1995). Pediatric peripherally inserted central catheter program report: A summary of 4,536 catheter days. *Journal of Intravenous Nursing, 18,* 280–291.

*Frey, A.M. (1997). Tips for pediatric IV insertion. *Nursing, 27*(9), 32.

*Frey, A.M. (1998a). Success rates for peripheral IV insertion in a children's hospital: Financial implications. *Journal of Intravenous Nursing, 21,* 160–165.

*Frey, A.M. (1998b). When a child needs peripheral IV therapy: Use these suggestions to choose the right site. *Nursing, 38*(4), 18.

*Frey, A.M. (1999). Pediatric and neonatal PICC complications. *Journal of Vascular Access Devices, 4*(Suppl. 2), 4.

*Frey, A.M. (2001). Intravenous therapy in children. In: J. Hankins, R.A. Waldman,-Lonsway, C. Hedrick, & M.B. Perdue (Eds.). *Intravenous therapy: Clinical principles and practice* (2nd ed., pp. 561–591). Philadelphia: W.B. Saunders.

*Frey, A.M. (2002). Peripherally inserted central catheters in neonates and children: modified Seldinger (microintroducer) technique. *Journal of Vascular Access Devices, 7*(2).

*Garland, J.S., Dunne, W.M., Jr., Havens, P., & Hintermeyer, M. (1992). Peripheral intravenous catheter complications in critically ill children: A prospective study. *Pediatrics, 89,* 1145–1150.

*Gauderer, M.W.L. (1992). Vascular access techniques and devices in the pediatric patient. *Surgical Clinics of North America, 72,* 1267–1284.

*Glaeser, P.N. & Losek, D. (1986). Emergency intraosseous infusions in children. *American Journal of Emergency Medicine, 4,* 35.

*Graef, J., & Cone, T. (1977). *Manual of pediatric therapeutics.* Boston: Little, Brown and Company.

*Greenberg, C. (2002). Practice applications of research: a sugar-coated pacifier reduces procedural pain in newborns. *Pediatric Nursing, 28*(3): 271–277.

*Guhlow, L., & Kolb, J. (1979). Pediatric IVs: Special measures you must take. *RN, 42,* 40–52.

*Guyon, G. (1989). Pharmacokinetic considerations in neonatal drug therapy. *Neonatal Network, 7,* 9–12.

*Gyr, P., Burroughs, T., Smith, K., Mahl, C., Pontious, S., & Swerczek, L. (1995). Double blind comparison of heparin and saline flush solutions in maintenance of peripheral infusion devices. *Pediatric Nursing, 21,* 383–389, 366.

*Hadaway, L. (1998). Catheter connection. *Journal of Vascular Access Devices, 3*(3), 40.

*Hanrahan, K.S., Kleiber, C., & Fagan, C.L. (1994). Evaluation of saline for IV locks in children. *Pediatric Nursing, 20,* 549–552.

*Hazinski, M.F. (1988). Understanding fluid balance in the seriously ill child. *Pediatric Nursing, 14*(3), 231–236 .

*Heilskov, J., Kleiber, C., Johnson, K., & Miller, J. (1998). A randomized trial of heparin and saline for maintaining intravenous locks in neonates. *Journal of the Society for Pediatric Nursing, 3,* 111–116.

*Heird, W.C. (1993). Parenteral support of the hospitalized child. In: R.M. Suskind & L. Lewinter-Suskind (Eds.). *Textbook of pediatric nutrition* (2nd ed., pp. 225–238). New York: Raven Press.

*Herrera, J.M., Krebs, A., Harris, P., & Barriga, F. (2000). Childhood tumors. *Surgical Clinics of North America, 80*(2) 747–760.

*Hill, S.E., Heldman, L.S., Goo, E.D.H., & Whippo, J.C. (1996). Fatal microvascular pulmonary emboli from precipitation of total nutrient admixture solution. *JPEN Journal of Parenteral and Enteral Nutrition, 20,* 81–87.

*Hockenberry, M. (2003). *Wong's nursing care of infants and children* (5th ed.). Philadelphia: Elsevier.

*Hodge, D. (1997). Intraosseous infusion. In: F. Henretig & C. King (Eds.). *Textbook of pediatric emergency procedures* (pp. 289–298). Baltimore: Williams & Wilkins.

*Holiday, M.A., & Segar, W.E. (1957). The maintenance need for water in parenteral fluid therapy. *Pediatrics, 14,* 698–704.

*Hutchinson, D.B. (1991). Pediatric IV therapy: Starting the line. *RN, 54*(12), 43–48.

*Infusion Nurses Society. (2005). *Infusion nursing standards of practice.* Cambridge, MA: Author.

*Ioli, J., & Gilday, M. (2002). Diseases & problems: Sickle cell disease. In: J.A. Fox (Ed.). *Primary health care of infants, children & adolescents* (2nd ed., p. 829). New York: Mosby.

*Jacobs, B.R. (2003). Central venous catheter occlusion and thrombosis. *Critical Care Clinics, 19,* 489–514.

*Jew, R. (Ed.). (2000–2001). *Pharmacy handbook and formulary, the Children's Hospital of Philadelphia.* Hudson, OH: Lexi-Comp, Inc.

*Jones, G.R. (1998). A practical guide to evaluation and treatment of infections in patients with central venous catheters. *Journal of Intravenous Nursing, 21*(Suppl. 5), 134–142.

*Kanter, R.K., Zimmerman, J.J., Straus, R.H., & Stoeckel, K. (1986). Pediatric emergency intravenous access: Evaluation of a protocol. *American Journal of Diseases of Children, 140,* 133.

*Kasprisin, C.A. (1985). Transfusion therapy for the pediatric patient. In: R. Rutman & W. Miller (Eds.). *Transfusion therapy* (pp. 179–185). Rockville, MD: Aspen.

*Kaste, S.C., & Young, C.W. (1996). Safe use of power injectors with central and peripheral venous access devices for pediatric CT. *Pediatric Radiology, 26,* 469–501.

*Keller, S. (1995). Small gauge needles promote safe blood transfusions. *Oncology Nursing Forum, 22,* 718.

*King, C.K., Glass, R., Bresee, J.S., & Duggan, C. (2003). Managing acute gastroenteritis among children: Oral rehydration, maintenance, and nutritional therapy. *Morbidity and Mortality Weekly Report: Recommendations and Reports, 52*(RR-16).

*Korth-Bradley, M. (1991). A pharmacokinetic primer for intravenous nurses. *Journal of Intravenous Nursing, 14,* 124.

*Kotter, R., (1996). Heparin vs. saline for intermittent intravenous device maintenance in neonates. *Neonatal Network, 15*(6), 43–47.

*Krueger-Paisely, M., Stamper, M., Brown, J., Brovan, N., & Ganong, L. (1997). The use of heparin and normal saline flushes in neonatal intravenous catheters. *Pediatric Nursing, 23,* 521–527.

*Kupensky, D.T. (1998). Applying current research to influence clinical practice: Utilization of midline catheters. *Journal of Intravenous Nursing, 21,* 271–274.

*Lal, M., McClelland, J., Taub, N., & Beattie, R. (2001). Comparison of EMLA cream versus placebo in children receiving distraction therapy for venepuncture. *Acta Paedia, 90*(2), 154–159.

*Landers, S., Moise, A.A., Fraley, J.K., & Smith, E.O. (1991). Factors associated with umbilical catheter-related sepsis in neonates. *American Journal of Diseases of Children, 145,* 675–680.

*Landier, W.C., Barrell, M.L., & Styffe, D.J. (1987). How to administer blood components to children. *Maternal and Child Nursing, 12,* 178–184.

*Lavelle, J., & Costarino, A. (1997). Central venous access and central venous pressure monitoring. In: F.M. Henretig & C. King (Eds.). *Textbook of pediatric emergency procedures* (pp. 251–278). Baltimore: Williams & Wilkins.

*LeDuc, K. (1997). Efficacy of normal saline solution versus heparin solution for maintaining patency of peripheral intravenous catheters in children. *Journal of Emergency Nursing, 23,* 306–309.

*LeRoy, K.E. (1999) Bacterial meningitis in infants and children: Standards of care. *Journal of Legal Nurse Consulting, 10*(3), 3–10.

*Lesser, E., Chhabra, R., Brion, L.P., & Suresh, B.R. (1996). Use of midline catheters in low birth weight infants. *Journal of Perinatology, 16,* 205–207.

*Lipton, J.D., & Schafermeyer, R.W. (1997). Umbilical vessel catheterization. In: F.M. Henretig & C. King (Eds.). *Textbook of pediatric emergency procedures* (pp. 515–522). Baltimore: Williams & Wilkins.

*Loeff, D.S., Matlak, M.E., Black, R.E., Overall, J.C., Dolcourt, J.L., & Johnson, D.G. (1982). Insertion of a small central venous catheter in neonates and young infants. *Journal of Pediatric Surgery, 17,* 941–948.

*Luban, N., & Keating, L. (Eds.). (1983). *Hemotherapy of the infant and premature.* Arlington, VA: American Association of Blood Banks.

*Manley, L., Haley, K., & Dick, M. (1988). Intraosseous infusion: Rapid vascular access for critically ill or injured infants and children. *Journal of Emergency Nursing, 14,* 63.

*Marcoux, C., Fisher, S., & Wong, D. (1990). Central venous access devices in children. *Pediatric Nursing, 16,* 123–133.

*Mattson, D., & O'Connor, M. (1986). Transilluminator assistance in neonatal venipuncture. *Neonatal Network, 4,* 43.

*Matyskicla-Frey, A.M. (1985). Pediatric dosage calculations. *Journal of the National Intravenous Therapy Association, 8,* 373–379.

*McCurdy, D., & Arnold, M. (1995) Development and implementation of a pediatric/neonatal i.v. syringe pump delivery system. *Neonatal Networks, 14*(3), 9–18.

*McGee, W.T., & Mallory, D.L. (1988). Cannulation of the internal and external jugular veins. *Problems in Critical Care, 2,* 217–241.

*McMullen, A., Fioravanti, I.D., Pollack, V., Rideout, K., & Sciera, M. (1993). Heparinized saline or normal saline as a flush solution in intermittent intravenous lines in infants and children. *Maternal Child Nursing, 18,* 78–85.

*Meyer, H.M. (1982). *Letter to hospital pharmacists.* Rockville, MD: U.S. Department of Health and Human Services, Federal Drug Administration.

*Miccolo, M.A. (1990). Intraosseous infusion. *Critical Care Nurse, 10,* 35–47.

*Mofenson, H.C., Tascone, A., & Caraccio, T.R. (1988). Guidelines for intraosseous infusions. *Journal of Emergency Medicine, 6*(2), 143–146.

*Nathan, D.G., & Orkin, S.H. (Eds.). (1998). *Nathan and Oski's hematology of infancy and childhood* (5th ed.). Philadelphia: W.B. Saunders.

National Institutes of Health. (1990). *Transfusion therapy guidelines for nurses.* National Blood Resource Education Program, Public Health Service. Washington, DC: U.S. Department of Health and Human Services.

*Nelson, D.B., & Garland, J.S. (1987). The natural history of Teflon catheter-associated phlebitis in children. *American Journal of Diseases of Children, 141,* 1090–1092.

*Oellrich, R.G., Murphy, M.R., Goldberg, L.A., & Aggarwal, R. (1991). The percutaneous central venous catheter for small or ill infants. *Maternal Child Nursing, 16,* 92–96.

*Oishi, L.A. (2001) The necessity of routinely replacing peripheral intravenous catheters in hospitalized children: a review of the literature. *Journal of Intravenous Nursing, 24*(3), 174–179.

*Pettit, J., & Hughes, K. (1999). Neonatal intravenous therapy practices. *Journal of Vascular Access Devices, 4*(1), 7–15.

*Phillips, S.K. (2004). Pediatric parenteral nutrition. *Journal of Infusion Nursing, 27*(3), 166–170.

*Piercy, S. (1981). Children on long term IV therapy. *Nursing 81, 11,* 66–69.

*Poole, M.A., Ross, M.N., Haase, G.M., & Odom, L.F. (1991). Right atrial catheters in pediatric oncology: A patient/ parent questionnaire study. *American Journal of Pediatric Hematology/Oncology, 13,* 152–155.

*Reiser, D.J. (1999). Intensive care nursery eliminates solusets. *Infusion Management Update, 8*(2), 6–8.

*Ringel, M. (1995a). For pediatric infusion, there's no place like home. *Infusion, 2*(1), 10–16.

*Ringel, M. (1995b). Providing pediatric infusion therapies: Putting the pieces together. *Infusion, 2*(2), 20–25.

*Rivitz, S.M., & Drucker, E.A. (1997). Power injection of peripherally inserted central catheters. *Journal of Intravenous Radiology, 8*(5), 853–863.

*Rosetti, V.A., Thompson, B.M., & Miller, J. (1985). An alternative route of pediatric intravascular access. *Annals of Emergency Medicine, 14,* 885–888.

*Roth, D. (1997). A comprehensive review of blood transfusion therapy, pt. 2. *Journal of Vascular Access Devices, 2*(4), 13–21.

*Roulston-Betts, K. (1998). Pediatric growth hormone deficiency. *Journal of Intravenous Nursing, 21,* 143–147.

*Ruble, K., Long, C., & Connor, K. (1994) Pharmacologic treatment of catheter-related thrombus in pediatrics. *Pediatric Nursing, 20,* 553–557.

*Ruess, L., Bulas, D.I., Rivera, O., & Markle, B.M. (1997). In-line pressures generated in small-bore central venous catheters during power injection of CT contrast media. *Radiology, 203,* 625–629.

*Sater, K.J. (1998). Treatment of sepsis in the neonate. *Journal of Intravenous Therapy, 21,* 275–281.

*Schuman, A. (1990). Homeward bound: The explosion of pediatric home care. *Contemporary Pediatrics, 7,* 26–29, 32–47, 50–54.

*Shaw, J.C. (1973). Parenteral nutrition in the management of sick low birthweight neonates. *Pediatric Clinics of North America, 20,* 333–354.

*Sherman, M.P. (1982). Percutaneous and surgical placement of fine silicone elastomer central catheters in high-risk newborns. *Journal of Pediatric Surgery, 7,* 75–78.

*Sickle Cell Disease Association of America, Inc. (2005). What is sickle cell disease? Available at www.sicklecelldisease. org. (Accessed 8/31/2005.)

*Sigda, M., Speights, J.T., & Thigpen, J. (1992). Pericardial tamponade due to umbilical venous catheterization. *Neonatal Network, 11*(2), 7–9.

*Simmons, C., Johnson, N.E., Perkin, R.M., & Van Stralen, D. (1994). Intraosseous extravasation complication reports. *Annals of Emergency Medicine, 23,* 363–366.

Sperling, M.A., & Menon, R.K. (2004) Differential diagnosis and management of neonatal hypoglycemia. *Pediatric Clinics of North America, 51*(3), 703–723.

*Stanford, A. (1990). Umbilical artery and venous catheters. In: J.L. Blumer (Ed.). *A practical guide to pediatric intensive care* (pp. 846–849). Philadelphia: Mosby–Year Book.

*Stenzel, J.P., Green, T.P., Fuhrman, B.P., & Carlson, R.P. (1989). Percutaneous femoral venous catheterizations: A prospective study of complications. *Journal of Pediatrics, 114,* 411–415.

*Stiehm, E.R. (1991). New pediatric indications for IVIG. *Contemporary Pediatrics, 8,* 29–52.

*Swanson, A. (2004). Pediatrics. In: M. Alexander & A. Corrigan (Eds.). *Core curriculum for infusion nursing* (3rd ed., pp. 247–297). Philadelphia: Lippincott Williams & Wilkins.

*Thiagarajan, R., Ramamoorthy, C., Gettmann, T., & Bratton, S. (1997). Survey of the use of peripherally inserted central venous catheters in children. *Pediatrics, 99,* 1–8.

*Thompson, V. (1994). An IV therapy teaching tool for children. *Pediatric Nursing, 20,* 351–355.

*Tocantins, L.M., & O'Neil, J.F. (1945). Complications of intraosseous therapy. *Annals of Surgery, 122,* 266–277.

*Trotter, C.W. (1996). Percutaneous central venous catheter-related sepsis in the neonate: An analysis of the literature from 1990 to 1994. *Neonatal Network, 15*(3), 15–28.

*Tully, J.L., Friedland, G.H., Baldini, L.M., & Goldman, D.A. (1981). Complications of intravenous therapy with steel needles and Teflon catheters: A comparative study. *American Journal of Medicine, 70,* 702–706.

*Turkel, H. (1983). Intraosseous infusions (Letter to the editor). *American Journal of Diseases of Children, 137,* 706.

*Vallino, L. (1998). IV house: Pediatric nurses contribute to refinement of IV protector. *Journal of Pediatric Nursing, 13,* 196–198.

*Van Cleve, L., Johnson, L., & Pothier, P. (1996). Pain responses of hospitalized infants and children to venipuncture and intravenous cannulation. *Journal of Pediatric Nursing, 11,* 161–168.

*Viall, C.D. (1990). Your complete guide to central venous catheters. *Nursing, 20,* 34.

*Von Meyenfeldt, M., Stapert, J., Deong, P., et al. (1980). TPN catheter sepsis: Lack of effect of subcutaneous tunneling of PVC catheters on sepsis rate. *JPEN Journal of Parenteral and Enteral Nutrition, 4,* 514–517.

*Weeks-Lozano, H. (1991). Clinical evaluation of Per-Q-Cath for both pediatric and adult home infusion therapy. *Journal of Intravenous Nursing, 14,* 246–252.

*Wickham, R.S. (1990). Advances in venous access devices and nursing management strategies. *Nursing Clinics of North America, 25,* 345–364.

*Wiener, E.S., & Albanese, C.T. (1998). Venous access in pediatric patients. *Journal of Intravenous Nursing, 21*(Suppl. 5), S122–S133.

*Williams, J., Smith, H.L., & Weller, P.H. (1988). Silastic catheters for antibiotics in cystic fibrosis. *Archives of Diseases in Children, 63*, 654–655.

*Winci, R.J. (1997). Venous cutdown catheterization. In: F.M. Henretig & C. King (Eds.). *Textbook of pediatric emergency procedures* (pp. 279–287). Baltimore: Williams & Wilkins.

*Wolfram, W., Turner, E.D., & Philput, C. (1997). Effects of parental presence during young children's venipuncture. *Pediatric Emergency Care, 13*, 325–328.

*Zanni, R.L., Shutack, J.G., Schuler, P.M., Christie, D., & Holsclaw, D.S., Jr. (1985). Peripherally inserted central venous catheters for treatment of cystic fibrosis. *Pediatric Pulmonology, 1*, 328–332.

Review Questions

1. For skin cleaning in premature neonates, the Association of Women's Health, Obstetric and Neonatal Nurses (AWOHNN) recommends which of the following?

   A. Alcohol prep for 30 seconds twice

   B. Povidone iodine for 30 seconds

   C. Chlorhexidine for 30 seconds twice

   D. Chlorhexidine for 30 seconds

2. An IV in the frontal vein might be the site of choice in which of the following children?

   A. 2-month-old with hydrocephalus

   B. Neonate with sepsis on 3 days of antibiotic therapy

   C. 20-month-old with leukemia

   D. 16-month-old in respiratory arrest

3. What size peripheral IV catheters are recommended for use in children?

   A. 18 and 20 gauge

   B. 14 and 16 gauge

   C. 5 and 7 French

   D. 24 and 22 gauge

4. The ideal location to place an IV in a hospitalized child is:

   A. At the bedside

   B. In the treatment room

   C. In the playroom

   D. In the home of the patient

5. After two attempts at IV access during resuscitative efforts, the following site should be used:

   A. Intracardiac

   B. Intra-arterial

   C. Intrathecal

   D. Intraosseous

6. The vascular access site unique to the newborn population is the:

   A. Umbilicus

   B. Anterior fontanel

   C. Subclavian area

   D. Antecubital fossa

7. What type of vascular access device would you recommend for an adolescent with cystic fibrosis who receives intermittent IV antibiotics several times annually?

   A. Broviac catheter

   B. Subclavian catheter

   C. Implanted port

   D. Hickman catheter

8. The best method for calculating maintenance fluid requirements for a child is:

   A. Caloric method

   B. Weight method

   C. Age method

   D. Meters-squared method

9. In parenteral nutrition solutions, which component provides energy for body tissue function?

   A. Amino acids

   B. Selenium

   C. Dextrose

   D. Fatty acids

10. The purpose of neonatal exchange transfusion is to:

    A. Elevate neutrophil count

    B. Prevent congestive heart failure

    C. Change blood type

    D. Lower bilirubin level

CHAPTER 22

Infusion Therapy in an Older Adult Patient

KEY TERMS

Cellular

Centenarians

Fluid Volume Assessment

Homeostasis

Medication Reaction Changes

Nurse Competence in Aging
(NCA)

Occlusion

Older Adult

Organic

Physiologic Changes

Systemic

Demographics: An Aging Population

Although people age at different rates, changes to the human body are a hallmark of aging. As a result of such changes, disease can present differently in a person older than 65 years than it does in a younger adult or child. (Amella, 2004). Advances in medical science and technology have resulted in an increased life span; older patients today represent 13% of the U.S. population. Along with the growth of the general elderly population has come a remarkable increase in the number of Americans reaching age 100. The 1990 census found that there were 37,306 **centenarians** in the United States. Current projections estimate that the number will reach 131,000 in the year 2010. By 2030, the older adult patient population will reach about 70 million.

The number of people 65 and over in the United States who were counted in Census 2000 reached 35 million. That is about 12% of the total population. Older adults are the primary recipients of care provided, and the statistics are compelling. Currently, 48% of hospital days are used by older adults, and 45% of direct care provided by nurses in both the community and public health settings is for persons aged 65 to 85 years. The burgeoning elderly population will continue to place great strains on the health care resources of the United States, which will need to expand its services to those older adults who have chronic diseases.

Effects of the Baby Boom Among People 45 to 54 Years Old

The baby boom propelled the largest percentage increases of any age group in the 1990-to-2000 decade, according to a recent analysis of Census 2000 data by the Commerce Department's Census Bureau. (The baby boom refers to people born in the post–World War II period from 1946 through 1964.)

People born during the early years of the baby boom (1946 through 1950) fueled the 55% increase of 50- to 54-year-olds, the largest percentage growth between 1990 and 2000 of any 5-year age group, the Census Bureau said. The second fastest-growing was the 45- to 49-year-old group, which registered a 45% increase.

Nurse Competence in Aging

Nurse Competence in Aging (NCA) is a serious concern. A 5-year initiative funded by The Atlantic Philanthropies (USA) Inc., awarded to the American Nurses Association (ANA) through the American Nurses Foundation (ANF), represents a strategic alliance between ANA, the American Nurses Credentialing Center (ANCC), and the John A. Hartford Foundation Institute for Geriatric Nursing in the Division of Nursing of New York University's Steinhardt School of Education. NCA works with specialty nursing associations to bring geriatric knowledge to their membership and to enhance members' competence in caring for the older adult patient.

These older citizens have age-related health problems requiring medications and treatment, many of which are given IV. This chapter addresses the important considerations in initiating, delivering, and maintaining IV therapy in the older adult patient. The term **older adult** describes a broad category that ranges from 50 to 80 years of age because many **physiologic changes** associated with the older adult begin in the sixth decade of life. Variations do exist among individuals. Principles of **fluid volume assessment**, patient teaching, and available resources are provided.

The Older Patient as a Health Care Consumer

The older adult patient may require administration of complex IV therapies to treat a multitude of clinical conditions that may occur simultaneously. The older patient may be more acutely ill for a longer time than a younger patient, and he or she may need additional resources to regain strength and health status. As a health care consumer, the older adult patient has special needs associated with the aging process that challenge the health care system and health care providers.

For example, an 82-year-old patient with chronic pulmonary disease and congestive heart failure is in need of complicated inpatient treatment. Her children live out of state and must travel frequently to her Florida home to deal with one medical crisis after another. During each hospitalization, a phalanx of case managers besieges the patient and confers about her care. These professionals represent the hospital, the insurer, and the skilled care facility where she has been residing. A new level of case manager may be added to the picture: one representing the patient and her long-distance family. Professionals with an understanding of the economics and medical aspects of providing care for the elderly are entering this field (Greene, 1999). The National Association of Professional Geriatric Care Managers offers a directory of advocates.

Although to the health care system the patient may be a product, such as a covered life, a patient day, or an encounter, patients see it differently. They view health care as the product and themselves as the consumer (Haugh, 1999). Estimates are that caregivers spend an average of 50% more time on health care Web sites than do other types of Internet health users (Haugh). Caregivers for the elderly generally are women in their 40s with children (Haugh). Caregiver Zone.com is a site specifically aimed at seniors (Katzman, 2000).

Physiology of Aging

Aging occurs at the cellular, organic, and systemic levels. **Cellular** refers to the changes in cell structure that affect the cells' ability to respond to illness. **Organic** changes are those that affect specific organs, such as the liver's ability to detoxify medications or the kidney's propensity to slow down with aging. Major **systemic** changes affecting IV therapy practice and delivery to the older patient include those related to homeostasis, the immune and cardiovascular systems, and skin and connective tissue. Details regarding the aging of the body's systems are presented in Table 22–1.

Homeostasis

Homeostasis is the ability of the body to maintain a balance of volume and composition of body fluids within normal ranges (see Chap. 7). The kidneys, heart and blood vessels, lungs, skin, adrenal glands, hypothalamus, pituitary gland, parathyroid gland, and gastrointestinal tract are the regulatory organs associated with maintaining the body's homeostasis. Recall from Chapter 7 that the kidneys are a primary force in homeostasis because they work to adjust the amount of water and electrolytes that exit the body in an amount equal to the quantity of solution entering the body, either through IV or oral feedings. Circulating blood reaches the kidneys in sufficient volume to regulate water and electrolytes, and the pumping action of the heart provides circulation through the kidneys, which produce and excrete urine. The lungs are involved in homeostasis through ventilation. Antidiuretic hormone

TABLE 22–1   The Aging of the Body's Systems

Body System	Physiologic Changes	Signs/Symptoms
Skin	• Loss of subcutaneous tissue and thinning of dermis	• Underlying tissue more fragile; inability to respond to heat or cold quickly; proneness to heat stroke; loss of moisture; wrinkling
Sensory	• Loss of lid elasticity • Ocular changes in cornea, iris, pupil, lens • Auditory canal narrows • Calcification of ossicles • Changes in organ of Corti • Olfactory bulb and cells decrease	• Eyelids droop or turn inward • Increased astigmatism; need for more light; glare problems; need for eyeglasses • Cataracts • Increased cerumen • Hearing loss • Impaired sound transmission; tinnitus • Inability to discriminate odors
Cardiovascular	• Decreased stress response • Stiffer valves • Conductivity altered • Vessels less elastic	• Diminished cardiac output • Diastolic murmurs • More ectopic beats; less ability to respond to changes in blood pressure • Poorer perfusion to vital organs with resulting hypoxia; varicosities; peripheral pulses not always palpable
Pulmonary	• Enlargement and rigidity of chest wall • Airway collapse	• Poor expansion with less efficient air exchange; shallow breathing; less effective cough • Less efficient oxygen exchange
Gastrointestinal	• Increase in incidence of hiatal hernia • Decrease in abdominal strength • Reduced gastric acid • Slowed neural transmission • Weakened intestinal walls	• Reflux • Peptic ulcers • Vitamin deficiencies • Constipation • Incontinence • Diverticulosis
Renal	• Decrease in blood flow, glomeruli, renin, and filtration	• Increased creatinine clearance • Decreased ability to concentrate urine and conserve water • Poor response to stress
Musculoskeletal	• Shrinkage of vertebral discs • Loss of bone mass • Muscle atrophy	• Loss of height by 1.5 to 3 in. • Tendency toward fractures • Decreased strength • Decreased stamina
Neurologic	• Diminished REM sleep • Altered pain sensation • Tactile sense decreases • Sleep disorders	• Difficulty with balance and position changes • Decreased perception of pain • Loss of sensation in extremities
Immune	• Decrease in thymus mass • Increase in immunoglobulins	• Decline in cell-mediated immunity with possible reactivation of herpes, tuberculosis • Autoimmune response not associated with disease

(Continued)

TABLE 22–1   The Aging of the Body's Systems *(Continued)*

Body System	Physiologic Changes	Signs/Symptoms
Endocrine	• Loss of sensitivity to insulin • Decrease in sex hormones	• Blood glucose does not return to normal as rapidly • BPH, testicular firmness; vaginal dryness and atrophy • Longer time to orgasm

BPH, benign prostatic hypertrophy; REM, random eye movement.
(Adapted from Ebersole, P. [2004]. Age-related changes. In: Ebersole P, Hess P. & Luggen A. *Toward healthy aging: Human needs and nursing responses* [pp. 74–80]. St. Louis: Mosby.)

(ADH), which causes fluid retention, is manufactured in the hypothalamus and stored in the pituitary gland. ADH also is involved in controlling blood volume. When blood volume is increased, ADH secretion is decreased and water is excreted through the kidneys. Parathyroid hormone affects calcium and phosphate concentrations and influences reabsorption of calcium, a key factor in maintaining fluid and electrolyte monitoring and replacement. The gastrointestinal tract also plays a major role in homeostasis by absorption and reabsorption through the small intestine, or "great absorbing organ." For the body to maintain homeostasis, all these organs must work in synchronicity.

Normal homeostatic mechanisms in aging become less efficient in the face of external trauma, surgical intervention, disease process, or infection. The older patient is vulnerable to complications associated with routine IV therapy.

The Immune System

In aging, the normal immune system becomes hyporesponsive to foreign antigens and hyperresponsive to self (Metheny, 2000). These changes may contribute to decreased resistance to infection, increased autoimmunity, and development of other immune disorders. The immunocompromised patient is at increased risk for IV-associated infection.

The Cardiovascular System

Cardiovascular changes are profound, contributing to a slower response to the stress of blood loss, fluid depletion, shock, and acid–base imbalances. Changes in renal and cardiac status have the potential to place the patient at great risk for development of infusion-related complications (see Table 22–1).

Skin and Connective Tissue

The skin, the body's first defense against disease, changes in texture, depth, and integrity as the person ages. After age 60 years, epidermal cell replacement decreases, resulting in a marked thinning of the epidermis and an increased fragility of the skin's surface. The result is dry, transparent, paper-thin tissue that tears easily and heals slowly. Changes in the dermis create a loose, wrinkling effect. The skin becomes pale, and nerve endings are less sensitive. The patient is at risk for thermal injuries. Subcutaneous fat cells decrease, resulting in changes to the superficial fascia, including decreased production of sebum and sweat (Metheny, 2000). Loss of subcutaneous tissue and resultant thinning of the skin present a venous access challenge. Purpura and ecchymoses may appear because of dermal fragility; minor trauma may inflict bruising.

Fluid Balance

Physiologic changes of aging affect the older adult's fluid balance. Fluid reserves are limited, and total body water is reduced by 6%, creating a potential for fluid volume deficit. Gastrointestinal changes such as decreased volume of saliva and gastric juice and decreased calcium absorption cause the mouth to be drier and increase potential for sodium and potassium deficit during episodes of vomiting and gastric suction. Assessment guidelines are presented in Box 22–1.

The usual assessment measures to determine fluid balance should be adjusted when providing care to the older adult. For example, testing skin turgor on the forearm is no longer a valid measure because skin loses elasticity with age. Skin turgor is best assessed in the older patient by tenting the tissue on the forehead or over the sternum. Alterations in skin elasticity are less marked in those sites (Metheny, 2000).

Senses

Changes in sensation affect the patient's response to treatment; changes in vision, hearing, and tactile sensation may alter communication. After age 50 years, subtle changes in the hearing process result in difficulty in differentiating sounds. For

---

BOX 22–1   Fluid Volume Assessment Parameters in the Older Adult Patient

Skin turgor of forehead/sternum
Temperature <98.6°F
Decreased rate/filling of hand veins
Intake and output
Daily weight
Tongue—center should remain moist
Blood pressure—possibility of orthostatic hypotension
Swallowing function
Functional assessment of patient's ability to obtain fluids

(Adapted from Metheny, N.M. [2000]. *Fluid and electrolyte balance* [4th ed., p. 352]. Philadelphia: Lippincott Williams & Wilkins.)

example, the older patient often cannot hear someone speaking within an otherwise normal range because of the outside influence of loud music or traffic (Metheny, 2000; S. Weinstein, personal communication, March, 1998). Older patients may need assistive devices, such as hearing aids, eyeglasses, and visual aids, to learn the skills associated with infusion therapy. Because of decreased tactile sensation, infiltration might go unnoticed, contributing to the potential for development of tissue necrosis, infection, or compartment syndrome (Metheny, 2000; see Chap. 9).

Vascular System

Chronic disease, such as asthma, chronic obstructive pulmonary disease, hypertension, and the changes associated with atherosclerosis and arteriosclerosis affect the blood vessels in the older patient. Vessels are fragile, with small, thin-walled surface capillaries easily observed across the extremities and chest of the older patient. Vascular fragility is a potential problem for IV access; a tourniquet sometimes is not used to decrease the potential for bruising.

Psychologic Changes

A confused patient or one experiencing the ill effects of senile dementia will respond differently to treatment. Teaching may become complicated because the patient has difficulty in differentiating between recent and remote memory. For example, the patient forgets what he or she learned the previous day, but remembers all the details of early childhood.

Access and Equipment

Medication Reaction Changes

In otherwise healthy adults, physiologic changes cause **medication reaction changes**—that is, they influence the absorption, distribution, and clearance of medications. Absorption in older adults is complete, yet slower. Age-related changes also affect the rate and extent of absorption. As people age, they lose lean body mass and gain adipose tissue. With less fluid available, water-soluble medications can reach toxic levels more quickly. Vigilant monitoring is needed with potentially nephrotoxic agents, H2-antagonists, hypoglycemics, and nonsteroidal anti-inflammatory agents. With decreases in kidney and liver function, clearance and excretion of drugs also takes longer. Monitoring serum protein and albumin levels as well as renal and liver functions is essential to help the older patient avoid toxicity or undertreatment (Amella, 2004).

When providing IV therapy to older adult patients, careful consideration should be given to the type of treatment ordered, the duration of therapy, and availability of IV access. A biocompatible catheter material is preferred, including products manufactured from silicone, elastomeric hydrogels, and others (see Chap. 11); these products are nonthrombogenic. The smallest gauge possible for the therapy being delivered should be used. Consideration must be given to the type of catheter–tubing connection used; some products are more irritating to frail skin and usually must be padded to prevent injury to the skin surface and underlying tissue.

When a central venous access device is needed for long-term therapy, the type of device should be determined carefully. Consideration should be given to the patient's living circumstances, availability of family or other support systems, and ability to manipulate the equipment involved and to maintain a secure, intact dressing (Infusion Nurses Society [INS], 1998, 2000, 2005).

Flow Control

Electronic flow control devices (electronic infusion devices) should be used liberally in the older adult to prevent overhydration and resultant fluid imbalances. Pump infusion pressures should be monitored carefully. As with all patients, the device used should be biomedically safe and meet and exceed standards developed by ECRI, formerly the Emergency Care Research Institute, and internal safety committees (see Chap. 11). ECRI publishes a diversity of information helpful in the selection of products for all patient populations, but especially those significant for older adults.

An electronic flow control device should be an accessory to quality patient care and not a substitute for ongoing monitoring. The nurse should refer to technical information provided by the manufacturer of equipment and institutional guidelines for use. The alarm on a pump with a fixed pressure of 4 psi activates when the peripheral venous pressure reaches 200 mm Hg (1 psi = 50 mm Hg). This setting can seriously harm the patient when infiltration occurs; the alarm will sound only after the damage has been noted. An infiltrated site exerts a mean pressure gradient at 100 mm Hg or 2 psi. Pumps that continue to infuse or that do not have a free-flow alarm system pose potential risks to the older patient (ECRI, 1999).

Site Selection

Principles of site selection applied to the younger patient (see Chap. 21) also may be used to determine appropriate venous access in the older patient. Assessment of available peripheral venous access is necessary. Avoiding bruised, fragile veins and conserving veins for future use are major considerations. The nurse should secure adequate lighting and ensure patient comfort.

Technique

Although a tourniquet may be used, it also may not be necessary. Excessive distention of the veins may contribute to bruising and subsequent tearing of the venous wall and hematoma. The veins should be palpated carefully to determine state of health and condition. Corded veins may indicate thickening, occluded vein walls, and valve blockage. Threading a catheter into such vessels may be difficult; venous stasis and dependent edema may result (Metheny, 2000).

Table 22–2 lists the special techniques required in an older adult. Skin tension is determined by assessing the direction or axis of the vessel. Traction is ensured by placing the thumb directly along the vein axis 2 to 3 inches below the intended venipuncture site. The palm and fingers of the hand used to apply traction hold and stabilize the patient's extremity. Traction is maintained throughout the procedure (INS, 1998, 2000, 2005).

The directional line of the vessel is determined. If the vein is very small, venous distention may be inadequate, and imaging techniques may be used. Imaging uses magnetic light to visualize hard-to-find veins.

A small-gauge IV catheter should be selected and positioned with the bevel up. The catheter should be aligned parallel to the vein track and brought close to the skin directly above the insertion site. A lower angle decreases vein trauma on insertion (INS, 1998, 2000; 2005; Metheny, 2000).

TABLE 22–2   Special Techniques in the Older Adult Patient

Intervention	Rationale
Avoid tourniquet in patients with fragile veins or who are taking anticoagulants or steroids.	Tourniquet may not be needed; use of tourniquet may contribute to hematoma formation.
If tourniquet is used, release it quickly.	Quick release decreases backflow of blood.
Multiple-tourniquet technique may be an option to facilitate venous distention:	
Grasp the patient's mid-upper arm and stroke the arm downward toward the hand. Place a tourniquet on the extremity.	Stroking promotes venous filling.
Wait 1–2 min and then place a second tourniquet below the antecubital fossa and continue to stroke the lower forearm.	Placement of the second tourniquet stimulates venous pressure and forces venous distention to small veins that otherwise would not be visible.
A third tourniquet may be placed after an additional 1–2 min at a point just above the wrist.	The third tourniquet promotes additional venous distention, particularly in the very small veins of the digits and lower wrist.
Release the first tourniquet and evaluate inner wrist, thumb, knuckle, and fingers for distention.	Although not *ideal* for infusion purposes, the veins in this area will fill owing to venous pressure and provide adequate hemodilution for infusion purposes.
In edematous patient, use anatomic landmarks.	Facilitates location of appropriate veins
Gently tap the vein to distend; do not slap.	Avoids hematoma formation and bruising
Use transillumination.	Assists in visualizing veins
Insert catheter with steady, firm motion.	Prevents bruising associated with difficult venipuncture
Consider preflushing catheter in patients with spidery, capillary-type veins.	Avoids trauma associated with sudden flushing
Use a one-handed approach.	Allows you to secure patient's extremity.

The direct or indirect technique may be applied (see Chap. 12); however, for patients with small, fragile veins, the clinician may find the two-step technique more beneficial. If the veins are extremely fragile and if a tourniquet has been used, it may be helpful to release the tourniquet as soon as blood return is evident. Doing so prevents damage from high-pressure backflow of blood from the catheter insertion point. The hooded technique also may help reduce vein damage. In this approach, the clinician advances the catheter forward over the bevel tip into the vein. This action retracts the stylet tip inside the catheter. Then, the clinician threads the catheter into the vein by grasping the hub of the catheter and advancing the catheter and stylet as a unit up the vein. This procedure minimizes the possibility of perforating the vein during threading. The clinician must maintain stabilization and skin tension throughout the process.

Maintenance and Monitoring

Securing, dressing, and stabilizing the IV catheter are unique challenges when providing infusion care to the elderly patient. Although the catheter should be secure, use of excessive tape is discouraged because of the fragility of the patient's skin. Adaptations to taping technique should be used as needed. The use of additional protection such as a skin polymer solution should be considered. The polymer solution is best applied in a concentric circle from the center to the periphery and allowed to air dry before the dressing is applied (INS, 1998, 2000, 2005). The elderly patient may be confused owing to physiologic reasons or medications, and the nurse should make every effort to ensure safety with the infusion device. Patient education is essential to ensure compliance with the plan of care. See Box 22–2 for principles of patient teaching.

Care should be taken when securement devices or restraints are used. The IV tubing should be long enough to provide adequate range of motion, but not so long as to dangle on the floor or get caught on the bedside or IV pole. A Luer-locking device provides added protection. Surgical stretch mesh gauze also may be used to cover the IV site, providing stability and protecting the catheter from snagging bed garments. Roll-type gauze should be avoided, consistent with institutional guidelines and established practice standards (INS, 1998, 2000, 2005).

BOX 22–2   Principles of Patient Teaching for the Older Adult Patient Receiving Infusion Therapy

- Speak slowly, clearly, and directly to the patient.
- Hearing impairment and sensitivity to outside sounds require patience.
- Address the patient by his or her proper name.
- Explain steps in logical order.
- Take steps to decrease anxiety.
- Use familiar terminology.

The IV site should be evaluated at regularly established intervals and as needed to ensure patency. Site rotation is recommended every 72 hours; however, deviations may be acceptable (see Chaps. 4, 9, and 12). If a routine site change is not performed because of limited access or the patient's clinical condition, a full description of the site, dressing change, and reasons for not completing the site rotation should be documented in the clinical records.

Occlusion

Catheter **occlusion** is the complete or partial obstruction of a vascular access device, preventing or limiting the infusion of solution or medication. Occlusion may occur if

TABLE 22–3   Occlusion Assessment and Nursing Interventions

Type of Occlusion	Appropriate Intervention
Fibrin	• Notify physician. • Obtain treatment orders for use of thrombolytic agent. • Complete catheter clearance.
Mechanical	• Notify physician. • Assess for kinking or clamp and correct. • If in-line filter is clogged, replace filter. • If sutures securing the device are constricting catheter, obtain order to remove sutures; reapply stabilizing device. • If noncoring needle is not in septum, remove and replace correctly.
Pinch off	• Notify physician. • If radiograph is ordered, notify radiologist of potential for pinch-off. • Determine appropriate intervention consistent with grade of catheter path.
Rupture	• Notify physician. • Follow procedures for catheter or air embolism.
Malposition or migration	• Notify physician. • Reposition patient to alter direction of catheter tip. • Inject fluid through catheter as ordered. • Catheter may be repositioned fluoroscopically as ordered. • Catheter may be partially withdrawn using aseptic technique. • If unsuccessful at repositioning catheter, notify physician for orders to remove device.
Drug and mineral precipitation	• Notify physician. • Obtain orders for instillation of thrombolytics to rule out occlusion. • Obtain orders for catheter clearance. • Clear catheter using hydrochloric acid, cysteine hydrochloride, sodium bicarbonate, ethanol, or sodium hydroxide as indicated.
Lipid residue	• Notify physician. • Obtain orders for catheter clearance using 70% ethanol or sodium hydroxide. • Complete catheter clearance.

(INS [2004]).

blood is permitted to flow back—or reflux—into the lumen of the catheter, owing to improper flushing technique or infrequent monitoring of the infusion site and the patient's activity. Types of occlusion and appropriate interventions are presented in Table 22–3.

References and Selected Readings

Asterisks indicate references cited in text.

*Amella, E.J. (2004). Presentation of illness in older adults. *American Journal of Nursing, 104*(10), 40–51.

American Association of Retired Persons. (2004). *A profile of older Americans.* Washington, DC: U.S. Department of Health and Human Services.

Bulger, R. (1999). What will health care look like in the future? In: E. Sullivan (Ed.). *Creating nursing's future* (pp. 16–17). St. Louis, MO: Mosby.

Chyna, J.T. (2000). The consumer revolution: An age of changing expectations. *Healthcare Executive, 15*(1), 7–9.

*Ebersole, P., Hess, P., & Luggen A. (2004). Age-related changes. In: *Toward healthy aging. Human needs and nursing responses* (pp. 74–80). Philadelphia: Mosby.

*ECRI. (1999). *Continuing care risk management system* (pp. 28–30). Plymouth Meeting, PA: Author, Health Devices.

Elsner, R.J., Quinn, M.E., & Fanning, S.D. (1999). Ethical and policy considerations for centenarians—the oldest old. *Image: Journal of Nursing Scholarship, 31,* 263–267.

Gordon, S. (1997). *Life support: Three nurses on the front lines.* Boston: Little, Brown and Company.

*Greene, J. (1999). Case management: Consumer consultant. *Hospitals and Health Networks, 73*(12), 24–25.

*Hankins, J. (1998). Aging adult. In: Infusion Nurses Society. *Core curriculum for intravenous nursing* (pp. 165–166). Philadelphia: Lippincott Williams & Wilkins.

*Haugh, R. (1999). The new consumer. *Hospitals and Health Networks, 73*(12), 30–32.

Herr, K. (2002). Chronic pain: Challenges and assessment strategies. *Journal of Gerontology Nursing, 28*(1), 20–27, quiz 54–55.

Hoechst, M.R. (1999). *Managed care digest series: Nursing home industry summary/institutional digest* (pp. 24–27).

Horgas, A., & McLennon, S. (2004). Pain management. In: Ebersole P, et al. (Eds.). *Toward healthy aging. Human needs and nursing responses* (pp. 229–250). St. Louis: Mosby.

*Infusion Nurses Society. (1998). *Revised standards of practice.* Philadelphia: Lippincott Williams & Wilkins.

*Infusion Nurses Society. (2005). *Standards of practice.* Philadelphia: Lippincott Williams & Wilkins.

*Infusion Nurses Society. (2004). Policies and procedures for infusion nursing of the older adult, INS Author. Norwood, MA

*Katzman, C.N. (2000). Catching the eldercare wave. *Healthcare Business, 3*(4), 22.

*Metheny, N.M. (2000). *Fluid and electrolyte balance* (4th ed.). Philadelphia: Lippincott Williams & Wilkins.

Payne, K. (2004) Total serum protein. Available at http://my.webmd.com/hw/health_guide_atoz/hw436 14.asp. (Accessed 9/01/2005.)

Sansivero, G.E. (1998). Venous anatomy and physiology. *Journal of Intravenous Nursing, 21*(Suppl. 5), S207–S209.

Thurlow, K.L. (2002). Infections in the elderly, pt. 2. *Emergency Medical Services, 31*(4), 44.

*U.S. Census Bureau. (2000). Resident population of the United States: Middle series projections, by age and sex. Available at http://www.census.gov/main/www/cen2000.html. (Accessed 2/15/2006.)

Review Questions

Note: Questions below may have more than one right answer.

1. Principles of education in the older adult patient include which of the following?
   A. Speak slowly, clearly, and directly.
   B. Address the patient by name.
   C. Use familiar terminology.
   D. All of the above

2. Which of the following skin layers is associated with development of dry, transparent surfaces?
   A. Deep fascia
   B. Dermis
   C. Epidermis
   D. Superficial fascia

3. Skin turgor in the adult patient should be measured at what location?

   A. Forehead

   B. Sternum

   C. Abdomen

   D. Inner aspect of forearm

4. All the following are true when determining skin tension *except*:

   A. Assess direction of vessel

   B. Assess axis of vessel

   C. Eliminate traction

   D. Determine direction line of vessel

5. The alarm on an electronic infusion device with fixed pressure of 4 psi activates when peripheral venous pressure reaches how many mm Hg?

   A. 100

   B. 150

   C. 200

   D. 250

6. The technique used to reduce vein damage is referred to as:

   A. Retraction

   B. Hooded

   C. Threaded

   D. Advanced

7. Total body water in the older patient is reduced by what percentage?

   A. 2%

   B. 5%

   C. 6%

   D. 8%

8. Respiratory function in the adult patient is associated with which of the following?

   A. Decreased elasticity of lung tissue

   B. Increased number of alveoli

   C. Decreased compliance of chest wall

   D. All of the above

9. Which of the following statements is true concerning skin turgor in the adult patient?

   A. It is a poor indicator of hydration.

   B. It is a good indicator of hydration.

   C. It diminishes ability to conserve sodium.

   D. It is more effective at cooling body temperature.

10. A primary cause of change in mental status, particularly confusion, in older adults, is which of the following:

    A. Stress

    B. The aging process

    C. Drug toxicity

    D. Visual changes

CHAPTER 23

Infusion Therapy in Alternate Clinical Settings: Cost Factors and Treatment Modalities

KEY TERMS

Ambulatory Infusion Centers
Home Health Care
Hospice
ICD9 Code

Long-term Care
Medicare
Subacute Care

The Changing Health Care Environment

In today's complex health care industry, hospitals have strong financial incentives to discharge patients as soon as possible. Hospitals and other health care providers face an increasingly complex dilemma: how to provide the highest quality care at the lowest price. Because of continuing advances in medical science and technology and the influence of managed care insurance contracts, patients discharged from hospitals now can receive complex, high-level services, once available only in hospitals, in alternate care settings. The patient population receiving treatment outside the hospital ranges from critically ill newborns to chronically ill older adults. The nurse needs an array of clinical and critical thinking skills to care for these patients, often while working within an autonomous practice setting.

Cost-cutting measures have enhanced the growth of new ways to provide infusion therapy services. The growth of infusion therapy in the home and alternate clinical settings has created countless opportunities for infusion nurses nationwide. Infusion nurse specialists must assess the level of skills and services currently being provided and determine venues where they can best use their skills, including, but not limited to settings such as the following:

- Hospitals
- Physicians' offices
- Home care
- Long-term care facilities
- Infusion pharmacies
- Subacute settings
- Teaching for other professionals
- Ambulatory infusion centers
- Insertion of peripherally inserted central catheters (PICCs) and midline catheters
- Hospice settings

This chapter examines alternate settings for the delivery of infusion therapy. It discusses the influence of managed care and cost-containment efforts. It thoroughly explores home infusion therapy, along with the parameters mandated by Medicare, patient selection, the role of various health care team members, and typical infusion therapies provided in the home. It also explores additional sites for infusion therapy delivery, including hospice, subacute care, ambulatory infusion centers, and long-term care.

Influence of Managed Care

Managed care is a system of controls to manage access, costs, and quality of health care services. The controls may include any or all of the following:

- Preferred provider contracts
- Prior approval/authorization
- Patient education/incentives
- Use review/quality assurance

Two other controls used in managed care include case management and capitation. Case management is a program to manage high-cost health care cases by exploring alternative care options to achieve the same patient outcomes while better controlling costs. Case management requires the insurance company and the provider of services (ie, home care agency and infusion pharmacy) to discuss the necessary infusion therapy orders for the patient before the initiation of services. Usually, the parties determine and agree on a number of nurse visits necessary for the infusion therapy ordered. Periodic updates and communication continue throughout the duration of the therapy. Patients and caregivers are taught to administer the ordered therapy with limited nursing monitoring, which results in decreased nursing visits and costs.

Capitation is a system of prepayment for health care in which a provider receives a flat monthly fee for agreeing to provide specified services to members of health maintenance organizations (HMOs) assigned to the provider for a contracted time (usually a year). Unlike traditional fee-for-service (FFS) systems, capitated systems pay providers, either individually or collectively, the same amount per member each month, in advance, regardless of how many times the members use their services. Usually, risk sharing is involved, meaning that the HMO and contracted provider share the financial risks and rewards to provide cost-effective care.

Under the auspices of the managed care umbrella,

- Payers are changing.
- New delivery systems are designed around risk sharing.
- Payers/providers are competing for managed care savings (profits).
- Competition is increasing.
- Risk is shifting (in both directions).
- Attitudes of providers, payers, and employers are changing.

Under the prior system, providers were paid on a fee-for-service basis; they are now paid on a discounted fee-for-service basis or by capitation. The patient base was the local community; now it is covered members/patients. The philosophy of care was to treat the disease and restore wellness; however, now the main focus is to maintain health. When providers are reimbursed under bundling or capitated contracts, the incentive is to keep members healthy, provide care in the least costly setting, and decrease total costs. The members are scheduled to have infusion therapy care and procedures performed in alternative clinical settings such as in the home, outpatient clinics, or ambulatory infusion centers, rather than in the hospital to avoid the higher costs.

Home Health Care

Home health care originally was conceived as a stage in the continuum of care after hospitalization, during which recovery and rehabilitation could continue effectively in the patient's home at a lower cost than if furnished in a hospital. Today, home care services often are used as low-cost alternatives for in-patient hospital care. Provision of services in the home decreases health care costs across the board and improves access to health care to all age groups in the community. The National Voluntary Consensus Standards for Home Health Care provided by the National Quality Forum (NQF) defines home health care as:

> "any healthcare services provided to clients in their homes, including but not limited to skilled nursing services, home health aide services, palliative and end-of-life care (e.g., in-home hospice services), therapies (i.e., physical, speech-language, and occupational), homemaker services/personal care, social services, infusion and pharmacy services, medical supplies and equipment and in-home physician services" (NQF, 2004 p. 4).

The NQF reports in the *Consensus Standards* that more than 4 million patients receive care from more than 20,000 home health agencies. Seven thousand of these agencies are Medicare-certified. The *Consensus Standards* also reports that in 2001 home health

TABLE 23–1   Home Infusion Coverage

Payer	Antibiotic	Chemotherapy	Hydration	Pain	Total Parenteral Nutrition
Medicare A (hospital)	No	No	No	No	—
Medicare B	Select antifungal/ antiviral	Yes	No	Yes	Very specific criteria *must* be met.
Medicaid	Yes	Yes	Yes	Yes	Yes
HMO/PPO	Yes	Yes	Yes	Yes	Yes
Commercial	Yes	Yes	Yes	Yes	Yes
CHAMPUS	Yes	Yes	Yes	Yes	Yes

HMO, health maintenance organization; PPO, preferred provider organization; CHAMPUS, Civilian Health and Medical Programs for Uniformed Services.

care services, which included public and private insurance and out-of-pocket payments, exceeded $45 billion; Medicare and Medicaid were reported to have covered half of these costs.

Reimbursement for Home Care Services

Third-party payers for home care therapies include Medicare, Medicaid, commercial insurance, HMOs, preferred provider organizations, and managed care companies. Managed care payers, HMOs, and preferred provider organizations determine payments on a case-by-case basis and usually do not go out of network unless absolutely necessary. Medicaid, third-party payers, and managed care programs have various payment methods along with specific criteria. An overview of various payment plans for therapies is presented in Table 23–1.

Combined with a working knowledge of precisely what types of therapy that various payer sources cover, it is essential that the written record of care, including the diagnosis, be consistent with the type of therapy provided. As in the tertiary care setting, a series of codes has been developed to reflect procedures (current procedural terminology [CPT]) and diagnoses (International Category of Disease [ICD9]). In the physician's office, application of the appropriate CPT code combined with a *correct* diagnosis ensures third-party payment. In home care, the ICD9 descriptors are applied. The **ICD9 code** filed by the infusion provider should match the diagnosis and the type of therapy provided. For example, blood transfusion is appropriate for a diagnosis of anemia; the ICD code is 285.9. Antibiotics are appropriate for a diagnosis of osteomyelitis; the ICD code is 730.2. Refer to Table 23–2 for more information.

Specific Considerations Related to Medicare

Home care has been one of the fastest growing benefits in the **Medicare** program, which is the largest purchaser of home health services in the United States (Disbrow, 1999). The number of Medicare beneficiaries has been expanding by approximately

TABLE 23–2 Potential Home Infusion Diagnosis and Suggested Therapies

Diagnosis	ICD9 Description Code	Suggested Therapy
Abscess, general	682.9	Antibiotic
Acquired immunodeficiency syndrome	279.3/D43	Anti-infective/TPN
Anemia	285.9	Blood
Arthritis, infective	711.9	Antibiotic
Bacteremia caused by organism	038.8	Antibiotic
Cellulitis	682.9	Antibiotic
Colitis	558.9	TEN/TPN
Congestive heart failure	428.9	Dobutamine
Crohn's disease	555.9	TEN/TPN
Deficiency, growth hormone	253.3	Growth hormone
Deficiency, immunoglobulin	279.0	Gamma globulin
Dehydration	276.5	Hydration
Diabetes with gangrene	250.7	Antibiotic
Endocarditis, infectious	421.0	Antibiotic
Fibrosis, cystic	277.0	Antibiotic/TEN/TPN
Fungal disease	117.9	Anti-infective
Hemophilia	286.0	Blood products
Hyperemesis gravidarum	643.0	TPN/hydration
Hypogammaglobulinemia	279.0	Gamma globulin
Infection, bacterial	041.9	Antibiotic
Labor, premature	644.2	Tocolytics
Leukemia	208.9	Chemotherapy
Malabsorption	579.9	TEN/TPN
Malnutrition	263.9	TEN/TPN
Meningitis	322.9	Antibiotic
Neoplasm	199.1	Chemotherapy
Osteomyelitis	730.2	Antibiotic
Pain, bone	733.9	Pain
Pulmonary disease, chronic obstructive	416.9	α_1-Proteinase inhibitor
Septicemia	038.9	Antibiotic
Short-bowel syndrome	579.2	TPN
Thrombophlebitis	451.9	Anticoagulants
Wound, complicated	879.8	Antibiotic

TEN, total enteral nutrition; TPN, total parenteral nutrition.

2% each year (Disbrow) and is expected to accelerate even more rapidly with the enrollment of the baby-boomer generation. Eligibility for the home care benefit within the Medicare program requires that the following conditions be met (Disbrow):

- The patient must be at least 65 years of age and have received acceptance for Medicare coverage.
- The patient must be homebound. In other words, the patient must be confined to the home in such a way that leaving requires considerable effort and the assistance of another person or an adaptive device such as a cane, walker, or wheelchair. Absences from the home must be infrequent, of short duration, and for the purposes of receiving additional medical care.
- Home care services must be provided under a Plan of Care established and reviewed by a licensed physician directly involved in the patient's care. Written physician orders are required for home care.
- The home care services the patient needs must be skilled intermittent nursing, physical therapy, occupational therapy, or speech therapy.
- A certified Medicare program provider who agrees to adhere to the extensive Medicare Conditions of Participation regulations and requirements and accepts Medicare's reimbursement for the provision of those services must provide home care (Health Care Financing Administration [HCFA], 1999).

The following are the requirements of Medicare Conditions of Participation (HCFA, 1999):

1. Nursing services must require the skills of a registered nurse.
2. Intermittent care is defined as consisting of up to 35 hours total per week by all professional disciplines combined.
3. No more than 8 hours of combined services may be provided per 24-hour day. Daily visits are not to last longer than a specified number of days per month.

Services eligible for Medicare reimbursement fall under Part A or B (Table 23–1). Congress decided in the 1980s to eliminate cost-based reimbursement to hospitals to reduce health care costs. Medicare introduced its prospective payment system (PPS) in the form of diagnosis-related groups (DRGs; Disbrow, 1999). Implementation of PPS reduced the costs of hospitalization by shifting the end point of care to the home, thereby contributing to the growth of the alternative care delivery system. Before January 1, 1998, Medicare-certified home health agencies were reimbursed retrospectively for the costs they incurred in providing services to patients. On January 1, 1998, reimbursement provisions for Medicare home health services underwent significant changes in legislation and regulations. Prospective payment for home care made the transition to an interim payment system in October, 2000. This form of prospective payment results in lump-sum payments for services provided to home care patients, a system similar to the DRG system used for hospital care.

Medicare has begun to redefine benefits it previously covered by limiting access to services, tightening eligibility requirements, and re-examining homebound status. As the government continues to struggle with rising costs, further changes are anticipated. A major problem that exists is when the home health care agency determines that a patient is no longer homebound and the patient is discharged. If the patient is receiving a long-term infusion therapy such as total parenteral nutrition (TPN) but is no longer homebound, the patient will be discharged and no further nursing assessment and care will be provided in the home. Who takes care of any problems that arise? The infusion pharmacy providing the therapy and equipment will not be reimbursed for any nursing provided.

REIMBURSEMENT FOR HOME INFUSION THERAPY

Reimbursement for home infusion therapy is very complex and depends on the nature of the home infusion business itself. For example, a Medicare-certified home health agency may bill for supplies associated with a Medicare Part A visit, but the same agency may not bill under Part A for TPN. Usually, a licensed infusion pharmacy provides the TPN and supplies. When a managed care company or private insurance is involved, services are provided on a per diem basis.

Patient Criteria for Home Care Infusion Therapy

In addition to meeting Medicare criteria for home care, patients must meet other criteria to qualify as candidates for home infusion therapy (Box 23–1). Patients are responsible for specific aspects of their infusion therapy, including administration of the ordered therapy, monitoring, catheter line management, operation of electronic infusion equipment (if necessary), and other duties. The patient, caregiver, or both are taught to identify signs and symptoms of complications that must be reported to the nurse, and are also taught how to identify any other situations that require immediate attention. A 24-hour emergency phone number is provided to patients and families, should they need any help.

APPROPRIATE DIAGNOSIS

Often the type of drug therapy ordered determines a patient's appropriateness for home infusion therapy. Many drugs given in the inpatient setting are acceptable for

---

BOX 23–1   Criteria for Patient Selection for Home Infusion

1. Appropriate diagnosis
2. Medical stability
3. Appropriate venous access device for ordered therapy
4. Evaluation of drug therapy
5. Laboratory profile
6. Presence of a caregiver
7. Learning ability of patient/caregiver
8. Appropriate home environment
9. Financial resources

home infusion programs. Table 23–2 listed some common home infusion diagnoses and suggested therapies.

The home infusion therapy ordered must be consistent with the patient's diagnosis and ability to receive therapy in the home. Common diagnoses for antibiotic therapy include osteomyelitis, otitis media, sinusitis, cryptococcal meningitis, pneumonia, subacute bacterial endocarditis, primary bacteremia, cellulitis, urinary tract infections, pyelonephritis, septic arthritis, histoplasmosis, peritonitis, toxic shock syndrome, Lyme disease, rickettsial infection, opportunistic infections related to acquired immunodeficiency syndrome, and many others. All types of patients with cancer are appropriate candidates for home infusion of antineoplastic agents, especially combination protocols. Fluorouracil (5FU) is a common antineoplastic agent infused in the home setting. Additional infusion therapies for the oncology patient may include nutritional support, pain management, antiemetics, antibiotics and leucovorin rescue regimens.

MEDICAL STABILITY

Medical stability is necessary of patients regardless of their ability to perform the ordered therapy including infusions. A family member or other caregiver may assume full responsibility for performing all procedures. Another person may be needed as a backup, depending on the home situation. Ideally, the patient should have a comprehensive assessment before discharge from the hospital. This allows the home health agency/home infusion pharmacy to assess the patient's needs and ability to provide the care. However, last minute referrals make this step difficult. The hospital needs to assist in this very important step.

VENOUS ACCESS

Appropriate vascular access is essential for home infusion therapy. Some patients may be discharged with an infusion device in place that was used in the hospital, including a jugular vein catheter, subclavian vein catheters (triple lumens), tunneled catheters (Hickman/Broviac, Groshong), implanted ports (chest or arm), PICCs, midline catheters, or peripheral catheters. Other times, the skilled and competent home nurse initiates the vascular access device placement in the home, such as a peripheral catheter for short-term therapy or a midline catheter for long-term therapy. Teaching protocols for catheter care management and flush procedures for the type of access are required and must be patient specific to address all areas of maintenance for self-care.

Certain drugs and infusions require the insertion of a central venous access device. The Infusion Nurses Society *2000 Infusion Nursing Standards of Practice* are very specific about appropriate venous access. Standard 43 *Site Selection* states:

> "Therapies not appropriate for peripheral-short catheters and midline catheters include continuous vesicant chemotherapy, parenteral nutrition formulae exceeding 10% dextrose and/or 5% protein, solutions and/or medications with pH less than 5 or greater than 9, and solutions and/or medications with osmolarity greater than 500 mOsm/l" (Infusion Nurses Society, 2000, p. 65).

Some of the most common drugs that must be given through a PICC line or other central access device include vancomycin, oxacillin, penicillin, dopamine, and dilantin, just to name a few. It is very important for the patient to receive the appropriate line prior to the initiation of therapy.

EVALUATION OF DRUG THERAPY

Each drug ordered is evaluated for all aspects of the administration: length of time required for the administration; dosing frequency; duration of therapy; insurer approval of the method of administration, and patient risks. For example, antibiotics may be administered over 30 minutes to 2 hours, depending on the drug and volume of solution. Dosing may be every 4, 6, 8, 12, or 24 hours. Duration may be 4 to 8 weeks or even longer. Certain drugs such as morphine and chemotherapy must be administered with an electronic pump or device. It is common to place a patient on an ambulatory infusion pump when the dosing schedule of the drug is every 4 to 6 hours. Oxacillin and penicillin are common drugs frequently dosed every 4 hours, and the pump allows the patient and caregiver to get some rest. Some drugs require close monitoring and the presence of a nurse in the event of an anaphylactic reaction.

LABORATORY PROFILE

Procedures must be established for routine laboratory studies and transmission of reports to the physician, home infusion pharmacist, and home care agency. The nurse should report changes in laboratory values immediately to the physician so that adjustments can be made in the treatment plan consistent with the patient's clinical condition. Laboratory testing of blood levels including complete blood counts (CBC) and metabolic panels may be performed weekly or biweekly for patients receiving total parenteral nutrition (TPN), antineoplastic therapy, and antibiotics or antifungal agents. Certain drugs, such as vancomycin, gentamicin, and tobramycin, may require routine peak and trough levels to avoid toxicity. The infusion pharmacist is vital in monitoring the patient and an excellent resource for the physician and nurse involved in the care of the patient.

PRESENCE OF A SUPPORT SYSTEM

Even if the patient meets the criteria for home care as discussed earlier, many adjustments need to be made in the home. The patient often is very ill and still recovering from whatever condition necessitated the hospitalization. The infusion therapy orders usually are a continuation of the therapy the patient received as an inpatient. Planning is necessary to provide 24-hour support from a family member or other caregiver until the patient can assume the procedures and self-care. The home care nurse/infusion nurse makes the initial visit and teaches the patient and/or caregiver to provide the ordered therapy. In most cases this can be accomplished on the first visit; sometimes, however, the nurse must make extra visits until the patient and/or caregiver is competent. A nurse is always available on call should any problems arise. A home health aide may be available to help the patient with personal care.

TECHNICAL CRITERIA

The compliant patient or caregiver administers drugs and treatments as ordered, follows aseptic technique, reports signs and symptoms of complications, and monitors and records intake and output, weights, temperature, blood glucose, and other parameters as indicated. The elderly patient must be evaluated for manual dexterity to perform the required procedures. Many patients have arthritis in their fingers and hands and are unable to assemble and manipulate the infusion equipment to participate in their care. Some patients have a limited educational background and are unable to learn the procedures they are taught. Some patients experience dementia, depression, or mental illness and are incapable of assuming responsibility for their care. In addition, the home environment must be evaluated for basic needs (ie, telephone, electricity, hot and cold water, refrigeration). When these basic needs are unmet, the physician must be notified so that another plan of care that is safe for the patient can be considered.

FINANCIAL RESOURCES

Before acceptance to home care, the patient's insurance benefits are assessed. Although many patients have outstanding health care benefits for inpatient care, they may have limited or no benefits for home care. Some patients may have insurance coverage for home care services, but no prescription coverage. Some patients may be able to pay out of pocket for the cost of the drugs and supplies needed to receive IV therapy in the home. If the patient is unable to pay, the physician is notified, and he or she must consider alternate plans or place the patient in a subacute facility paid for by insurance.

Role of Health Care Professionals in Home-Based Infusion Therapy

The home infusion program must be full service, available 24 hours a day, and able to meet the patient's total needs for nursing, supplies, delivery, inventory, and storage. Qualified professional personnel must be responsible for the direction, coordination, and supervision of all professional services. Care should be consistent with the highest standards of the three accrediting organizations that provide guidelines: the Joint Commission on Accreditation of Healthcare Organizations (JCAHO), Accreditation Commission for Health Care (ACHC), and the Community Health Accreditation Program (CHAP) of the National League for Nursing (NLN). Table 23–3 compares JCAHO, ACHC, and CHAP.

Policies and procedures for the provision of home infusion services must be consistent with published practice standards. The Infusion Nurses Society (INS) has published Infusion Standards for all patients regardless of their clinical setting (INS, 2005). The procedures must be comprehensive and address all the infusion therapies provided. The home infusion therapy program must be consistent with the organization's philosophy and purpose.

Positive outcomes should be the treatment goal for restoring the patient to a functional capacity and enabling the patient and family to return to a level consistent with the stage of disease and its process. Outcome measurements, based on those

TABLE 23-3 Comparison of JCAHO, ACHC, and CHAP

	JCAHO	ACHC	CHAP
Number of accredited providers			
Home care organizations	5,200	98	100
Infusion providers	1,500	263	0
Cost of accreditation (single entity)	$3,565–$12,125	$3,800–$8,700	$1,300–$24,000
Accredits networks	Yes	Yes	Yes
Accredits ambulatory centers	Yes	Yes	Yes
Year accrediting for home care facilities began	1988	1986	1965

ACHC, Accreditation Commission for Health Care; CHAP, Community Health Accreditation Program; JCAHO, Joint Commission on Accreditation of Healthcare Organizations.
(Adapted with permission from Epstein, D. [1995]. Struggling for recognition. *Infusion, 1*[7], 36–37.) Updated information obtained from each organization's website.

developed by JCAHO, ACHC, and CHAP, enhance the level of care provided and help ensure excellence.

THE DISCHARGE PLANNER/HOME CARE COORDINATOR

Discharge planning begins during hospitalization. The home care coordinator may be involved in identifying appropriate candidates for home infusion therapies. The discharge orders must be consistent with the type of infusion therapy, medication, dose, route, duration, frequency interval, and method of administration. The discharge planner arranges final coordination with the supplier before the patient is discharged from the hospital to ensure the safe and timely arrival of medications and related supplies and equipment. Open lines of communication enable the infusion provider to meet the patient's current and ongoing needs for care and ensure a high degree of confidence.

THE PHYSICIAN

The physician orders the referral to the appropriate alternate care setting. He or she writes the plan of treatment for the patient in need of home infusion therapy. In addition to routine infusion orders and other treatments, the individualized plan also should define functional limitations, goals, and duration of treatment. For some modalities, a letter of medical necessity is required. The physician also maintains the role of "gatekeeper," providing recertification for ongoing care, reviewing progress notes, and coordinating the home care plan.

THE NURSE AS HOME CARE INFUSION PROVIDER

The home care infusion nurse maintains ongoing communication with the physician regarding the patient's status and changes in orders. The nurse continues to assess the patient, and whenever the patient's condition changes or deteriorates, he or she notifies the physician and may send the patient to the physician's office or to the hospital.

Once the referral to home care has been completed and insurance coverage or other reimbursement is verified, the nurse should complete a referral checklist (Fig. 23–1). The nurse should review the Patient's Bill of Rights, Responsibilities for Participation in the Home Infusion Program, and the assignment of benefits document. Then the nurse performs an initial patient assessment that includes review of body systems, review of current and past medical history, psychosocial assessment, evaluation of available support systems, and assessment of functional limitations, environment, and cognitive and technical skills. He or she clarifies the orders if needed; develops the patient's plan of care; coordinates interdisciplinary communication for physical therapy, occupational therapy, speech therapy, social worker, or nurse aide as needed; and orients the patient to the services being provided.

A designated nurse case manager must coordinate services for each patient. The infusion therapy nurse case manager is selected for his or her expertise and experience, and preferably is a Certified Registered Nurse in Infusion Therapy (CRNI). A list of case manager responsibilities is provided in Box 23–2. This nurse is the home care nurse who is assigned as a case manager to the patient and is responsible for coordinating care among all disciplines: nursing, physical therapy, occupational therapy, speech therapy, social work, and home health aides. Also, the nurse case manager monitors the patient's progress toward goals, independence, and discharge from home care.

The plan of care should include patient teaching for the ordered therapy, including managing the catheter, using aseptic technique, changing dressings, flushing the IV line and heparin-locking the catheter, hooking up and disconnecting continuous or intermittent administration, changing tubings and other devices, handling infusion equipment, performing emergency interventions, observing for signs and symptoms of possible complications, handling inventory, and managing the pump if necessary.

SAFE PRACTICE ALERT The nurse should provide teaching with return demonstrations until the patient or caregiver is confident, independent, and competent. Even then, the nurse provides ongoing support and monitoring. However, some patients may be discharged at this point depending on the insurance.

BOX 23–2   Responsibility of the Case Manager

- Initial assessment of the patient, family, and home environment
- Development of a plan of care
- Appropriate referral and follow-up
- Coordination of services
- Implementation of the plan of care
- Ongoing evaluation
- Plan for termination of home care

Home Infusion Referral Checklist

Home Care Provider:

[ ] _____

[ ] _____

	DATE/INITIAL
INFORMATION TO:	
A. DISCHARGE PLANNER INFORMED	_____
B. IV TEAM INFORMED	_____
C. HOME AGENCY INFORMED:	_____

Name of agency _____

Address _____

Phone # _____ FAX # _____

Local contact _____

D. LOCAL PHYSICIAN IDENTIFIED (if applicable)   _____

Name _____

Address _____

Phone # _____ FAX # _____

TYPE OF REFERRAL:

A. Parenteral nutrition   _____

B. Enteral nutrition   _____

C. IV antibiotics   _____

D. Pain management   _____

E. Nupogen   _____

F. Chemotherapy   _____

G. Catheter care   _____

H. Other _____   _____

TEACHING COMPLETED:

A. HOME INFUSION _____   _____

B. SUBCLAVIAN/CATHETER CARE   _____

[ ] Port   Type _____

[ ] Hickman/Groshong   [ ] Subclavian   [ ] Other _____

Lumens _____

SUPPLIES NEEDED FROM HOSPITAL ON DISCHARGE:

_____

_____

_____

_____

DELIVERY DATE _____   START OF INFUSION _____

DATE OF REFERRAL FROM PHYSICIAN _____   DATE OF DISCHARGE _____

SIGNATURE/INITIAL _____ _____   TITLE _____

_____ _____   _____

_____ _____   _____

FIGURE 23–1. Home infusion referral checklist.

¿Cómo está? Soy la enfermera encargada de administrarle el suero intravenoso.

▲ **HELLO, I AM YOUR I.V. NURSE. (FEMALE)**

Como esta? Soy el enfermero encargado de administrarle el suero intravenoso.

▲ **HELLO, I AM YOUR I.V. NURSE. (MALE)**

Vengo a revisarle la aguja del suero intravenoso.

▲ **I AM HERE TO CHECK YOUR I.V.**

Voy a aplicarle el suero intravenoso.

▲ **I AM HERE TO START YOUR I.V.**

Le cambiaremos la aguja intravenoso de lugar cada (2) - (3) dias.

▲ **WE CHANGE THE I.V. SITE EVERY (2) - (3) DAYS.**

Le duele en donde tiene inyectada la aguja intravenosa?   Si   No

▲ **DO YOU HAVE PAIN AT YOUR I.V. SITE?**   **YES**   **NO**

Tengo que cambiarle el lugar de la aguja intravenosa debido a que:

▲ **I NEED TO   CHANGE YOUR I.V. TODAY BECAUSE OF:**

(a) le duele,	(b) tiene inflamacion,	(c) tiene la piel roja,	(d) es un procedimiento de rutina.
▲ **(A) PAIN**	**(B) SWELLING**	**(C) REDNESS**	**(D) ROUTINE**

Si le duele o si se le inflama el lugar donde tiene la aguja del suero intravenoso, hagaselo saber a la enfermera.

▲ **IF PAIN OR SWELLING BEGINS, TELL YOUR NURSE.**

SPANISH

FIGURE 23–2.   Language for IV patient teaching: Spanish. (Courtesy of Jaclyn Tropp, CRNI, Evanston, IL.)

The nurse should provide specific teaching packets with pictures and individualize the teaching plan to the patient's specific needs. Once therapy is initiated in the home, the nurse must take adequate time to ensure the patient's competence with the therapeutic regimen. Language barriers often inhibit a successful teaching program. Every effort should be made to address the patient in the language he or she best understands. Figure 23–2 provides an example of infusion teaching in Spanish.

The nurse should develop, review, and sign the teaching plan for the patient. A copy should become part of the patient's clinical record, with a second copy given to the patient and kept in the place of residence.

Home care providers should offer infusion classes for nurses before patient assignment to enhance skills and learning with verification and documentation of infusion competencies. Ongoing education is necessary to keep abreast of the latest technologies, equipment, and infusion therapy procedures. Competency of infusion skills for nurses should be documented and validated on an annual basis. The resources of professional societies and the role that such organizations play in development of the nurse's knowledge base cannot be overlooked. These societies provide the collegiality and professional camaraderie that enable nurses to grow in this

---

BOX 23–3   Resources for Ongoing Education

Accreditation Commission for Health Care (ACHC)
American Association of Blood Banks (AABB)
American Hospital Association (AHA)
American Society of Health-System Pharmacists (ASHP)
American Society for Parenteral and Enteral Nutrition (ASPEN)
Association for Practitioners in Infection Control (APIC)
Case Management Society of America (CMSA)
Centers for Disease Control and Prevention (CDC)
Community Health Accreditation Program (CHAP)
Infusion Nurses Society (INS)
Joint Commission on Accreditation of Healthcare Organizations (JCAHO)
National Association of Vascular Access Networks (NAVAN)
National Association for Home Care (NAHC)
National Home Infusion Association (NHIA)
National Hospice Organization (NHO)
National Subacute Care Association (NSCA)
Oncology Nursing Society (ONS)

---

rapidly changing field. Infusion nursing professionals should be encouraged to publish case studies about their success stories in home infusion care and to share their knowledge and expertise with others. Box 23–3 lists available resources.

THE PHARMACIST

The roles and responsibilities of the pharmacist vary in different parts of the country. In general, the pharmacist is responsible for reviewing medical records for current and past medical history and nutritional and medication history; obtaining and correlating physician orders; checking allergies and drug compatibilities; and facilitating delivery of medications, solutions, supplies, and equipment to the patient's place of residence. The pharmacist also reviews laboratory data and monitors pharmacokinetic dosing with the physician for certain drugs and therapies.

Types of Home Infusion Therapy

Home infusion therapies are diverse and encompass many modalities. Such modalities include antibiotics and anti-infectives, hydration, antiemetics, antineoplastics, nutritional support, pain management, blood and blood component therapy, cardiovascular drugs, drugs to prevent transplant rejection, and venous sampling.

Some health care providers prefer that the first dose of some drugs be administered in a monitored clinical setting, but many first doses are now administered in the patient's residence in the presence of a nurse. This change may be attributed to changes in technology and pharmaceuticals as well as to the increased availability of professional nurses with appropriate IV therapy credentials.

> ⚖ **LEGAL ISSUES:**   First Dosing
>
> The patient who is scheduled to receive the first dose in the home should have a thorough allergy profile and history, including a risk assessment for first dosing.

An appropriate order for emergency anaphylaxis should be provided. The medication should be available immediately and sent to the home before the first administration of the medication. Components of the anaphylactic kit may include epinephrine, diphenhydramine, hydrocortisone, acetaminophen, sodium chloride solution, IV administration set, needles, and syringes. Allergic reactions may occur with subsequent doses of medication as well. The home care infusion nurse must be able to identify and differentiate allergic responses from anaphylactic reactions and teach the patient and caregiver.

In the home care program, provision must be made for handling infectious patient waste. The U.S. Environmental Protection Agency (EPA), a federal regulatory board, has developed many advisories regarding infectious waste. With the passage of the Medical Waste Tracking Act of 1988, Congress mandated to the EPA the investigation and development, if needed, of guidelines for handling home-generated waste. Prepackaged kits are available from various manufacturers and include sharps disposal systems and several types of spill kits. Today's emphasis on safety in the workplace has enhanced these efforts (see Chaps. 11 and 19).

ANTIBIOTICS AND ANTI-INFECTIVES

The delivery of antibiotics and anti-infective agents in the home is a rapidly growing home care service. To qualify, the patient should be medically stable and compliant, the infection should be treatable in the home, and a reliable venous access should be available. Disease conditions amenable to home care IV antibiotic therapy include long-lasting and deep-seated infections. Awareness of a patient's medication history and allergic reactions allows guided monitoring before, during, and after IV antibiotic administration. Recognition of potential adverse drug reactions associated with each class of antibiotics and anti-infectives is an important part of safe and effective infusion therapy (Barrio, 1998).

NUTRITIONAL SUPPORT

The advent of TPN in the 1960s enabled physicians to support intestinally compromised patients indefinitely. Technical barriers have diminished over time. Advanced products, catheters, and technologies have enabled advanced nutritional support to be provided to patients with the appropriate diagnoses. If the patient is under the Medicare program, he or she must require TPN for 90 days or more to qualify. For diagnoses associated with TPN, see Box 23–4.

In the home setting, the patient usually receives TPN as a cyclic administration rather than a continuous 24-hour infusion. With the cyclic infusion, the patient receives a full day's prescribed requirement of fluid, glucose, protein (amino acids),

---

BOX 23–4   Applicable Diagnoses for Total Parenteral Nutrition

Kwashiorkor
Cystic fibrosis
Nutritional marasmus
Disorders involving the immune mechanism
Severe protein-calorie malnutrition
Anorexia nervosa
Malnutrition
Nutritional and metabolic cardiomyopathy
Unspecified vitamin deficiency or other nutritional deficiency
Obstruction of duodenum
Disorders of amino acid transport and metabolism
Regional enteritis
Intestinal disaccharidase deficiencies
Idiopathic proctocolitis
Malabsorption
Disorders of lipid metabolism
Chronic liver disease and cirrhosis
Disorders of fluid, electrolyte, and acid–base balance
Postsurgical nonabsorption
Cancer cachexia

---

lipids, and other additives over 12 to 18 hours. The pharmacist prepares the TPN solution, but the nurse, patient, or caregiver must add some drugs to the solution just before administration. Home monitoring must be done, including weekly to daily weights, temperature, blood glucose monitoring, intake and output, and weekly blood sampling.

Many patients begin their TPN solution in the evening, to be administered while they are sleeping, and disconnect in the morning. The patient, caregiver, or both learn to flush the IV catheter and perform catheter maintenance to keep the line patent. This allows the patient to be free from using the infusion pump during the day. When it is necessary to visit the physician's office, the patient does not have to deal with TPN administration and equipment, especially when nonambulatory equipment is supplied (see Chap. 16).

HYDRATION

Elderly patients often become dehydrated, especially during very hot weather, the influenza season, or periods of inadequate fluid intake. The goal for home hydration is to maintain the patient's fluid balance by providing multiple electrolytes, supplemental vitamins, or plain IV solutions (without additives), and also to avoid hospitalization for those people who resist admission for this therapy. This can be done either intravenously or subcutaneously (hypodermoclysis).

PAIN MANAGEMENT

Continuous or intermittent administration of analgesics in the home allows those in need of pain relief to remain with their families while experiencing a degree of comfort not previously available. Manufacturers have developed sophisticated equipment to ensure safe administration of these drugs in an unmonitored environment. Pain medications may be administered by a patient-controlled analgesia pump through IV, epidural, intrathecal, subcutaneous, or other routes of administration. The most frequently ordered medications are morphine sulfate and hydromorphone. A common concern among patients and families is addiction. Health care providers should assure patients and caregivers that addiction is a minimal concern and that doses should be administered as needed (see Chap. 20).

ANTIEMETICS

Antiemetic protocols aimed at intermittent infusion facilitate the care of the patient receiving antineoplastic therapy and ensure patient comfort. Protocols may call for antiemetic infusions as a single-agent treatment or combined with TPN therapies. Patients with a diagnosis of hyperemesis gravidarum may also benefit from home IV antiemetic therapy.

ANTINEOPLASTICS

Chemotherapeutic agents are administered by various infusion systems to patients in their homes. Vesicant and nonvesicant agents are administered through centrally placed IV catheters, PICCs, implanted chest or arm ports, tunneled catheters, and implanted pumps. In some patients, the chemotherapeutic agents may be initiated in a chemotherapy clinic or physician's office. The infusate is connected to an ambulatory infusion pump and sent home. The home care infusion nurse monitors the patient, changes tubings and dressings, and disconnects the equipment at the end of therapy (see Chap. 19).

BLOOD AND COMPONENT THERAPY

Transfusion of blood and blood components may be performed in the home whenever the policies and procedures required by the American Association of Blood Banks can be followed and the procedure itself is cost-effective. See Chapter 17 for more information.

LEGAL ISSUES: Transfusion Parameters

The availability of the physician *as well as paramedic services* should be determined before the transfusion. Policies should be written for safe administration and compatibility checks, identification checks and verification, transportation of the blood unit or component, emergency measures, registered nurse monitoring (including remaining with the patient for the duration of the procedure and for approximately 90 minutes after the completion of the transfusion), and signs and symptoms of various types of blood reactions.

VENOUS SAMPLING

Venous sampling for all types of laboratory testing is available in home infusion programs. Peak and trough levels, chemistry panels, complete blood counts, and other tests may be performed depending on the therapy. Venous samples may be drawn through peripheral venipuncture or central line sampling. Procedures should be established for blood draws from central line catheters, including the amount of blood to discard before the sampling, the volume at which to flush the catheter after the draw, and change of any equipment.

Hospice

Hospice is a specialized program of care for any person with a limited life expectancy. Available through a national network (1-800-658-8898; www.nho.org), hospice seeks to enhance, preserve, and encourage the dignity of life for patients and families by providing medical care, supportive care, and grief educational services. Hospice emphasizes the management of pain and other symptoms, so the patient is comfortable, alert, and able to maintain the highest quality of life possible. One of the major fears of the seriously ill is pain (Flores, 1998). In a hospice program, medications are prepared for any patient with pain to achieve constant pain control without impairing alertness. A team of physicians, nurses, pharmacists, psychologists, dietitians, social workers, clergy, and volunteers provides 24-hour care. The hospice team develops an individualized plan of care for each patient. Hospice care may be provided in the home with a primary caregiver, or in a hospice center when no primary caregiver is available or for short-term acute symptom management that cannot be given at home. Each eligible Medicare patient must decide whether to choose the hospice benefit, which means that the hospice will provide all care related to the terminal illness. Regular Medicare coverage can be used for any services provided by a personal physician or for illnesses or accidents unrelated to the terminal illness. Hospice care also is provided under other insurances, HMOs, and Medicaid. Currently, many Hospice organizations are servicing residents in the long-term care facilities.

Subacute Care Facilities

Subacute programs are a new level of care for patients in various stages of an acute illness or injury, usually after, but sometimes instead of, hospitalization for an acute episode (Levenson, 1998). **Subacute care** is sometimes called *transitional care*. Two organizations developed the definition: the National Subacute Care Association (NSCA) and JCAHO (Griffin, 1998). Subacute care facilities respond to the need for the treatment of patients with complex medical conditions and rehabilitation needs and provide for a more cost-effective approach.

Beginning in the 1980s, the earliest subacute care units were located in skilled nursing facilities. Later, hospitals began to add subacute units and called them *extended acute care* or *specialty hospitals*. These specialty hospitals typically have 40 beds or more and usually are located in a separate wing or floor of the host hospital. They have an independent admission and discharge function, are licensed separately as a long-term acute care hospital, and are accredited by JCAHO. Their costs are 30% to 60% lower than general acute care hospitals.

The extended acute care hospital provides high-quality, cost-effective, long-term care for high-acuity patients. These specialty hospitals manage patients with medically complex conditions who require extended stay, and whose medical condition will resolve sufficiently for transfer to lower levels of care within a few days with an achievable positive outcome for the patient. The types of patients admitted are those who have multiple body system complications with difficult medical and therapeutic needs: patients with challenges of pulmonary care, ventilator dependency, cardiovascular complications, complicated wounds, major multiple trauma, disease management problems, burns, or other special needs. Infusion therapy treatments include antibiotic or anti-infective therapy, pain management, nutritional support, hydration, and various other infusions, including PICC/midline insertions and central venous catheter care management.

Ambulatory Infusion Centers

Ambulatory infusion centers (AICs) are another alternative site for delivering infusion therapies. Ideally, the physical layout of an AIC is in a medical office building, either adjacent to or near an inpatient hospital. The standard components are a small laboratory, infusion admixture room, education and training area, medical record station, nourishment area, and individualized patient rooms. The patient is seated in a recliner-type chair, with access to infusion teaching videotapes or other movies during treatment. Laboratory parameters are reviewed, along with the physician's orders. If needed, additional laboratory studies are obtained and processed. The patient is offered juices and appropriate snacks during the visit. A nurse assigned to and familiar with the patient performs a complete assessment (including vital signs) and initiates treatment, which may take from 30 minutes to more than 4 hours.

Ambulatory infusion centers may be physician practice based or hospital based. Some organizations provide a stand-alone infusion center, but this model has faced many reimbursement constraints, limiting its viability and growth. With the introduction of the prospective payment system (PPS) in long-term care and home care, the need for AICs will be even greater as the pressure to lower costs continues, and the AIC may help patients to avoid rehospitalization.

Under Medicare Part B reimbursement, physician practice–based infusion centers are reimbursed for medications and clinical nursing time spent on medication administration. Hospital-based infusion centers are able to bill Medicare through the outpatient billing modality. Traditionally, Medicare has reimbursed hospitals for outpatient services based on their costs. The Balanced Budget Act of 1997, however, required Medicare to begin paying for hospital outpatient services on a prospective basis. The program began in 2000 (Hallam, 2000). Stand-alone (independent) infusion centers are not covered. When Medicare is not the main payer source and reimbursement billing is through private insurers, stand-alone infusion centers may be the most effective model (Flores, 1998).

BOX 23–5   Types of Infusion Therapy Provided at Ambulatory Infusion Centers

Antibiotics/anti-infectives and first dosing
Anticoagulants–heparin therapy
Biologics
Blood transfusion and component therapy
Catheter placement and maintenance (peripheral, peripherally inserted central catheter/midline insertion)
Chemotherapy
Drug monitoring (peak and trough)
Hydration
Intravenous immune globulin
Pain management
Parenteral nutrition
Steroids
Venous sampling

Patient selection for the AICs depends on reimbursement. The types of patients appropriate for AICs are those who do not have a caregiver in the home or who are unable to learn or perform self-administration. Another appropriate referral is a patient who is not homebound, does not qualify for home care, or does not have insurance coverage for home health care services. Patients can still recover at home and schedule visits for their infusions as prescribed by the physician.

Other benefits of AICs include teaching, monitoring, follow-up, quality assurance, patient satisfaction, and outcomes (Liebert & Bryant-Wimp, 1997). Types of infusion therapy provided at AICs are addressed in Box 23–5. Because this model focuses on positive patient outcomes, other therapies provided may include allergy desensitization injections; diabetes education; hormone therapy; immunizations; protease inhibitors; vaccines for influenza and pneumonia; respiratory therapy (aerosolized pentamidine); and wound care (Liebert & Bryant-Wimp). Patient care, education, continuity of care, and positive patient outcomes are the keys to patient satisfaction, physician satisfaction, and the success of AICs.

Long-Term Care

Long-term care, often provided in skilled nursing facilities or nursing homes, is part of the continuum of care and an ongoing element of integrated health care. Long-term care services are intended for people of all ages with chronic disabilities and functional deficits to maintain their physical, social, and psychologic functioning. The initiation of long-term care services may be preceded by an acute medical illness or the inability to perform activities of daily living (ADL) independently for 90 days or more (Nazarko, 1998). The care ranges from skilled nursing care, to supportive services provided in the home, to informed assistance given by family and friends.

Many residents of long-term care facilities have complex medical problems and receive skilled care for tracheostomies, gastric feeding tubes, ventilators, mobility disabilities, impaired nutrition, IV medications, and deficits in ADL associated with Alzheimer's disease. Acute care and subacute care hospitals, nursing homes, and assisted living centers are the only places that offer 24-hour nursing services with the exception of private duty nursing. Professional nurses are essential to care for the residents by assessing and coordinating patients' needs for care, focusing on rehabilitation and convalescence, providing high-quality care, reducing complications and mortality, and being cost effective.

Infusion therapy is frequently required for the long-term resident. Commonly used modalities include antibiotic/anti-infective therapy, TPN, pain management, blood products, immune globulin, central venous catheter care and management, and PICC and midline catheter insertion. Credentialed infusion nurse consultants offer educational in-service sessions for the staff to enhance resident care and reduce complications.

As the population ages, chronic illness and disability also will increase, thus creating a growing need for long-term care. The greatest surge in the aging population will occur as the baby boomers reach old age. Estimates are that 20% of the U.S. population will be 65 years or older by 2020 (Nazarko, 1998). Demographic increases also are expected in the segment of the population aged 85 years and older. Based on such projections, the number of people needing long-term care services will triple within the next 30 years (Beck & Chumbler, 1997; see Chap. 22).

Future Infusion Technology for Alternate Care Programs

Technology is one of the most important factors affecting infusion therapy for alternate care programs. In the future, patient care will change to accommodate new technologies, new drug therapies, and new equipment. The greatest obstacle will be reimbursement. Many professionals recognize that patients have multiple, medically complex needs that will necessitate more intensive clinical monitoring of the therapy, requiring improvements in staff and caregiver education.

Health care providers are being challenged to become more efficient and cost-conscious about what they do and how they do it. The delivery of antibiotics and anti-infectives is one of the fastest-growing therapies in alternative care programs. Over the years, tremendous changes have occurred in how these therapies are administered. Both high- and low-technology devices and methods are available for these therapies: gravity infusion, stationary infusion pumps, ambulatory electronic pumps, IV push, syringe delivery, and elastomeric devices with rate-restricted IV systems (Saladow, 1999).

As pressure builds to contain costs, studies are being done to evaluate techniques and procedures. Providers are using IV push administration for selected therapies as a safer and more efficient means of delivery than the traditional piggyback method (Poole & Nowobilski-Vasilios, 1999). Some drugs that are commonly (and safely) administered by IV push are cefazolin (Ancef/Kefzol), Rocephin, and Fortaz. Positive patient outcome monitoring remains essential.

References and Selected Readings

*Barrio, D. (1998). Antibiotic and anti-infective agent use and administration in home care. *Journal of Infusion Nursing, 21,* 50–58.

*Beck, C., & Chumbler, N. (1997). Planning for the future of long-term care: Consumers, providers, and purchasers. *Journal of Gerontological Nursing, 23*(8), 6–13.

Benco, L.B. (2000). The exodus escalates: Medicare market pullouts to double in 2001. *Modern Healthcare, 30*(27), 14.

Bowers, M. (1999). *The JCAHO home health mock survey made simple.* New York: Opus Communications.

*Disbrow, R. (1999). *The impact of prospective payment implementation on Medicare beneficiary access to home health services.* Unpublished master's thesis. Flint: University of Michigan.

*Epstein, D. (1995). Struggling for recognition: Meet CHAP—the "other" accrediting body. *Infusion, 1*(7), 36–37.

*Flores, K. (1998). AIC—What's your role in the most talked about delivery model? *Infusion, 4*(11), 35–38.

*Griffin, K. (1998). Evolution of transitional care settings: Past, present, future. *AACN Clinical Issues, 9,* 398–408.

*Health Care Financing Administration. (1999). *Medicare health insurance manual (HIM).* U.S. Department of Health and Human Services. Washington, DC: Author.

*Infusion Nurses Society. (1998). Revised infusion nursing standards of practice. *Journal of Infusion Nursing, 21*(Suppl. 1), 51–59.

*Infusion Nurses Society. (2000). Revised infusion nursing standards of practice. *Journal of Infusion Nursing, 23,* 65.

*Infusion Nurses Society. (2000). Revised infusion nursing standards of practice. *Journal of Infusion Nursing, 23* (Suppl. 1).

*Infusion Nurses Society. (2005). Revised infusion nursing standards of practice. *Journal of Infusion Nursing, 28* (Suppl. 1).

*Levenson, S. (1998). Subacute settings: Making the most of a new model of care. *Geriatrics, 53,* 69–74.

*Liebert, L., & Bryant-Wimp, J. (1997). Ambulatory infusion centers: Hospitals' survival in an outpatient world. *Infusion, 4*(3), 25–29.

Malone-Rising, D. (1994). The changing face of long-term care. *Nursing Clinics of North America, 29,* 417–426.

*National Quality Forum. (2004). *National voluntary consensus standards for home health care.* Available from the NQHF. www.qualityforum.org

*Nazarko, L. (1998). Continuing to care. *Nursing Management, 5*(5), 29–33.

*Poole, S.M., & Nowobilski-Vasilios, A. (1999). To push or not to push. *Infusion, 5*(9), 53–55.

*Saladow, J. (1999). History in the making: Health care delivery and pump technology continue to evolve. *Infusion, 5*(9), 15–48.

Review Questions

Note: Questions below may have more than one right answer.

1. The fastest-growing alternate clinical setting for infusion is:
   A. Home care
   B. Hospice
   C. Ambulatory infusion center
   D. Long-term care

2. The plan of treatment in a home care program is written by the:
   A. Pharmacist
   B. Nurse
   C. Physician
   D. Branch manager

3. A case manager is responsible for which of the following activities?
   A. Initial assessment
   B. Development of a care plan
   C. Appropriate referral and follow-up
   D. All of the above

4. Frequently prescribed home infusion therapies include:
   A. Antibiotics
   B. Parenteral nutrition
   C. Hydration
   D. All of the above

5. The managed care system imposes limits including which of the following?
   A. Preferred provider contracts
   B. Prior approval/authorization
   C. Use review
   D. All of the above

6. Capitation is a system of prepayment in which providers receive:
   A. Prepayment on a monthly basis
   B. Prepayment on a quarterly basis
   C. Payment based on utilization
   D. Increased payment on utilization

7. Types of patients admitted to subacute care facilities include those:

   A. With multiple body system complications

   B. Who are ventilator dependent

   C. With complicated wounds

   D. With endocarditis

8. Which of the following might appropriately receive services at an ambulatory infusion center?

   A. A patient with inadequate insurance coverage

   B. A patient who is homebound

   C. A patient who is not homebound

   D. A patient who is totally independent

9. One type of infusion therapy administered for the long-term patient is:

   A. Enteral food supplements

   B. TPN

   C. Pain drug patches

   D. Antibiotic intramuscular injections

10. Because of their credentialing and high skill level, the need for infusion nurses in alternate clinical settings will increase in:

   A. Subacute hospitals

   B. Ambulatory infusion centers

   C. Long-term care facilities

   D. All of the above

The Future of Infusion Nursing

KEY TERMS

Brain Drain
Credentialing
Dual Missions

Globalization
Interdisciplinary Education
Strategic Partnering

Strategic Partnering

Strategic partnering enables infusion nurses to extend their scope of practice and professional network. Collaboration with like-minded professionals enables each of us to grow as health care professionals (Weinstein, 2004). Partnering and collaboration are the hallmark of many successful models implemented in practice and academic health care settings worldwide.

Impression of the Profession

Nursing suffers badly from the contagion of negative perspective that comes from nurses themselves as often as from others. We hear only of all that is wrong with nursing and rarely of what is really great about the field. The general public is aware of the many reasons nursing is considered a hard job, but few could describe why nurses love their work. As nurses, we need to communicate this positive and gratifying part of our experience to balance negative messages. The impression of nursing is improving as a result of programs that celebrate nursing's successes and accomplishments—for example, the Magnet Recognition Program of the American Nurses Credentialing Center.

Safe Working Environment

Every day, nurses in all clinical settings are faced with the challenges of a changing patient population, a changing work environment, and changing tools with which to do their jobs. Patient and worker safety are key concerns, especially for those who specialize in infusion nursing.

Health care workers are exposed to pathogens primarily via contaminated needlestick and sharps injuries. At least 1,000 health care workers are estimated to contract serious infections annually from needlestick and sharps injuries. You may be aware of a colleague who has sustained an injury, or perhaps you have been stuck yourself. It is important that you fully understand these risks, including possible infection with hepatitis B virus (HBV), hepatitis C virus (HCV), and human immunodeficiency virus (HIV), the virus that causes AIDS. Each of these viruses poses a serious health risk, and more than 20 other infections, including syphilis, malaria, and herpes, can be transmitted through needlesticks.

Workforce Shortage and Safe Staffing

Opportunities abound for the nursing profession to intervene and make changes to address current staffing and patient safety problems and the growing nursing shortage. According to Geolot (2000), it is estimated that the available supply of registered nurses will fall short of demand by 2010. At that time, if the registered nurse supply has not improved, no incentives or workforce redistribution will resolve the problem. *Nursing's Agenda for the Future* (2002) outlines priorities for the nursing profession, its practice, and patient and nurse safety. Many of those priorities have been reinforced by subsequent reports and recommendations across the health care field.

At a national level, nursing organizations need to standardize a strategic plan to address priorities. Professional societies such as the Infusion Nurses Society, supporting and advocating on behalf of professional **credentialing**, will educate the public to recognize the value of the credentialed nursing professional and will empower us as certified nurses to seek and gain recognition. Employers increasingly recognize the value of the credential and the enhanced outcomes that result from a certified workforce.

International Migration

Brain drain, or taking the best health professionals from other countries to compensate for U.S. nursing shortages, is not always the right answer. Organizations such as the International Council of Nurses (ICN) and the World Health Organization (WHO) have stated their concerns publicly. Brain drain deprives developing nations of quality care, whereas global nursing organizations support and advocate on behalf of ethical recruitment of foreign nursing professionals.

A Universal Perspective

So what are the issues facing nurses and nursing today? **Globalization,** the sociopolitical system, the economy, and safety are key concerns. Within our health care system, we worry about economics, the role of government, quality, access to care, patient safety, patient satisfaction, ethics, and bioterrorism. Academic health centers face their own challenges in the form of **dual missions**, health disparities, sick care versus integrative care, an aging population, competition, and succession (see Chap. 23).

Nurses all face similar problems, regardless of the environment in which they work and the area where they reside. Within their workforce, nurses are concerned with undersupply, knowledge work, the work environment, and culturally competent care. Models of care delivery that affect outcomes are also a concern, including continuum of care, cost and efficiency, evidence-based outcomes, best practices, sustainability, and wellness incentives.

The professional nurse is a knowledge worker and knowledge manager (Table 24–1). Through continuous learning, the nurse seeks **interdisciplinary education**, technology training, marketing acumen, global mentoring, and emotional intelligence.

This is a great time for nursing. In the future, the public will recognize our vision, our voice, and our vitality. We have the unique opportunity to leverage our talents, skills, and abilities and seek abundant results for ourselves and for our patients.

Professional nursing is at a crossroads, and for those professionals involved in infusion nursing, the future has never been brighter. Value the skills and talents that you have developed as an infusion specialist. Become an active member of the nursing councils within your organization, and promote the future of the nursing profession.

TABLE 24–1   Terminology Associated With Knowledge Management

Knowledge manager
A role with developmental and operational responsibility for promoting and implementing knowledge management principles and practices.

Knowledge mapping
A process for determining where knowledge assets are within an organization and how knowledge flows. Evaluating relationships between holders of knowledge will then illustrate the sources, flows, limitations, and losses of knowledge that can be expected to occur.

Knowledge repository
A place to store and retrieve explicit knowledge. A low-tech knowledge repository could be a set of file folders. A high-tech knowledge repository might be a database.

Knowledge worker
An employee whose role relies on his or her ability to find and use knowledge.

References and Selected Readings

Asterisks indicate references cited in text.

American Nurses Association. (1995). *Nursing care report card for acute care.* Washington, DC: Author.

*American Nurses Association. (2002). *Nursing's agenda for the future: A call to the nation.* Available at www.nursingworld.org/naf.

Arnold, L., Bakhtina, I., Brooks, A.M., et al. (1998). Nursing in the newly independent states of the former Soviet Union: An international partnership for nursing development. *Journal of Obstetric and Gynecologic Neonatal Nurseries, 27*(2), pp. 203–208.

*Geolot, D. (2000, May). *Resources and funding.* Paper presented at the Nurse Staffing Summit of the American Nurses Association, Washington, DC.

Joint Commission on Accreditation of Healthcare Organizations. (2002). *Health care at the crossroads: Strategies for addressing the evolving nursing crisis.* Available at www.jcaho.org/about+us/public+policy+initiatives/emergency.htm

Kimball, B., & O'Neil, E. (2002). *Health care's human crisis: The American nursing shortage.* Princeton, NJ: The Robert Wood-Johnson Foundation. Available at http://www.rwjf.org/research/researchdetail.jsp?id=1108&ia=137

Page, A. (Ed.). (2003). *Keeping patients safe: Transforming the work environment of nurses.* Committee on the Work Environment for Nurses and Patient Safety, Washington, DC: Institute of Medicine. Available: http://books.nap.edu/catalog/10851.

Weinstein, S. (2000). Certification and credentialing to define competency-based practice. *Journal of Intravenous Nursing, 23*(1), 21–28.

Weinstein, S. (2002). A nursing portfolio: Documenting your professional journey. *Journal of Infusion Nursing, 25*(6).

*Weinstein SM. (2004). Strategic partnering. *Journal of Infusion Nursing, 26*(5).

www.hospitalconnect.com/ahanews/jsp/display.jsp?dcrpath=AHANEWS/AHANewsNowArticle/data/ann_051213_nursing&domain=AHANEWS

Review Questions

Note: Questions below may have more than one right answer.

1. Which of the following is true of strategic partnering as it relates to infusion nursing?

    A. Allows one to extend scope of practice

    B. Facilitates professional networking

    C. Limits implementation of advanced practice

    D. A and B only

2. All of the following statements are true concerning professional nursing except:

    A. We need to communicate positive experiences

    B. We need to communicate the intensity of our jobs

    C. We should celebrate our successes

    D. We must have Magnet recognition

3. Which of the following statements is true concerning a strategic plan?

    A. Advocating on behalf of credentialing supports our practice

    B. Professional societies support our growth

    C. A and B

    D. A only

4. Terminology associated with knowledge management includes all of the following except:

    A. Manager

    B. Mapping

    C. Depository

    D. Worker

5. Key issues facing professional nursing today include:

    A. Globalization

    B. Dual missions

    C. Economics

    D. All of the above

ANSWERS TO QUESTIONS

CHAPTER 1

1. C
2. A, B, C, D
3. A
4. B
5. B, C

CHAPTER 2

1. B
2. C
3. C
4. A
5. A
6. C
7. B
8. D
9. A, B, C
10. A, B, C

CHAPTER 3

1. D
2. D
3. A
4. A, B
5. B
6. A
7. D
8. D
9. D
10. C

CHAPTER 4

1. D
2. A
3. C
4. A, B, C, D
5. D
6. A, B, C
7. D
8. C
9. C

CHAPTER 5

1. B
2. A, B, C, D
3. C
4. A
5. D
6. A, B, C
7. C
8. D
9. D
10. A

CHAPTER 6

1. A, B, C, D
2. A, B, C
3. A, B
4. A, B
5. C
6. A, B
7. D
8. D
9. C
10. C

CHAPTER 7

1. A
2. D
3. A
4. A
5. A, B
6. A
7. A, B, C, D
8. A, B, C
9. A
10. B

CHAPTER 8

1. B
2. A
3. A
4. B, C

5. A
6. A
7. D
8. B
9. A, B
10. D

CHAPTER 9

1. A
2. A
3. C
4. B
5. D
6. A, B
7. D
8. D
9. D
10. B

CHAPTER 10

1. C
2. B
3. A
4. D
5. A, B
6. D
7. A, B, C, D
8. B
9. A
10. B

CHAPTER 11

1. D
2. A
3. D
4. A, B, C
5. A, C
6. C
7. D
8. A
9. D
10. B, C, D

CHAPTER 12

1. A
2. D
3. A
4. A
5. A
6. C, D
7. D
8. D
9. B
10. A

CHAPTER 13

1. D
2. A
3. C
4. C
5. A
6. B
7. A
8. B
9. B
10. C

CHAPTER 14

1. B, C
2. A
3. B
4. B
5. D
6. D
7. A
8. D
9. B, D
10. A, B

CHAPTER 15

1. A
2. A
3. B, C
4. D
5. D
6. D
7. A
8. B
9. C
10. A, B, C

CHAPTER 16

1. C
2. B

3. D
4. C
5. A
6. D
7. B
8. D
9. A
10. D

CHAPTER 17

1. A
2. C
3. A, B
4. A
5. B
6. C
7. C
8. B
9. D
10. A

CHAPTER 18

1. D
2. C
3. A, B, C, D
4. B
5. A, B, C
6. D
7. D
8. C
9. D
10. D

CHAPTER 19

1. B
2. D
3. B
4. A
5. C
6. D
7. C
8. B
9. C
10. C

CHAPTER 20

1. D
2. A
3. A
4. B
5. B
6. D

7. A
8. C
9. D
10. A
11. D
12. C

CHAPTER 21

1. C
2. B
3. D
4. B
5. D
6. A
7. C
8. B
9. C
10. D

CHAPTER 22

1. D
2. B
3. A, B
4. C
5. C
6. B
7. C
8. D
9. A
10. D

CHAPTER 23

1. A
2. C
3. D
4. D
5. D
6. A
7. A, B, C
8. C
9. B
10. D

CHAPTER 24

1. D
2. D
3. C
4. C
5. D

GLOSSARY

ABO system — a basic hereditary blood group system used to classify a person's blood group

Absorption — process by which medication moves from drug administration sites to vasculature

Acidosis — blood pH below normal (<7.35)

Active transport — the passage of a substance across a cell membrane by an energy-consuming process, permitting diffusion to occur

Adjuvant chemotherapy — the addition of drug therapy to surgery and/or radiation therapy to eradicate metastatic disease

Admixture — combination of two or more medications

Adsorption — attachment of one substance to the surface of another

Agglutination — clumping of red blood cells when incompatible bloods are mixed

Agglutinin — an antibody causing agglutination with its corresponding antigen

Alkalosis — blood pH above normal (>7.45)

Alkylating agents — agents that kill cells by cross-linking DNA strands (ie, disturbing the normal structure) in the DNA molecule

Alopecia — the loss of hair from the body and/or the scalp

Alpha (α) — (a) the level of statistical significance designating the probability of committing a type I error. Also known as the *p* value; (b) a reliability coefficient, such as Cronbach's alpha, to estimate internal consistency

Alternate site care — care that is delivered beyond the confines of an inpatient facility

Ambulatory infusion device — electronic infusion device specifically designed to be worn on the body to promote patient mobility and independence in the home or work environment

Analgesia — freedom from nociceptive stimuli; absence of pain

Analogue — a compound that resembles another in structure (eg, fluorouracil is an analogue of uracil)

Anorexia — absence or loss of appetite for food

Antibody — a substance present in the plasma that incites immunity and that can react with the specific antigen that caused its production

Antidiuretic hormone (ADH) — hormone secreted from a pituitary mechanism that causes the kidneys to conserve water

Anti-free-flow administration set — an IV administration device that stops when removed from the electronic infusion device, yet allows gravity flow when the user takes action

Antigen — an immunizing agent capable of inducing the body to form antibodies

Antimetabolites — anticancer drugs that substitute for or block the use of an essential metabolite

Antimicrobial — an agent that destroys or prevents development of micro-organisms

Antimicrobial ointment — a semisolid preparation used to prevent the pathogenic action of microbes

Antineoplastic agent — a medication or treatment for cancer

Antitumor antibiotics — anticancer drugs that interfere with cellular production of DNA and/or RNA

Arterial pressure monitoring — monitoring of arterial pressure through an indwelling arterial catheter connected to an electronic monitor

Arteriovenous (AV) fistula — the surgical anastomosis of an artery and vein

Arteriovenous (AV) grafts — the insertion of a synthetic device connecting a vein and an artery

Aseptic technique — mechanism used to reduce potential contamination

Assay determination — decision based on an analysis and/or examination

Auscultation — process of listening to or for sounds in the body

Autologous — products or components of the same individual

Bacteria — micro-organisms that may potentiate disease and infection

Benchmarking — comparing one's systems to others

Beta (β) — (a) statistical testing term referring to the probability of making a type II error; (b) the standardized regression coefficient in the regression equation indicating the relative weights of the independent variables

Biotransformation-metabolism — the enzymatic alteration of a drug molecule

Blood grouping — the testing of red blood cells to determine antigens present and absent

Body surface area — surface area of the body determined through use of a nomogram; important when calculating drug dosages

Bone marrow — the inner spongy tissue of a bone in which red blood cells, white blood cells, and platelets are formed

Cancer — the general name for more than 100 diseases in which abnormal cells grow out of control; a malignant tumor

Cannula — a hollow tube made of plastic or metal used for accessing the vascular system

Catheter — a hollow tube made of plastic used for accessing the vascular system

Cell kill — the number of cancer cells killed at a given dose by an antineoplastic drug

Cellular kinetics — study of mechanisms and rates of cellular changes

Chemical incompatibility — a change in the molecular structure or pharmacologic properties of a substance, which may or may not be visually observed

Chemotherapy — the chemical treatment for cancer patients with agents designed to kill cancer cells

Cognitive — behaviors that place primary emphasis on mental or intellectual processes

Cold agglutinin — a red blood cell agglutinin that acts at a relatively low temperature; part of a disease process caused by a transient infectious disease; may be idiopathic

Color coding — system developed by manufacturers that identifies products/medications by color. These color code systems are not standardized and may vary with manufacturer.

Compartment syndrome — compression of circulation evidenced by impaired pulses, compromised circulation, and pain

Compatibility — capacity for being mixed and administered without undergoing undesirable chemical and/or physical changes or loss of therapeutic action

Compatibility test — all tests performed on donors and recipients to determine compatibility of blood; also known as *cross-matching*

Complement — a group of proteins in normal blood serum and plasma that, in combination with antibodies, cause the destruction of particular antigens

Contamination — introduction of pathogens or infectious material from one source to another

Corrective action — a defined plan to eliminate deficiencies

Cross-contamination — movement of pathogens from one source to another

Curative — healing or corrective

Cutdown — surgical procedure for exposure and catheterization of a vein

Cytoprotectant — drug to minimize toxicities of chemotherapy without compromising the cytotoxic effects of drugs on cancer cells

Delayed reaction — in relation to blood transfusions, adverse effect occurring after 48 hours and up to 180 days after the transfusion

Delivery system — product that facilitates administration of drug(s); can be integral or have component parts. Delivery systems encompass all products used, from the solution container down to the cannula.

Dermatomes — segmental distribution of the spinal nerves. Dermatomes are labeled according to their exit point on the spinal cord. The spinal canal has 31 dermatomes. Dermatome pathways are not defined or determined through dissection, but by observation of patients with spinal cord injuries for the resultant neurologic effects.

Diffusion — passage of molecules of one substance between the molecules of another to form a mixture of the two

Disinfectant — an agent that eliminates all micro-organisms except spores; generally used on inanimate objects

Distal — farthest from the heart; farthest from point of attachment; below previous site of catheterization

Distention — expansion owing to pressure within

Document — a written or printed record that contains original, official, or legal information

Documentation — a recording in written or printed form containing original, official, or legal information

Dome — a plastic component used in hemodynamic monitoring

Dose-limiting toxicity — the degree of toxicity that dictates the maximum amount of drug that safely can be administered

Drug-nutrient interaction — an event that occurs (a) when nutrient availability is altered by a medication or (b) when a drug effect is altered or an adverse reaction is caused by the intake of nutrients

Ecchymoses — bruising resulting from escape of blood from injured vessels

Electronic infusion device (EID) — an electronic instrument that regulates the flow rate of the prescribed therapy

Embolus — a blood clot or other foreign substance that is carried in the blood stream and has the potential to impede and/or obstruct circulation

Enteral nutrition — nutrition provided via the gastrointestinal tract

Epidemiology — the division of medical science concerned with defining and explaining the interrelationships of the host, agent, and environment in causing disease

Epidural — a potential space that is part of the spinal canal outside the dura mater. This space contains a network of large and thin-walled veins as well as fat that is proportional in volume to a person's body fat.

Epithelialization — the growth of epithelial cells over a wound or over and around a catheter site

Erythema — redness

Extravasation — inadvertent escape of a solution or medication (usually a vesicant) into surrounding tissue

Factor V Leiden — the most common hereditary blood coagulation disorder in the United States; causes blood to have an increased tendency to clot (also called factor 5 Leiden)

Filter — a porous device used to prevent the passage of undesired substances

Filtration — process of passing fluid through a filter using pressure

Free flow — referring to nonregulated, inadvertent administration of fluid

Fungi — vegetable cellular organisms that subsist on organic matter

Gram-negative bacteria — organisms that remain unstained by Gram's method, including *Klebsiella, Escherichia coli, Pseudomonas, Serratia,* etc.; associated with infusate contamination and arterial catheters

Gram-positive bacteria — organisms holding the dye after being stained by Gram's method, including *Staphylococcus aureus, S. epidermidis,* and others; associated with venous catheter contamination

Grounded theory — theory that is constructed from theoretical propositions based on data obtained in the real world

Hematocrit — an expression of the volume of red cells per unit of circulating blood

Hematogenous — produced by or derived from the blood; disseminated through the bloodstream or via circulation

Hematoma — usually refers to uncontrolled bleeding at a venipuncture site, generally creating a hard, painful lump

Hemodynamic pressure monitoring — the measurement of pulmonary artery pressure, arterial pressure, cardiac output, and so forth, via an electronic monitor and internally placed catheter

Hemoglobin — the iron-containing pigment of red blood cells; functions primarily in transporting oxygen from the lungs to the body tissues

Hemolysis — rupture of the red blood cell membrane causing the release of hemoglobin

Hemorrhage — abnormal discharge of blood, either external or internal

Hemostasis — cessation of the flow of blood through a port or vessel

HLA system — human leukocyte antigens; a complex array of genes that are involved in immune system regulation and cell differentiation

Homeostasis — ability to restore equilibrium under stress

Hypercalcemia — serum calcium concentrations above normal levels

Hyperkalemia — excess of potassium in the blood

Hypertonic — solution more concentrated than that with which it is compared; a fluid having a concentration greater than the normal tonicity of plasma

Hyperuricemia — uric acid blood concentrations above normal levels

Hypodermoclysis — use of the subcutaneous route as a vehicle for absorption of IV isotonic

Hypokalemia — low potassium concentration in the blood

Hypotonic — solution less concentrated than that with which it is compared; a fluid having a concentration less than the normal tonicity of plasma

IgA — immunoglobulin A; a class of immunoglobulins in body secretions

IgG — immunoglobulin G; a class of immunoglobulins or circulating antibodies in the blood that frequently causes sensitization

IgM — immunoglobulin M; a class of immunoglobulins or circulating antibodies in the blood that is capable of binding complement

Immediate reaction — in blood transfusions, an adverse effect occurring immediately or up to 48 hours after the transfusion

Immunocompromised — having decreased resistance to disease

Immunoglobulin — a protein with antibody activity

Immunohematology — the study of blood and blood reactions

Implanted port or pump — vascular access device placed totally beneath the skin surface by surgical procedure

Incident — an unusual occurrence that requires documentation and action because of potential or implied consequences

Incompatible — incapable of being mixed or used simultaneously without undergoing chemical or physical changes or producing undesirable effects

Infection — invasion of the body by living micro-organisms

Infiltration — the inadvertent administration of a nonvesicant solution or medication into surrounding tissues

Infusate — parenteral solution administered into the vascular system

Integumentary — cutaneous; dermal

Interferons (IFNs) — cytokines that initiate immune responses that are antiviral, antitumor, and immunomodulatory

Interleukins — cytokines that stimulate the migration of active immune cells to the tumor

Intermittent intravenous therapy — IV therapy administered at prescribed intervals with periods of infusion cessation

International normalized ratio (INR) — the PT (prothrombin time) ratio that would have been obtained using the World Health Organization reference PT reagent

Interval variables — an ordered set of categories if categories form a set of intervals that are all exactly the same

Intraosseous — within the cavity of a bone that is filled with marrow

Intrathecal — a space that contains cerebral spinal fluid and bathes the spinal cord. The intrathecal space runs parallel to the epidural space. The two spaces are separated by the dura mater.

Intrinsic contamination — contamination during product manufacture

Isolation — the separation of potentially infectious persons and/or materials

Isotonic — solution having the same concentration as that with which it is compared (ie, plasma)

Laminar flow hood — a contained work area in which the air flow within the area moves with uniform velocity along parallel flow lines with a minimum of eddies

Latex injection port — a resealable rubber cap designed to accommodate needles for administration of solutions into the vascular system

Leukopenia — total number of leukocytes in the circulating blood less than normal, the lower limit of which generally is regarded as $5,000/\mu L$

Lumen — the interior space of a tubular structure, such as a blood vessel or cannula

Lymphedema — swelling of an extremity caused by obstruction of the lymphatic vessel(s)

Malignancy — uncontrolled growth and dissemination of a neoplasm

Malnutrition — any disorder of nutritional status including those resulting from a deficient intake of nutrients, impaired nutrient metabolism, or overnutrition

Medical act — procedure performed by a licensed physician

mEq — the measure of the chemical-combining power of an ion with hydrogen

Metastasis — the spread of cancer to sites distant from the site of origin

Microabrasion — break in skin integrity, which may predispose the patient to infection

Microaggregate — microscopic collection of particles, such as platelets, leukocytes, and fibrin, that occurs in stored blood

Microaggregate blood filter — device that removes potentially harmful microaggregates and reduces non-hemolytic febrile reactions

Micro-organisms — extremely minute living matter that can be seen only with the aid of a microscope

Midline — peripherally inserted catheter with tip terminating in the proximal portion of the extremity, usually 6 inches long

Monoclonal antibody — antibody produced by a clone of cells derived from a single cell in large quantities for use against a specific antigen

Morbidity — number of infected persons or cases of infection in relation to a specific population

Mortality — ratio of number of deaths in a population to number of individuals in that population

Multiple-dose vial — medication bottle that is hermetically sealed with a rubber stopper and designed to be entered more than one time

Nadir — the lowest level; in chemotherapy, the nadir is the lowest level to which the blood count drops in response to an antineoplastic agent.

Needle — a slender, pointed, hollow metal device

Neo-adjuvant — the use of chemotherapy prior to treatment for localized cancer when the local therapy is less than completely effective

Neoplasm — a new growth or tumor, either benign or malignant

Nitrosoureas — anticancer drugs that produce metabolites that attack DNA in a manner analogous to alkylating agents

Nominal variables — names of categories

Nonpermeable — able to maintain integrity

Nonvesicant — intravenous medications, including, but not limited to, medications administered for cancer; these medications generally do not cause damage or sloughing of tissue

Nutrients — proteins, carbohydrates, lipids, vitamins, minerals, trace elements, and water

Nutritional assessment — a comprehensive evaluation to define nutritional status; includes medical history, dietary history, physical examination, anthropometric measurements, and laboratory data

Nutritional screening — the process of identifying characteristics known to be associated with nutrition problems, particularly in individuals who are at risk for malnutrition or who are malnourished

Nutritional support — provision of specially formulated and/or delivered parenteral or enteral nutrients to maintain or restore optimal nutrition status

Occlusion — a blockage, which may result from precipitation or clot formation

Oncology — the study of tumors

Oncotic — within the tissue; relating to tissue pressure

Opiate receptor sites — cells that receive only one particular kind of drug. These are located in the dorsal horn of the spinal cord and the periaquaductal gray region of the brain. The discovery of spinal opiate receptors in 1973 led to the development of selective spinal opiate analgesia.

Opioids — narcotics that stimulate the opiate receptor site to produce analgesia

Ordinal variables — sets of ordered categories

Osmolarity — number of solutes contained in solution measured in milliosmoles per liter

Outcome — the interpretation of documented results; educational goal

Palliative — treatment that may be provided for comfort and/or temporary relief of symptoms, but that does not cure

Palpable cord — a vein that is rigid and hard to the touch

Palpation — examination by touch

Parenteral — denoting any route other than the alimentary canal, such as intravenous

Parenteral nutrition — nutrients that are administered intravenously, comprising carbohydrates, proteins, and/or fats, and additives, such as electrolytes, vitamins, and trace elements

Paresthesia — abnormal spontaneous sensations (eg, burning, prickling, tingling, or tickling without physical stimulus)

Particulate matter — relating to or composed of fine particles

Pathogens — disease-producing micro-organisms

PCA — patient-controlled analgesia

Percutaneous puncture — puncture performed through the skin

Peripheral — pertaining to veins of the extremities, scalp, and external jugular; not central

Peripheral neuropathy — dysfunction of postganglionic nerves, ranging from paresthesia to paralysis

Peristalsis — progressive wave-like movement that occurs involuntarily

Phlebitis — inflammation of a vein; may be accompanied by pain, erythema, edema, streak formation, and/or palpable cord; rated by a standard scale (see phlebitis topic); a possible precursor to sepsis

Phlebotomy — withdrawal of blood from a vein

Physical incompatibility — an undesirable change that is visually observed

Plant alkyloids — anticancer drugs derived from plants, such as the periwinkle (vincristine and vinblastine) in the vinca family

Port — port of entry

Positive pressure — maintaining a constant, even force within a lumen to prevent reflux of blood; achieved while injecting by clamping or withdrawing needle from cannula

Postinfusion phlebitis — inflammation of a vein occurring after cannula removal

Pounds per square inch (psi) — a measurement of pressure; 1 psi equals 50 mm Hg or 68 cm H_2O

Preservative-free — containing no added substance capable of inhibiting bacterial contamination

Priming — initial filling of the administration set with infusate

Process — actual performance and observation of performance based on compliance with policies, procedures, and professional standards

Product integrity — state of product that is intact and uncompromised; condition suitable for intended use

Proximal — nearest to the heart; closest to point of attachment; above previous site of cannulation

Pruritis — itching

Psychomotor — referring to behaviors that place primary emphasis on the various degrees of physical skills and dexterity as they relate to the thought process

Purpura — condition in which spontaneous bleeding occurs in subcutaneous tissue resulting in purple patches visible on the skin

Purulent — containing or producing pus

Push — direct injection of a medication into a vein or access device

Quality indicator — a systematic process for monitoring, evaluating, and problem-solving

Radiopaque — able to be detected by radiography

Ratio variables — interval variables with an absolute zero point, indicating absence of a point being measured

Reflex sympathetic dystrophy (RSD) — a condition of burning pain, stiffness, swelling, and discoloration of the hand

Rh system — a blood group system denoting the presence or absence of the D (Rh) red blood cell antigen

Risk management — process that centers on identification, analysis, treatment, and evaluation of real and potential hazards

Roller bandage — a roll of gauze or other material used for protecting an injured part, for immobilizing a limb, for keeping dressings in place, and so on

Sclerotic — referring to fibrous thickening of the wall of the vein resulting in decreased lumen size; on palpation, usually feels hard to the touch

Semi-quantitative culture technique — a laboratory protocol used for isolating and identifying micro-organisms

Sensitization — the initial exposure of an individual to a specific antigen that results in an immune response

Sentinel event — an unexpected occurrence involving death or serious physical or psychologic injury, or the risk thereof

Sepsis — infectious micro-organisms or their toxins in the blood stream

Septum — a wall dividing two or more cavities

Single-use vial — medication bottle intended for one-time use that is hermetically sealed with a rubber stopper

Skin-cannula junction — point at which the cannula enters the skin

Spike — insertion of the administration set into the solution container

Statistics — the science of collecting, classifying, and interpreting information based on the numbers of things

Stomatitis — sores on the inside of the mouth

Structure — describes the elements on which a program is based. Elements may include resources such as federal and state laws, professional standards, position descriptions, patient rights, policies and procedures, documentation forms, quality controls, corrective action programs, and so on.

Stylet — a rigid metal object within a catheter designed to facilitate insertion

Surfactant — material whose properties reduce the surface tension of fluid

Surveillance — the active, systematic, ongoing observation of the occurrence and distribution of disease within a population and of the events or conditions that increase or decrease the risk of such disease occurrence

Sympathetic — referring to the part of the autonomic nervous system responsible for the fight-or-flight response. The sympathetic system is dominant when a person experiences pain. The effects on the body are from a release of norepinephrine in the body, resulting in increased heart rate, blood pressure, and respiration.

Systemic — pertaining to the whole body rather than one of its parts

Tamper-proof — impossible to alter

Thrombocytopenia — decrease in thrombocyte or platelet count

Thrombolytic agent — a pharmacologic agent capable of dissolving blood clots

Thrombophlebitis — inflammation of the vein with clot formation

Thrombosis — formation of a blood clot within a blood vessel

Total nutrient admixture — parenteral nutrition formulation containing carbohydrates, amino acids, lipid, vitamins, minerals, trace elements, water, and other additives in a single container

Trace elements — minute amounts of essential elements present in the body

Transfusion reaction — any adverse effect to the transfusion of whole blood or its components or derivatives

Transitional feeding — progression from one mode of feeding to another, while continuously administering estimated nutrient requirements

Transparent semipermeable membrane (TSM) — a sterile dressing that allows visualization, repels water, and allows air to permeate it

Trendelenburg — a position in which the head is lower than the feet, used to increase venous distention

Tunneled catheter — a central catheter designed to have a portion lie within a subcutaneous passage before exiting the body

Valsalva maneuver — the process of making a forceful attempt at expiration with the mouth, nostrils, and glottis closed

Vascular access — means of approaching or entering the vascular system

Vascular access devices — catheters placed directly into the venous system for infusion therapy and/or phlebotomy

Venipuncture — puncture of a vein for any purpose

Ventricular reservoir — a device that, once implanted, provides direct access to the cerebrospinal fluid (CSF) without the need to perform a spinal tap

Vesicant — caustic intravenous medication that causes blisters and tissue injury when it escapes into the surrounding tissue(s)

Volumetric — relating to measurement of a substance by its volume

INDEX